Genitourinary Radiology THE REQUISITES

SERIES EDITOR   **James H. Thrall**, M.D.
Radiologist-in-Chief
Department of Radiology
Massachusetts General Hospital
Juan M. Taveras Professor of Radiology
Harvard Medical School
Boston, Massachusetts

Genitourinary Radiology

THE REQUISITES

RONALD J. ZAGORIA, M.D.
Associate Professor of Radiology
The Bowman Gray School of Medicine
Wake Forest University
Winston-Salem, North Carolina

GLENN A. TUNG, M.D.
Associate Professor
Brown University
Rhode Island Hospital
Women and Infants' Hospital
Providence, Rhode Island

with 701 illustrations

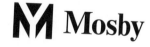

Mosby

St. Louis Baltimore Berlin Boston Carlsbad Chicago London Madrid
Naples New York Philadelphia Sydney Tokyo Toronto

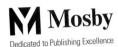

Mosby
Dedicated to Publishing Excellence

A Times Mirror Company

THE REQUISITES
THE REQUISITES
THE REQUISITES
THE REQUISITES
THE REQUISITES ™

THE REQUISITES is a proprietary
trademark of Mosby–Year Book, Inc.

Vice President and Publisher: Anne S. Patterson
Executive Editor: Robert A. Hurley
Managing Editor: Elizabeth Corra
Associate Developmental Editor: Mia Cariño
Project Manager: Chris Baumle
Project Specialist: David Orzechowski
Designer: Nancy McDonald
Manufacturing Manager: William A. Winneberger

First Edition
Copyright © 1997 by Mosby–Year Book, Inc.

Printed in the United States of America
Composition by Bi-Comp Incorporated
Printing/binding by R.R. Donnelley & Sons

Mosby–Year Book, Inc.
11830 Westline Industrial Drive
St. Louis, Missouri 63146

Library of Congress Cataloging-in-Publication Data

Zagoria, Ronald J.
    Genitourinary radiology : the requisites / Ronald J. Zagoria,
Glenn A. Tung.
        p.   cm.—(Requisites series)
    Includes bibliographical references and index.
    ISBN 0-8016-7482-4
    1. Genitourinary organs—Imaging. I. Tung, Glenn A.
    II. Title. III. Series.
    [DNLM: 1. Urogenital Diseases—radiography. WJ 141 Z18g 1997]
RC874.Z34 1997
616.6'0757—dc21   97-5013
DNLM/DLC   CIP
for Library of Congress

98 99 00 01 / 9 8 7 6 5 4 3 2

*I dedicate this book to my dear wife, **Kathy**, and our wonderful sons, **David** and **Michael**. The love and pleasure they have given me have fulfilled me throughout my career.*

*To my parents, **Sam** and **Sylvia**, who taught me the importance of helping others and the power of the pen.*

*And finally to **Raymond Dyer**, my friend and mentor, whose enthusiasm and knowledge drew me to the rewarding field of Genitourinary Radiology.*

R.J.Z.

Ask nothing more of me, sweet;
   All I can give you I give.
Heart of my heart, were it more,
   More would be laid at your feet:
Love that should help you to live,
   Song that should spur you to soar.

ALGERNON CHARLES SWINBURNE
The Oblation

*I dedicate this book to my wife, **Nadine**. Your love sustains me.*

Who is the happy Warrior? Who is he
That every man in arms should wish to be?
It is the generous spirit, who, when brought
Among the tasks of real life, hath wrought
Upon the plan that pleased his childish thought:
Whose high endeavors are an inward light
That makes the path before him always bright:
Who, with a natural instinct to discern
What knowledge can perform, is diligent to learn.

WILLIAM WORDSWORTH
Character of the Happy Warrior

*I also dedicate this book to my parents, **Lillian** and **C.C.**, who have given me the inward light, and to my sons, **Matthew** and **Eric**, who make the path before me forever bright.*

G.A.T.

Foreword

Genitourinary Radiology: THE REQUISITES is the eighth book in a series designed to provide core material in major subspecialty areas of radiology for use by residents during their training and by practicing radiologists and clinicians seeking to review or expand their knowledge.

The contemporary practice of genitourinary radiology reflects the richness and diversity of methods available for diagnostic imaging and image-guided therapy. Only a generation ago, the practice of genitourinary radiology was limited to plain films, intravenous urography, and cystourethrography. Today, the field requires a comprehensive knowledge of computed tomography and ultrasonography, with magnetic resonance imaging applications gaining momentum. Image-guided interventions have expanded in parallel. Drs. Ron Zagoria and Glenn Tung have succeeded brilliantly in creating a text that presents the full spectrum of the diagnostic and image-guided therapy armamentarium.

Drs. Zagoria and Tung have structured their book so that material is presented in a logical manner that parallels the presentation of clinical disease to the radiologist. The book's organization by anatomy facilitates the discussion of differential diagnosis by grouping diseases and conditions that affect respective components of the genitourinary system. Drs. Zagoria and Tung start with the kidneys and then continue to the lower urinary tract and the female and male genital tracts.

All of the volumes in THE REQUISITES™ in Radiology series use tables and boxes to restate and summarize essential information in concise form. In this way, the corresponding narrative discussion is reinforced. Drs. Zagoria and Tung have done an outstanding job of making use of these features to outline differential diagnoses and to highlight the key findings of important diseases and conditions. These summaries almost serve as a subtext for the book that permits rapid review of the fundamentals. Busy residents and clinical practitioners will especially appreciate this feature.

THE REQUISITES™ in Radiology series includes one book specifically written for each of the major subspecialties. The length and format of each volume are dictated by the material being covered, but the principal goal is to equip the resident with a text that might reasonably be read within several days at the beginning of each subspecialty rotation and perhaps reread several times during subsequent rotations. Not intended to be exhaustive, the volumes instead provide the basic conceptual, factual, and interpretive material required for clinical practice. Each book is written by nationally recognized authorities in the respective subspecialties who, because THE REQUISITES™ is a completely new series, are able to present material in the context of today's practice of radiology rather than graft information about new imaging modalities onto a preexisting text.

Drs. Zagoria and Tung have done an excellent job of sustaining the philosophy of THE REQUISITES™ in Radiology series and have produced a truly contemporary text for genitourinary imaging. I believe that *Genitourinary Radiology: THE REQUISITES* will serve residents in radiology as a concise and useful introduction to the subject, and as a very manageable text for review by fellows and practicing radiologists. Further, I hope that urologists, nephrologists, obstetricians, gynecologists, and internists, as well as their resident and fellowship trainees, will consider this a user-friendly vehicle for exploring imaging of the genitourinary tract.

James H. Thrall, M.D.

Radiologist-in-Chief
Massachusetts General Hospital
Juan M. Taveras Professor of Radiology
Harvard Medical School
Boston, Massachusetts

Preface

Genitourinary radiology encompasses nearly all technologies used in diagnostic radiology. Knowledge of and experience with interventional radiologic techniques also are crucial to the practice of the field. Working closely with urologists and other specialists, the genitourinary radiologist plays a central role in diagnosis and treatment planning. The radiologist's interpretation of diagnostic studies often is the main factor in determining whether a patient will undergo surgery. The recognition of specific radiologic features of benign and malignant entities in the genitourinary system will greatly impact patient treatment decisions. Finally, interventional techniques such as nephrostomy tract creation, ureteral occlusion, stent placement, and fallopian tube recanalization will produce immediate therapeutic impact on patients, a most gratifying result. These aspects of genitourinary radiology make it an exciting, stimulating field and motivated us to author this book.

We had been cautioned about taking on the task of writing a book. We are told that precious academic time is better spent on original research. However, we would not have accepted Dr. Thrall's invitation to write this genitourinary volume if we did not believe in the concept of THE REQUISITES™ in Radiology series and its value as a pedagogical tool. Preparing *Genitourinary Radiology: THE REQUISITES* has given us the opportunity to reach many more students of radiology than we ordinarily have the privilege to teach. Further, it has allowed us to distill from original research what we believe is the most clinically useful information: the required, necessary, indispensable, or, in short, the requisite.

Thus, in 10 chapters, we present the essentials of genitourinary radiology. Our book describes the imaging techniques and diseases commonly encountered in the field. We intend for the reader, after completing the book, to be familiar with most pathology affecting the genitourinary system and to be equipped with a practical approach for detecting and characterizing these abnormalities.

We have crafted this book in the style that has become the trademark of THE REQUISITES™: complete but not exhaustive text; many figures, tables, and "pearls" listed in boxes; and easy readability. David C. Kushner, M.D., taught one of us how to read a chapter from a textbook of radiology, and we hope he will be flattered if we share his wise suggestion with you. First, read the chapter title and the outline of headings featured at the beginning of the chapter. Glancing at this list will alert you to the major topics that are explored in the chapter. Then, study the figures, tables, and boxes twice, the first time *before* you read any of the text, because we (and most authors) try to encapsulate key points in these summary features. Then, read the chapter from start to finish. We think it becomes easier to digest written material when you do not have to dart between text, figures, tables, and boxes. Finally, review these figures, tables, and boxes again, having acquired an enlightened perspective from reading the text. Dave's approach can be applied to the study of journal articles as well.

The first and last chapters are overviews of imaging methods and interventional uroradiology, respectively. Chapter 1 begins with a discussion of iodinated contrast media, adverse reactions to these media, and the management of these reactions. It summarizes radiologic methods, from urography to magnetic resonance imaging, commonly used to investigate genitourinary disease. Chapter 10 is a review of procedures that are commonly performed by the interventional uroradiologist, including percutaneous interventional procedures, interventional techniques used to manage infertility, and renal angioplasty and embolotherapy. It also addresses extracorporeal shock wave lithotripsy and transrenal endoscopic procedures.

Chapters 2 through 9 each focus on an organ or a functional unit of organs. We believed that a pattern-oriented approach best enabled us to present a large body of information in the most useful form. As a result, these chapters are organized by radiologic patterns, problem-oriented patterns, or both.

In Chapter 2, congenital renal diseases are classified and discussed in terms of abnormalities of renal number, position, fusion, vasculature, and structure. This chapter includes a section on the normal anatomy and diseases of the retroperitoneal spaces around the kidney. Chapter 3 takes a "balls" versus "beans" approach, classifying renal mass lesions by morphology. The chapter discusses ball-shaped masses, multiple exophytic masses, and infiltrating masses, and concludes with an approach to the indeterminate renal mass. In Chapter 4, diffuse abnormalities of the kidney are discussed in terms of the size and shape of the kidney. Sections on nephrocalcinosis, renal failure, and renal trauma are included in the discussion of this subject. The renal sinus and the collecting system of the upper urinary tract are the subjects of Chapter 5. Diseases are classified in terms of familiar radiologic patterns of disease: masses, filling defects, and abnormalities of ureteral position or caliber. Chapter 6 classifies diseases of the bladder and urethra by similar radiologic

patterns: masses, wall thickening, filling defects, displacement, mural air or calcification, and outpouchings. In Chapter 7, diseases of the female genital tract are addressed using a problem-oriented approach. This chapter is divided into sections on congenital anomalies, pelvic pain, the ovarian cyst, infertility, and gynecologic oncology. The male genital tract is the subject of Chapter 8, and again, we use a problem-oriented approach to discuss common diseases of the scrotum and prostate gland. This chapter concludes with a discussion of the radiologic evaluation of erectile dysfunction. Chapter 9 begins with a systematic review of diseases of the adrenal gland and ends with a discussion of approaches to the patient with an incidental adrenal mass, adrenal hyperfunction, or adrenal insufficiency.

We hope our work serves you well and that you enjoy *Genitourinary Radiology: THE REQUISITES.*

Ronald J. Zagoria, M.D.
Glenn A. Tung, M.D.

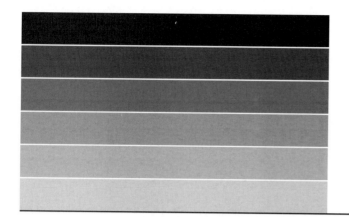

Acknowledgments

I am greatly indebted to many people in the Department of Radiology at The Bowman Gray School of Medicine of Wake Forest University for their help with this book. I feel blessed to have such superb staff and colleagues. Secretaries Karen Watson and Miriam Vernon have helped me keep my sanity throughout. Their skills and work habits are superb, and they kept a good sense of humor throughout this demanding project. Donna Garrison and her able assistants, Nancy Ragland and Terry Poovey, gave indispensable help on this book. Their assistance with editing, linguistics, and references has greatly improved the readability and flow of the text. I am indebted to Ray Dyer for his expertise, support, and the many figures that he shared with me for this book. I also thank the entire Abdominal Imaging Section for allowing me the time to complete this writing project. The excellent artwork was contributed by AnneMarie Johnson, who did a wonderful job converting my scribbles to understandable diagrams.

Finally, I am thankful to C. Douglas Maynard, the Chair of our department. As a role model and leader, he has encouraged my work and created an environment that supports academic excellence.

R.J.Z.

An undertaking of this magnitude cannot be completed without the assistance and support of many talented professionals. First and foremost, I sincerely thank Ronald J. Zagoria, M.D., for his dedication to this book. Struggling to complete a project that had begun to falter, I called on Ron to breathe new life into this endeavor. He came through with inimitable vigor and talent.

I also would like to acknowledge the residents, fellows, and staff of the Departments of Diagnostic Imaging at the Rhode Island Hospital and at the Women and Infants' Hospital, and the Department of Radiology at the Massachusetts General Hospital. In particular, I want to thank the following talented radiologists, who, with their knowledge and friendship, helped me to complete this book: Jeffrey M. Brody, M.D., John J. Cronan, M.D., William W. Mayo-Smith, M.D., Timothy P. Murphy, M.D., Richard B. Noto, M.D., Nicholas Papanicolaou, M.D., Richard C. Pfister, M.D., Mark S. Ridlen, M.D., Jeffrey M. Rogg, M.D., Juan M. Taveras, M.D., and Isabel C. Yoder, M.D.

I also would like to acknowledge the following individuals for their artistic and secretarial talents: Debbie Desjardins, John LaRiviere, Gayle Pascetta, Kassie Randall, and Hank Randall. I want to give very special thanks to Donna Garrison for her outstanding editorial talents and to Mia Cariño, David Orzechowski, and Elizabeth Corra at Mosby–Year Book, Inc., for their expertise, patience, and encouragement.

Finally, I am indebted to James H. Thrall, M.D., for his unwavering support from start to finish. Thank you for having faith in me.

G.A.T.

Contents

CHAPTER 1

An Introduction to Radiologic Methods

Table 1-1   Classification of Radiographic Contrast Media

Ionicity	Monomer or dimer	Ratio*	Relative osmolality†‡	Examples
Ionic	Monomer	1.5	~5	Diatrizoate
				Iodamide
				Ioglicate
				Iothalamate
				Ioxithalamate
				Metrizoate
Ionic	Dimer	3	~2	Ioxaglate
Nonionic	Monomer	3	1.5–1.8	Iohexol
				Iopamidol
				Iopentol
				Iopromide
				Ioversol
				Ioxilan
Nonionic	Dimer	6	1	Iodixonal
				Iotrol

*Ratio between the number of iodine atoms per molecule and the number of osmotically active particles produced by that molecule in solution.
†Relative osmolality expressed as a multiple of serum osmolality, 278–305 mOsm/kg serum water.
‡Data from product package inserts, product brochures, or technical information services.

Optimal radiologic investigation of the genitourinary system requires a combination of diverse but complementary examinations that evaluate form and function. In this chapter, we present an overview of diagnostic tests that are commonly used to evaluate genitourinary disease. In the first section, the pharmacology of iodinated contrast media is reviewed. Adverse effects and an approach to the management of common adverse reactions are also discussed. In the second section, we turn to the individual radiologic examinations and discuss the general indications for the test and guidelines for interpretation. The penultimate section reviews the cross-sectional imaging methods (ultrasonography, computed tomography [CT], and magnetic resonance imaging [MRI]), angiography, and nuclear medicine. In the final section, recommended methods for performing these examinations are presented in a series of appendices.

RADIOGRAPHIC CONTRAST MEDIA

Radiographic contrast media (RCM) were developed to increase differences in the attenuation (absorption) of radiation by soft tissues. As a result, all commercially available radiographic contrast agents are triiodinated derivatives of benzoic acid. The other chemical constituents of the contrast molecule carry the iodine so that it can

be delivered in large volumes, in high concentrations, and with as little toxicity as possible. Some contrast materials are ionic, which means these agents dissociate into cations and anions in water. The osmolality of a solution is a measure of the number of dissolved particles in each liter of solution. Some of the adverse effects of RCM are related to their hyperosmolality, which ranges between two and five times that of plasma. The density of RCM is related to the number of iodine atoms per milliliter of solution and directly correlates with x-ray attenuation. RCM can be subdivided into three classes, which are based on a ratio between the number of iodine atoms in the molecule and the number of osmotically active particles produced by that molecule in solution (Table 1-1 and Fig. 1-1). At present, ratio 1.5 (high osmolar contrast media [HOCM]) and ratio 3 (low osmolar contrast media [LOCM]) are in active use.

All ionic contrast media are salts of iodinated, organic salts that dissociate completely in blood. Thus, these

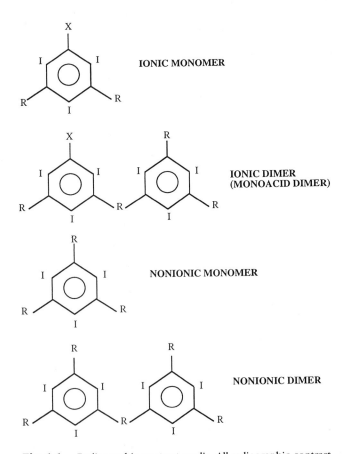

Fig. 1-1   Radiographic contrast media. All radiographic contrast media are based on a 2-, 4-, 6-substituted triiodobenzoic acid molecule. High-osmolar contrast media (ratio 1.5) are ionic monomers. Low-osmolar contrast media are either ionic dimers (ratio 3), nonionic monomers (ratio 3), or nonionic dimers (ratio 6). [R = hydrophilic, nonionizing side chains; X = ionic moiety: —COO⁻ and either a sodium or methylglucamine cation].

molecules consist of a positively charged cation and a negatively charged anion. The diagnostically useful contrast molecule itself is the organic anion, which consists of an iodine-substituted benzene ring, with sodium or meglumine serving as the cation. The cation provides no radiographically significant information but contributes half of the osmotic effect of the medium. Diatrizoate and its derivatives are ionic monomeric salts of triiodinated, fully substituted benzoic acids. As ratio 1.5 agents, ionic monomeric salts are also referred to as HOCM because for every three iodine atoms in solution, there are two osmotically active particles in the solution. The ionic dimeric salts are ratio 3 contrast agents, consisting of an anionic moiety with two triiodinated benzene rings. Ioxaglate is an example of a monoacidic dimeric salt that is intended for intravascular use but not for myelography.

The nonionic compounds were developed to reduce the osmolality of contrast agents while preserving excellent image contrast. The addition of a nonionizing glucose moiety to the carboxyl group transforms the iodinated benzoic acid derivative into a nonionic compound. The nonionic monomer class of RCM consists of ratio 3 agents because for every three iodine atoms, there is only one particle in solution. Iopamidol and iohexol are two examples of second generation nonionic monomers. These agents, along with the ionic dimer class of contrast medium, are referred to as low osmolar contrast media because the osmolality of these compounds is about twice that of serum osmolality. The third class of RCM is made up of nonionic dimers that do not dissociate in solution. Iotrol and iodixanol provide six iodine atoms for every osmotically active molecule. These ratio 6 agents have the lowest osmolalities but also the greatest viscosity of all RCM because of the large molecular size.

Pharmacokinetics

All radiographic contrast media are hydrophilic and have low lipid solubility. Having little affinity for proteins and membrane-bound receptors, RCM also have minimal pharmacologic action. After intravenous administration, the decline in the plasma concentration of contrast material results from diffusion into the extravascular space, vascular mixing, and renal excretion. The kidneys normally excrete more than 99% of the intravenous dose of ratio 1.5 or ratio 3 contrast media. Less than 1% is excreted through nonrenal routes, including the hepatobiliary system and sweat, tears, and saliva. All of the currently available contrast media are excreted via the kidney by glomerular filtration with no significant tubular excretion or resorption. HOCM cause significant osmotic diuresis, which secondarily decreases the tubular concentration of contrast medium. By comparison, LOCM cause less

osmotic diuresis, and as a result, the concentration of ratio 3 contrast media in the urine is significantly higher.

Contrast Nephropathy

Contrast-associated nephropathy (CN) is defined as an acute impairment of renal function after exposure to a radiographic contrast medium. Although there are various specific definitions, a common definition of renal impairment is a rise in the serum creatinine of at least 1.0 mg/dL within 2 to 5 days of exposure to RCM. Creatinine levels usually return to normal by 7 to 12 days. Contrast nephropathy is typically reversible, but rare cases of permanent nephrotoxicity, which is more common when renal failure is oliguric, have necessitated dialysis or transplantation. A delayed, persistent nephrogram at 24 hours has been observed in the majority of patients with CN. Various mechanisms have been suggested to explain the adverse effect of contrast media on renal function. Some putative mechanisms include prerenal effects from dehydration or hypotension, direct effects on intrarenal hemodynamics, direct nephrotoxic effect on tubular cells, intratubular obstruction from proteinuria, uricosuria, and indirect nephrotoxic effects from an altered immunologic response.

The most important risk factor for the development of CN is preexisting renal insufficiency, practically defined as a serum creatinine level greater than 1.5 mg/dL. Unsuspected azotemia caused by hypertensive nephropathy or vascular disease is especially prevalent in the elderly. Preexposure dehydration, whether inadvertent or intentional, may exacerbate nephrotoxicity, particularly in patients with azotemia. Patients with insulin-dependent diabetes mellitus and secondary renal disease are at a particularly high risk for development of CN; the frequency of CN is 50% to 100% when serum creatinine is more than 3.5 mg/dL in these patients. However, patients with diabetes mellitus or multiple myeloma and normal renal function do not appear to be at an increased risk. Repeated administration of contrast material over a short period of time (within 72 hours) increases the risk of developing CN. In general, a total iodine dose of 80 g in a 24-hour period is safe. With a total iodine dose of more than 100 g in a 24-hour period, the patient is at high risk for irreversible renal failure.

Compared with ionic counterparts, nonionic monomers cause fewer changes in the glomerular filtration rate and less tubular damage. However, some studies of patients with normal or slightly decreased renal function report no statistical difference in the prevalence of contrast-induced nephrotoxicity between patients receiving ionic compounds and those receiving nonionic compounds. Other studies suggest that patients who have preexisting renal insufficiency, defined as serum creatinine levels between 1.4 mg/dL and 2.4 mg/dL, may be at higher risk for nephrotoxicity with HOCM than with LOCM. In 1993, Barrett et al concluded from a meta-analysis of 24 trials that the use of LOCM may be beneficial in patients with preexisting renal failure because the mean postexposure change in serum creatinine level was 0.2 to 6.2 μmol/L less with LOCM than with HOCM.

The prevention of CN first involves determining if the requested examination is appropriate for the given clinical question. Directing the work-up away from an examination requiring contrast material administration is appropriate when the potential risks of adverse reaction might be serious or life-threatening. Careful screening of patients for well-defined high-risk factors, known renal disease, treatment with nephrotoxic drugs, renal insufficiency, diabetes mellitus, and dehydration is mandatory. If any of these high-risk factors is present, an assessment of renal function is prudent. In patients with none of these risk factors, the likelihood of suffering permanent renal damage from CN is so remote that routine measurement of renal function is unnecessary. Preparation protocols that involve intentional dehydration or catharsis should be avoided. If multiple examinations requiring contrast material are indicated, they should be performed over an extended period of time, for example, longer than 72 hours.

Adverse Reactions

Like other drugs, radiographic contrast media are associated with untoward reactions attributable to their physicochemical structure, direct toxic effects on sensitive organs, and allergy-like reactions (anaphylactoid, idiosyncratic, or pseudoallergic). These adverse side effects occur after 5% to 8% of all intravenous injections with ionic HOCM and in 1% to 3% of injections with nonionic or LOCM. Fortunately, most of these adverse reactions are minor in severity; they include sensations of body warmth, pruritus, urticaria, nausea, and vomiting.

A practical way to classify untoward reactions to RCM is to group them by nature and clinical severity. *Mild* contrast reactions include pruritus, hives, nausea, warmth, altered gustatory sensations, swelling of the face, conjunctival injection, and vomiting. In the majority of patients, no treatment beyond reassurance is necessary. However, like all untoward effects, these mild reactions require close observation because they rarely do progress or are prodromal to more serious reactions. About 1% to 2% of patients receiving conventional HOCM have a non–life-threatening, *moderate* reaction. Examples of these types of reactions include bradycardia or tachycardia (especially when associated with acute changes in blood pressure), dyspnea, laryngospasm, and bronchospasm. Patients with moderate reactions require close monitoring and often require treatment. Any reaction may be classified as *severe* when it is potentially life-threatening. Often, the patient loses consciousness or has clinically significant dysrhythmia. Patients with severe reactions not only must be treated promptly, but almost always require hospitalization for optimal treatment. Severe, life-threatening reactions occur after 0.05% to 0.10% of injections of HOCM. Reported fatalities attributable to reactions to contrast media are estimated to occur in one of every 75,000 administrations.

The majority of adverse effects are evident immediately after injection, and all life-threatening reactions occur within 15 minutes after injection. Rarely, delayed reactions can occur 24 to 48 hours after exposure. However, these delayed reactions are almost exclusively mild in character and include rash or pruritus and pain near the injection site. "Iodine mumps" refers to delayed parotid swelling caused by trace levels of free iodide in contrast media. Specific management of the more commonly encountered mild and moderate adverse reactions is outlined in Tables 1-2 and 1-3.

The frequency and severity of reactions to contrast material may be influenced by the type, dose, route, and rate of delivery. Experimental and clinical data suggest

Table 1-2 Management of Common Adverse Reactions to Radiographic Contrast Media			
Adverse reaction	**First line**	**Second line**	**Third line**
Urticaria (hives)	Reassurance	Diphenhydramine	Epinephrine SC
Vagal reaction	Elevate legs; consider volume expansion*	Atropine sulfate	—
Laryngeal edema	Oxygen	Epinephrine SC	Intubation
Bronchospasm	Oxygen	Inhaled beta$_2$-agonist†	Epinephrine SC‡
Hypotension and tachycardia	Elevate legs; consider volume expansion*	Epinephrine IV	—

*Volume expansion with 0.9% saline or Ringer's lactate.
†Inhaled beta$_2$-agonists, such as metaproterenol, albuterol, or nebulized terbutaline.
‡Alternatives to subcutaneous epinephrine in the management of bronchospasm include aminophylline drip or terbutaline SC or IM.
SC = subcutaneous; IV = intravenous; IM = intramuscular.

Table 1-3   Drugs Used in the Management of Common Adverse Reactions

Drug	Trade name	Dose	Route of administration
Albuterol	Proventil®, Ventolin®	—	Inhaled
Aminophylline drip	—	6 mg/kg loading dose, 0.5-1.0 mg/kg/hr IV drip	Intravenous
Atropine sulfate	—	1-mg doses to a total of 2 mg	Intravenous
Diphenhydramine	Benadryl®	25-50 mg	Oral/intramuscular/intravenous
Epinephrine	—	1:10,000 dilution, 3-mL doses to a total of 10 mL	Intraveneous
Epinephrine	—	1:1,000 dilution, 0.3-mL dose to a total of 1 mL	Subcutaneous
Metaproterenol	Alupent®, Metaprel®	—	Inhaled
Terbutaline	—	0.25-0.5 mg	Subcutaneous/intramuscular

that LOCM produce fewer chemotoxic adverse side effects than do HOCM. The prevalence of anaphylactoid reactions may also be lower. Multicenter surveillance studies have estimated that the relative risk of any adverse reactions is reduced by a factor of 3 to 8, and the risk of severe reaction is reduced by a factor of 4 to 12 when LOCM are used. The prevalence of most reactions is greater with the intravenous route than with the intraarterial route. Exposure of mast cell–rich pulmonary capillary beds to relatively higher concentrations of contrast may explain this observation. However, the prevalence of severe reactions is greater after intraarterial injections. Bolus intravenous injection produces fewer reactions than drip infusion does.

Nonionic radiocontrast media are approximately 10 to 12 times as expensive as ionic contrast agents, and in the era of cost-containment, universal use is waning. If the use of nonionic or other LOCM is selective, the prevention of adverse reactions to HOCM depends on identifying those patients at higher risk for these reactions. In these patients, the selective use of LOCM, medical pretreatment, or both is logical and advised (Box 1-1). For patients with a history of allergy or asthma, the relative increased risk of any adverse reaction is about twice that for the general population. In any patient who is debilitated or has a history of severe cardiopulmonary disease, the effects of even a moderate reaction may be poorly tolerated. For patients who have a history that includes an adverse reaction after RCM exposure, the reaction prevalence is 17% to 35%, or three to eight times the risk for the general population.

Several studies have concluded that medical pretreatment can reduce the re-treatment prevalence of adverse side effects in high-risk patients to that observed in the general population. Most of these premedication regimens include a corticosteroid administered alone or together with either an H1- or an H2-antihistamine. Steroids exert a salutary effect through stabilization of membranes and therefore may impede release of critical mediators of anaphylactoid reactions. In a group of patients with a history of adverse reaction to RCM, Lasser et al concluded that pretreatment with an oral regimen of methylprednisolone, 32 mg, taken 12 and 2 hours before the

Box 1-1   Considerations for the Selective Use of Low Osmolar Contrast Media*

UROGRAPHY, BODY COMPUTED TOMOGRAPHY, NEURORADIOLOGY, AND PEDIATRIC ANGIOGRAPHY

Previous contrast reaction (if previous contrast reaction was moderate or severe and required treatment)

Severe allergy, asthma, reactive airways disease, or atopy

History of heart disease (e.g., unstable or daily angina pectoris, within 1 week of myocardial infarction, borderline or overt congestive heart failure, or pulmonary artery hypertension)

PEDIATRIC RADIOLOGY (IN ADDITION TO ABOVE)

Phlebitis or difficult access to small vessels
Neonatal gastrointestinal evaluation

ANGIOGRAPHY (IN ADDITION TO ABOVE)

Pain or spasm associated with the examination
Pulmonary angiography in a patient with pulmonary hypertension

NEURORADIOLOGY (IN ADDITION TO ABOVE)

Myelography
Spinal angiography
Selective arteriography for severe occlusive carotid and vertebral artery disease
Selective angiography for arteriovenous malformation and aneurysm angiography
Selective external carotid arteriography
If any patient specifically requests that low osmolar contrast medium be used for the examination, it should be provided.

*Modified from the Procedure Manual, Department of Radiology, Massachusetts General Hospital.

intravenous administration of HOCM, decreased the occurrence of all classes of reactions. Other studies delivering a three-dose oral regimen of prednisone, 50 mg, taken every 6 hours beginning at least 13 hours before exposure to HOCM, and diphenhydramine, 50 mg, administered orally or intramuscularly at least 1 hour before exposure to HOCM, have also demonstrated reduced reaction prevalence. The acceptance of pretreatment protocols is hampered by inconvenience. Unless the need for pretreatment is recognized in advance, examinations or procedures must be delayed at least 12 hours. The resulting logistic problems have favored the use of LOCM over medical pretreatment.

INTRAVENOUS UROGRAPHY

Intravenous urography (IVU) is the test of choice when a screening examination of the upper and lower urinary tracts is indicated (Appendix A). This test is primarily used to investigate a suspected or known congenital anomaly of the urinary tract, ureteral obstruction, or upper tract mucosal neoplasm. IVU is used frequently to evaluate the patient with flank, pelvic, or groin pain that might be caused by an obstructing renal or ureteral calculus. It is also one of the principal tests used for the evaluation of hematuria.

Because the appearance of contrast medium in the renal tubules depends on glomerular filtration, renal visualization may be suboptimal in patients with moderate and severe renal failure. In general, urography is unlikely to be useful in patients with serum creatinine levels above 3.5 to 4.0 mg/dL. In addition, the risk of contrast nephropathy is increased with serum creatinine levels above 1.5 mg/dL.

Normal Intravenous Urogram

A careful evaluation of the preliminary or scout film is mandatory. This preliminary film is not only important for the subsequent interpretation of the IVU, but it may provide important ancillary information about the axial skeleton, abnormal calcifications, visceral enlargement, soft tissue masses, and bowel gas pattern, i.e., "bones, stones, mass, gas." Renal shadows and the pubic symphysis must be included on the preliminary film.

Sixty to 90 seconds after the bolus administration of contrast medium, a cortical nephrogram can be seen. The nephrogram represents contrast material within the tubules and depends on the plasma concentration of contrast and the glomerular filtration rate. The peak nephrogram density after bolus administration of contrast

occurs earlier and is somewhat greater, but it decreases more rapidly than when contrast medium is given by intravenous drip infusion. The lower limit of normal renal length can be approximated by the distance between the superior endplate of L1 and the inferior endplate of L3. Renal length should not exceed the span of the first four lumbar vertebrae. Peak opacification of the intrarenal collecting system and true pelvis occurs approximately 2 to 3 minutes after contrast material administration (Fig. 1-2). Ureteral filling with contrast begins at about this time, and peak opacification occurs 5 to 10 minutes after intravenous contrast material is given (Fig. 1-3). As contrast medium slowly appears in the bladder, it preferentially collects against the dependent posterior wall in the patient positioned supine. In the patient positioned prone, contrast is seen along the anterior bladder wall, which is in a relatively more cephalad position than the posterior wall (Fig. 1-4). The mucosal pattern of the bladder is best assessed on the post-void film, because dense contrast in the filled bladder may obscure a lesion (Fig. 1-5B on p. 10). Furthermore, a radiograph obtained after voiding that shows complete emptying suggests normal bladder function. The converse is not true, however, because a moderate amount of residual urine may be explained by causes other than dysfunctional micturition.

CYSTOGRAPHY AND URETHROGRAPHY

Retrograde cystography is the radiologic evaluation of the bladder after instillation of contrast material by catheter, either transurethral or suprapubic, or by needle puncture. Voiding cystourethrography (VCUG) is contrast radiography of the urinary bladder and urethra during spontaneous micturition (Appendix B). Dynamic retrograde urethrography (RUG) is radiography of the urethra while it is being distended by instillation of contrast through a catheter (Appendix C).

The main indications for cystography are the evaluation of acquired disorders of micturition, vesicoureteral reflux, and traumatic injury of the bladder. Injury to the bladder should be suspected in a patient with difficulty voiding, pelvic fracture, or gross hematuria after trauma. Radiologic evaluation of the bladder frequently is performed before renal transplantation and in patients with spinal cord injury. Cystography has been used to distinguish a mechanical obstructive cause of micturition dysfunction from a neurogenic cause. VCUG in children is used to determine whether vesicoureteral reflux or a congenital anomaly of the urinary tract is responsible for urinary tract infection or collecting-system dilatation. In adults, reflux should be suspected in the patient with an upper urinary tract infection when no other cause is

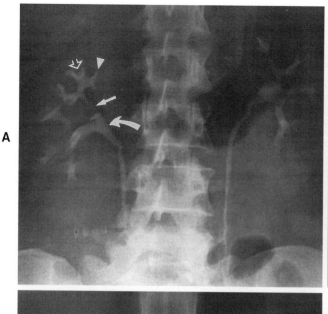

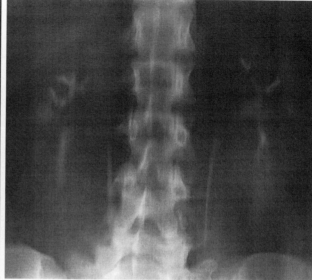

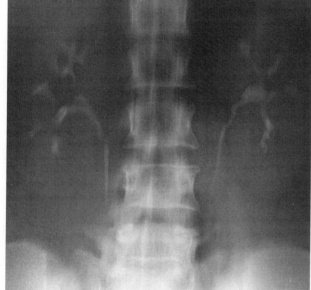

Fig. 1-2   Normal pyelogram and nephrotomograms. **A,** Normal 5-minute urogram. The renal pelvis (curved arrow) branches to form the infundibula. There is a filling defect at the base of the right superior infundibulum (arrow) that is typically caused by a crossing vessel. The cupped calyx (open arrow) is formed by the impression of the papilla, and the fornix (arrowhead) is the side of the calyx. There are between 10 and 25 calyces in each kidney. **B and C,** In many patients, the kidneys are rotated obliquely. As a result, three or four contiguous nephrotomograms are necessary to image the kidneys. The upper pole of the kidney is situated more posteriorly, and therefore, a lower nephrotomogram **(B)** usually defines the upper pole, and a higher cut **(C)** will define the lower pole of the kidney.

plausible or when reflux nephropathy is noted on urograms. In women, cystourethrography frequently is used to evaluate stress incontinence or suspected urethral diverticulum. In men, benign prostatic hyperplasia and urethral stricture are common reasons why cystourethrography is performed.

In boys or men, the main indication for dynamic RUG is suspected injury or stricture of the anterior urethra. If no trauma to the urethra is documented by urethrography, the catheter can be advanced safely into the bladder. As necessary, cystography may follow. Urethrography with a double-balloon catheter is performed in women primarily when a urethral diverticulum is suspected but cannot be confirmed by VCUG.

Normal Cystogram and Urethrogram

The wall of the distended bladder is smooth and thin. In men, the height (vertical dimension) of the bladder may be greater than the width (horizontal dimension); the opposite is often true in women. The base of the bladder is normally at or just below the level of the superior pubic ramus. The base is slightly convex in the supine position, but it is funnel-shaped when the patient voids in an upright position (Figs. 1-5, 1-6 on p. 10).

The male urethra consists of the anterior and posterior urethrae (Fig. 1-6). The posterior urethra is divided into the prostatic and membranous parts and extends from the internal sphincter (at the bladder neck) to the exter-

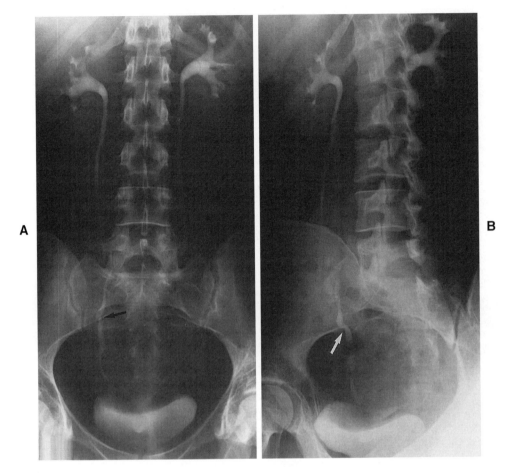

Fig. 1-3   The normal ureter on intravenous urogram anteroposterior **(A)** and oblique **(B)** 15-minute urograms demonstrates the normal morphology of the collecting system. The abdominal part of the ureter begins at the renal pelvis. In general, a ureter that is medial to the ipsilateral lumbar pedicle is abnormally deviated medially, and a ureter that lies more than 1 cm lateral to the tip of the ipsilateral lumbar transverse process is deviated laterally. The abdominal ureters should be separated by 5 cm or more. The pelvic part of the ureter begins where it crosses the iliac vessels at the pelvic brim (arrow). The level of the ureterovesical junction is approximated by the ipsilateral ischial spine. Normal areas of ureteral narrowing are expected at the ureteropelvic junction, at the pelvic brim, and at the ureterovesical junction.

nal sphincter (at the urogenital diaphragm). The prostatic part is normally wide and passes through the transitional zone of the prostate gland. The verumontanum (urethral crest) is an elongated oval filling defect on the posterior wall of the prostatic urethra; the prostatic urethra ends at the distal end of the verumontanum. The external sphincter is distal to the verumontanum and creates a narrowing on the retrograde urethrogram; this is the membranous part of the posterior urethra. The anterior urethra is divided into the bulbar and penile parts. The bulbous part of the anterior urethra extends from the external sphincter to the penoscrotal junction, where the penile urethra is angled by the suspensory ligament of the penis. Cowper's glands are embedded in the mus-

cle of the urogenital diaphragm, and its ducts enter the floor of the bulbar urethra. The penile or pendulous urethra is the most distal part of the anterior urethra and ends at the external meatus. Just proximal to the external meatus, there may be a slight widening of the penile urethra, the fossa navicularis.

The female urethra is approximately 4 cm in length and extends from the internal urethral orifice (at the bladder neck) to the external orifice (anterior to the vagina). The urethra is widest at the bladder neck and tapers distally; it has an oblique anterior course (Fig. 1-7 on p. 11).

Further discussion of the anatomy of the male urethra and other examples of normal radiographic examinations of the bladder and urethra can be found in Chapter 6.

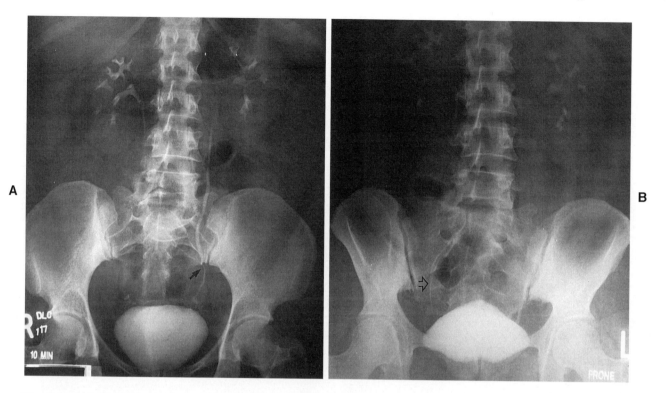

Fig. 1-4   Supine and prone intravenous urograms. **A,** On this supine urogram, the distal right ureter is not seen well. The entire ureter may not be opacified because of peristalsis. Normal peristalsis may be stalled where the ureter crosses the iliac vessels (arrow); a focal dilatation just above the iliac vessel crossover is called the ureteral spindle. The posterior part of the bladder is opacified. **B,** The prone urogram is useful because there is often filling of ureteral segments that are not seen on the supine film. On this prone urogram, the distal right ureter (open arrow) is well demonstrated. The prone film is also excellent for demonstrating filling defects on the anterior bladder wall. The sacrum appears larger; the iliac wings are foreshortened, and the apex of the anterior bladder wall is tapered on a prone urogram.

RETROGRADE PYELOGRAPHY

Retrograde pyelography (RP) is radiography of the ureter and renal collecting system after direct injection of contrast material into the ureter. The technique requires cystoscopy. A 4 to 7 F ureteral catheter with a round, bulb, or spiral tip is used to cannulate and obstruct the ureteral orifice. Many of the current catheters have open ends that allow passage of a guidewire for further endo-urologic manipulation. Contrast medium is instilled slowly by syringe or by gravity flow. Alternatively, a flexible catheter can be passed over a guidewire to the upper ureter or renal pelvis, and contrast is instilled through the catheter.

Retrograde pyelography is not an adequate screening examination of the urinary tract because the renal parenchyma is not directly opacified. For this reason and because it is an invasive procedure, RP is usually performed after preliminary urography, sonography, or CT, which

may suggest the presence of a filling defect, mass, or obstruction of the collecting system. Indications for RP include evaluation of the ureter when not adequately visualized on IVU, evaluation of a filling defect in the renal pelvis or ureter detected on IVU, and evaluation of the collecting system in patients with hematuria and no clear cause after urography, sonography, or CT. RP is also performed as a preliminary examination before selective collection of urine from each kidney or before ureteral brushing and biopsy of a lesion suspected of being malignant.

Test Interpretation

When filming is not supervised directly by a radiologist, it is important to confer with the urologist if any questionable radiographic finding is discovered. For a study result to be considered normal, the entire collecting system must be demonstrated. If present, the entire length of a ureteral filling defect should be shown. The

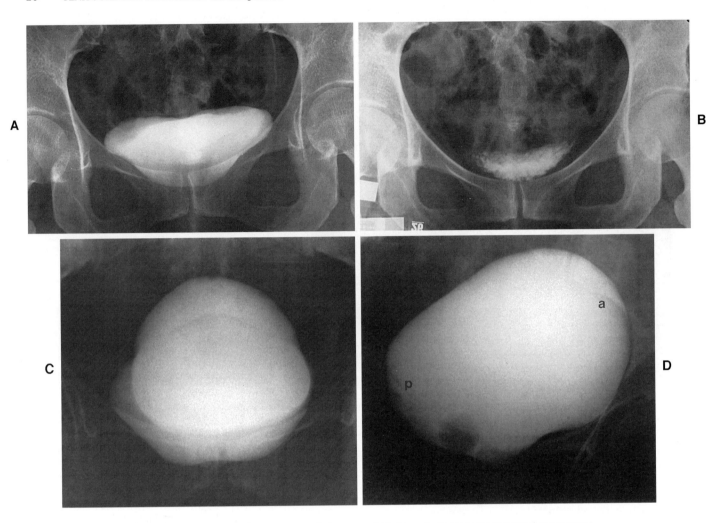

Fig. 1-5   Urograms and cystograms of the normal bladder. **A,** Supine anteroposterior urogram demonstrates the normal bladder wall. **B,** The postvoid film shows the normal mucosal pattern of the empty bladder. **C,** On the cystogram, the anterior and posterior margins of the bladder overlap. The walls of the bladder are smooth. **D,** On this oblique cystogram with a Foley catheter at the bladder neck, the superior surface and apex or anterior part of the bladder are more cephalad than the base and neck or posterior part of the bladder (a = anterior, p = posterior).

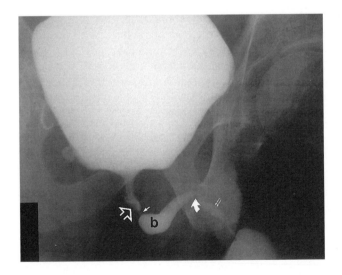

Fig. 1-6   Left posterior oblique voiding cystourethrogram demonstrates the normal appearance of the male urethra. The verumontanum (open arrow) is a mound of tissue that causes a focal filling defect along the posterior wall of the prostatic urethra. The focal narrowing (small arrow) distal to the prostatic urethra is caused by the external urethral sphincter and denotes the membranous part of the posterior urethra. Another normal narrowing (curved arrow) can be seen at the penoscrotal angle. The anterior urethra consists of the bulbous (b) and the penile or pendulous (small double arrows) urethra.

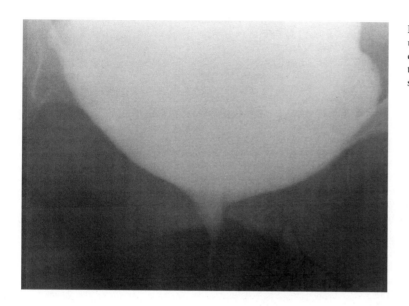

Fig. 1-7 Voiding cystourethrogram shows the normal urethra in a woman. The urethra is 4 cm long and tapers distally; its length corresponds to the male posterior urethra. The base and neck of the bladder assume a funnel shape during micturition.

calyces are blunted frequently on retrograde pyelograms because contrast material is injected under positive pressure. Backflow occurs when there is rupture at the calyceal fornices or retrograde opacification of the collecting ducts (pyelotubular backflow). With pyelosinus backflow, there is opacification of renal sinus tissues around the calyces, renal pelvis, or proximal ureter after forniceal rupture (Fig. 1-8). The arcuate veins and hilar lymphatic vessels are opacified with pyelovenous and pyelolymphatic backflow, respectively.

Complications

The most commonly reported complication of RP is perforation of the ureter or renal pelvis. Spasm or edema of the ureter may cause transient obstruction. Contrast medium can be absorbed during RP, and moderate or severe reactions may occur, although they are rare. Fulminant sepsis may complicate an injection of contrast material proximal to a site of pelvoureteral obstruction.

URODYNAMIC ANTEGRADE PYELOGRAPHY

Dilatation of the collecting system does not always result from mechanical obstruction. Residual ectasia from previous obstruction, vesicoureteral reflux, congenital malformation, or high urine-flow states are common disorders that can cause dilatation of the collecting system in the absence of obstruction. Evaluation of a dilated collecting system with a renal scan or by measuring contrast material excretion rates after antegrade or RP may

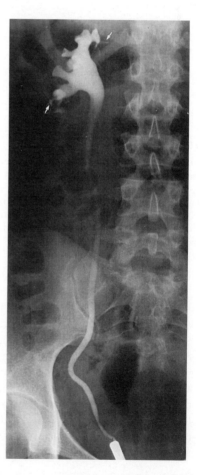

Fig. 1-8 Pyelosinus backflow. A retrograde pyelogram demonstrates the normal course and contour of the right ureter; blunting of the calyces can be normal. Streaks of contrast material extend from an upper and a lower pole calyx (arrows). Pyelosinus backflow results from microtears of the calyceal fornix caused by the positive pressure of the retrograde injection.

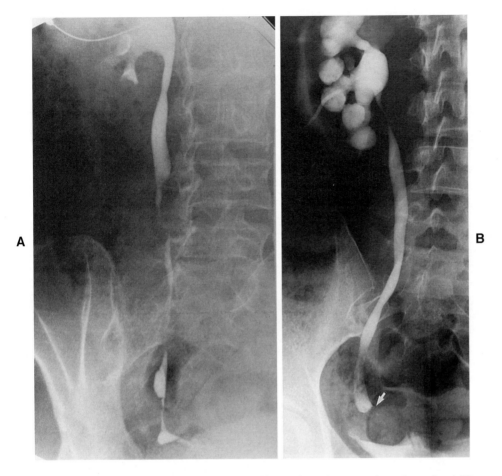

Fig. 1-9   Distal ureteral stricture demonstrated by urodynamic antegrade pyelography. A 22-year-old woman with recurrent urinary tract infections was referred for a Whitaker test because minimal dilatation of the right ureter was seen on an intravenous urogram. **A,** The opening pressure was 10 cm water, and the antegrade pyelogram shows multiple ureteral narrowings that were attributed to peristalsis. **B,** At a perfusion rate of 10 cc per minute, the differential pressure increased to 32 cm water (normal < 13 cm water). Pyelogram demonstrates ureteropyelocaliectasis caused by a focal stricture of the distal ureter (arrow).

not be optimal in patients with poor renal function, a markedly dilated or tortuous ureter, or a urinary bladder diversion. For patients in whom it is unclear whether collecting system dilatation is associated with a pressure gradient between the upper collecting system and bladder, urodynamic antegrade pyelography (ureteral perfusion test or pressure–flow examination of Whitaker) is indicated. This study quantifies resistance within the collecting system by measuring the pressure gradient between the kidney and bladder at known rates of flow.

Technique

Urodynamic antegrade pyelography is an invasive examination, requiring antegrade pyelography. VCUG is performed first to exclude vesicoureteral reflux. The vesi-

cal catheter is left in place, and the patient is turned to a prone position on the fluoroscopy table. Standard needle puncture of the kidney is performed with a 20- to 22-gauge needle. The antegrade needle and the vesical catheter are attached to separate manometers, which are positioned at the level of the urinary bladder. The opening or resting pressure of the kidney is recorded. An antegrade pyelogram is performed. Next, dilute iodinated contrast medium is instilled through the antegrade pyelography needle, and an infusion pump is used to regulate the flow. Perfusion of the collecting system at a rate of 10 cc per minute is continued until the entire pyeloureteral system is opacified, usually after approximately 5 minutes. At this time, the infusion pump is stopped, and the pressure within the collecting system and urinary bladder is measured and recorded (Fig. 1-9).

Examination Interpretation

With chronic hydronephrosis, elevated intrarenal pressure gradually decreases as renal function decreases and as the compliance of the dilated collecting system increases. The opening pressure of the renal collecting system may be normal or only slightly elevated, particularly in the setting of chronic obstruction. For this reason, the opening intrarenal pressure is significant only when it is substantially elevated (i.e., ≥ 50 cm water). A more meaningful assessment of pyeloureteral resistance is the differential pressure (DP) between the bladder and the kidney. As the bladder fills, intravesical and renal pelvis pressures increase, but the DP decreases. At a perfusion rate of 10 cc per minute, the normal DP is less than 13 cm water. Mild, moderate, and severe mechanical obstruction are suggested by differential pressures of 14 to 20 cm water, 21 to 34 cm water, and more than 34 cm water, respectively. When the DP is in the high normal or low abnormal range, the infusion rate can be increased from 10 cc per minute to 15 cc per minute or even 20 cc per minute. At these higher rates of flow, the normal range of values for the DP increases. At an infusion rate of 15 cc per minute in a patient with an empty bladder, the normal upper-limit value for the DP is 18 cm water, and at 20 cc per minute, it is 21 cm water.

ILEOSTOURETEROGRAPHY (ILEAL LOOPOGRAM)

Excretory urography, radionuclide studies, and sonography are used commonly to evaluate the cutaneous ureteroileostomy. The urogram is probably the simplest way to evaluate the collecting system and ileal loop, and in the majority of patients, it provides the necessary anatomic and functional information. Radionuclide imaging can be used to quantify upper urinary tract function and provides some anatomic information. Sonography is used to evaluate the size of the intrarenal collecting system, particularly in patients with poor renal function or contraindications to urography, but it is not well suited to evaluate the ureters. If poor renal function precludes optimal anatomic evaluation of the collecting system by excretory urography or if there is a contraindication to performing IVU, a retrograde contrast examination of the ileal loop and renal collecting system (ileostoureterogram or ileal loopogram) may be performed (Appendix D).

Ileostoureterography is usually performed if the patient has progressive hydronephrosis and the cause is not apparent after intravenous urography or radionuclide renography. Causes of mechanical obstruction include urolithiasis, ureteroileal anastomotic strictures, midloop stenosis, and stomal stenosis. Although urography is usually diagnostic in patients with ureteroileal leak, an ileal loopogram can also confirm this diagnosis.

Test Interpretation

The ileal conduit should be evaluated for size and shape. The ileal conduit is usually constructed in the right lower quadrant and is 12 to 15 cm in length. It is important to evaluate for segmental narrowings attributed to loop ischemia. These stenoses may cause obstruction.

Free reflux of contrast material through the ureteroileal anastomoses permits evaluation of the collecting system of the upper urinary tract. However, in approximately 10% of patients, reflux of contrast material is not possible and the antegrade flow of urine through the ureteroileal anastomosis is normal. The course and contour of the ureters must be evaluated. The left ureter may opacify later than the right ureter because the left ureter is tunneled beneath the mesentery. Mild dilatation of the ureter and blunting of the calyces is normal because contrast material is instilled under positive pressure (Fig. 1-10). Any filling defect or stenosis should be filmed in multiple projections.

Complications

Because the vigorous instillation of contrast medium can result in bacteremia, preprocedure medication with antibiotics is recommended. A rare complication of loopography is the development of autonomic dysreflexia in patients with spinal cord injuries. This complication is thought to result from overdistension of the ileal loop and may result in severe hypertension.

HYSTEROSALPINGOGRAPHY

Hysterosalpingography is a radiographic method of examining the endometrial cavity and the lumen of the fallopian tubes after instillation of contrast material into the cervical canal (Appendix E). The main indication for hysterosalpingography is the evaluation of the endometrial cavity and fallopian tubes in patients with primary or secondary infertility. Patients who have had tubal reconstructive surgery may undergo hysterosalpingography to evaluate tubal patency and morphology and to assess the development of paratubal adhesions. Hystero-

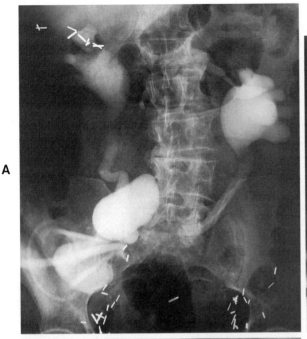

A

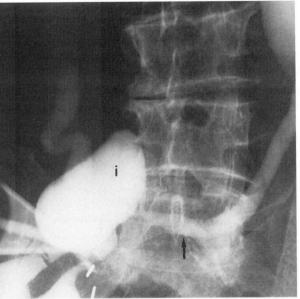

B

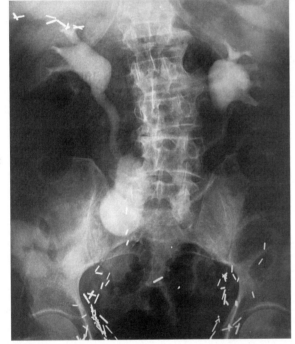

C

Fig. 1-10   Radiography of the ileal loop conduit. **A,** Retrograde ileostoureterogram (ileal loopogram) shows a nonobstructed collecting system. Distension of the collecting system can be a normal finding on retrograde urograms. **B,** On a magnified, coned view, the left ureter (arrow) crosses the midline to reach the ileal conduit (i) in the right lower quadrant. **C,** Compare the appearance of the collecting system on this intravenous urogram with its appearance on the ileal loopogram.

salpingography is also performed on patients with known or suspected müllerian anomalies, which may manifest as infertility, multiple miscarriages, premature labor, or fetal malpresentation. Hysterosalpingography may also be used to determine the location of a uterine leiomyoma relative to the endometrial cavity. Three contraindications to hysterosalpingography are pregnancy, acute pelvic infection, and active menstruation.

Normal Hysterosalpingogram

The opacified endometrial and endocervical cavities have the shape of a triangle with an elongated apex. The base of the triangle is the fundus; with anteflexion of the uterus, a common position when the bladder is empty, the fundus may be located inferior to the lower corpus and cervix. The elongated apex of the triangle is the

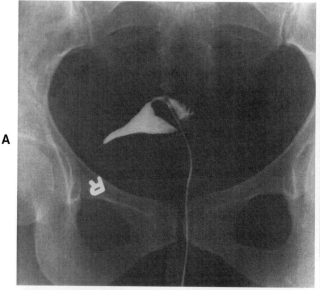

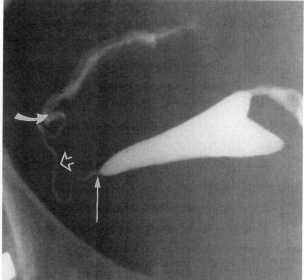

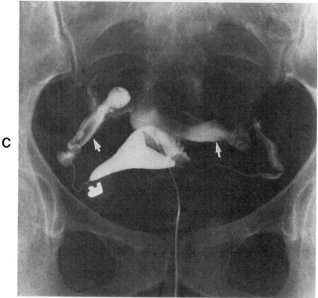

Fig. 1-11 Catheter hysterosalpingograms demonstrate the normal uterus and fallopian tube. **A,** The normal endometrial and endocervical cavities of an anteflexed uterus are shown. The tip of the catheter is in the endocervical canal, which has a feathery contour. **B,** The interstitial part of the right fallopian tube (long arrow) is contained in the myometrium. The gracile part of the tube, the isthmus (open arrow), inserts at the uterine cornua. The tube flares laterally, forming the ampulla (curved arrow) and the infundibulum. The infundibulum opens into the peritoneal cavity at the fimbriated end of the tube. **C,** Contrast material is seen in the pelvic peritoneal space around the left and right tubes (arrows); this "spill" of contrast medium indicates that the fallopian tubes are patent.

endocervical cavity, which has a jagged contour because of the cervical mucosa (Fig. 1-11A). The shape and size of the endometrial cavity should be assessed, and any displacement of the cavity or filling defects within it should be reported.

The fallopian (uterine) tubes insert at the cornua of the uterus. From medial to lateral, there are four named parts of each fallopian tube: interstitial (intramural), isthmus, ampullary, and infundibulum (Figs. 1-11B, 1-11C). The patency, size, and shape of the fallopian tubes should be evaluated. The examination is concluded when contrast material can be seen around loops of small bowel or if tubal occlusion is demonstrated. When there is tubal obstruction, the site of the blockage should be reported.

It is also important to report if there is pooling of contrast material around the patent fallopian tube, which suggests adhesions.

Complications

Complications of hysterosalpingography include pain and infection. Pelvic pain, similar to menstrual cramps and typically mild or moderate, may begin during the procedure and continue for as long as several hours afterward. As many as 80% of patients may experience varying degrees of pelvic pain, which is not related to the type of contrast material administered. Fever, which complicates hysterosalpingography in 0.3% to 3% of patients, may be the harbinger of infection and requires prompt evaluation. Patients with tubal obstruction and hydrosalpinx or those with a history of pelvic inflammatory disease appear to be at higher risk for the development of infection after hysterosalpingography; such an infection is most often the result of retrograde introduction of cervical flora.

SONOGRAPHY

Kidneys and Upper Urinary Tract

Renal and upper urinary tract sonography is a commonly performed examination because it is accurate and safe and because it does not require normal renal function for image production. With modern instrumentation, bedside imaging and imaging-directed procedures can be performed on even the most seriously ill patients. Several of the more common indications for urinary tract sonography include:

1. Evaluation of collecting system obstruction. Ultrasonography is used not only to evaluate the presence and significance of upper collecting system dilatation but also to determine if there is urine flow at the ureterovesical junction;
2. Evaluation of suspected or known nephrolithiasis;
3. Evaluation of renal cystic disease;
4. Detection of a renal, adrenal, or perinephric mass lesion;
5. Characterization of a renal mass lesion as solid, cystic, or fat-containing; and
6. Guidance for aspiration or biopsy of a renal or adrenal mass.

Normal sonographic anatomy

Renal parenchyma is anatomically and functionally divided into the peripheral cortex and central medulla. Normal invaginations of cortical tissue, called septa of Bertin, separate adjacent medullary pyramids. On sonograms, normal renal cortex is hypoechoic compared with liver parenchyma. The renal pyramids, which represent that portion of the renal medulla cupped by the calyces, are hypoechoic compared with adjacent renal cortex (Fig. 1-12). This sonographic corticomedullary differentiation or definition is accentuated in children aged up to 6 months, in whom the pyramids may appear echo-free. The relative size ratio of cortex to medulla is 1.6 : 1.0 in children, but 2.6 : 1.0 in adults. The arcuate arteries mark the true corticomedullary junction and can be seen as punctate, echogenic foci in approximately 25% of patients.

The renal sinus contains the calyces, infundibuli, and a portion of the renal pelvis, and fibrous tissue, fat, vessels, and lymphatics. On sonograms, the renal sinus appears typically as a central hyperechoic area, largely because of its fat content (Fig. 1-12). It contrasts with the hypoechoic renal pyramids that border the sinus. It is important to note the gradation of tissue echogenicity on an ultrasound examination. The order of decreasing tissue echogenicity in the adult is: renal sinus, pancreas, liver and spleen, renal cortex, and renal medulla.

The determination of renal size with ultrasonography is more accurate than with intravenous urography because the kidney is imaged without magnification and contrast-induced osmotic diuresis. The normal superomedial inclination or tilt of the kidney may create some factitious shortening on sonograms. As a result, renal size is approximately 15% smaller than that measured on a radiograph. Renal length decreases with age, although the volume of the renal sinus increases somewhat in the elderly. For a 30- to 50-year-old, the upper tenth percentile of renal length is 10 cm for the right kidney and 10.3 cm for the left kidney. For people aged 60 to 69 years, the upper tenth percentile of right renal length is 9.6 cm, and for those aged 70 to 79 years, this value is 9.2 cm; for the left kidney, 0.3 cm is added to the tenth percentile value of the right kidney.

Transabdominal and Endovaginal Sonography of the Female Pelvis

Transabdominal and endocavitary ultrasonography can be used to produce high-resolution images of the lower urinary tract and pelvis. Particularly in female patients of child-bearing age, it is the test of first choice for the evaluation of acute or chronic pelvic pain. Pelvic sonography can also be used to evaluate most pelvic masses, although large masses (i.e., those larger than 8 to 10 cm) are more effectively characterized with CT or MR imaging. Ultrasonography is also the test of choice in evaluating the patient with a suspected intrauterine or extrauterine gestation.

Transabdominal (transvesical) sonography is performed using the full urinary bladder as a sonic window. In most patients, transabdominal sonography is performed with a 3.5-MHz transducer; in some patients, a 5.0-MHz or even a 7.5-MHz transducer may be used to optimize imaging of the near field. In the majority of situations, endovaginal sonography supplements the transabdominal study (Appendix F). It is used to clarify ambiguities discovered on the transabdominal examination of the pelvis and is unnecessary if the transabdominal examination is technically satisfactory. Because its field of view is limited, endovaginal sonography is unsatisfactory for the evaluation of a large pelvic mass and can be misleading if performed without the orientation provided by a transabdominal study.

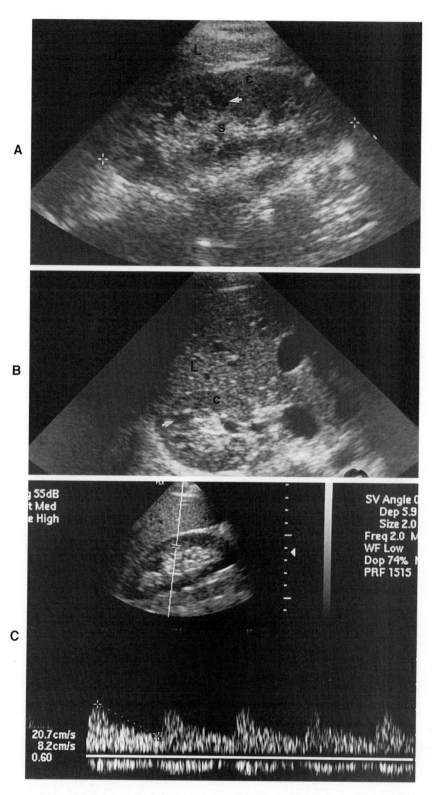

Fig. 1-12 Sonography of the normal kidney. Sagittal (**A**) and transverse (**B**) images of the right kidney demonstrate normal corticomedullary differentiation. The real sinus (s), liver parenchyma (L), renal cortex (c), and renal medulla (arrow) are seen, in decreasing order of echogenicity. **C,** The renal resistive index (RI) is determined from Doppler waveform analysis of the arcuate artery. The normal value for the RI (peak systolic frequency shift − end diastolic frequency shift ÷ peak systolic frequency shift) is less than 0.70, and in this patient, the RI is 0.60.

Normal sonographic anatomy

The uterine wall consists of an external serosa (perimetrium), a middle muscularis (myometrium), and an internal mucosa (endometrium). The perimetrium is not normally visible on ultrasound examination, although subserosal veins may be seen as a normal variant. By sonography, the myometrium has two, and sometimes three, distinct layers. The inner myometrium (subendometrial halo) appears as a thin hypoechoic area surrounding the echogenic endometrium (Fig. 1-13A). The

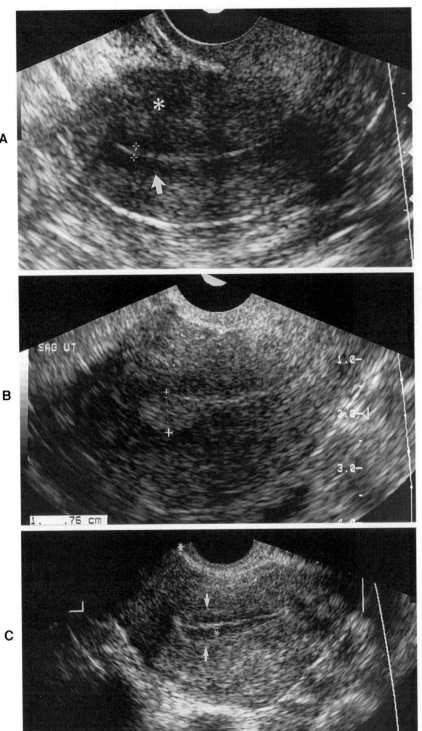

Fig. 1-13   Endovaginal sonograms of the normal uterus. **A,** Sagittal sonogram shows the central endometrial echo (between electronic markers), which measures 3 mm. The hypoechoic inner myometrium (arrow) is seen and can be differentiated from the middle and outer myometrium (*). **B,** On hormone replacement therapy, the endometrial echo may be thicker, as demonstrated in this patient. Measurement of the endometrial thickness should be performed in the sagittal plane and should include the endometrial layers anterior and posterior to the endometrial canal ("outer-to-outer" measurement). The hypoechoic inner layer of the myometrium should not be included in this measurement. **C,** Endovaginal sonogram of another patient shows the triple line sign (between arrows); the hypoechoic functional zone (*) is between the inner echogenic stripe and the hyperechoic basal endometrial layer. This appearance can be seen during the late proliferative phase of the menstrual cycle.

outer myometrium is relatively hyperechoic compared with the inner myometrium and may have a bilaminar appearance.

The endometrium appears as a central echogenic zone that varies during the menstrual cycle. In the early proliferative phase, the endometrium appears as a single, echo-genic line (Fig. 1-13A). In the midfollicular phase, three longitudinal lines can be seen in the center of the uterus; these characterize the proliferative endometrium. The outer lines represent the echo-interface between the myometrium and endometrium, and the central line is the uterine canal. The hypoechoic region between these

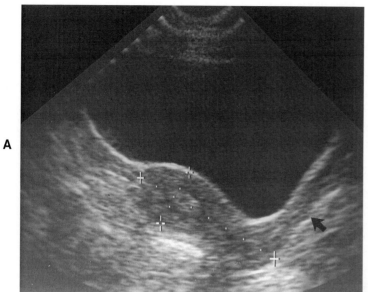

A

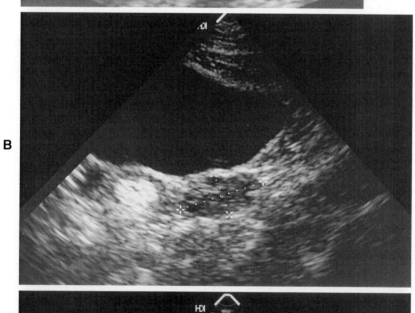

B

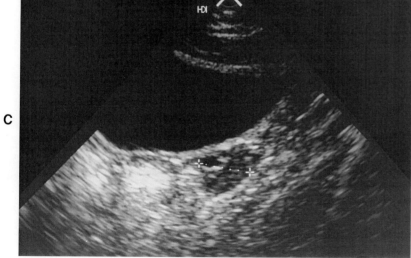

C

Fig. 1-14   Transabdominal sonograms of the normal uterus and ovary. **A,** The length and height (anteroposterior) of the uterus should be measured on a sagittal sonogram in which the maximal length of the central endometrial echo complex is seen. The width of the uterus is measured on the orthogonal transverse sonogram. The vagina (arrow) curves inferiorly. **B,** In a similar manner, the dimensions of the ovaries are measured. The length of the ovary is the maximal dimension in a parasagittal plane, and the height is measured perpendicular to the length on the same image. **C,** The width of the ovary is measured perpendicular to the height in the orthogonal transverse plane. The volume of the ovary can be estimated using the formula for a prolate ellipse; volume equals the product of length, height, width, and $\pi/6$.

linear borders represents the functional endometrial layer, which thickens as endometrial development progresses in the late proliferative phase (Fig. 1-13C). Within 48 hours of ovulation, this hypoechoic layer gradually becomes more hyperechoic, and the triple-line sign disappears, signaling the onset of the secretory endometrium. The distance between the outer lines of the endometrial echo complex can be measured (outer-to-outer border), and cycle-specific normal limits have been established for each phase: menstrual, 2 to 3 mm; early proliferative, 5 ± 1 mm; periovulatory, 10 ± 1 mm; and late secretory, up to 16 mm.

On a sagittal image through its long axis, the maximal length of the uterus is measured from the top of the uterine fundus to the external cervical os. The uterine height is measured perpendicular to the length measurement on the same sagittal image (Fig. 1-14A on p. 19). The width of the uterus is measured in a transverse plane orthogonal to the sagittal plane in which the height was measured. For the nulliparous woman, the normal upper limits of uterine dimensions are: length, 9 cm; height, 4 cm; and width, 5 cm. Parity will increase the normal dimensions of the uterus.

The adnexa consists of the ovaries, uterine tubes, ligaments, and vessels. In nulliparous women, the ovaries are situated in the ovarian fossa. The ovarian (Waldeyer's) fossa is bounded by the internal iliac artery posteriorly, the external iliac vein superiorly, and the obliterated umbilical artery anteriorly. However, in parous patients or in those with a pelvic mass, the ovary is often displaced from the ovarian fossa. The ovaries are hypoechoic ellipsoid structures and have a thin hyperechoic rim. Using the formula for a prolate ellipse (length × height × width × 0.52 = volume [cc]). Cohen et al report a mean ovarian volume of 9.8 cm³ (95% confidence value, 21.9 cm³) in adult menstruating women (Figs. 1-14B, 1-14C). The mean for postmenopausal women was 5.8 cm³ (95% confidence value, 14.1 cm³). The ovaries are distinctive because of the presence of developing follicles in the cortex. Graafian follicles become visible as fluid accumulates in the antrum of the follicle. With endovaginal sonography, follicles can be seen when they reach 1 to 2 mm in diameter. Nondominant follicles are usually less than 14 mm in diameter, and dominant follicles reach a maximum diameter of approximately 20 to 25 mm (Fig. 1-15).

The interstitial part of the fallopian tube is occasionally seen on an endovaginal sonogram as a thin echogenic line extending to the wall of the uterus from the endometrium. However, unless dilated or surrounded by pelvic ascites, the isthmus and ampulla of the fallopian tube are not seen routinely. Similarly, the suspensory ligament of the ovary and the broad ligament are usually not visualized with sonography unless there is free intraperitoneal fluid.

Bladder

Some of the more common indications for ultrasonography of the bladder include:

1. Determination of the existence and rate of urine flow through the vesicoureteral junction in subjects with dilated ureters (Fig. 1-16);
2. Determination of pre- and post-void bladder volume;
3. Detection of bladder stone or bladder wall mass;
4. Detection and quantitation of bladder wall thickening; and
5. Direction for bladder aspiration or cystostomy.

Normal sonographic anatomy

The normal distended bladder is an anechoic structure that occupies the midline of the true pelvis. It is triangular in the sagittal plane and oval in the transaxial plane. Normally, the wall of the bladder is uniform and 3 to 4 mm in thickness. The capacity of the bladder can be estimated by the product of its length, width, and height.

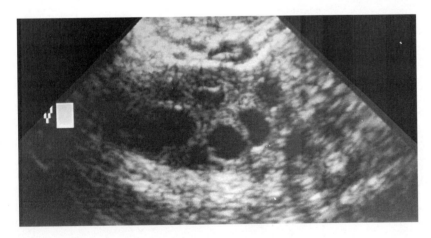

Fig. 1-15 Endovaginal sonogram of a normal ovary in a 19-year-old woman. The cortex of the ovary contains several follicles and corpora lutea. The medulla contains loose connective tissue and numerous blood vessels.

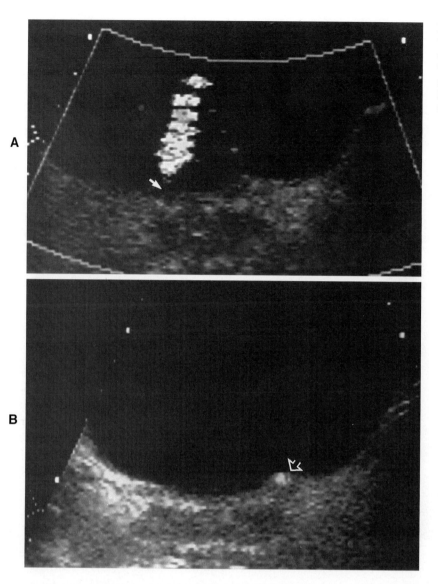

Fig. 1-16 Color Doppler sonogram of an ureteral jet. **A,** A transverse sonogram of the bladder demonstrates a stream of color from the right ureterovesical junction (arrow) as a result of the normal flow of urine. **B,** An echogenic calculus is lodged in the left ureterovesical junction (open arrow), and no jet is seen.

Transrectal Sonography of the Prostate

Transrectal sonography of the prostate is used as an adjunct to the digital rectal examination to quantify prostate volume, assess a palpable nodule, guide prostate biopsy, and evaluate the infertile patient (Appendix G). Less commonly, it is used to investigate perirectal masses or collections, particularly when biopsy is contemplated.

Normal sonographic anatomy

The normal prostate gland is a triangular ellipse that is surrounded by a thin capsule. The glandular tissue or parenchyma of the prostate is composed of the peripheral zone, central zone, and transitional zone (Fig. 1-17A). The parenchyma is bounded anteriorly by fibromuscular stroma. The prostatic "capsule" is seen as a bright echogenic structure posteriorly and laterally, but it is thin or absent at the apex of the gland. The normal prostate measures approximately 4 cm in length (cephalocaudal), 4 cm in transverse diameter, and 3 cm in height (anteroposterior); the normal volume ranges from 20 to 25 cc, and the normal weight is approximately 20 g.

Seminal vesicles are cephalad to the prostate gland and posterior to the bladder. The paired structures are imaged in long axis on transverse images and cross-sectional on sagittal images. The seminal vesicles are well-defined, saccular structures that are most often symmetric in size and shape. The normal seminal vesicle measures 3 cm ± 0.5 cm in length and 1.5 cm ± 0.4 cm in width. Seminal vesicles are usually hypoechoic and contain scattered fine internal echoes. The vasa deferentia are located medially to the seminal vesicles and just cephalad to the prostate gland (Fig. 1-17B). The dilated terminus of the vas deferens is called the ampulla. On

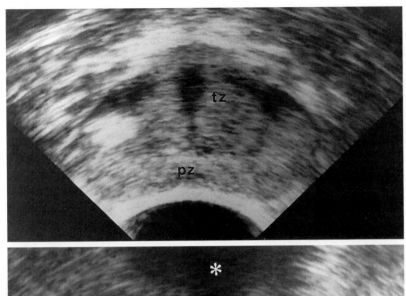

Fig. 1-17   Transrectal sonograms of the normal prostate, seminal vesicles, and vas deferens. **A,** The size of the prostate gland is normal. The echogenicity of the peripheral zone (pz) is slightly greater than that of the transitional zone (tz). **B,** A transverse image cephalic to the prostate demonstrates normal hypoechoic seminal vesicle (curved arrow) and ampullary part of the deferent duct (open arrow). The vas deferens and duct of the seminal vesicle join to form the ejaculatory duct * = bladder lumen.

the transaxial plane, the paired vasa deferentia appear as a pair of oval, convoluted tubular structures and are isoechoic to the seminal vesicles. The confluence of the seminal vesicle and ampullary portion of the vas deferens form the ejaculatory duct. The neurovascular bundle consists of paired cords of nerves and vessels that extend along the posterolateral margins of the prostate. The neurovascular bundles, which are frequently identified on sonograms, are important routes for extraprostatic spread of cancer. The periprostatic venous plexus is seen anteriorly and can be prominent. Vessels can be identified entering the gland laterally, most often near the apex, where they can simulate a hypoechoic tumor.

Scrotum

Ultrasonography of the scrotum is used to evaluate a palpable mass or scrotal enlargement because it can accurately distinguish an intratesticular lesion from one that originates from extratesticular tissues (Appendix H). This distinction is important because the majority of lesions that originate in an extratesticular location are benign (e.g., hydrocele, varicocele, or epididymitis), unlike testicular neoplasm, the most common intratesticular mass. The integrity of the traumatized testis can also be evaluated quickly with sonography. Duplex sonography of the "acute scrotum" can be used to distinguish testicular torsion from epididymoorchitis. Finally, ultrasonography has been used to identify the undescended inguinal testicle but is less accurate than CT, MR imaging, and testicular phlebography for locating the abdominal testis. Other indications for scrotal sonography include the evaluation of infertile man, the follow-up evaluation of sexual precocity, and the evaluation of occult primary tumors in patients with metastatic disease.

Normal sonographic anatomy

The normal testis is an ovoid structure, measuring 3.5 cm in length and 2.5 cm to 3 cm in width and height

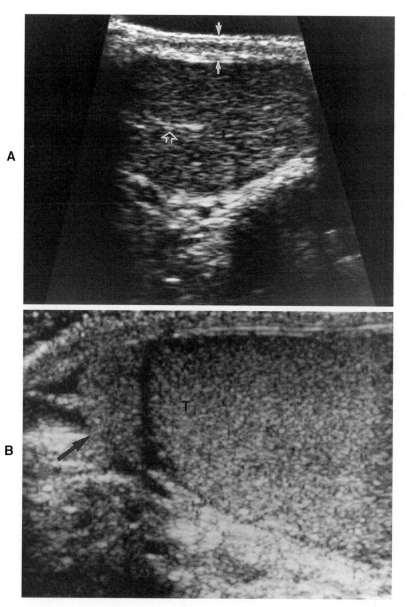

Fig. 1-18 Sonograms of the normal testicle and epididymis. **A,** This sagittal sonogram demonstrates normal echogenicity of the testicular parenchyma and the linear, hyperechoic mediastinum (open arrow). Also note the normal thickness and echogenicity of the scrotal wall (between small arrows). **B,** The globus major or head of the epididymis (arrow) is seen cephalad to the upper pole of the testis (T).

(anteroposterior diameter). The echogenicity of the two testes should be similar and should consist of uniform, medium level echoes. The mediastinum represents an invagination of the tunica albuginea along the posterior aspect of the testis and appears as an echogenic line parallel to the epididymis (Fig. 1-18). Septations within the testis may be visualized as linear echogenic or hypoechoic structures and may divide the testicle into lobules.

Of the normal extratesticular structures, the epididymis is most commonly identified with sonography. The epididymal head (globus major) is the largest component. It measures 5 to 15 mm in diameter and is found laterally and superiorly to the upper pole of the testicle. The head of the epididymis is usually slightly more echogenic than the body and tail and isoechoic to testicular parenchyma (Fig. 1-18B). The body and tail (globus minor) extend

inferiorly along the posterior margin of the testicle and appear as a thin cord approximately 1 to 3 mm in thickness on sonograms. Color Doppler sonography shows no detectable flow in the normal epididymis. On occasion, small protuberances from the head of the epididymis and superior aspect of the testicle can be identified; these protuberances represent the appendices of epididymis and testicle, respectively.

The scrotum is composed of several layers that are derived from the skin, abdominal wall muscles, and peritoneum. Sonographically, the scrotal wall is 5 mm to 7 mm thick and is hyperechoic compared with the testicle (Fig. 1-18A). The tunica vaginalis is derived from peritoneum and applies the testicle to the posterior scrotal wall. Bursa-like, the tunica vaginalis envelops the testicle and normally contains 1 to 2 cc of fluid. The spermatic cord contains the testicular and deferential arteries and the pampiniform plexus of veins. Normal vessels are no more than 1 to 2 mm in diameter, and the presence and direction of flow can be ascertained by using color Doppler sonography.

Doppler Ultrasonography

Principles

In medical ultrasonography, images are produced by tissue reflection of a beam of sound at a frequency of 2 to 15 MHz. For a moving point reflector, such as an erythrocyte, the frequency of sound received by the transducer will differ from that of the transmitted frequency. This frequency difference, or shift, can be used to determine the direction and velocity of reflector movement. Johann C. Doppler is credited with the elucidation of this principle and the relationship between frequency shift and flow velocity.

Information about the Doppler shift frequency is displayed graphically as a series of spectra in real time. These spectra are vertical line graphs showing the relative strength of frequency shifts with respect to time, which is represented on the horizontal axis. Thus, four variables are displayed on the Doppler spectra: frequency shift (velocity), distribution of frequency shifts by a population of point reflectors, direction of flow, and time. A number of different indices have been used to quantitate impedance, the total resistance to flow. The pulsatility index is equal to $(S - D)/M$, where S is the peak systolic frequency, D is the peak diastolic frequency, and M is the mean frequency shift. Other such indices include the resistive index, $S - D/S$, and the systolic–diastolic ratio, S/D. In duplex Doppler sonography, the pulsed Doppler system is interfaced with a real-time image so that the source of the shifted frequency can be user-selected from a gray scale image. Color Doppler uses colors to encode directional and velocity information about flow.

Indications

Doppler sonography has been used to evaluate normal flow of urine into the urinary bladder (Fig. 1-16), testicular parenchymal perfusion to exclude spermatic cord torsion, renal parenchymal perfusion to identify glomerulotubular disease (Fig. 1-12), and cavernosal artery flow to investigate vasculogenic causes of impotence.

COMPUTED TOMOGRAPHY

Computed tomography creates a two-dimensional image of the body from measurements of relative linear attenuation collected from multiple projections around a thin tomographic slice. This technique can demonstrate density differences between tissues of 1% or less. The reconstructed image is displayed as a matrix of pixels. The numerical value of each pixel is the relative linear attenuation coefficient of the volume of tissue represented by that pixel. The attenuation value assigned to each pixel is based on a reference scale in which −1000 Hounsfield units (HU) are assigned to air, +1000 HU to dense bone, and 0 HU to water. The relative linear attenuation coefficient assigned to each pixel is correlated with a shade of gray in the image. User selection of the number of shades of gray (window width) in the image and the central hue of gray (window level) permits modification of image contrast.

Spiral, helical, or volume-acquisition CT is a technique that permits continuous acquisition of data by constant rotation of a slip-ring x-ray tube-detector system while the patient moves through the gantry. Most spiral CT scanners rotate at a fixed rate of 360° per second, but the rate of patient movement through the gantry and the collimation of the beam are selected by the radiologist. Pitch is defined as the ratio of the rate of table movement (per 360° tube rotation) to beam collimation; if the scan time is 1 second, pitch is equal to the rate of table movement in mm/sec divided by the beam width in millimeters. The trade-off in selecting the appropriate pitch is between spatial resolution (optimized with a smaller pitch) and coverage (optimized with a larger pitch). Recent work suggests that the optimal pitch for spiral CT of the abdomen is 1.5 to 1.6. There are several advantages of spiral CT over conventional CT. First, spiral CT data can be manipulated through post-processing, which permits targeted image reconstruction to an area of interest. For instance, overlapping images could be reconstructed in narrow intervals to increase the sensitivity for smaller lesions. Second, because of shortened scan times, less contrast material is needed for some studies, and scanning can be optimized to specific phases of contrast enhancement. Finally, CT angiography is possible because three-dimensional data acquisition is combined with an imaging method that optimizes the detection of contrast enhancement in vessels.

Renal CT is used to characterize masses and can evaluate the perinephric spread of primary renal disease or the secondary involvement of the kidneys by primary intraperitoneal or retroperitoneal disease. CT is also the imaging procedure of choice in patients with suspected or known renal trauma because it accurately characterizes injuries to the parenchyma and vascular pedicle. The more common genitourinary indications for abdominal and pelvic CT include:

1. Detection and characterization of an adrenal, renal, or pelvic soft-tissue mass;
2. Staging of kidney, adrenal, ureter, and bladder malignancy;

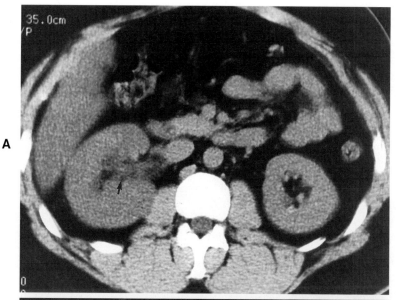

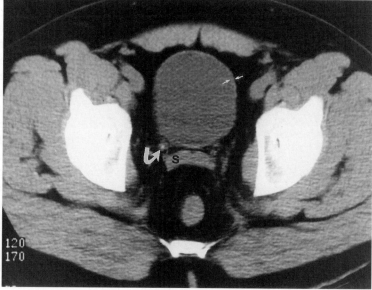

Fig. 1-19   Uninfused (noncontrast) computed tomography (CT) of the kidneys and bladder. **A,** Uninfused CT of the normal left kidney shows the image contrast provided by the perinephric and renal sinus fat. There is increased attenuation of the right renal sinus fat (arrow) and, as a result, relatively reduced image contrast. **B,** This finding results from acute ureteral obstruction caused by a calculus (curved arrow) in the distal right ureter (s = seminal vesicle). The wall of the urinary bladder (between small arrows) is seen because of the image contrast created by unopacified urine and perivesical fat.

3. Staging of gynecologic malignancy (ovary and uterus);
4. Staging of male genital malignancy (testis and prostate);
5. Evaluation of known or suspected retroperitoneal disease;
6. Evaluation of chronic pelvic pain;
7. Evaluation of cryptorchidism; and
8. Directed aspiration, biopsy, or drainage.

See Appendices I and J.

Normal Anatomy

The renal parenchyma is homogeneous on nonenhanced CT, and measured attenuation ranges from 30 HU to 60 HU. Renal sinus and perinephric fat provide intrinsic contrast for the renal parenchyma on noncontrast- and contrast-enhanced CT (Fig. 1-19). After administration of contrast material, there is gradual enhancement of the large vessels, renal parenchyma, and collecting system. During the vascular phase, there is opacification of the aorta and major arteries. Sequential enhancement of the renal cortex and medulla follow during the nephrogram phase. Normal corticomedullary differentiation is demonstrated during the early nephrogram phase (approximately 20 to 100 seconds after the administration of contrast material); one can miss small medullary tumors on CT during this phase (Fig. 1-20A). The exact timing of the early nephrogram phase depends on the dose and method of intravenous contrast administration and on the cardiac output and renal function of the pa-

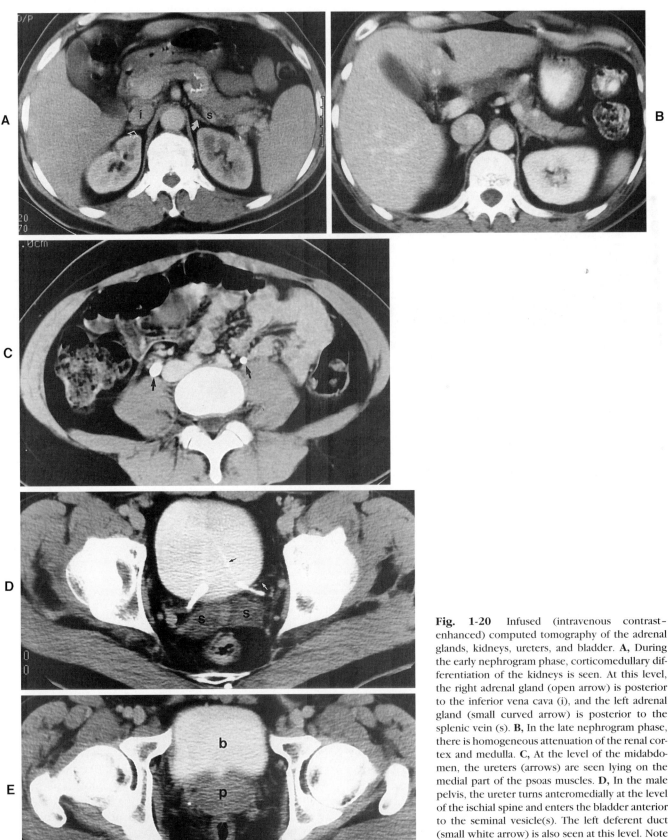

Fig. 1-20 Infused (intravenous contrast–enhanced) computed tomography of the adrenal glands, kidneys, ureters, and bladder. **A,** During the early nephrogram phase, corticomedullary differentiation of the kidneys is seen. At this level, the right adrenal gland (open arrow) is posterior to the inferior vena cava (i), and the left adrenal gland (small curved arrow) is posterior to the splenic vein (s). **B,** In the late nephrogram phase, there is homogeneous attenuation of the renal cortex and medulla. **C,** At the level of the midabdomen, the ureters (arrows) are seen lying on the medial part of the psoas muscles. **D,** In the male pelvis, the ureter turns anteromedially at the level of the ischial spine and enters the bladder anterior to the seminal vesicle(s). The left deferent duct (small white arrow) is also seen at this level. Note the ureteral jet of contrast material (small black arrow) in the bladder. **E,** At a more caudal level, the prostate gland (p) indents the base of the bladder (b).

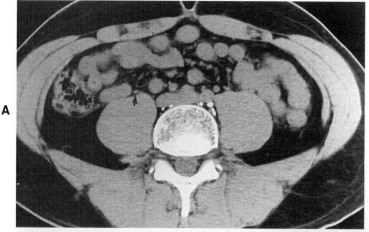

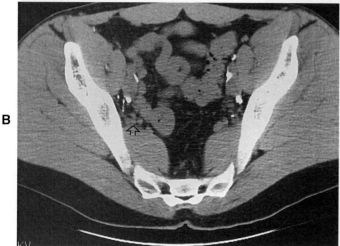

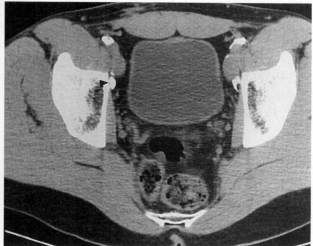

Fig. 1-21   Pelvic lymph nodes on computed tomography after bipedal lymphangiography. **A,** Normal small common iliac lymph nodes are opacified with contrast material. The right ureter (arrow) is seen at the medial aspect of the psoas muscle. **B,** At the level of the upper sacroiliac joint, normal external iliac nodes are opacified, but internal iliac nodes (open arrow) are not opacified. The upper limit of normal for maximum short-axis diameter of the iliac nodes is 10 mm. **C,** The medial group of external iliac lymph nodes includes the surgical obturator node (arrowhead), which is an important sentinel node for bladder and prostate cancers. Also note that the normal wall of the bladder is uniformly thin.

tient. Scans obtained approximately 120 to 240 seconds after intravenous contrast administration demonstrate more homogeneous attenuation of the parenchyma during the equilibrium phase (Fig. 1-20B). After contrast-material injection, the attenuation value of the normal renal parenchyma will increase to 80 to 120 HU. During and after the equilibrium or pyelographic phase, there is enhancement of the renal collecting system.

The adrenal glands are variable in shape, although the posterior limbs are usually uniform in width. The normal width of the adrenal limbs, measured perpendicular to the long axis, is less than 8 mm (Fig. 1-20A).

In the abdomen, the nondilated ureter may be difficult to distinguish from gonadal vessels or other retroperitoneal vessels and can be identified on the medial part of the psoas muscle (Fig. 1-20C). In the pelvis, the ureter descends posterolaterally, and opposite the ischial spine, it turns anteromedially in front of the seminal vesicles or vaginal fornices to reach the base of the bladder (Fig. 1-20D). The bladder is identified in the midline of the true pelvis; on noncontrast CT, its wall is uniformly thin and is outlined by urine and perivesical fat. The presence

of dense contrast material in the bladder may create artifacts and obscure the bladder wall (Figs. 1-19B, 1-20D).

Lymph nodes are routinely identified on CT; normal lymph nodes have the attenuation of soft tissue, are homogeneous, and measure 4 to 10 mm in diameter. Abdominal and pelvic lymph nodes are abnormal if they are larger than 15 mm; retrocrural nodes are enlarged if more than 6 mm in diameter. The pelvic nodes are grouped around the common iliac, external iliac, and internal iliac vessels; the inguinal nodes lie medial and anterior to the femoral vessels (Figs. 1-21A, 1-21B). The "surgical" obturator nodes are particularly important because cancer of the prostate and bladder frequently spreads to these nodes first (sentinel nodes). These nodes actually form the medial chain of the external iliac lymph nodes and can be identified adjacent to the lateral pelvic wall at the level of the acetabulum (Fig. 1-21C).

The seminal vesicles are oblong, tubular structures that lie at the superior aspect of the prostate, posterior to the lower urinary bladder, and anterior to the rectum. A plane of fat separates the seminal vesicles from the bladder (Figs. 1-19B, 1-20D). The prostate gland is identi-

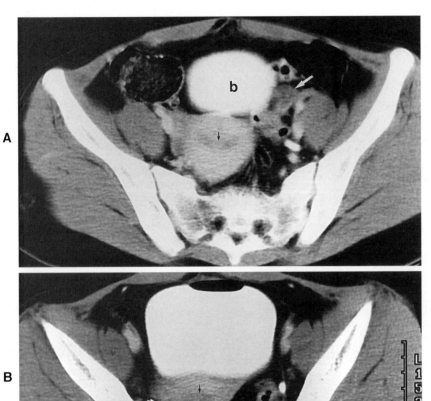

Fig. 1-22   Contrast-enhanced computed tomography of the uterus and ovary. **A,** The endometrium (small black arrow) is relatively hypodense because of enhancement of the myometrium. The left ovary (white arrow) is slightly hypodense compared with skeletal muscle. Often, it is not possible to separate the wall of the bladder (b) from hyperdense urine. **B,** At a more caudal level, the hypodense endometrium (small black arrow) is demonstrated. Note the proximity of the right ureter (white arrow) to the uterine parametrium in this patient.

fied posterior and inferior to the bladder neck, anterior to the rectum, and posterior to the pubic symphysis. When healthy, it is homogeneous in attenuation but may contain punctate calcifications (Fig. 1-20E). The spermatic cord is formed at the internal inguinal ring by the confluence of the vas deferens with vessels and nerves. The spermatic cord is seen medial to the ipsilateral femoral vein and anterolateral to the symphysis pubis. The vas deferens leaves the cord at the inguinal ring and continues posteriorly and medially toward the ipsilateral seminal vesicle (Fig. 1-20D).

The uterus is located between the urinary bladder and the rectosigmoid colon in the true pelvis. The fundus and corpus of the uterus have a triangular shape, and the cervix has a rounded contour. The attenuation of the uterus is usually homogeneous on noncontrast CT, although the normal endometrial cavity may appear slightly hypodense if it contains secretions. The endometrium appears relatively hypodense after administration of intravenous contrast medium because of intense enhancement of the myometrium (Fig. 1-22). The ovaries may be slightly hypodense, particularly if follicles are prominent. The ovaries can be identified by following the ovarian ligament from the cornua of the uterus to the ovary. The broad ligaments are peritoneal folds that connect the lateral margin of the uterus to the pelvic sidewalls.

MAGNETIC RESONANCE IMAGING

For most radiologic problems in genitourinary radiology, MR imaging is used as a supplementary examination to further investigate or characterize disease detected with urography, ultrasonography, or CT. It is often performed as a carefully targeted study (Appendix K). Hence, MR imaging is not intended to be a screening study or a substitute for biopsy because with a few notable exceptions, specific tissue characterization is not possible.

Biophysics of Proton Relaxation

Proton MR images are based on the signal intensity from hydrogen nuclei in molecules that are hydrogen rich: water and fat. Image contrast is based on inherent properties of tissues. Specifically, signal intensity depends on hydrogen content or hydrogen spin density and on relaxation times, T_1, T_2, and T_2^*. Most soft tissues have similar proton density but vary greatly in relaxation times. Spin–lattice relaxation time (T_1) involves the transfer of energy from spins to their environment, the lattice. Spin–spin relaxation (T_2) occurs because of the loss of phase coherence, also described as phase dispersal, among excited nuclei. Phase dispersal is hastened by the dipole interactions that disrupt local magnetic field homogeneity.

Conventional Spin–Echo Pulse Sequence

For MR imaging of the male and female pelvis, the spin–echo pulse sequence remains the standard. This pulse sequence uses a 90° radiofrequency pulse to nutate the longitudinal magnetization into the transverse plane, and a 180° radiofrequency pulse refocuses the transverse magnetization for signal readout at the echo time (TE). The repetition time (TR) is the time between iterations of the 90° to 180° readout sequence.

Gradient–Echo Pulse Sequence

Gradient- or field-echo pulse sequences produce images with T_1- or T_2^*-weighting in a short acquisition time, especially when compared with the spin–echo sequence. Although the spin–echo sequence produces a refocused echo with 90° and 180° radiofrequency pulses, gradient echoes are formed by a single radiofrequency pulse in conjunction with gradient reversals. Gradient-recalled-echo imaging refocuses spins with magnetic gradients rather than with radiofrequency pulses. In addition, the radiofrequency pulse is used to tip the longitudinal magnetization through a flip angle that is usually less than 90°. Refocusing by gradient reversal corrects only for those phase shifts induced by the gradient itself. Phase shifts caused by static tissue susceptibility, magnetic field inhomogeneity, and chemical shifts are not reversed and contribute to the loss of transverse magnetization, along with the inherent T_2 of the tissue. As opposed to T_2, the transverse decay of the gradient–echo signal is termed T_2^*, the effective spin–spin relaxation time. Gradient-echo sequences require TRs of 20 to 500 msec, and because acquisition time is related directly to TR, gradient-echo imaging has been one viable method of reducing scan time.

Fast (Turbo) Spin–Echo Pulse Sequence

One of the salient disadvantages of T_2-weighted conventional spin–echo (CSE) imaging is a relatively long acquisition time, which can lead to degradation of image quality as a result of patient motion. Fast spin–echo (FSE)

is a pulse sequence designed to provide the contrast characteristics of a spin–echo pulse sequence from two to four times as fast as the CSE pulse sequence. In FSE, a 90° radiofrequency pulse is followed by a series of 180° refocusing pulses, numbering between two and 16, each acquired with a different phase-encoding value and TE. Each echo exhibits different degrees of T_2 decay, depending on where it occurs in the echo train. In FSE, image contrast is determined through the reordering of phase-encoding views so that views with the lowest spatial frequency are obtained in the echoes nearest the desired TE or the "effective" TE. The decrease in acquisition time achieved with FSE imaging can be exchanged for a longer TR (increasing the signal-to-noise ratio [SNR]), a larger matrix (increasing spatial resolution), more signal averaging (increasing SNR), and implementing fat-suppression techniques.

Studies comparing FSE with CSE have shown that overall image quality and the conspicuity of pelvic pathology are equivalent. In FSE, unlike CSE imaging, fat remains hyperintense on T_2-weighted images. A typical full-echo train FSE protocol for T_2-weighted imaging of the pelvis is TR = 4000 to 6000 msec, effective TE = 80 to 120 msec, echo train length = 8 or 16, echo spacing = 20 msec, matrix = 256 × 256 or 256 × 192, two signals averaged, superior and inferior spatial saturation pulses, and fat saturation. Use of either a pelvic binder or intramuscular glucagon may reduce respiratory- and peristalsis-related motion artifacts, respectively.

Fat Saturation and Chemical Shift MR Imaging

A method that is commonly used for negating the signal from fat is lipid proton frequency-selective presaturation, which can be applied before each section-selective pulse of a CSE sequence. This technique is based on chemical shift, or the observation that aliphatic hydrogen protons in fat precess at a frequency of approximately 220 Hz lower than water protons at 1.5 T. The selective fat-suppression technique begins with a low-amplitude, long-duration radiofrequency pulse centered on the frequency of lipid proton resonance, which converts the z magnetization of fat into xy magnetization. Application of a spoiling gradient dephases this lipid-specific transverse magnetization. Subsequently, the spin–echo sequence is performed with signal reception centered on the resonance frequency of water. When the 90° excitation pulse of the spin–echo pulse sequence is applied, the time elapsed will not be sufficient to permit significant recovery of longitudinal relaxation for fat protons, and little or no transverse magnetization will exist for signal detection. In-phase and opposed-phase T_1-weighted gradient-echo imaging is another chemical shift MR imaging method that has been used to characterize adrenal

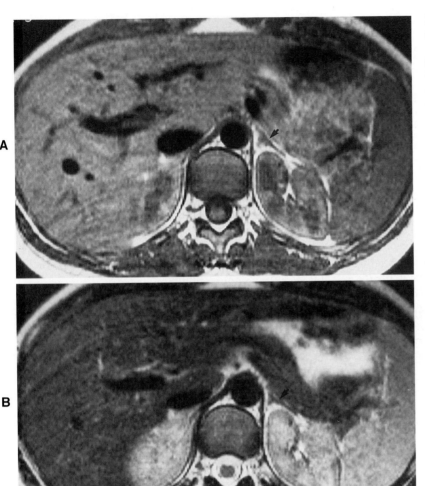

A

B

Fig. 1-23 MR imaging of the normal adrenal gland. **A,** On a T_1-weighted image (repetition time = 529 msec; echo time = 15 msec), the left adrenal gland (arrow) is isointense compared with skeletal muscle and slightly hypointense relative to liver parenchyma. **B,** The left adrenal is isointense compared with liver on a fast spin–echo T_2-weighted image (repetition time = 4,000 msec; effective echo time = 120 msec).

masses. This chemical shift imaging method is discussed in Chapter 9.

Normal Anatomy

On T_1-weighted images, the adrenal glands are of intermediate signal intensity and can be identified because of periadrenal fat. On T_2-weighted images, normal adrenal gland tissue decreases in signal intensity and becomes isointense with liver parenchyma (Fig. 1-23).

Renal corticomedullary image contrast can be identified on T_1- and T_2-weighted images, but it is usually more conspicuous on T_1-weighted images (Figs. 1-24A, 1-24B). The renal cortex is of relatively higher signal intensity than the medulla on T_1-weighted images. After the intravenous administration of gadopentetate, the vasculointerstitial phase begins immediately after the contrast medium reaches the kidneys. There is increased signal

intensity of the cortex, followed by enhancement of the medulla (Figs. 1-24C, 1-24D). The tubular phase begins approximately 60 to 90 seconds after contrast administration; there is decreased signal intensity at the corticomedullary junction, which progresses centripetally toward the medullary papillae. Stable low signal intensity in the inner medulla occurs during the ductal phase, which occurs approximately 2 minutes after contrast administration. This last phase is accompanied by contrast excretion in the collecting system, which can be seen approximately 4 minutes after injection (Fig. 1-24E).

The wall of the urinary bladder is best seen on T_2-weighted images, where it appears as a thin (2 to 3 mm) stripe of intermediate signal intensity (Figs. 1-25, 1-26A). The bladder wall is separable from paravesical fat and urine, which are of relatively higher signal intensity. On T_2-weighted images, it is also important to distinguish the bladder wall from the hypointense line produced at one edge of the bladder by chemical shift artifact. On T_1-

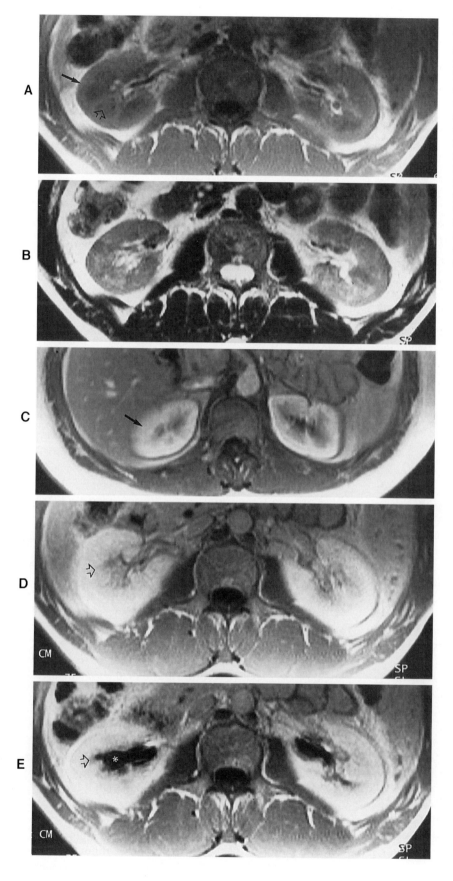

Fig. 1-24   MR imaging of the kidneys. **A,** On a T₁-weighted image (two-dimensional fast low angle shot; repetition time = 140 msec; echo time = 4.8 msec; flip angle = 75°), the renal cortex (arrow) has a higher signal intensity than the medulla (open arrow). **B,** This corticomedullary differentiation is usually not as apparent on a T₂-weighted image (turbo spin–echo; repetition time = 5028 msec; effective echo time = 138 msec). After the administration of gadopentetate, a normal temporal pattern of enhancement of the renal parenchymal and collecting system has been described on T₁-weighted images. **C and D,** During the vasculointerstitial phase, there is increased signal intensity of the cortex (arrow in *C*), followed by enhancement of the medulla (open arrow in *D*). **E,** Stable low signal intensity in the inner medulla (open arrow) occurs during the ductal phase, which is accompanied by contrast excretion in the collecting system (*).

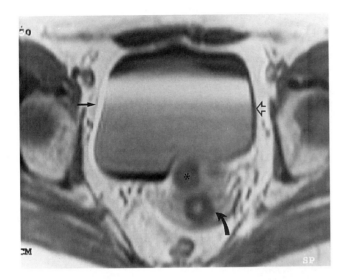

Fig. 1-25   Normal bladder and cervix on a transverse axial T₁-weighted image after the intravenous administration of contrast material. The pseudolayering of urine in the bladder results from different concentrations of gadopentetate. The top layer of fluid represents pure urine. The bottom pseudolayer represents urine with a relatively high concentration of gadopentetate, and the middle hyperintense pseudolayer has a lower concentration. The linear hyperintense (arrow) and hypointense (open arrow) walls of the bladder are caused by chemical shift artifact. The normal stroma of the cervix (curved arrow) is hypointense and surrounds the endocervical canal (* = leiomyoma).

weighted images, the wall may not be clearly distinguishable from urine within the bladder, which has a relatively long T₁ relaxation time (Fig. 1-27B). However, when compared with T₂-weighted images, the signal intensity contrast between paravesical fat and bladder is more on T₁-weighted images.

Normal lymph nodes are best evaluated on T₁-weighted images because detection is aided by contrast with surrounding fat (Fig. 1-28). Malignant or inflammatory nodes are indistinguishable from normal nodes using signal intensity as a criterion. Thus, as in CT, size remains the important differentiating feature.

Zonal anatomy of the prostate gland is seen on T₂-weighted images in most patients older than 25 years. The peripheral zone is hyperintense, and the central gland tissue is hypointense or isointense compared with skeletal muscle (Figs. 1-26B, 1-27C, 1-27D). The capsule of the gland may be distinguished as a thin hypointense border and is more consistently identified with endorectal surface coil imaging (Fig. 1-26B). On T₁-weighted images, the zonal anatomy is less apparent, although glandular hyperplasia may create a heterogeneous signal intensity pattern in transitional zone tissue. Image contrast between the prostate and periprostatic fat is greater on T₁-weighted images than on T₂-weighted images, although improved contrast between peripheral zone and

periprostatic fat is achieved with the implementation of frequency-selective fat saturation on T₂-weighted images (Figs. 1-27C, 1-27D).

The seminal vesicles appear as multicystic tissue of high signal intensity on T₂-weighted images and can be readily differentiated from periprostatic fat, which is of relatively lower signal intensity (Figs. 1-26A, 1-27E). This contrast pattern is reversed on T₁-weighted images, where the seminal vesicles are of intermediate signal intensity compared with the relatively higher intensity of surrounding fat (Fig. 1-27B).

The corporal bodies of the penis demonstrate increased signal intensity on T₂- and T₁-weighted images and are surrounded by the tunica albuginea, a low signal intensity stripe (Fig. 1-27D). The collapsed male urethra cannot be distinguished as a separate structure.

On T₂-weighted images, the testis and epididymis are readily differentiated. The uniform high signal intensity of the testes contrasts with the intermediate signal intensity of the epididymis (Fig. 1-29). The mediastinum testis normally can be identified as a focal area of relatively decreased signal intensity in the superoposterior testicle. The testicular artery and pampiniform plexus can also be identified in the scrotum, superolateral to the epididymis. On T₁-weighted images, the testis and epididymis are isointense with muscle.

Like the testes, the ovaries are most conspicuous on T₂-weighted images because compared with T₁-weighted images, there is an increase in signal intensity because of antral fluid in developing Graafian follicles (Fig. 1-30A on p. 36). On T₁-weighted images, the intermediate signal intensity of the ovaries may not permit separation from loops of small bowel unless contrast material is administered (Figs. 1-30B, 1-30C). The ovaries may appear as a single solid structure or as an agglomeration of multiple small follicular cysts. Given mobility, the normal ovaries can be found at variable sites within the pelvis.

The concentric, zonal anatomy of the uterus in women of child-bearing age is identified on images with T₂-weighting (Fig. 1-31 on p. 37). The signal intensity of the endometrium is high and typically isointense to slightly hypointense, relative to urine in the bladder. Compared with the endometrium, a zone of much lower signal intensity is seen peripheral to the endometrium and represents the junctional zone or inner myometrium. The outer myometrium has a higher signal intensity than the junctional zone but has a lower signal intensity than endometrium. The lower signal intensity of the junctional zone has no histologic explanation, although it has been conjectured that the junctional zone has a slightly lower water content and relatively sparse vascularity. In premenarchal and postmenopausal women, the junctional zone may not be distinguished from the outer myometrium. Variations in the width of the outer myometrium occur during the menstrual period. During the secretory

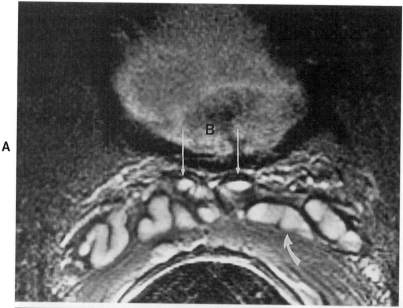

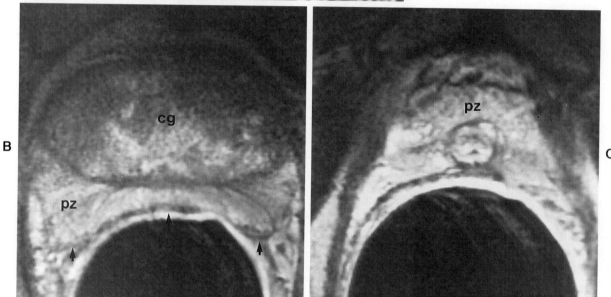

Fig. 1-26   Fast spin–echo T$_2$-weighted MR images of the seminal vesicles, deferent ducts, and prostate gland obtained with an endorectal surface coil. **A,** On this transaxial image, the folded and tubular seminal vesicle (curved arrow) and the ampullary part of the deferent duct (arrows) are hyperintense compared with saturated perivesical fat (B = bladder lumen). **B,** Zonal differentiation is demonstrated on this transaxial image through the middle of the prostate gland. The peripheral zone (pz) appears higher in signal intensity than the central gland (cg), which consists of the transitional and central zone glandular tissue. The prostatic capsule is a thin hypointense line (arrows). **C,** At the apex of the prostate gland, the parenchyma is almost entirely composed of peripheral zone tissue.

phase, the outer myometrium may double from a width of 1 to 3 mm during the proliferative phase. The junctional zone, by contrast, does not change in size during the menstrual cycle.

The zonal anatomy of the uterus, cervix, and vagina can be seen on contrast-enhanced T$_1$-weighted images (Fig. 1-32 on p. 38). Compared with nonenhanced T$_1$-weighted images, the outer myometrium and endometrium are more conspicuous because of contrast enhancement. A small teardrop-shaped region of low signal intensity fluid may be seen in the endometrial canal. The junctional zone demonstrates less enhancement than either the outer myometrium or endometrium.

Normal bizonal anatomy of the uterine cervix is visual-

ized on T$_2$-weighted images (Fig. 1-31B). There is a central area of high signal intensity representing cervical mucosa and mucus. Cervical stroma appear as a rim of decreased signal intensity against the relatively high signal intensities of the cervical mucosa centrally and the paracervical fat peripherally. In contrast with T$_2$-weighted images, the zonal anatomy of the cervix and supracervical uterus on T$_1$-weighted images is not apparent. The cervix is of uniform intermediate signal intensity on T$_1$-weighted images, although the endometrium and cervical canal may be relatively hypointense.

Like the cervix, the normal vagina can be seen as a central area of increased signal intensity surrounded by fibromuscular tissue on T$_2$-weighted images. Identifica-

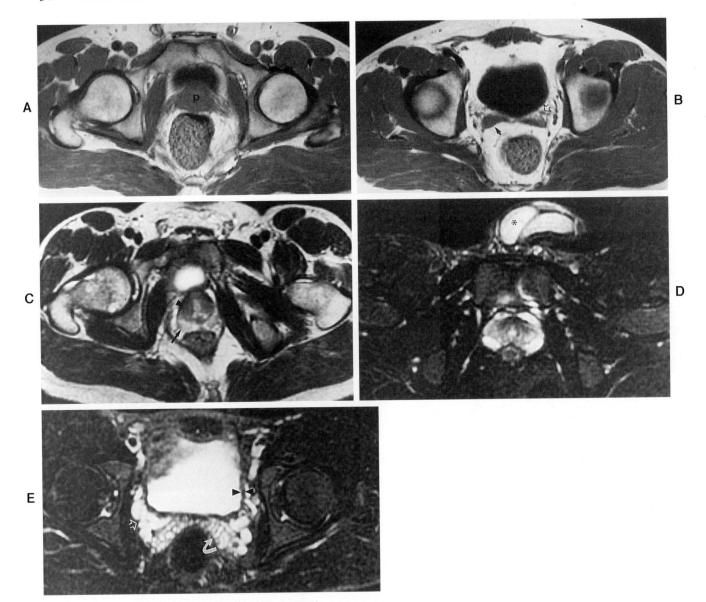

Fig. 1-27   Body coil MR imaging of the normal male pelvis. **A,** On a transaxial spin–echo T_1-weighted image (repetition time = 600 msec; echo time = 15 msec), the prostate gland (p) has a homogeneous low signal intensity, similar to that of skeletal muscle; there is no zonal differentiation. **B,** At a more cephalic level, the thin wall of the normal bladder is slightly hyperintense compared with urine. Like the prostate gland, the seminal vesicle (solid arrow) is homogeneously hypointense. Periprostatic veins (open arrow) are seen in a normal wedge of fat between the seminal vesicle and the bladder. **C,** On a fast spin–echo T_2-weighted image, the peripheral zone (arrow) has a higher signal intensity than the central gland (arrowhead). **D,** This prostatic zonal differentiation is accentuated when fat saturation is implemented. Note the hyperintense corporal bodies of the penis (*). **E,** On another fast spin–echo T_2-weighted image with fat saturation, the seminal vesicle (curved arrow) appears as a collection of small, hyperintense cystic spaces. The periprostatic venous plexus (open arrow) consists of larger, hyperintense curvilinear structures. The wall of the urinary bladder (between arrowheads) appears as a low intensity line.

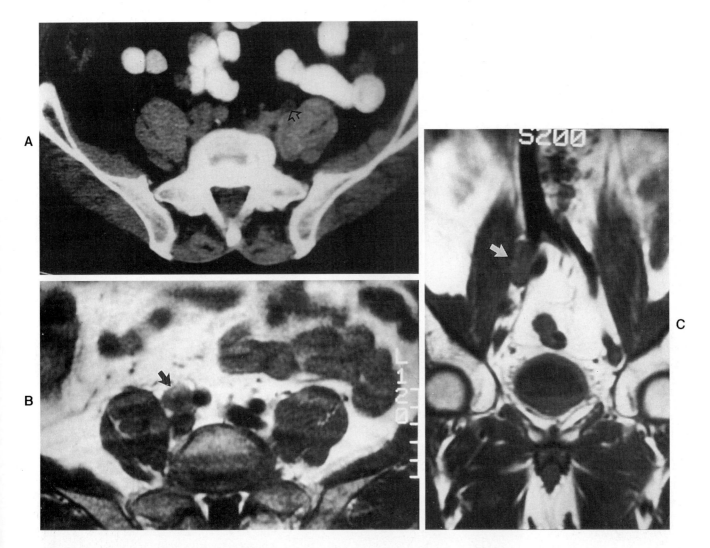

Fig. 1-28   Computed tomography and MR imaging of the lymph nodes. **A,** Is this computed tomography scan normal? The left ureter (open arrow) lies on the medial aspect of the psoas muscle (arrow). T_1-weighted MR images in the transaxial **B,** and coronal **C,** planes demonstrate an enlarged right common iliac node (arrow). On T_1-weighted MR images, vessels can be distinguished from lymph nodes because of the signal void of moving protons.

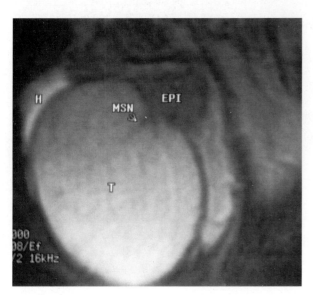

Fig. 1-29   MR imaging of the scrotum. Sagittal T_2-weighted fast spin–echo (repetition time = 4000 msec; effective echo time = 108 msec) image demonstrates uniform hyperintense signal of the normal testis (T). The hypointense mediastinum (MSN) is identified along the superoposterior pole of the testicle next to the head of the epididymis (EPI). A small hydrocele (H) is also demonstrated.

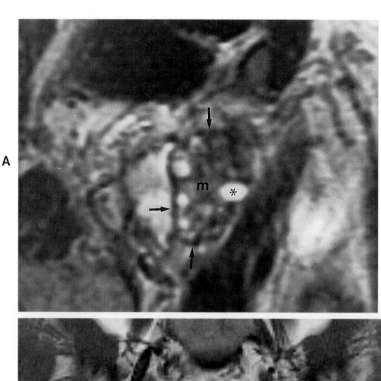

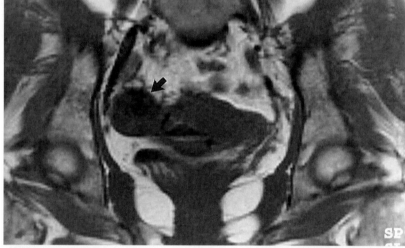

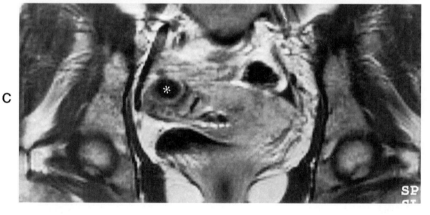

Fig. 1-30   MR imaging of the normal ovary in a premenopausal woman. **A,** A magnified sagittal T₂-weighted fast spin–echo image (repetition time = 5000 msec; effective echo time = 98 msec) demonstrates higher signal intensity of the medulla (m) compared with the cortex of the ovary (arrows) and the stromal rim around developing follicles (*). The Graafian follicles in the cortex of the ovary are hyperintense because, as they develop, fluid accumulates in the follicular antrum. **B,** On a coronal T₁-weighted image (repetition time = 500 msec; echo time = 15 msec), the right ovary (arrow) is isointense compared with skeletal muscle and may not be distinguished from loops of small bowel. **C,** After gadopentetate administration, the medulla and the follicular wall (granulosatheca) enhance. Developing follicles (*) are identified because fluid in the follicular antrum does not enhance.

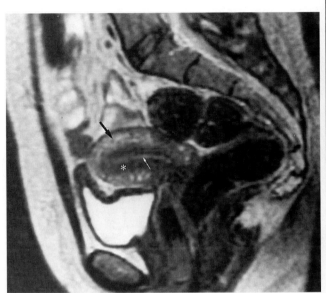
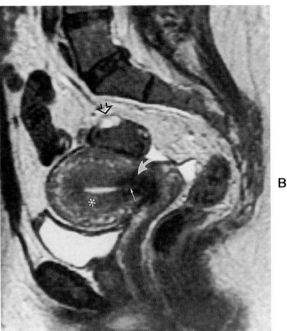

A

B

Fig. 1-31   Zonal anatomy of the normal uterus on T$_2$-weighted images. **A,** A sagittal fast spin–echo T$_2$-weighted image (repetition time = 3200 msec; effective echo time = 104 msec) of the uterus shows the trilaminar appearance of the normal uterus. The endometrium (small white arrow) has a high signal intensity similar to or greater than that of fat. The outer myometrium (black arrow) has an intermediate signal intensity, and the inner myometrium or junctional zone (*) has a lower signal intensity similar to that of skeletal muscle. **B,** In another patient, the sagittal fast spin–echo T$_2$-weighted image shows a normal but thicker junctional zone (*). The cervical epithelium and mucus (small white arrow) have a high signal intensity. The cervical stroma (curved white arrow) surrounds the endocervix and has a homogeneously low signal intensity. Normal ovarian follicles (open arrow) are also seen.

tion of the vagina on T$_1$-weighted images can be facilitated by the insertion of a tampon.

ANGIOGRAPHY

Angiography has been relegated to a secondary role in the evaluation of most genitourinary tract disease because of the advent of cross-sectional imaging. Nevertheless, there are still well-defined indications for angiography of the genitourinary tract.

Indications for Arteriography

Renal arteriography
1. Evaluation of renal artery occlusion or stenosis;
2. Evaluation of renal arteriopathy (e.g., vasculitis, aneurysm, fibromuscular dysplasia, arteriovenous malformation (AVM), arteriovenous or arteriocalyceal fistula, or hemangioma);

3. Evaluation of suspected renal mass when the diagnosis is unclear after noninvasive radiologic workup, aspiration or biopsy, or both; and
4. Preoperative or palliative ablation of a hypervascular neoplasm.

Adrenal arteriography rarely is performed in the era of cross-sectional imaging and imaging-directed biopsy. Occasionally, it can be used to demonstrate the arterial supply of a large retroperitoneal mass and to identify the adrenal gland as the organ of origin.

Gonadal arteriography is also performed rarely. Occasionally, testicular arteriography is needed to localize a maldescended testicle and, rarely, to study a testicular mass.

Selective internal pudendal arteriography is performed for the evaluation of vasculogenic impotence. Hemodynamically significant stenosis of the internal iliac, internal pudendal, penile, or cavernosal arteries may be the cause of arteriogenic vascular impotence.

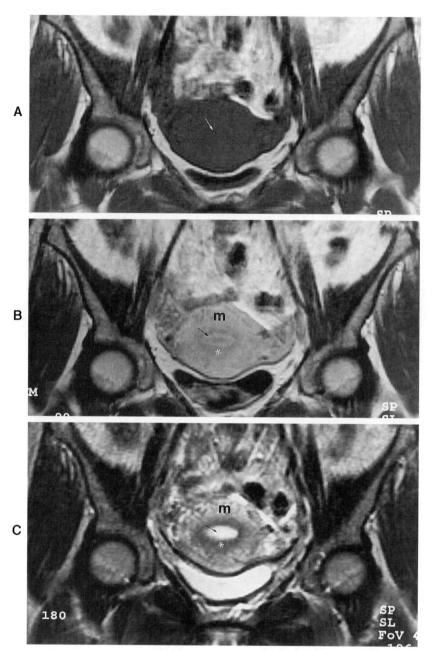

Fig. 1-32 Contrast-enhanced MR imaging of the uterus. **A,** On a coronal spin–echo T_1-weighted image, the endometrium (white arrow) is slightly hypointense compared with the myometrium, but, in general, there is little tissue contrast. **B,** After the administration of gadopentetate, increased signal intensity of the endometrium (small black arrow) and outer myocardium (m) improves tissue contrast on a T_1-weighted image. There is relatively less enhancement of the junctional zone (*). Compare the zonal anatomy shown on the postcontrast T_1-weighted image with that demonstrated on a fast spin–echo T_2-weighted image **C.**

Indications for Venography and Venous Sampling

Renal venography

1. Evaluation of suspected renovascular hypertension (renal vein sampling for renin concentration); and
2. Evaluation of occlusive disease of the renal vein or inferior vena cava after a nondiagnostic work-up.

Adrenal vein sampling is most often performed to identify small, hyperfunctional adrenal neoplasms (e.g., aldosteronoma) that cannot be localized with CT or MR imaging.

Sampling may be followed by adrenal phlebography because small adrenal tumors may be identified by mass effect or displacement. A complication of venography is adrenal hemorrhage or contrast extravasation, which may present clinically as progressive back pain and low-grade fever and may result in permanent dysfunction of the affected adrenal gland.

Testicular and ovarian venography have been superseded by sonography and CT, with a few exceptions. The most common indication for testicular phlebography is the identification and transcatheter occlusion of varicocele in infertile patients. Testicular phlebography is still required in some patients to identify the pampiniform plexus in patients with testicular nondescent when sonography, CT, or MR imaging is nondiagnostic. Sampling of the ovarian venous effluent may be used to identify a rare functional neoplasm of the ovary.

Technique for Conventional Angiography

Renal and pelvic arteriography is performed by a transfemoral route, with the Seldinger method of catheter insertion. For selective renal arteriography, an endhole visceral catheter, 5 to 6.5 F shepherd's crook, or cobra catheter is used (Fig. 1-33). A multiple sidehole catheter is used for renal venography. Selective pelvic arteriography usually can be performed from an ipsilateral or bilateral approach. Selective catheterization of the internal iliac branches can be performed with a cobra catheter or shepherd's crook catheter. The type of iodinated contrast, injection rate and volume, and filming technique

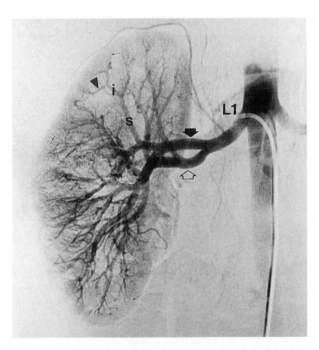

Fig. 1-33 Normal right renal arteriogram. The main renal artery typically originates near the inferior endplate of L1. In 20% to 30% of patients, a supplementary renal artery originates distal to the main renal artery. The ventral ramus (solid arrow) is the major continuation of the renal artery and is dominant, sending segmental branches to the cranial, caudal, and middle poles (hollow arrow = dorsal ramus). Segmental arteries (s) course through the renal sinus and, beyond the papillae, are termed interlobar arteries (i). The arcuate arteries (closed triangle) are the terminal branches of the interlobar arteries and demarcate the corticomedullary junction. Interlobular arteries (small arrows) originate from and course perpendicular to the arcuate arteries toward the renal capsule. About 20 afferent glomerular arterioles originate from each interlobular artery.

for selected genitourinary tract angiographic examinations are summarized in Appendix L.

Digital Subtraction Angiography

Digital subtraction angiography (DSA) is a computer-assisted vascular imaging method that requires only about one half of the intraarterial concentration of contrast material to depict vessels of similar size by conventional angiography. The main advantage of DSA over conventional angiography is the ability to postprocess digitized images to maximize contrast resolution. The DSA technique calls for exposure of several precontrast images immediately after contrast medium injection but before the contrast appears in the target vessels. These images serve as subtraction masks. Multiple images are obtained during contrast opacification of the vascular anatomy of interest. Computer subtraction of the postcontrast images from the precontrast masks yields an image with high vascular conspicuity. Postprocessing manipulation of images improves mask registration, magnifies the image, zooms to a part of the image, or changes window and level settings.

Digital subtraction technology can be performed with injections of contrast material into either a central vein or artery. For intravenous DSA of the kidney, 40 cc of 76% contrast medium is injected via power injector at a rate of 20 to 30 cc per second through a pigtail catheter in the right atrium. Areas of interest are filmed at 2 frames per second. Although the main renal artery is demonstrated well by this technique, renal intravenous DSA is limited in the visualization of renal branch vessels compared with conventional angiography. To visualize renal branch vessels, intraarterial DSA is necessary. With this technique, contrast material is injected directly into the aorta or selectively into the renal artery. Using 43% contrast medium injected at a rate and volume less than that for cut-film arteriography, excellent opacification of main and branch renal arteries can be attained with filming at either 1.5 or 3 frames per second.

NUCLEAR MEDICINE

Renal Scintigraphy

Radiopharmaceuticals

Tc-99m diethylenetriaminepentaacetic acid (DTPA) The accurate measurement of glomerular filtration rate (GFR) requires an agent that is filtered completely by the glomerulus but is not reabsorbed, metabolized, or secreted by the renal tubules. DTPA is one of the agents that can be used to accurately measure GFR. Its clearance is typically a few percent lower than inulin, the traditional standard for measuring GFR. The relative GFR of each kidney can be determined from the net counts that accumulate in the kidneys during the 2 to 3 minutes after tracer injection. The extraction fraction is the percentage of the radiopharmaceutical removed by the kidney with each pass. In patients with impaired renal function, Tc-99m DTPA may not be as useful because the extraction fraction is approximately 20%. Tc-99m mercaptoacetyltriglycine (MAG$_3$) has an extraction fraction of 40% to 50% and provides better quality scintigrams in patients with poor renal function.

I-131 orthoiodohippurate (OIH) To measure effective renal plasma flow, the ideal radiopharmaceutical should be removed completely from arterial plasma during a single pass through the kidney. OIH is similar in structure to paraaminohippurate, and approximately 80% is extracted during a single pass through the kidney; 85% is removed by tubular secretion, and the remaining 15% is removed by glomerular filtration. The major use of OIH scintigraphy is for the evaluation of total and individual renal function. The main disadvantage of I-131 OIH is the suboptimal imaging characteristics of I-131 compared with Tc-99m. Patients with impaired renal function may receive high doses of radiation to the kidney.

Tc-99m mercaptoacetyltriglycine (MAG$_3$) Tc-99m MAG$_3$ is a radiopharmaceutical with imaging properties similar to those of OIH. However, image quality with this agent is better than that of either I-131 OIH or Tc-99m DTPA. This is attributed to the superior imaging characteristics of Tc-99m relative to I-131 and to the smaller volume of distribution and more rapid clearance of MAG$_3$ compared with DTPA. MAG$_3$ is excreted in the kidney primarily through secretion by proximal renal tubule cells, and its clearance is only about 40% to 50% that of OIH. However, because it is highly protein-bound, a larger proportion of MAG$_3$ remains in the plasma. A higher plasma concentration compensates for the relatively lower extraction fraction, and the renogram curve and the 30-minute urinary excretion of MAG$_3$ are nearly identical to those of OIH (Fig. 1-34).

Tc-99m dimercaptosuccinic acid (DMSA) and glucoheptonate (GHA) The ideal renal cortical imaging agent should accumulate in the cortical tubules and be retained in cortical tissue exclusively so that interference from pelvocalyceal activity is minimized. Approximately half of the administered dose of DMSA accumulates in the distal tubules within 1 hour and remains in the renal cortex for up to 24 hours. Glucoheptonate is cleared primarily by glomerular filtration; a small amount is extracted and concentrated in the cytosol of proximal renal tubule cells. Up to 45% is excreted in the urine within 1 hour, and 10% remains bound to the renal tubular cells for up to 2 hours. These agents serve to indicate functioning tubular mass and can be used to elucidate renal morphology.

Renogram curve

The renogram curve is a graph of summated activity over a targeted region of interest with respect to time. The region of interest may be the entire kidney or one of its constituents (i.e., the renal cortex or the renal pelvis). This time–activity curve can be subdivided into periods of tracer appearance or accumulation, extraction, and elimination (Fig. 1-34A). Depending on the radiopharmaceutical, tracer extraction is proportional to effective renal plasma flow (MAG$_3$ and OIH) or GFR (DTPA).

Quantitative measurements of renal function based on the time–activity data can aid the interpretation of images. The relative renal uptake is a comparative measurement of tracer accumulation by each kidney and is determined on an image made 1 to 2 minutes after tracer injection; normal differential function can be as great as 56%/44%. The time-to-maximum activity is used to assess the extraction of radiotracer by each kidney. In general, the peak height of radioactivity should occur by 5 minutes after injection. The rate of radiotracer washout can be measured by the T 1/2, which is determined during the steep part of the washout curve (Fig. 1-34A). Normal values for the T 1/2 depend on the radiopharmaceutical, but as a general rule, a value less than 10 minutes is normal, and a value more than 20 minutes is abnormal. A general measure of tracer transit through the renal cortex is the 20-minute/maximum activity ratio. In the absence of pelvic or caliceal retention, a normal ratio for Tc-99m MAG$_3$ or I-131 OIH is less than 0.3.

Indications

Evaluation of renal parenchyma
1. Determination of relative renal blood flow (renovascular hypertension, trauma);
2. Determination of relative renal function (unilateral obstruction, previous renal surgery, trauma); and
3. Evaluation of renal cortical disease (pyelonephritis, reflux nephropathy, or renal pseudomass); cortical agents may still have a role in the rare patient with an absolute contraindication to iodinated contrast, in a patient with diabetes with severe renal insufficiency, or in the evaluation of a renal pseudomass (cortical column of Bertin).

Collecting system
1. Evaluation of collecting system dilatation; and
2. Evaluation of vesicoureteral reflux.

Adrenal Scintigraphy

Adrenal scintigraphy complements cross-sectional imaging methods in the evaluation of an adrenal mass lesion. Scintigraphy with the cholesterol analogue NP-59 pro-

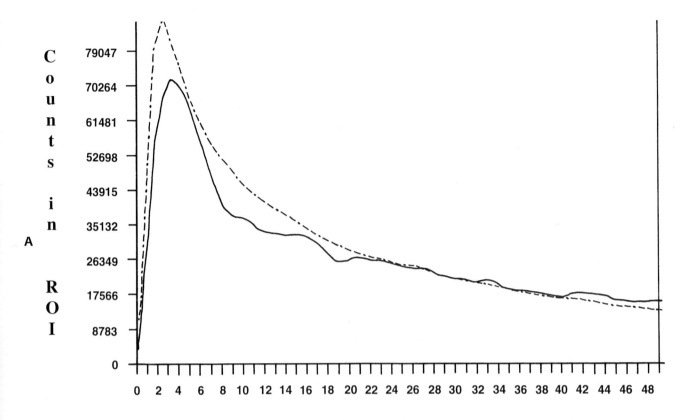

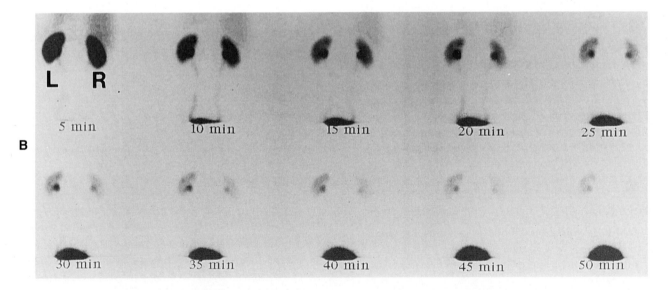

Fig. 1-34   Normal Tc-99m MAG₃ renogram. **A,** Time-activity curve. **B,** Static images. Quantitative measurements of tracer accumulation and excretion aid the interpretation of images. The relative renal uptake provides a measure of relative renal function and can range to 56%/44%. The peak activity should occur by 5 minutes after injection. The T 1/2 quantifies tracer washout, and a value of less than 10 minutes is normal. As renal function deteriorates, the transit time through the kidney increases, which is reflected in an elevated value for the 20 minute/maximum activity ratio; a normal ratio for Tc-99m MAG₃ is 0.3.

vides functional localization of adrenocortical disease. Imaging with or without dexamethasone suppression is used to evaluate hypofunctional adrenal disease and diseases of adrenocortical hyperfunction, such as Cushing's syndrome, primary aldosteronism, and adrenogenital syndrome. Sympathoadrenal imaging is performed with I-131 metaiodobenzylguanidine (MIBG). MIBG scintigraphy is useful for the detection of extraadrenal and metastatic disease, particularly when CT or MR imaging is not helpful in localizing a suspected pheochromocytoma.

Scrotal Scintigraphy

Color Doppler sonography and radionuclide imaging have been used to differentiate testicular torsion from epididymoorchitis in the patient with an acutely painful and enlarged hemiscrotum. Tc-99m pertechnetate, DTPA, or human serum albumin can be used to assess the perfusion of the acute scrotum. After a radioactive string is positioned between the testicles, the radiotracer is injected and rapid sequential images are obtained over the scrotal region. Relative decrease or nonperfusion of the symptomatic testicle suggests acute torsion as the cause of the "acute scrotum." Preservation of flow or increased flow in the symptomatic testicle suggests an inflammatory cause of unilateral scrotal pain or swelling.

APPENDIX A: INTRAVENOUS UROGRAPHY*

BOLUS INFUSION UROGRAPHY
Contrast

The dose of iodinated contrast that is administered depends on the size of the patient, the method of contrast administration, and the nature of the contrast. The average adult dose is between 20 and 30 g of iodine or about 200 mg iodine per pound body weight. Using the bolus technique, 100 to 120 mL of a 30% contrast material is administered over 30 to 60 seconds.

Procedure

1. Before the injection of contrast material, a preliminary film of the abdomen is always obtained.
2. 1-minute coned film of both kidneys or nephrotomograms.
3. 5-minute coned film of both kidneys. Apply abdominal compression.
4. 10-minute abdominopelvic plain film with abdominal compression; then release compression.

*Modified from the Procedure Manual, Department of Radiology, Massachusetts General Hospital.

5. 15-minute abdominopelvic plain film.
6. Post-void abdominopelvic plain film.

DRIP INFUSION PYELOGRAPHY

The advantage of drip infusion is that the nephrogram and ureterogram are visualized for a longer period of time, which reduces the stringency of filming.

Contrast

The drip infusion technique delivers larger doses of contrast material, typically 40 to 45 g of iodine, over a longer period of time: 300 mL of an ionic contrast medium, such as diatrizoate (14%) or iothalamate (30%), or 100 to 150 mL of a nonionic contrast medium, such as iopamidol (40.8%) or iohexol (38.8%). Use an 18- or 19-gauge needle in an antecubital vein whenever possible.

Procedure

1. Supine scout film: check film for position, technique, and renal stones; obtain oblique views if indicated. After the administration of contrast material, secure temporary venous access for use should management of an adverse reaction become necessary.
2. 5-minute coned film of the kidneys.
3. 10-minute coned film of the kidneys.
4. 15-minute KUB with bilateral oblique films.
5. At this point, review all films, and if supplemental views are not necessary, obtain a post-void film.

Comments

1. If infusion of contrast medium is slow, delay oblique views until end of infusion.
2. For solitary kidneys and renal transplantations, use half the amount of contrast medium.
3. Supplementary films are requested as necessary after each routine film is reviewed. Prone and erect films are used for viewing portions of the ureter that are not seen optimally in the supine position, i.e., the distal third of the ureter. These views are also useful for demonstrating bladder hernias and renal ptosis. Delayed views are used in patients with obstruction when the collecting system is not imaged on the routine series of films but when a delayed nephrogram is seen.
4. In a patient with ureteral obstruction, acquire either prone or supine KUB films after 10-minute ambulation by the patient to expedite opacification of the distal third of the ureter.

5. Should there be a catheter in the bladder or ureter, drain any urine within the catheter, and then clamp the catheter before contrast injection.
6. Abdominal compression is used to distend the ureters to facilitate the visualization of small tumors or papillary necrosis. Compression of the ureters is usually applied after the 5-minute film. Immediately after the anteroposterior 10-minute "overhead" film, compression is released. It is important to remember that compression rarely causes contrast extravasation because of forniceal rupture. Thus, abdominal compression is contraindicated in patients with suspected ureteral obstruction or calculi, recent surgery, severe hypertension, or abdominal aortic aneurysm. Finally, compression is usually unnecessary when contrast material is administered by the drip infusion technique.

DRIP INFUSION PYELOGRAPHY WITH NEPHROTOMOGRAPHY

Contrast

The volume of ionic contrast medium (14% to 30% solution) that is administered ranges from 100 to 500 mL. The drip infusion pyelography (DIP) contrast medium is available in a 300-cc bottle; hang the bottle high on an IV stand so that this mixture is infused rapidly. Use either an 18-gauge or 19-gauge needle or scalp vein tubing; secure the venous access device in place for future access.

Procedure

1. Acquire preliminary radiographs including an abdominal plain film and a preliminary tomogram at about 8 cm from the table top.
2. Begin drip infusion of iodinated contrast material. After 200 cc are infused (i.e., when only 100 cc is left in bottle), nephrotomography is begun. Tomograms are obtained in an anteroposterior position to include both kidneys; usually four cuts are required (e.g., 8 to 11 cm from the table top). Low kidneys have a more anterior position, so tomographic cuts should begin more anteriorly. The kidneys of extremely thin patients with "flat back" are more posterior. As supplemental views, oblique nephrotomograms (15° to 20°) of the side in question may be performed.
3. Finish the DIP procedure, as enumerated previously.
4. Perform post-infusion KUB with bilateral oblique films.
5. At this time, review all films. If supplemental views are not necessary, obtain a post-void film.

APPENDIX B: VOIDING CYSTOURETHROGRAPHY*

Contrast

The meglumine salts of diatrizoate and iothalamate are used for cystography and urethrography. In general, 15% solutions are used for cystography because higher concentrations may cause a chemical cystitis.

Procedure

The routine voiding cystourethrogram is performed with spot films and fluoroscopy; overhead films routinely are not required unless atypical anatomy or high-grade vesicoureteral reflux is demonstrated.

1. After cleansing the glans penis or introitus with sterile iodine solution, the urethra is catheterized with a 14 F to 18 F straight rubber catheter. The catheter is advanced until urine is obtained. The bladder is drained of residual urine, and contrast material is instilled slowly under gravity. If transurethral catheterization of the bladder is not possible, percutaneous cystostomy with an 18-gauge or 20-gauge needle can be performed.
2. Obtain spot films of the urinary bladder and both renal fossa.
3. As the bladder fills with contrast material, anteroposterior and bilateral oblique spot films of the urinary bladder are acquired. The bladder is filled gradually, and intermittent fluoroscopy is used to evaluate for vesicoureteral reflux. Should reflux or diverticula be detected fluoroscopically, spot films should be taken for documentation. The bladder is filled until capacity is reached and the urge to void occurs. Any spontaneous micturition should be filmed, and in men, films should be exposed in the steep oblique position to profile the urethra.
4. If the patient feels ready to void, gently remove the catheter. If the patient is voiding into a radiolucent receptacle, care should be exercised not to compress the urethra at the penoscrotal junction, causing extrinsic obstruction. Manual compression of the penile meatus by the patient can facilitate opacification of the urethra during spontaneous micturition. In women, start in the oblique position and slowly turn the patient to an anteroposterior position. In men, a steep oblique position will image the urethra in profile. Multiple spot films of the urethra are obtained while the patient voids.

*Modified from the Procedure Manual, Department of Radiology, Massachusetts General Hospital.

5. After micturition is completed, estimate the residual urine volume, and fluoroscopically evaluate the pelvis and abdomen for ureteral reflux. Repeat spot films of the urinary bladder and both renal fossa.

APPENDIX C: URETHROGRAPHY

DYNAMIC RETROGRADE URETHROGRAPHY*
Contrast

Retrograde urethrography commonly is performed with a 30% contrast solution, although a 60% concentration may be necessary to opacify the adult male urethra adequately.

Procedure

Spot filming is performed with the objective of demonstrating the morphology of the male urethra.

1. Insert a Foley catheter with a 5-mL balloon into the distal urethra after cleansing the glans penis with povidone-iodine solution. Then, gently inflate the balloon of the Foley catheter in the fossa navicularis until the patient senses pressure and the catheter is secure.
2. Attach an adapter, extension tube, and 50-mL syringe with contrast medium in sequence to the Foley catheter. The entire system should be flushed in advance to avoid instillation of air bubbles.
3. Position the patient in a 45° oblique position with the dependent thigh flexed.
4. Tape extension tubing to the inner aspect of the thigh.
5. Inject contrast gently but firmly to overcome resistance of the external sphincter. Volitional relaxation of the internal sphincter can be achieved by asking the patient to simulate pelvic relaxation of micturition.
6. Acquire multiple spot films to document the morphology of the anterior and posterior urethra.
7. Because the external urethral orifice is more difficult to occlude, the double balloon catheter technique frequently is used for urethrography in a woman. A proximal balloon occludes the external meatus of the urethra, and a distal balloon occludes the vesical neck. Intraurethral pressure increases as contrast material is instilled and suffices to fill a urethral diverticulum, if one exists.

*Modified from the Procedure Manual, Department of Radiology, Massachusetts General Hospital.

PERICATHETER RETROGRADE URETHROGRAPHY*

Procedure

The examination is performed with spot films to demonstrate part or all of the urethra when an intraurethral catheter is present. This study is most typically requested after pelvic trauma or urethroplasty.

1. Advance a 5 to 7 F pediatric feeding tube, lubricated with anesthetic jelly, into the urethra adjacent to a preexisting catheter. The tip of the catheter should be positioned in the distal urethra when investigating patients with recent urethroplasty but should be advanced near the external urethral sphincter when studying the traumatized urethra.
2. Complete remaining sequences as in steps 2 to 6 of the dynamic retrograde urethrogram.

APPENDIX D: ILEOSTOURETEROGRAPHY (ILEAL LOOPOGRAPHY)*

Contrast

Cystographic contrast solution is recommended. Undiluted 15% or 30% iodinated contrast medium in a syringe may be used if there is inadequate definition of the collecting system resulting from ureteropelvocaliectasis.

Procedure

1. Obtain a preliminary plain film of the abdomen and pelvis.
2. Use a 14 F Foley catheter with 5-cc balloon. Insert the tip of the catheter well beyond the inner abdominal wall. Inflate the balloon of the Foley catheter, and withdraw gently to ensure tamponade of loop.
3. Connect bottle containing contrast material to a three-way stopcock, manometer, connecting tube, Colby adaptor, and Foley catheter, in that order. Instill cystographic contrast material by gravity; it is important not to exceed a manometric pressure of 40 cm water when instilling contrast medium.
4. Under fluoroscopy, document retrograde filling of collecting systems, and acquire spot films of any unusual findings. Include one spot film of the ileal or colon conduit in profile. It is important to observe the presence of ureteral and loop peristalsis.
5. Obtain overhead anteroposterior and bilateral oblique films.
6. Deflate the balloon of the Foley catheter, and, after 10 to 15 munutes, obtain a post-drainage overhead anteroposterior film.

APPENDIX E: BALLOON CATHETER HYSTEROSALPINGOGRAPHY*

There are two different methods of hysterosalpingography. The balloon catheter technique is favored by the majority of radiologists because it is a more versatile technique, facilitating filming in oblique and prone positions. Gynecologists favor the tenaculum–cannula technique, which does not entail intubation of the cervical canal. Use of the tenaculum and cannula allows the physician to opacify a scarred uterine cavity, a condition in which the balloon catheter often is expelled.

Contraindications

1. Menses.
2. Active pelvic inflammatory disease.
3. Within 4 days after dilatation and curettage.
4. Pregnancy.

Contrast

Either an oil-soluble or a water-soluble contrast material can be used for hysterosalpingography. Water-soluble contrast material is preferred because mucosal detail is depicted more clearly and because it is promptly resorbed by peritoneal epithelium. Oil-soluble contrast material gained popularity because higher pregnancy rates initially were reported. However, the major disadvantage of oil-soluble contrast material is relatively poor mucosal detail. Because of delayed absorption, retention of oil-soluble contrast material may incite fibrosis and granuloma formation.

Technique

1. Acquire a preliminary anteroposterior spot film of the pelvis.
2. Perform bimanual pelvic examination to determine the position of the uterus and cervix and to palpate any uterine or adnexal masses.
3. Insert a speculum, and open as wide as possible for complete visualization of the cervix. A uterine sound may be used to dilate the external cervical os. Fascial dilators may be required to enlarge a stenotic endocervical os or canal.
4. Connect in sequence a syringe filled with contrast material, extension tubing, three-way stopcock, plastic or metal adaptor, and an 8 F Foley catheter. Air should be expelled completely from the system. The Foley catheter balloon is tested, and a 3-cc

*Modified from the Procedure Manual, Department of Radiology, Massachusetts General Hospital.

syringe, filled with 1 cc of sterile saline, is attached to the balloon port. The three-way stopcock is then closed to the Foley catheter, and the extension tubing and syringe are separated from the rest of the system.
5. Grasp the end of the Foley catheter with long forceps just proximal to the balloon. Insert the catheter into the cervical canal; gently inflate the balloon just beyond the external cervical os until the catheter cannot be withdrawn with moderate tension.
6. Carefully remove the speculum, and position the patient on the fluoroscopy table in a supine position.
7. Reattach the extension tubing and syringe to the system, and open the three-way stopcock.
8. Slowly inject contrast medium, observing the sequential opacification of the endometrial cavity and uterine tubes. Expose selected, coned spot films in the anteroposterior and oblique positions. The initial anteroposterior film is a view of the underfilled uterine cavity to demonstrate contour. Next, obtain shallow oblique views of the uterine tubes. Finally, acquire an anteroposterior view showing both uterine tubes and free dispersion of contrast medium around pelvic loops of small bowel.
9. If the uterine tubes cannot be opacified with the patient in a supine position, acquire spot films in the prone position while contrast material is instilled. Alternatively, glucagon or terbutaline may be administered if nonopacification is attributed to tubal spasm.

APPENDIX F: ENDOVAGINAL SONOGRAPHY

Preparation and Positioning

1. The urinary bladder should be empty to prevent displacement of pelvic organs by a distended bladder. With an empty bladder, the procedure is far better tolerated by the patient.
2. A modified lithotomy position facilitates manipulation of the transducer. The head and upper body of the patient are elevated to cause pooling of any abdominal fluid in the pelvis. If a flat examining table is used, a thick foam cushion should be inserted below the pelvis to facilitate free movement of the examiner's hand in tilting the transducer probe in the vertical plane.
3. The typical endovaginal transducer operates at 5 to 7.5 MHz, may be either end- or side-firing, and has focal zones between 1 to 8 cm. Many tranducers can perform duplex and color Doppler sonography as well. A 90° to 115° sector scan format is typical.

The transducer is prepared for insertion by lubricating it with coupling gel and covering it in a condom.

Imaging Technique

The fundamental transducer orientations are longitudinal (sagittal) and coronal. Systematic examination of the uterine fundus, corpus, cul-de-sac, cervix, ovaries, and adnexa is suggested.

1. The uterine fundus and corpus are examined in the longitudinal plane. The uterus assumes a more anteverted position when the bladder is not distended. To image the fundus, the transducer may have to be angled anteriorly. As with the transabdominal study, the myometrium and endometrium can be readily distinguished.
2. Posterior angulation of the transducer permits sequential evaluation of the lower uterine segment, cervix, and cul-de-sac.
3. Rotating the transducer 90° shifts the image into a coronal plane. After the uterus is reexamined in the coronal plane, the adnexa and ovaries are studied.
4. The ovaries are imaged by angulating the transducer to the side and then slowly scanning in an anterior-to-posterior direction. Several anatomic landmarks can be used to localize the ovaries. The first is location. In the nulliparous patient, the ovaries are usually found in the ovarian fossa, just anterior to the internal iliac artery and vein. Second, the ovary usually is identified in women who are menstruating by the presence of multiple, peripheral follicles. Unless dilated, the fallopian tubes are not usually visualized.

APPENDIX G: TRANSRECTAL SONOGRAPHY OF THE PROSTATE GLAND

Preparation and Positioning

1. The optimal transducer permits imaging in the transverse and parasagittal planes at a frequency of 5 to 7 MHz. End-viewing transducers are designed such that the imaging plane is directed along the long axis of the transducer; thus, any plane between the standard orthogonal planes can be selected readily.
2. The patient is scanned in either the left lateral or semiprone (Sims') position. The examination begins with a digital rectal examination; the prostate gland should be examined for firmness, size, and nodularity.

3. An excess of fecal material in the rectum may create artifacts and compromise the transmission of sound. An enema immediately before scanning will minimize this problem but is optional unless biopsy is planned.

Imaging Method

1. A lubricated and condom-sheathed transducer is introduced into the rectum.
2. A series of four to six transaxial images of the prostate gland and seminal vesicles is obtained in the midline, followed by a series of four to six laterally angled transaxial images of the left and right margins of the gland. Recalling that peripheral zone tissue comprises a major part of the apical prostate, particular attention to this area of the prostate is suggested.
3. The transducer is then rotated, and a series of six to eight sagittal images of the prostate is performed. Cephalocaudal angulation of the transducer when imaging in the parasagittal plane may be required.

APPENDIX H: SONOGRAPHY OF THE SCROTUM

Preparation and Positioning

1. The scrotal ultrasound examination begins with a review of the clinical history and a physical examination of the scrotum.
2. To optimize scanning, the scrotum is positioned so that it rests on a towel draped over the thighs. A second towel is placed over the ventral surface of the penis after it is positioned to rest on the lower abdominal wall.

Imaging

1. Scanning is performed with a 7.5-MHz or 10-MHz linear-array or sector-scanning transducer. If the physical examination indicates, scanning of the suspected area of focal abnormality is performed first.
2. Comparative transaxial images of both testes are important to accentuate subtle differences in parenchymal echogenicity that may occur with diffusely infiltrative disease. One image each through the upper pole, midpole, and lower pole of the testes should be recorded.
3. Sagittal and transaxial images of the upper, middle, and lower pole of each testicle are acquired next.

4. When indicated, routine gray-scale images can be supplemented by color Doppler sonography of the testis or epididymis.

APPENDIX I: CONVENTIONAL COMPUTED TOMOGRAPHY OF THE GENITOURINARY TRACT—ORAL AND INTRAVENOUS CONTRAST MEDIA

Oral Contrast Media

Oral contrast media include dilute Gastrografin and barium preparations. One oral contrast medium for abdominal and pelvic CT consists of a 2.5% solution of Gastrografin in water or juice (i.e., 0.25 ounce of Gastrografin in 10 ounces of water or juice) or a 2% suspension of barium. Optimal opacification of the colon is achieved after the patient consumes an 8-ounce cup of the dilute contrast suspension 12 hours and 6 hours before CT.

Intravenous Contrast Medium

The majority of renal and pelvic CT examinations are performed with intravenous contrast medium. In some patients, supplementary noncontrast CT will provide important information about nephrolithiasis and parenchymal or neoplastic calcification patterns. Particularly in patients who undergo CT for evaluation of a renal mass, CT before and after contrast enhancement is recommended because change in attenuation is an important diagnostic criterion.

Intravenous contrast material is administered by a variety of methods, depending on the organ of interest. The rapid-drip infusion technique calls for infusion of 100 to 150 cc of 60% contrast medium or 250 to 300 cc of 30% contrast medium. For the evaluation of a renal mass, dynamic scans after a bolus injection are particularly useful. A 50-cc bolus of contrast medium is injected, and after a pause of 15 to 20 seconds, a set of single-level dynamic scans is taken at the level of the renal mass. Additional contrast medium can be given by bolus or drip infusion to evaluate the rest of the kidneys. For staging of the liver and pelvic lymph nodes, a triple bolus technique has been advocated. This method calls for administering contrast medium through a power injector at three separate rates. Before scanning, contrast material is administered at 2 cc per second for 20 seconds. Scanning is initiated at the level of the hepatic dome, and the rate of contrast delivery is decreased to 0.5 cc per second as scanning through the liver is performed. The power injector is then stopped until the level of the true pelvic inlet is reached. At that time, contrast injection is resumed at a rate of 0.8 cc per second and continues until scanning of the pelvis is complete.

APPENDIX J: SUGGESTED CONVENTIONAL COMPUTED TOMOGRAPHY PROTOCOLS FOR SPECIFIC CLINICAL PROBLEMS

Adrenal Mass

After localizing the suprarenal area on a scout image, contiguous 3-mm to 5-mm sections are acquired through both adrenal glands. Unless a large mass is found, a noncontrast CT technique will suffice. Determining the attenuation value of an adrenal mass may be of value for characterization.

Renal or Perinephric Mass

Evaluation should include contiguous 5-mm sections through both kidneys with unenhanced and intravenous contrast–enhanced sequences. Staging of a known or suspected renal cell malignancy requires evaluation of the renal veins, the adrenal glands, and the liver.

Renal Trauma

Standard technique calls for contiguous 10-mm sections throughout both kidneys with contrast-enhanced technique.

Pyeloureteral Filling Defect

Computed tomography is used to differentiate a nonopaque stone from a tumor or clot if this cannot be accomplished by ultrasound examination. Suggested technique requires contiguous 5-mm sections through area of question with a noncontrast technique.

Disease of the Pyeloureteral and Retroperitoneal Region

Extrinsic displacement or obstruction of the ureter in the adult usually results from malignancy (metastasis) but occasionally results from a benign process (retroperitoneal fibrosis, abscess) or a primary mesenchymal tumor. Depending on the extent and location of the lesion, contiguous 5-mm or 10-mm sections with noncontrast- and contrast-enhanced sequences are recommended.

Cervical, Uterine, and Ovarian Cancer Staging

For characterization and staging of known or suspected malignancies of the ovary or uterus, contiguous 10-mm thin sections through the true pelvis immediately after intravenous bolus administration of 75 cc of iodinated contrast medium is recommended. Ten-millimeter slices every 15 mm through the abdomen to the xiphoid process are acquired after imaging of the pelvis is completed. Placement of a tampon before scanning helps to identify the vagina.

Staging of Prostate Cancer

To assess extraprostatic and seminal vesicle spread for staging prostate cancer, photographically magnified, 5-mm contiguous thin sections through the prostate are obtained. For nodal staging of prostate cancer, contiguous 10-mm sections or 5-mm sections with a 3-mm interslice gap from the prostate to the level of the xiphoid process are recommended. Use of intravenous contrast material is reserved for specific dilemmas (e.g., to distinguish lymph nodes from vessels or to detect rare liver metastases). Images should be acquired in soft-tissue and bone window formats.

Undescended Testicle

Noncontrast 5-mm contiguous sections from midscrotum to the aortic bifurcation are obtained. Asymmetry of soft tissues at and below the inguinal ligament is the focus of the evaluation.

Bladder Mass

To investigate a mass or thickening of the bladder wall, contiguous 5-mm sections through the bladder, immediately after a 50- to 100-cc intravenous bolus of iodinated contrast medium, are recommended. Contrast-enhanced CT is performed routinely. If nodal staging of a known bladder malignancy is the intent, contiguous 10-mm sections through the abdomen and pelvis are obtained. For distinguishing pelvic lymph nodes from vessels, contrast-enhanced imaging is begun at the symphysis pubis and is continued in a cephalad direction.

APPENDIX K: SUGGESTED PROTOCOLS FOR MR IMAGING OF THE KIDNEYS AND PELVIS

MR Imaging of the Kidney

1. For evaluation of a renal mass, pre-contrast and post-contrast T_1-weighted spin–echo or gradient–echo images in the transverse and coronal planes are recommended. An image section thickness of 5 to 7 mm is recommended. The body coil is used routinely to image the kidneys; in asthenic patients, a posterior surface coil can also be used to obtain high resolution images.
2. Fast spin–echo proton density-weighted and T_2-weighted images of the kidneys in the transverse

axial or coronal plane are also used to evaluate known or suspected renal masses.
3. For staging of a known renal malignancy, the liver, adrenal glands, and upper retroperitoneum should also be evaluated routinely.
4. Flow-compensated T_1-weighted spoiled gradient echo images are used to evaluate patency of the renal veins and inferior vena cava. This pulse sequence can be implemented alone or as a component of magnetic resonance venography.

MR Imaging of the Male Pelvis

1. If a body coil is used, spin–echo pulse sequences are used to generate T_1- and T_2-weighted images in the transverse axial plane. An image section thickness of 5 mm is recommended for evaluation of the bladder and prostate. Although contiguous sections are recommended, 1- to 2-mm interslice gaps may be implemented.
2. Regarding the imaging of disease of or related to the urinary bladder, coronal plane images are recommended when disease involves the lateral walls or base and for pathology of the muscular pelvic floor. Coronal plane images can also be valuable for evaluating the seminal vesicles and invasion of periprostatic fat by cancer in patients with disease of the prostate. For the staging of prostate cancer, sagittal views can be used to evaluate invasion of the bladder base or rectum. Sagittal plane images are used to evaluate disease involving the bladder base or dome and the urethra.
3. Imaging of the prostate with an endorectal surface coil, phased-array multicoil, or both has been an improvement over body coil MR imaging. Recommended sequences for endorectal surface coil imaging of the prostate include transaxial T_1-weighted and transaxial and sagittal FSE T_2-weighted images. Typical CSE T_1-weighted images in the transaxial plane are performed with 12-cm field of view, 3-mm slice thickness with 1-mm interslice gap, and 256×256 matrix. FSE T_2-weighted images in the transaxial and sagittal planes can be performed with TR = 4,000 msec, TE = 100 msec, 8- to 12-cm field of view, 3-mm slice thickness (interleaved), 2 acquisitions, and 256×256 matrix. It is important that images are taken with the patient in the supine position and to use both antialiasing options (swap-phase and frequency) and surface coil correction filtering.

MR Imaging of the Female Pelvis

1. For most clinical problems, T_1-, proton density-, and T_2-weighted images in the transaxial and sagittal imaging planes will suffice. MR imaging is usually

performed with a body coil, an anterior and posterior Helmholtz coil, or a phased-array pelvic multicoil.

2. Sagittal plane images are used to evaluate the relationship or spread of adnexal disease to the bladder or rectum. Coronal imaging planes depict the muscular pelvic floor optimally and are also used to evaluate extension of tumor to the pelvic sidewall.

3. For the evaluation of myometrial disease or müllerian anomalies, coronal and transaxial oblique imaging is advised because the relationship between the endometrial canal and myometrial tissue is depicted more clearly. Coronal oblique planes are oriented orthogonally to the long axis of the endometrial canal and are prescribed from a sagittal image. Similarly, transaxial oblique images can be prescribed from either the axial or sagittal planes and are oriented parallel to the long axis of the endometrium.

4. A T_1-weighted sequence with fat saturation is useful to distinguish masses with fat from those that contain subacute blood products. Contrast-enhanced T_1-weighted images with fat saturation have also been used to improve the staging of endometrial carcinoma.

APPENDIX L: SELECTED GENITOURINARY ANGIOGRAPHY METHODS

Renal Arteriogram*

Catheter Position	Proximal renal artery
Contrast Medium	76% solution
Rate of Injection	5–6 cc/sec
Volume of Contrast Medium	10–12 cc
Filming Rate	2 fps × 3 sec; 1 fps × 5 sec†

*Magnification technique is recommended.
†A poorly vascularized neoplasm can be visualized with high-dose arteriography. (5 cc/sec for 30 cc total volume of contrast), epinephrine (5–8 μg)-augmented angiography, or renal venography; fps = films per second.

Renal Venography

Catheter Position	Main or segmental renal vein
Contrast Medium	76% solution
Rate of Injection	12–15 cc/sec*
Volume of Contrast Medium	25–30 cc*
Filming Rate	2 fps × 3 sec; 1 fps × 4–5 sec

*Injection rate and volume for main renal vein injection; injection rate will vary, depending on the location of the catheter.

Renal Vein Sampling for Renin Concentration

Catheter Position	Main renal vein*
Preparation	1 g salt diet; furosemide pretreatment; antihypertensive medications discontinued
Sample Volume of Blood*	6 cc

*Samples are obtained from inferior vena cava proximal and distal to renal veins; segmental renal vein sampling may be indicated with focal renal disease.

Adrenal Arteriography

Catheter Position*	Superior, middle, or inferior adrenal artery*
Contrast Medium	60% solution
Rate of Injection	1–2 cc/sec
Volume of Contrast Medium	4–8 cc
Filming Rate	1 fps × 8 sec

*Selective catheterization may be necessary if standard aortography does not provide sufficient information.

Adrenal Venography*

Catheter Position	Selective adrenal vein
Contrast Medium	60% solution
Rate of Injection	1–2 sec manually
Volume of Contrast Medium	2–5 cc
Filming Rate	3 fps/3 sec

*If performed, venous sampling should always be done before venography.

Gonadal Venography

Catheter Position	Selective gonadal vein*
Contrast Medium	60% solution
Rate of Injection	Manual
Volume of Contrast Medium	5–10 cc
Filming Technique	1–2 films centered in ipsilateral upper and lower abdomen

*Reflux of contrast material into testicular vein may occur during retrograde renal venography.

SUGGESTED READINGS

Barrett B, Carlisle E: Metaanalysis of the relative nephrotoxicity of high- and low-osmolality iodinated contrast media. *Radiology* 188:171–178, 1993.

Berkseth R, Kjellstrand C: Radiologic contrast-induced nephropathy. *Med Clin North Am* 68:351–370, 1984.

Cohen H, Tice H, Mandel F: Ovarian volumes measured by ultrasound: bigger than we think, *Radiology* 177:189–192, 1990.

Emamian S, Nielsen M, Pederson J, et al: Kidney dimensions at sonography: correlation with age, sex, and habitus in 665 adult volunteers. *AJR Am J Roentgenol* 160:83–86, 1993.

Greenberger P, Patterson R, Tapio C: Prophylaxis against repeated radiocontrast media reactions in 857 cases. *Arch Int Med* 145:2197–2200, 1985.

Harris K, Smith T, Cragg A, et al: Nephrotoxicity from contrast material in renal insufficiency: ionic versus nonionic agents. *Radiology* 179:849–852, 1991.

Katayama H, Yamaguchi K, Kozuka T, et al: Adverse reactions to ionic and nonionic contrast media: a report from the Japanese Committee on the Safety of Contrast Media. *Radiology* 175:621–628, 1990.

Lasser E, Berry C, Mishkin M, et al: Pretreatment with corticosteroids to prevent adverse reactions to nonionic contrast media, *AJR Am J Roentgenol* 162:523–526, 1994.

Lasser E, Berry C, Talner L, et al: Pretreatment with corticosteroids to alleviate reactions to intravenous contrast material, *N Engl J Med* 317:845–849, 1987.

Moore R, Steinberg E, Powe N, et al: Nephrotoxicity of high-osmolality versus low-osmolality contrast media: randomized clinical trial, *Radiology* 182:649–655, 1992.

Palmer F: The R.A.C.R. survey of intravenous contrast media reactions: final report, *Australas Radiol* 32:426–428, 1988.

Parfrey P, Griffiths S, Barrett BJ, et al: Contrast material-induced renal failure in patients with diabetes mellitus, renal insufficiency, or both: a prospective controlled study. *N Engl J Med* 320:143–149, 1989.

Schwab S, Hlatky M, Pieper C, et al: Contrast nephrotoxicity: a randomized controlled trial of a nonionic and an ionic radiographic contrast agent, *N Engl J Med* 320:149–153, 1989.

Shehadi W: Adverse reactions to intravenously administered contrast media, *AJR Am J Roentgenol* 124:145–152, 1975.

Wolf G, Arenson R, Cross A: A prospective trial of ionic vs. nonionic contrast agents in routine clinical practice: comparison of adverse effects, *AJR Am J Roentgenol* 152:939–944, 1989.

CHAPTER 2

The Kidney and Retroperitoneum: Anatomy and Congenital Abnormalities

Normal urinary structures develop as the result of a series of complex, staged embryologic processes. As a result of this complexity of urinary tract development, congenital abnormalities occur in up to 10% of individuals. Because normally the kidneys and ureters develop simultaneously, an in utero event causing one malformation often affects other areas of the urinary tract. Therefore, the presence of one urinary tract anomaly greatly increases the likelihood of coexistent genitourinary anomalies; if one congenital anomaly is detected in the urinary tract, there is a 75% chance of a coexistent anomaly. Many of these anomalies are clinically insignificant, but some are very important. In addition, development of the genitourinary tract spans the period of organogenesis, when other major organ systems are developed. Hence, genitourinary anomalies commonly are seen coexisting with congenital abnormalities of other organ systems, most commonly the musculoskeletal system, central nervous system, cardiovascular system, and gastrointestinal tract. Finally, because the urinary and the genital systems are closely related embryologically, their development is interdependent, and anomalies of the genital system often coexist with urinary tract anomalies and vice versa. This chapter concentrates on congenital abnormalities of the kidney and upper urinary tract and describes normal retroperitoneal anatomy as it pertains to the kidneys.

EMBRYOLOGY

In humans, mature kidneys develop as a result of evolution of three successive sets of primitive excretory structures (Box 2-1). These excretory organs, in order of development, are the pronephros, the mesonephros, and the metanephros. These develop in a cranial-to-caudal progression. The pronephros develops in the segmented mesoderm of the upper thoracic and cervical region of the fetus during the third week of fetal life. The pronephros is a transient structure with no adult correlate. However, its development is crucial for induction of the next major phase of kidney development: differentiation of the mesonephros into the mesonephric duct. The mesonephros, which originates caudal to the pronephros, forms in unsegmented nephrogenic cord during the fourth to eighth week of fetal development, just as the pronephros is regressing. Although the mesonephric

Box 2-1 Development of the Urinary Tract

Pronephros →	Induces mesonephric differentiation
Mesonephros →	Efferent ductules of testes, epioophoron, paroophoron
Ureteric bud →	Ureter, renal pelvis, calyces, collecting tubules
Metanephric blastema →	Bowman's capsule, proximal and distal convoluted tubules, loop of Henle, stromal tissue

duct forms the first functioning excretory duct of the fetus, it degenerates rapidly after the ninth week of gestation. Some segments of the mesonephric duct, also known as the Wolffian duct, persist and develop into segments of the genital system. In boys, the Wolffian duct forms the efferent ductules of the testes, the epididymis, and the vas deferens. In girls, the Wolffian duct develops into the epoophoron and the paroophoron. During the fifth week of gestation, the metanephros begins to develop into the definitive kidney.

The metanephros develops from two separate cell lines, each with different potential. These cell lines are the ureteric bud and the metanephric blastema. The ureteric bud develops as an outgrowth of the mesonephric duct proximally to the cloacal entry. The ureteric bud develops into the ureter, renal pelvis, calyces, and collecting tubules of the renal medulla. The metanephric blastema develops from the caudal portion of the nephrogenic cord and becomes the excretory part of the kidney. Development of the metanephric blastema into the excretory system must be induced by contact with the ureteric bud. Induction of the metanephric blastema occurs after growth of the ureteric bud and physical contact with the metanephric blastema. As the ureteric bud grows, the end approaching the metanephric blastema enlarges. This ampullary segment later develops into the renal pelvis, whereas the remainder of the ureteric bud will become the ureter. After the ampullary portion of the ureteric bud contacts the metanephric blastema, multiple divisions of this segment of the ureteric bud commence. Division of the ureteric bud is dichotomous but asynchronous, and this dividing process continues for 12 to 14 generations. Each generation of the ureteric bud invaginates deeper into the metanephric tissue. First- and second-generation divisions develop into the major calyces, and the minor calyces originate from the third through

fifth generations. All subsequent generations provide the basis for development of the collecting tubules. These tubules are arrayed radially around minor calyces, forming the renal pyramids. After final development, there should be 10 to 25 fully formed calyces. Divisions of the ureteric bud in the polar regions of the kidney temporally lag behind development in the interpolar segment of the kidney. This developmental delay often results in the development of fewer calyces and more incompletely divided compound calyces in the polar regions of each kidney.

Segments of metanephric blastema form a cap overlying the terminal ampullary segments of the ureteric bud. The metanephric blastema tissue is carried with the dividing and growing ureteric bud. Maturation of the blastema is induced by physical contact with the ureteric bud. The metanephric blastema differentiates into the excretory system of the kidney. Differentiation of the metanephric blastema leads to the development of Bowman's capsule, the proximal and distal convoluted tubules, the loop of Henle, and supporting tissue of the renal parenchyma. Development of the glomerulus induces angiogenesis. The developing glomerulus is supplied by branches of the renal artery and is connected to the developing convoluted tubules and the loop of Henle. Eventually, the tubules communicate with the ampullary segment of the ureteric bud, allowing for excretion of urine into the collecting tubules. The metanephric blastema surrounding this developing excretory system differentiates into the interstitial supporting tissue of the renal parenchyma. Because the ureteric bud development is dominant in the embryology of the kidney, its branching pattern and induction of metanephric blastema define the renal lobe. A single renal lobe consists of a calyx, collecting ducts, and its overlying renal cortex. As they develop, these renal lobes coalesce to form a normal kidney made up of approximately 14 renal lobes. In utero, renal lobar anatomy is evident as early as the fourth month of gestation. Renal maturation continues from birth until age 5 years. During maturation, cellular multiplication in the renal cortex continues and leads to obscuring of gross lobar anatomy in most individuals. Persistent fetal lobation, an anomaly of kidney maturation, is seen in up to 5% of adults (Fig. 2-1). After age 5 years, renal cellular multiplication is no longer possible. Renal hypertrophy can occur well into adulthood. Hypertrophy leads not to an increased number of glomeruli but rather to enlargement and increased capacity of the existing glomeruli. This enlargement can result in overall enlargement of the kidney, as is seen commonly in patients after unilateral loss of kidney function. The remaining kidney enlarges and increases its excretory capacity to compensate for the lost renal parenchyma, which is evident in adults up to approximately age 60 years. In older adults, potential for renal hypertrophy is minimal.

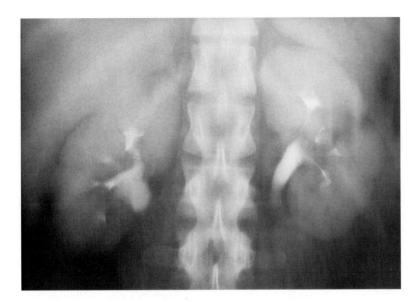

Fig. 2-1   Persistent fetal lobation. This nephrotomogram demonstrates typical radiographic features of this entity. There is normal renal parenchymal thickness without atrophy. The indentations are smooth, and the calyces are centered in the renal lobule between the parenchymal indentations.

The metanephros originally develops in the upper sacral region of the fetus. However, at birth, the kidneys lie in the upper lumbar region because of the differential migration of fetal tissues during gestation. This apparent ascent of the kidney results from the rapid longitudinal growth of the embryo in the lumbar and sacral regions caudal to the developing kidney. This cephalic migration to the adult position occurs during the fourth through eighth weeks of gestation. Concomitant with the cephalic migration is a 90° medial rotation of the kidney about its longitudinal axis, which brings the ureteral pelvic junction to a medial position in relation to the kidney. During ascent from the pelvis, vascular supply to the kidneys comes from progressively higher branches of the aorta, whereas the inferior branches regress. The primitive kidney is supplied originally from lateral sacral branches of the aorta, but as it ascends to the adult position, it is supplied by progressively higher lateral branches from the aorta until it reaches its adult position. The renal artery then originates laterally from the aorta at approximately L2. Although progressive ascent usually leads to regression of the inferior blood vessels, anomalous vessels commonly are seen supplying the kidney. In addition, failure of complete ascent, leading to anomalous renal position, is almost always associated with coexistent anomalous blood supply to the affected kidney, which reflects persistence of these inferior branches.

Obviously, kidney development involves a complex series of developmental processes during gestation. It is interesting to note that successive development and maturation of the primitive excretory organs—the pronephros, mesonephros, and metanephros—recapitulate the complex evolution of excretory organs in species of varying levels of sophistication. A primitive pronephros is the excretory organ of primitive fish. The mesonephros is the excretory organ of more advanced fish and amphibians. The metanephros is the excretory organ of reptiles, birds, and mammals.

CLASSIFICATION OF CONGENITAL RENAL ABNORMALITIES

It is helpful to classify congenital renal abnormalities as anomalies of (1) number, (2) position, (3) fusion, (4) vasculature, (5) structure, and (6) ureteropelvic junction (UPJ) obstruction. Abnormalities in each of these categories are outlined in Box 2-2.

Abnormalities of Number

Renal agenesis

Renal agenesis results from failure of the ureteric bud to reach the metanephric blastema because the ureteric bud fails to form or it degenerates prematurely, and the induction of the functional nephron does not occur. Associated ureteral abnormalities are present universally (Box 2-3). These include absence of the ipsilateral ureter and its associated hemitrigone or presence of a blind-ending ureteral stump, a remnant of the incompletely developed ureteral bud. In 20% of the men with renal agenesis, there is absence of the ipsilateral epididymis, vas deferens, or seminal vesicle, or presence of an associated ipsilateral seminal vesicle cyst (Fig. 2-2). In 70% of women with unilateral renal agenesis, associated genital anomalies are present (Fig. 2-3), including absence or atresia of the uterus or vagina, a unicornuate uterus with absence or atresia of the vagina and ovary, or duplication anomalies

Box 2-2 Congenital Renal Abnormalities

Abnormalities of number
  Agenesis
  Supernumerary
Abnormalities of position
  Nonrotation
  Malrotation
  Ectopia
    Underascent
    Overascent
Abnormalities of fusion
  Horseshoe kidney
  Cross-fused ectopia
Abnormalities of vasculature
  Anomalous renal arteries
  Anomalous renal veins
Abnormalities of renal structure
  Persistent fetal lobation
  Renal pseudotumors
    Column of Bertin
    Hilar lip
    Renal duplication
  Congenital cystic disease
    Multicystic dysplastic kidney
      Pelvoinfundibular type
      Hydronephrotic type
    Autosomal recessive polycystic kidney disease
      Perinatal
      Neonatal
      Infantile
      Juvenile
    Medullary sponge kidney
    Multilocular cystic nephroma
    Calyceal diverticulum
  Congenital solid masses
    Mesoblastic nephroma
    Nephroblastomatosis
Ureteropelvic junction obstruction

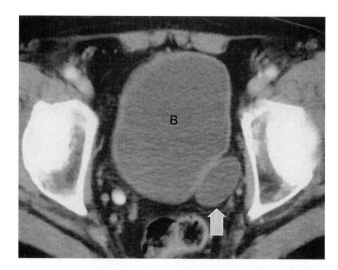

Fig. 2-2 Seminal vesicle cyst (arrow) adjacent to the bladder (B) in a patient with unilateral renal agenesis. Pelvic cysts commonly are seen ipsilateral to renal agenesis and often occur in the seminal vesicle in male patients.

of the genital tract. These complex müllerian duct anomalies are considered part of the Mayer-Rokitansky-Küster-Hauser syndrome. Absence of the ipsilateral adrenal gland is associated with renal agenesis in 10% of patients. Although renal agenesis can be diagnosed definitively with ultrasound, computed tomography (CT), or radionuclide renography, findings are often evident on plain radiographs of the abdomen. With absence of one kidney, the bowel (usually the colon) will fall into the empty renal fossa. When this occurs on the left, it is usually evident on a plain abdominal radiograph. The gas-distended splenic flexure demonstrates an unusual configuration; the splenic flexure is dislocated medially and looped (Figs. 2-4, 2-5; Box 2-4). This condition can be diagnosed defini-

tively if a portion of the splenic flexure is noted to be medial to the lesser curvature of the stomach on an anteroposterior abdominal radiograph. Medial dislocation of the hepatic flexure associated with right renal agenesis can sometimes be diagnosed, but the findings usually are less obvious than when renal agenesis occurs on the left.

Renal agenesis occurs in 1 per 1000 live births. Seventy-five percent of patients with renal agenesis are boys. Bilateral involvement is rare. It occurs approximately once in every 3000 live births. Bilateral renal agenesis is incompatible with life. With bilateral renal agenesis, intrauterine growth occurs because the placenta serves as the excretory organ for the fetus. Because no urine is excreted, oligohydramnios results, which causes pulmonary hypoplasia and facial abnormalities—features of the well-known Potter's syndrome (Fig. 2-6 on p. 58). Signs of Potter's syndrome include a typical facial pattern with low-set ears, a broad flat nose, and prominent skin folds below the lower eyelids, coupled with pulmonary hypoplasia and pneumothoraces. Unilateral renal agenesis re-

Box 2-3 Abnormalities Commonly Present with Renal Agenesis

Absent ipsilateral ureter
Absent ipsilateral hemitrigone
Absent ipsilateral vas deferens
Ipsilateral seminal vesicle cyst
Unicornuate uterus
Abnormal bowel gas pattern

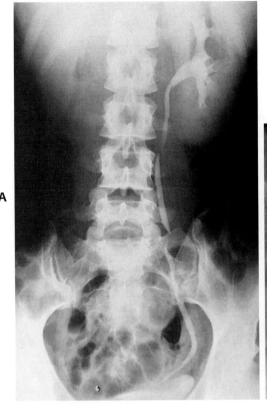
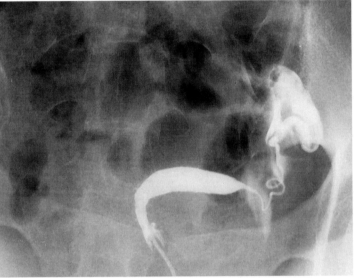

Fig. 2-3 Unicornuate uterus associated with unilateral renal agenesis. **A,** Intravenous urography demonstrates agenesis of the right kidney. Compensatory hypertrophy of the solitary left kidney is present. **B,** Hysterosalpingography demonstrates a left-sided unicornuate uterus. Ipsilateral müllerian duct abnormalities commonly occur in association with renal agenesis.

mains asymptomatic as long as the contralateral kidney functions normally. Usually, the contralateral kidney becomes hypertrophied and appears enlarged (Fig. 2-3), which is an expected development. Associated congenital malformations of the contralateral kidney are com-

mon. If these abnormalities depress renal function, symptomatic renal insufficiency can develop.

Supernumerary kidney

In extremely rare conditions, more than two discrete kidneys are present, probably as a result of formation of two ureteral buds on one side. Usually, the supernumerary kidney occurs on the left side caudal to the normal kidney and is hypoplastic. Supernumerary kidneys are of two basic types. In the first type, a bifid ureter also drains the second kidney on the ipsilateral side. In the second variety, a separate ureter drains the supernumerary kidney, and another ureter drains the second kidney on the ipsilateral side.

Abnormalities of Position

Rotational abnormalities

Malrotation and nonrotation of the kidneys are not uncommon congenital anomalies, which occur when the kidney fails to rotate about its vertical axis during ascent. Nonrotation results in an anteriorly positioned UPJ. Some of the calyces will be located medial to the renal pelvis,

---

Box 2-4   Causes of Unilateral Absent Kidney Opacification in Renal Fossa

Common: Previous nephrectomy
         Renal agenesis
         Renal ectopia
Uncommon: Renal artery occlusion
         Renal vein occlusion
         Ureteral obstruction
         Pyonephrosis
         Pyelonephritis
         Xanthogranulomatous pyelonephritis
Rare: Multicystic dysplastic kidney
      Tumor infiltration of kidney

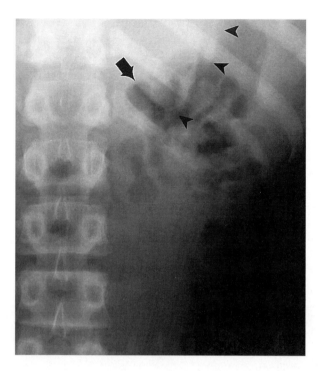

Fig. 2-4 Abnormal splenic flexure in association with left renal agenesis. A cone-down view of the left upper quadrant demonstrates medial dislocation of the splenic flexure. The splenic flexure (arrow) is dislocated medial to the lesser curvature of the stomach (arrowheads), which typically is seen with absence of a kidney in the left renal fossa.

a hallmark of rotational anomalies (Figs. 2-7, 2-8). Rarely, overrotation of the kidney around its vertical axis results in a malrotated kidney. In these patients, the UPJ is oriented posteriorly.

Renal ectopia

Renal ectopia describes arrest or exaggeration of normal caudal-to-cranial ascent of the kidneys. Underascent is more common than overascent of the kidney. Anomalous blood supply to the kidneys virtually is always associated with renal ectopia. Blood supply to an ectopic kidney usually is from adjacent vessels. For example, pelvic kidneys are supplied via branches of the lower abdominal aorta or from branches directly off the iliac arteries. Renal ectopia may also be associated with anomalies of fusion or lateral crossed anomalies. Depending on the degree of ascent, pelvic kidneys may lie in the true pelvis, in the iliac fascia opposite the iliac crest, or in the lower abdomen above the iliac crest but below L2. Ectopic kidneys are often associated with contralateral renal anomalies (Fig. 2-9), including contralateral agenesis (Fig. 2-10 on p. 60) or ectopia of the contralateral kidney. Bilateral pelvic kidneys may fuse (Fig. 2-11 on p. 60). If the medial segments of the kidney fuse, the combined

kidney mass forms a ring-like renal structure in the pelvis, which has been described as a discoid, lump, or pancake kidney. Either a single ureter or two separate ureters may be present to drain this mass of renal parenchyma.

Pelvic kidneys occur approximately once per 1000 live births. There is a 3:2 male-to-female predominance. Pelvic kidneys are usually asymptomatic, although they do seem to be less well protected from trauma than kidneys positioned normally in the retroperitoneal upper lumbar region. Because urinary tract anomalies tend to be multiple, pelvic kidneys also are associated with an increased incidence of UPJ obstruction, vesicoureteral reflux, and decreased function. The incidence of stone formation in ectopic kidneys may be higher as a result of stasis caused by the altered geometry of urinary drainage. Usually, pelvic kidneys are relatively small and are irregular in shape. They have variable degrees of rotation, extrarenal calyces, and multiple arteries supplying their parenchyma. Normal pelvic kidneys should not be expected to have the same radiographic appearance as the normally situated kidney.

Overascent of the kidneys is uncommon. In this situation, one or both kidneys come to lie in a position cranial to the normal expected position of the kidney (Fig. 2-12 on p. 60). The affected kidney is nearly always below the hemidiaphragm, however, its high position may lead to a focal eventration of the diaphragm overlying the kidney and may mimic a supradiaphragmatic renal position. The high intraabdominal kidney has been described as a thoracic kidney.

Abnormalities of Renal Fusion

Horseshoe kidneys

The horseshoe kidney is the most common renal anomaly, occurring once in every 400 live births (Box 2-5). There is a 2:1 male-to-female predominance of patients with horseshoe kidneys. Horseshoe kidneys develop after a midline connection forms between the two developing masses of renal tissue as a result of fetal contact of both metanephric collections. The midline connection, or isthmus, may consist of a fibrotic band

---

Box 2-5 Radiographic Abnormalities of Horseshoe Kidney

Renal nonrotation
Lower pole fusion
Low retroperitoneal position
Renal vascular anomalies

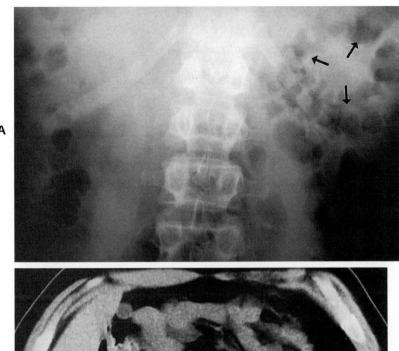

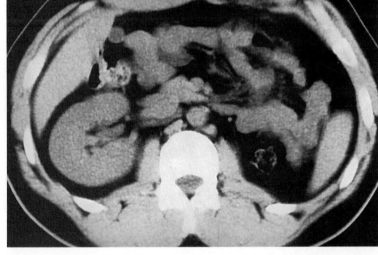

Fig. 2-5   Abnormal splenic flexure pattern with left-sided renal agenesis. **A,** The splenic flexure is dislocated medially and has an abnormal looping pattern (arrows) typical of left-sided renal agenesis or ectopia of the left kidney. **B,** Computed tomography scan demonstrates colon dislocated into the vacant left renal fossa.

(Fig. 2-13 on p. 61) or of functioning renal parenchyma representing a fusion of the caudal poles of both kidneys (Figs. 2-14, 2-15 on p. 61). The horseshoe kidney usually is positioned low in the abdomen as a result of arrest of normal ascent. Ascent of the horseshoe kidney ends prematurely when the horseshoe kidney becomes hooked under the origin of the inferior mesenteric artery. Numerous renal vascular anomalies associated with horseshoe kidneys result from anomalous development and incomplete ascent. The incidence of other urinary tract abnormalities also is increased in association with horseshoe kidney, including UPJ obstruction, duplication anomalies, and stone formation resulting from the abnormal geometry of the kidney, which leads to urine stasis in the renal pelvis. An increased incidence of horseshoe kidney has been noted in association with anomalies in other organ systems, including the gastrointestinal tract, the cardiovascular system, and the musculoskeletal sys-

tem. An increased risk of horseshoe kidney is associated with Turner's syndrome and Ellis-Van Creveld syndrome.

Crossed-fused ectopia

Crossed-fused ectopia is an uncommon congenital renal abnormality in which one kidney crosses the midline and fuses with the opposite kidney. The fused kidneys are noted to lie to one side of the spine. The ureters insert in their normal positions, therefore, the ureter from the crossed kidney extends across the midline to enter the bladder on the side opposite that of the fused kidney (Fig. 2-16 on p. 62). There are many variations of the pattern of renal parenchymal fusion. The resulting fused kidneys can be described as the usual pattern, "S"-shaped kidney, "L"-shaped kidney, disc kidney, and lump kidney. There are no specific pathologic processes associated with these variations of crossed-fused ectopia. Crossed-fused ectopia is more common in boys than in girls, and

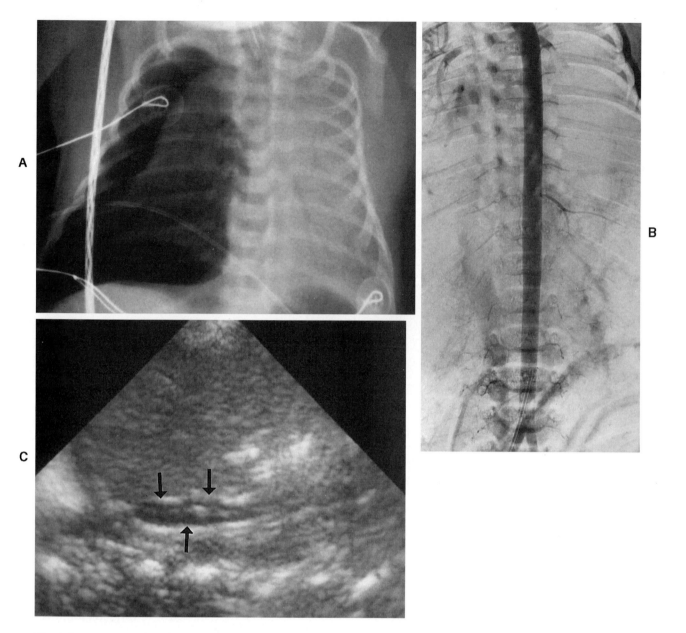

Fig. 2-6   Findings seen with bilateral renal agenesis. **A,** Chest radiograph in a newborn with renal agenesis demonstrates pulmonary hypoplasia with a small thorax, a right pneumothorax, and diffuse opacification of the left lung. **B,** An aortogram in this infant demonstrates absence of the renal arteries resulting from bilateral renal agenesis. **C,** Sonogram of the renal fossa demonstrates absence of the kidney. The adrenal gland is prominent and disk-shaped (arrows) in its normal position.

the left kidney more commonly crosses the midline to lie on the right than vice versa. The cross-fused kidney is usually asymptomatic, but it has an increased susceptibility to the same complications as other ectopic kidneys.

Abnormalities of Renal Vasculature

As described previously, the blood supply to the kidney follows a complex series of stages involving development, maturation, ascent, and rotation of the kidney. Vascular anomalies involving the kidney are very common. Most often, kidneys with anomalous vasculature have multiple renal arteries instead of a classic single renal artery supplying each kidney. This anomaly occurs in up to 25% of adults. The most common variety involves a second, diminutive renal artery supplying the lower pole of the kidney. However, the existence of two or more renal arteries is not uncommon (Fig. 2-17 on p. 62), or the renal parenchymal arterial supply may come from multiple renal arteries with no dominant vessel.

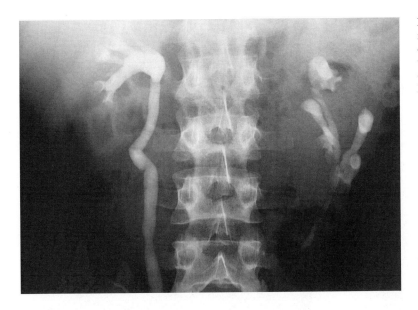

Fig. 2-7   Renal nonrotation. Findings typical of the nonrotated kidney are demonstrated, including calyces located medial to the renal pelvis, abnormal orientation of the calyces and renal pelvis, and deviant course of the upper ureter draining the nonrotated kidney.

Supernumerary veins also commonly are found draining the kidney, which occurs about half as commonly as supernumerary renal arteries do. Supernumerary renal veins often are retroaortic when present on the left.

Anomalies of renal vasculature are more common in ectopic kidneys. Horseshoe kidneys almost always have an anomalous blood supply. Most anomalous renal vessels are without clinical significance, although accessory arteries become significant in some common situations, including surgical bypass or reconstruction of the abdominal aorta, renal parenchymal surgery, or repair of a UPJ stricture. For surgery on the infrarenal abdominal aorta,

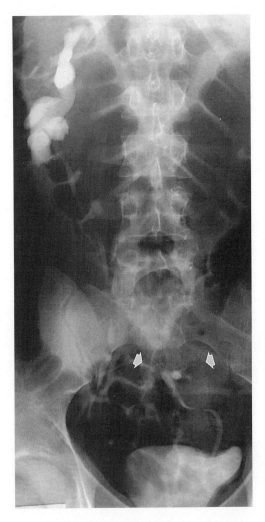

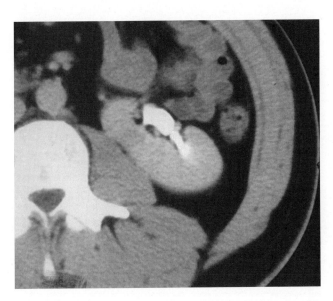

Fig. 2-8   Renal nonrotation. This computed tomography scan demonstrates the nonrotated kidney with the renal pelvis draining the kidney anteriorly rather than in its normal medial position.

Fig. 2-9   Pelvic kidney with contralateral renal malrotation. The left kidney is ectopic (arrows), being located low in the pelvis. The right kidney is normal other than the rotational anomaly. Multiple congenital urinary tract abnormalities often coexist.

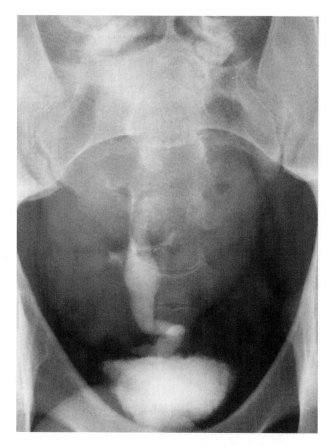

Fig. 2-10 Solitary pelvic kidney. Solitary pelvic kidney is drained by a single ureter. This represents renal ectopia with contralateral renal agenesis.

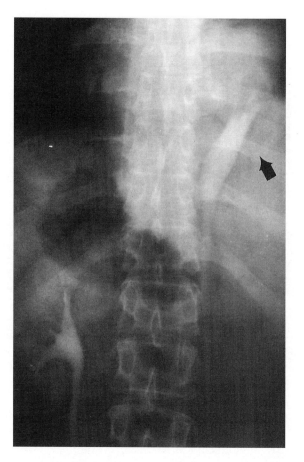

Fig. 2-12 Thoracic kidney. Urogram demonstrates an abnormally high position of the left kidney (arrow) caused by overascent of the kidney during development. These kidneys usually are subdiaphragmatic with overlying focal eventration of the diaphragm.

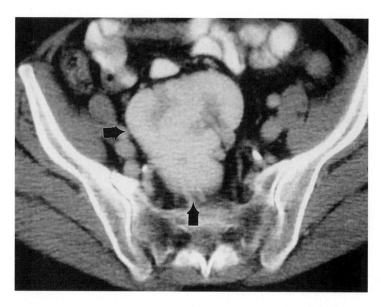

Fig. 2-11 Pelvic "lump" kidney. Bilateral pelvic kidneys are fused in the pelvis, forming a lump, discoid, or pancake kidney (arrows).

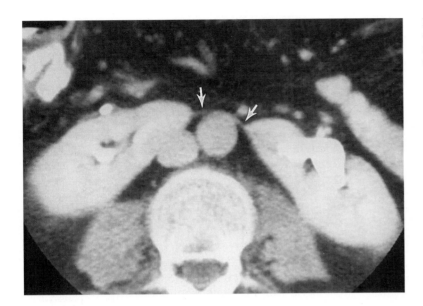

Fig. 2-13   Horseshoe kidney with fibrous isthmus. Computed tomography scan demonstrates a horseshoe kidney fused only by a thin band of fibrous tissue (arrows).

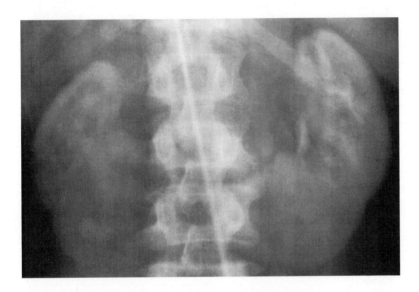

Fig. 2-14   Nephrographic findings of a horseshoe kidney. Radiograph taken during the nephrogram phase demonstrates the abnormal axis, medial fusion of the lower poles, and low position typical of a horseshoe kidney.

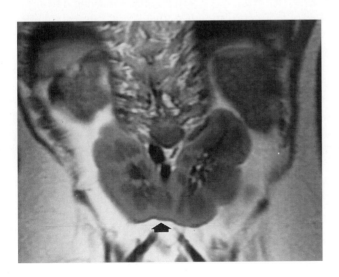

Fig. 2-15   Magnetic resonance (MR) imaging of a horseshoe kidney. Coronal MR imaging scan demonstrates medial fusion of the lower pole renal parenchyma (arrow) and low position of this horseshoe kidney.

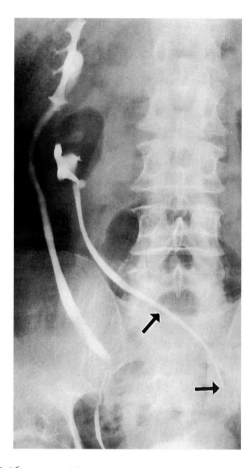

Fig. 2-16   Crossed-fused renal ectopia. Urogram demonstrates the typical appearance of crossed-fused ectopia. Both kidneys are fused together on one side of the spine. The ureter draining the lower kidney crosses the midline to enter the bladder in its normal position (arrows).

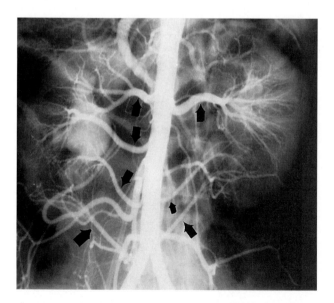

Fig. 2-17   Multiple renal arteries. Abdominal aortogram demonstrates four separate arteries supplying the right kidney (arrows) and three separate arteries supplying the left kidney (arrows). The caudal-most of these arteries bilaterally originates directly from the common iliac artery.

preoperative recognition of accessory renal arteries can help to avoid damage to or ligation of these accessory branches. The anomalous vessels are end arteries, and ligation of such a branch leads to infarction of a segment of kidney, which may diminish overall renal function and lead to hypertension because of oversecretion of renin by the ischemic renal parenchyma. When renal-sparing surgery is undertaken, previous knowledge of an anomalous renal blood supply can assist in avoiding inadvertent renal parenchymal damage during renal dissection.

Finally, recent advances in endoscopy have made endoscopic pyelostomy and pyeloplasty a commonly used procedure for the management of UPJ strictures. With this minimally invasive procedure, laceration of a renal artery can be devastating because access to that hemorrhaging vessel is not available during the procedure. In most patients, these endopyelotomy procedures are performed with transmural incision of the full thickness of the ureteral wall. This depth of incision inadvertently could lacerate an adjacent artery. Incisions traditionally are performed in the posterolateral aspect of the ureter to avoid anterior crossing arteries. Most accessory renal branches cross anteriorly to the UPJ and would be avoided with this approach. However, in up to 5% of patients with accessory renal arteries, the accessory polar branch is positioned behind the UPJ and is at risk for laceration during endopyelotomy. Optimal techniques for preoperative identification of these aberrant vessels currently are being explored. It appears that evaluation before surgery with CT angiography or magnetic resonance angiography will be useful in identification of these at-risk arteries (Fig. 2-18).

Abnormalities in Structure

Fetal lobation

Persistent fetal lobation can be identified in approximately 5% of adults undergoing renal imaging. The number of lobes corresponds to the overall calyceal number and represents a vestige of the lobar development of the kidney. Lobar anatomy is evident in all neonates at birth, but with cellular multiplication, lobar anatomy usually is obscured by age 4 to 5 years. Persistent fetal lobation is of no clinical significance, except when it is mistaken for another entity. With persistent fetal lobation, renal parenchymal thickness should be normal (14 mm or more) and the renal indentations should be smooth and regular (Fig. 2-1). A key to identifying persistent fetal lobation is that the indentations occur so that calyces are centered between indentations. This appearance is distinctly different from that seen with other causes of renal irregularity. Reflux nephropathy commonly causes indentations in the renal parenchyma. However, these indentations overlie subtending calyces. Similarly, papillary necrosis can lead to renal indentations, but these

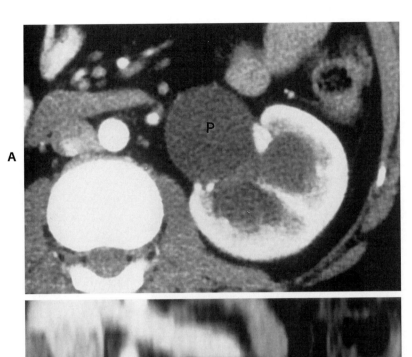

Fig. 2-18 Ureteropelvic junction (UPJ) obstruction caused by accessory renal artery branch. **A,** Axial computed tomography (CT) scan of the left kidney demonstrates marked dilatation of the left renal pelvis (P) and calyces. **B,** Coronal reconstruction of the CT scan demonstrates an accessory renal artery (arrows) crossing anterior to the UPJ obstruction just below the renal pelvis (P).

also overlie the necrotic renal papilla and its subtending calyx. Lobation also can be mimicked by multiple renal infarcts when interlobar vessels are involved, which is most commonly seen in patients with small-vessel disease, the prototype being chronic diabetes. In these patients, indentations in the renal parenchyma occur between calyces, but overall renal parenchymal thickness is diminished by atrophy.

Normal renal tissue masses

In several anomalies, prominent areas of normal renal tissue may lead to visible abnormalities with imaging studies. These anomalies include column of Bertin, hilar lips, dromedary humps (Fig. 2-19), and duplication anomalies.

Column of Bertin

The column of Bertin, also known as septum of Bertin or cloison, represents invagination of renal cortical tissue extending from the outer cortex to the renal sinus. It is normally functioning tissue that usually occurs at the junction of the upper and middle thirds of the renal parenchyma. A column of Bertin averages 3.5 cm in diameter. It is bilateral in 60% of patients with this abnormality. In addition, a bifid renal pelvis or other duplication anomaly commonly is associated. When present, a normal nephrogram is visualized with a column of Bertin (Fig. 2-20A). During the pyelographic phase, separation and splaying of normal calyces may occur around this invagination of cortical tissue. There commonly is a small, aberrant papilla subtending the cloison and draining to a longer major calyx or directly into the renal pelvis (Fig. 2-20B). The appearance of this subtending calyx has been described as the "teat and udder" sign. The column of Bertin has a conical shape similar to that of an udder, from which the subtending calyx with its short infundibulum emerges, mimicking the appearance of a cow's teat. Splaying of surrounding calyces can be prominent. On urography, the appearance of the splayed calyces draped around a column of Bertin has been described as the "factory siren" sign, because their urographic appearance is akin to that of a curved siren or musical horn. Column of Bertin is a normal variant, however, it can mimic abnormal masses on urography or pyelography.

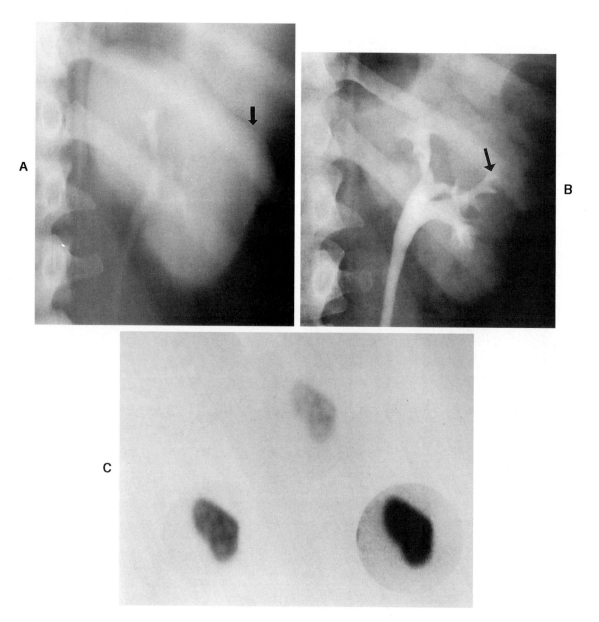

Fig. 2-19   Renal pseudotumor (dromedary hump). **A,** A nephrotomogram demonstrates a focal convex bulge (arrow) along the lateral margin of the left kidney. This location is typical for a dromedary hump, a common anomaly, thought to result from splenic impression on the kidney. **B,** During the pyelogram phase, a calyx (arrow) extends laterally paralleling the contour of the cortex, to subtend this pseudotumor formed by normal renal cortex. No calyceal deviation or other mass effect is noted. These features are diagnostic of a renal pseudotumor. **C,** A radionuclide scan of the left kidney confirms normal renal tissue in the area of the focal contour bulge.

Additional imaging should be performed to confirm this anomaly when it is suspected and to exclude a pathologic process. Renal sonography is a simple test that can be used to identify normal renal parenchyma as the cause of the mass effect and to exclude an abnormal mass. Other available confirmatory tests include radionuclide scanning, contrast-enhanced CT, and MR imaging. All of these techniques will demonstrate normal functioning renal parenchyma in the area of mass effect when a column of Bertin is present.

Hilar lips

Hilar lips are prominent collections of normal renal tissue that occur in areas of complex renal lobar fusion at the most medial aspect of the renal parenchyma surrounding the renal sinus. When prominent, the hilar lip

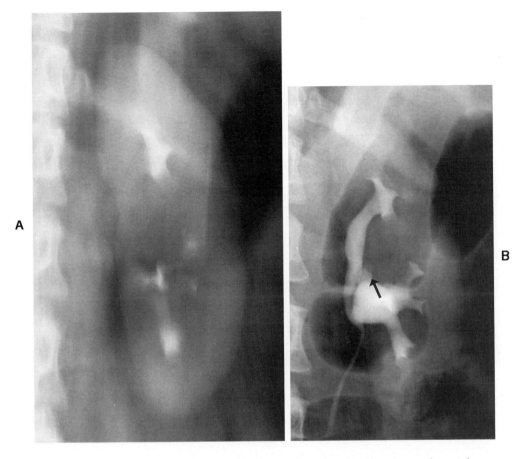

Fig. 2-20   Column of Bertin. **A,** This nephrotomogram demonstrates enhancing renal parenchyma separating the upper pole infundibulum from the remainder of the renal collecting system. **B,** An aberrant papilla drains directly into the subtending calyx (arrow), which is connected directly to the renal pelvis. This appearance is typical of a column of Bertin.

can protrude into the sinus and may distort the polar calyces (Fig. 2-21), which more often occurs in the upper pole than in the lower pole and is present more often in the left than in the right kidney. Hilar lips can mimic abnormal masses. Careful analysis of the imaging study should demonstrate a completely normal area of renal parenchyma, i.e., a normal nephrogram, normal echogenicity, and normal functioning renal tissue. The margin of the hilar lips should be smoothly contoured without focal irregularities or focal convex bulges. Confirmatory tests can be used if results of initial imaging studies are enigmatic. Renal sonography usually is satisfactory to evaluate the hilar region of both kidneys and to exclude a pathologic process.

Duplication anomalies

Duplication anomalies are defined by the presence of two or more pyelocalyceal elements. The spectrum of duplication anomalies extends from a bifid pelvis to a blind-ending, bifid ureter. Between these ends of the spectrum are incomplete ureteral duplication, complete duplication with a common entry into the bladder, and complete duplication with ectopic entry of the upper pole moiety. Duplication anomalies result from development of a second ureteric bud (complete duplication) or redundant duplication of the single ureteric bud, which is the single most common congenital urinary tract anomaly as some form is present in 10% of the population. Duplication anomalies frequently are bilateral. Ureteral duplications are discussed more thoroughly in a later chapter. It is important to know that duplication anomalies can lead to unusual configurations of the renal parenchyma, including renal enlargement and prominent areas of normal renal parenchyma dividing the renal sinus into two separate pyelocalyceal components (Fig. 2-22). The appearance often is similar to that of a column of Bertin. A focal area of normal renal cortex extends from the cortex medially to divide the renal sinus. Duplication anomalies of the kidney seldom present a diagnostic dilemma. Discrete renal sinuses and duplication of the pyelocalyceal system will be evident to indicate the etiology of these pseudomasses.

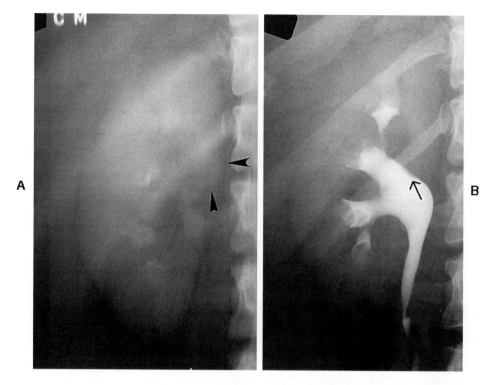

Fig. 2-21 Renal hilar lip. **A,** Nephrotomogram of the right kidney demonstrates a hilar lip arising from the upper pole of the kidney (arrowheads) and extending caudally. **B,** The pyelogram phase demonstrates a focal indentation on the upper aspect of the renal pelvis (arrow) caused by the adjacent hilar lip, another form of renal pseudotumor.

Congenital cystic disease

This diverse category of congenitally based abnormalities includes multicystic dysplastic kidney (MDK), autosomal recessive polycystic kidney disease (ARPKD), medullary sponge kidney (MSK), multilocular cystic nephroma (MLCN), and calyceal diverticulum.

Multicystic dysplastic kidney Multicystic dysplastic kidney is one of the most common causes of an abdominal mass detected during infancy. Other common causes of unilateral abdominal masses in this age group include the hydronephrotic kidney, Wilms' tumor, neuroblastoma, mesoblastic nephroma, adrenal hemorrhage, and renal vein thrombosis. The term *multicystic dysplastic kidney* encompasses a spectrum of renal abnormalities, includ-

ing the classic pelvoinfundibular type (Box 2-6) and the hydronephrotic type (Box 2-7) at the ends of the spectrum (Fig. 2-23). MDK is thought to result from failure in utero of the ureteral bud to adequately induce maturation of the metanephric blastema into nephrons. MDK is a common malformation, and it is often diagnosed when a palpable abdominal mass is detected in an infant. MDK is rarely bilateral, which is incompatible with life because renal function is impaired severely or absent. In MDK, the renal parenchyma is replaced with numerous simple cysts scattered throughout the kidney in place of normal renal parenchyma. Immature tissue elements, such as cartilage, may develop in areas of dysplastic metanephric blastema. Although renal function is usually ab-

---

Box 2-6 Radiographic Findings—Pelvoinfundibular Multicystic Dysplastic Kidney

Randomly distributed cysts
Noncommunicating cysts
Absent renal function
Atretic ureter

Box 2-7 Radiographic Findings—Hydronephrotic Multicystic Dysplastic Kidney

Dominant cyst in renal pelvis region
Radially arrayed cysts may intercommunicate
Minimal renal function possible
Ureter occluded at ureteropelvic junction

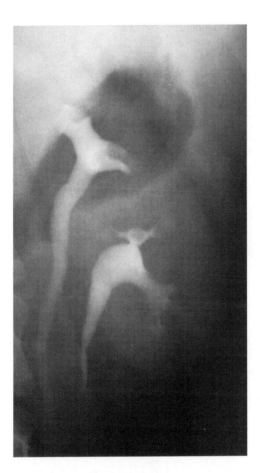

Fig. 2-22   Renal duplication anomaly. The kidney is enlarged with solid renal parenchyma separating two separate renal collecting systems in this patient with a complete duplication.

and nonfunctional. The ureter is occluded in the expected region of the UPJ.

In any form, MDK causes a benign mass that rarely becomes symptomatic. These lesions will remain unchanged in size or will regress with time (Fig. 2-24). There is no known increased risk of malignancy associated with MDK, therefore, lesions diagnosed as MDK need not be excised. Rarely, MDK can be complicated by cyst infection or by hypertension. A key element in the diagnosis of MDK is the evaluation of the contralateral kidney. Because MDK results in a nonfunctioning kidney, exclusion of remediable lesions in the contralateral kidney is crucial. MDK is associated with contralateral abnormalities, specifically with an increased risk of UPJ obstruction. Early diagnosis of an abnormality in the functioning kidney can lead to treatment to avoid the development of irreversible renal insufficiency.

Autosomal recessive polycystic kidney disease   Autosomal recessive polycystic kidney disease is a subtype of renal cystic disease in which innumerable radially oriented cysts 1 to 8 mm in diameter are present throughout the renal parenchyma (Box 2-8; Fig. 2-25). ARPKD is

sent, in a minority of patients, there may be minimal residual functioning renal parenchyma with urine excretion.

In the pelvoinfundibular form of MDK, the renal parenchyma is replaced with multiple, noncommunicating cysts of various sizes. These cysts occur with a random distribution throughout the kidney. No residual functioning renal mass is present. Where the renal pelvis would be expected, no dominant cystic lesion exists. An atretic ureter of variable length usually is present, reflecting incomplete formation of the ureteral bud. The hydronephrotic form of MDK likely results from ureteral bud abnormalities that develop later in gestation than in the pelvoinfundibular form of MDK. The hydronephrotic form of MDK can be thought of as a severe, in utero form of UPJ obstruction. In this form of MDK, a dominant cyst is seen in the expected location of the renal pelvis. Around this cyst are numerous other cysts that may intercommunicate. These cysts lie in the expected location of the calyces. Minimal renal function may be present, but the majority of the renal parenchyma is dysplastic

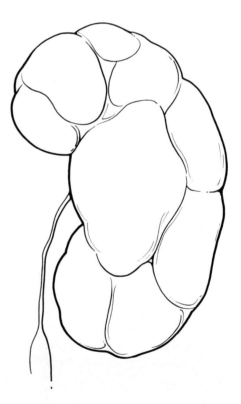

Fig. 2-23   Diagram illustrating the hydronephrotic type of multicystic dysplastic kidney. The renal parenchyma is dysplastic and replaced by numerous cystic areas. The upper ureter is atretic. There is a dominant central cyst in the area where the renal pelvis would be expected. This dominant cyst is surrounded by radially arranged smaller cysts.

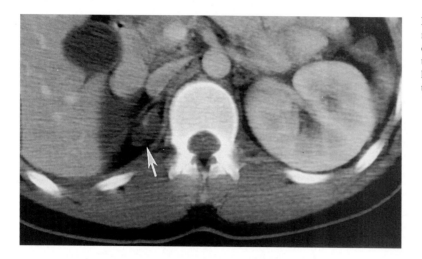

Fig. 2-24   Remnant of a multicystic dysplastic kidney. Computed tomography through the renal beds demonstrates a small multilocular cystic remnant in the right renal bed (arrow). There is compensatory hypertrophy of the left kidney in this adult with untreated right multicystic dysplastic kidney.

also known as Potter Type I cystic disease or infantile polycystic kidney disease. The most appropriate designation for this disorder is ARPKD because its presentation during infancy is less common than the perinatal and neonatal varieties.

In ARPKD, normal renal parenchyma is replaced to varying degrees by cystically dilated, nonfunctional tubular structures. Another element unique to ARPKD is the coexistence of hepatic disease. In patients with ARPKD, periportal hepatic fibrosis develops, leading, in severe cases, to hepatic failure, portal hypertension, splenomegaly, and bleeding varices (Fig. 2-26). The severity of hepatic disease in patients with ARPKD tends to be related inversely to the severity of renal disease. One classification system for describing the spectrum of disease in ARPKD subdivides this disorder into four separate categories: perinatal, neonatal, infantile, and juvenile. The perinatal variety is the most common form of ARPKD. In this form, more than 90% of normal renal collecting ducts are replaced by nonfunctional cystically dilated tubules. In utero, this causes oligohydramnios, which in turn causes pulmonary hypoplasia. The perinatal form of ARPKD leads to death in the perinatal period from pulmonary insufficiency. Autopsy studies demonstrate minimal

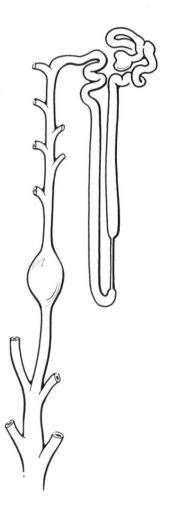

Fig. 2-25   Diagram illustrating cystic dilatation of a renal tubule as seen with autosomal recessive polycystic kidney disease (ARPKD). Small, focal cystic dilatations of the renal tubules occur in ARPKD as demonstrated in this diagram.

Box 2-8   Abnormalities with Autosomal Recessive Polycystic Kidney Disease

Oligohydramnios
Nephromegaly
Hyperechoic kidneys
Renal insufficiency inversely proportional to hepatic
　failure

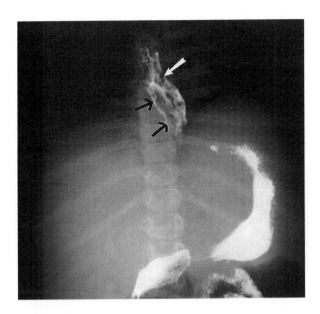

Fig. 2-26   Esophageal varices with autosomal recessive polycystic kidney disease (ARPKD). This film from an upper gastrointestinal series demonstrates serpiginous filling defects in the esophagus (arrows). These defects represent esophageal varices in this patient with ARPKD. Hepatosplenomegaly also is present, resulting from portal hypertension.

or absent periportal hepatic fibrosis in these patients. In the neonatal form, approximately 60% of renal collecting tubules are replaced by small cysts, and patients also have mild, usually asymptomatic, periportal hepatic fibrosis. These patients present clinically during the first month of life with severe renal insufficiency, which generally leads to death within a few months. Infantile ARPKD represents a form of the disease in which there is a balance between moderately severe renal disease and hepatic fibrosis. Infants with this form generally present clinically at age 3 to 6 months with renal insufficiency, nephromegaly, and hepatosplenomegaly. Without therapy, renal insufficiency usually leads to the patient's death during childhood. In juvenile ARPKD, hepatic disease predominates clinically. In this form, fewer than 10% of the renal collecting tubules are replaced by nonfunctional cysts. Severe periportal fibrosis and resulting hepatic insufficiency and portal hypertension are predominant. Patients with this form generally present during their teenage years with acute upper gastrointestinal bleeding from varices or with other signs of liver failure. Renal function is generally normal or only mildly impaired. Unless managed, this form causes death, usually during the second or third decade of life as a result of hepatic insufficiency and complications of portal hypertension.

Imaging is the key element in the diagnosis of ARPKD. Because the disease is inherited in an autosomal recessive pattern, parents of these patients inevitably are asymptomatic and unaware that they are carriers of this disease.

However, ARPKD is often diagnosed prenatally. Classically, oligohydramnios is detected, and additional evaluation of the fetus demonstrates large, echogenic kidneys. This finding is virtually diagnostic of ARPKD. Because of the innumerable cystically dilated tubules throughout the renal parenchyma, the kidneys appear hyperechoic and enlarged, and they demonstrate abnormal contrast enhancement. Renal sonography of patients with ARPKD inevitably demonstrates reniform enlargement of both kidneys with increased echogenicity (Fig. 2-27). The hyperechogenicity results from the multitude of specular echoes caused by the ectatic tubules, and also a hyperechoic periphery representing compressed cortical tissue is characteristic. Although renal sonography may demonstrate mildly hyperechogenic kidneys in healthy infants, in those with ARPKD, the kidneys also demonstrate enlargement. CT and urography of patients with ARPKD demonstrate nephromegaly with maintenance of the reniform shape of both kidneys. After the administration of intravenous contrast material, a striated nephrogram is usually demonstrated (Fig. 2-27). The striations result from normally functioning, contrast-filled tubules adjacent to the cystically dilated, urine-filled nonfunctional tubules. This pattern is very characteristic of ARPKD. On imaging studies, gross simple renal cysts (macrocysts) are not present in ARPKD. Their absence helps to distinguish this disorder from other polycystic kidney diseases. Later in life, findings of hepatic fibrosis will develop, including hepatosplenomegaly and the development of varices. Currently, hepatic fibrosis associated with ARPKD can be managed palliatively with portosystemic shunts, and it can be cured only with liver transplantation.

Medullary sponge kidney   Medullary sponge kidney is also referred to as benign renal tubular ectasia. MSK is common; it is diagnosed on 1 of every 200 urograms. MSK results from idiopathic ectasia of renal collecting tubules (Fig. 2-28).

Medullary sponge kidney is unusual in that its involvement of the kidneys is patchy. In some patients, as few as one renal pyramid may be involved, but in some patients, all renal pyramids may show evidence of MSK. MSK usually has a benign clinical course and remains asymptomatic. In most patients, it is an incidental finding on imaging studies. The major complication associated with MSK is the increased incidence of nephrolithiasis. The increased incidence of stone formation in patients with MSK is thought to result from urinary stasis occurring in the cystically dilated distal tubules. Stasis can lead to precipitation of minerals from the normally supersaturated urine. These minerals can serve as the nidus for stone formation. The fact that medullary nephrocalcinosis is commonly seen in association with MSK supports this theory (Fig. 2-29). The nephrocalcinosis results from punctate calcifications within the ectatic tubules of

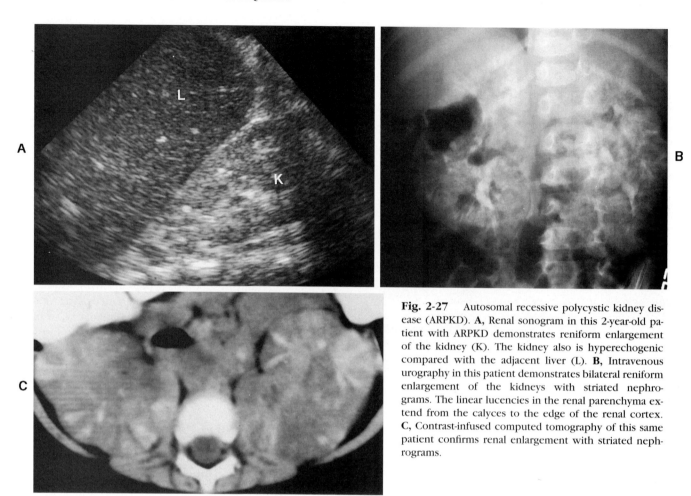

Fig. 2-27   Autosomal recessive polycystic kidney disease (ARPKD). **A,** Renal sonogram in this 2-year-old patient with ARPKD demonstrates reniform enlargement of the kidney (K). The kidney also is hyperechogenic compared with the adjacent liver (L). **B,** Intravenous urography in this patient demonstrates bilateral reniform enlargement of the kidneys with striated nephrograms. The linear lucencies in the renal parenchyma extend from the calyces to the edge of the renal cortex. **C,** Contrast-infused computed tomography of this same patient confirms renal enlargement with striated nephrograms.

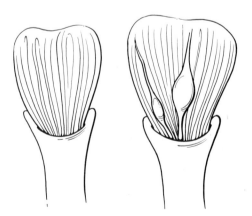

Fig. 2-28   Diagram of normal medulla and medullary sponge kidney. With medullary sponge kidney, focal areas of tubular ectasia are present within the renal medulla just peripheral to the subtending calyx.

the affected renal medulla. It is likely that some of these calcifications are excreted into the calyces and serve as a nidus for nephrolithiasis. Patients with MSK have a much higher incidence of nephrolithiasis than normally would be expected. There are several uncommon associations in MSK. A known association exists between MSK and hemihypertrophy syndrome. With hemihypertrophy syndrome, there is enlargement of one entire side of the body, including unilateral renal enlargement, which is often associated with scoliosis and leg-length discrepancies. Hemihypertrophy syndrome also is associated with an increased risk of several malignancies, including Wilms' tumor and pheochromocytoma. Also known to be associated with MSK is Caroli's disease, which is a form of idiopathic congenital intrahepatic biliary duct dilatation, and Ehlers-Danlos syndrome.

Radiographically, MSK can be recognized after the injection of intravenous contrast material. Focal cylindrical or saccular collections of contrast material are noted in the renal medulla adjacent to a calyx (Fig. 2-30). As few as one renal pyramid may be involved. The adjacent calyx is normal. Another finding that is often present in

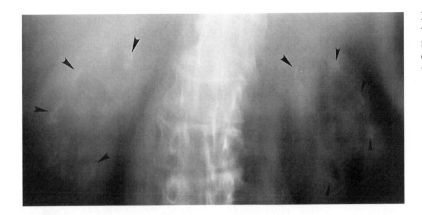

Fig. 2-29   Medullary nephrocalcinosis in a patient with medullary sponge kidney. Plain film nephrotomography demonstrates bilateral nephrocalcinosis (arrowheads) in the renal papilla resulting from medullary sponge kidney.

patients with MSK is medullary nephrocalcinosis. These calcifications are present within the cystically dilated collecting tubules. After contrast material administration, the iodinated contrast material pools within these dilated tubules and obscures the calcifications. Radiographically, this appears as enlargement of the calcifications that were seen on the scout radiograph and is referred to as the "growing calculus" sign, which is diagnostic of MSK.

Many radiologists prefer to reserve the diagnosis of MSK for patients who harbor medullary nephrocalcinosis or have a history of recurrent nephrolithiasis in association with radiographically demonstrated cystically dilated distal collecting tubules. Patients who demonstrate the

cystically dilated renal tubules as the only evidence of MSK are often classified as having benign renal tubular ectasia, a less ominous-sounding label.

Other considerations in the differential diagnosis for the radiographic appearance of MSK include papillary blush, papillary necrosis, and other causes of medullary nephrocalcinosis. Renal papillary blush, commonly seen in healthy individuals undergoing urography with low osmolar contrast agents, refers to hyperconcentration of iodinated contrast material in the distal portion of the collecting tubules. Papillary blush can be distinguished from MSK in that medullary nephrocalcinosis is absent, and the opacification pattern is different. In MSK, discrete cylindrical or saccular collections of contrast material are seen in the renal papilla adjacent to a normal calyx. With papillary blush, discrete or collections of contrast material are absent (Fig 2-31). Rather, there is homogeneous opacification of the entire papilla. Papillary necrosis can also lead to punctate pools of contrast material in the renal medulla. However, these pools freely communicate with the subtending calyx. The calyx itself does not appear normal, but it demonstrates changes of papillary necrosis (Fig. 2-32). On retrograde pyelography, medullary cavities resulting from papillary necrosis fill with contrast material, whereas the cavities present with MSK do not opacify under normal circumstances. Other causes of medullary nephrocalcinosis and their characteristics are discussed in a later chapter.

Multilocular cystic nephroma   Multilocular cystic nephroma is a rare neoplasm that is thought to result from a defect in embryogenesis of a segment of metanephric blastema. This benign cystic neoplasm occurs in a bimodal age distribution. Approximately half of the patients are boys in their first decade of life. The other half of MLCNs occur in women in their third and fourth decades of life. The lesions generally present as abdominal masses, and they often are detected incidentally. MLCNs appear radiographically as well-circumscribed renal masses with a thick pseudocapsule. The mass is composed of multiple cysts of varying sizes separated by septa. Hemorrhage

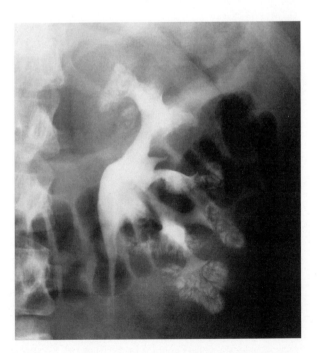

Fig. 2-30   Urographic features of medullary sponge kidney. The collecting system and renal pelvis appear normal. However, there are striated and saccular collections of contrast material in the renal papilla of the medulla. These features are diagnostic of medullary sponge kidney.

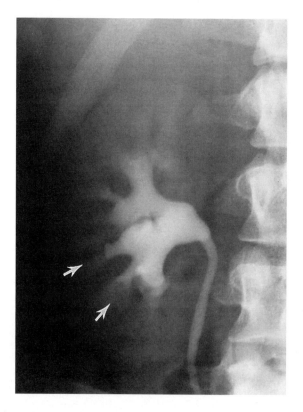

Fig. 2-31 Papillary blush. Urogram demonstrates features typical of papillary blush, a normal radiographic finding. There is homogeneous enhancement of the renal papillary tips (arrows) caused by concentration of the radiographic contrast material in the collecting tubules. Papillary blush is typified by homogeneous enhancement of the papilla without discrete linear or saccular contrast material collections. This finding commonly is seen when low-osmolar contrast material is used for urography.

and calcification usually are absent in MLCNs. A classic radiographic finding commonly associated with MLCN is evidence of herniation of this parenchymal mass into the renal pelvis (Fig. 2-33). Although this finding strongly suggests MLCN, it is not diagnostic. Other diagnostic considerations with similar radiographic findings include cystic Wilms' tumor, renal abscess, segmental MDK, cystic renal cell carcinoma, and rare inflammatory renal diseases, such as echinococcosis, segmental xanthogranulomatous pyelonephritis, and renal malakoplakia. Definitive diagnosis usually is impossible before surgery. However, when radiographic findings suggest MLCN, renal-sparing surgery can be attempted.

Calyceal diverticulum   Also known as a pyelogenic cyst, the calyceal diverticulum is an intraparenchymal cavity lined by transitional epithelium within the kidney. These cavities are urine-filled. Calyceal diverticula are detected in three to four of every 1000 urograms. Calyceal diverticula are thought to result from failure of a segmental ampulla of the ureteric bud to induce nephron development in overlying renal parenchyma. Although

these outpouchings communicate with calyces, they are not connected directly to renal collecting ducts. Three types of calyceal diverticula have been described (Box 2-9; Fig. 2-34). Type I, the most common, is a calyceal diverticulum directly connected to a calyx. Type II calyceal diverticulum has an infundibulum that communicates with a major calyx, more centrally in the collecting system. Type III calyceal diverticulum, the least common variety, communicates directly with the renal pelvis. The third type of diverticula are centrally located, tend to be larger, and produce symptoms from stasis more often than do the first two types of diverticula. All types of calyceal diverticula are smooth-walled outpouchings that fill with excreted radiographic contrast materials slightly later than normal calyces do. Calyceal diverticula tend to have narrow necks communicating with the normal collecting system, leading to urinary stasis, which predisposes patients to stone formation and urinary infection (Fig. 2-35). These complications are the most common causes of symptomatic calyceal diverticula. Radiographi-

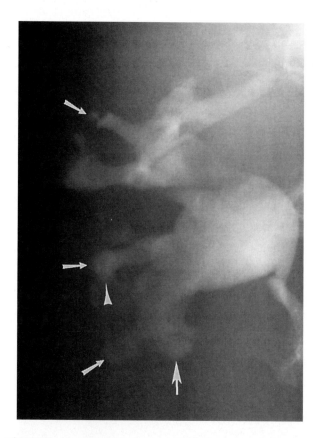

Fig. 2-32 Radiographic features of papillary necrosis. Urogram demonstrates focal papillary contrast material collections (arrows) typical of mild papillary necrosis. These collections are cystic, countable, and usually are associated with an abnormal appearance of the adjacent calyx (arrowhead). These features help distinguish papillary necrosis from the urographic features of medullary sponge kidney.

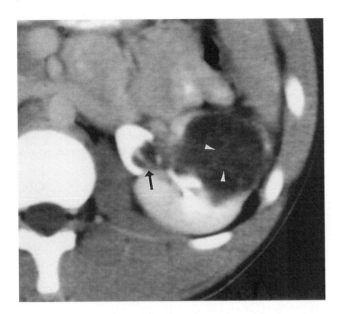

Fig. 2-33   Multilocular cystic nephroma. Computed tomography scan demonstrates an exophytic cystic mass originating from the left kidney. Thin enhancing septa (arrowheads) are present within this water density mass. A segment of this mass herniates into the renal pelvis (arrow), typical of this lesion.

cally, calyceal diverticula appear as rounded, smooth-walled, urine-filled outpouchings from the collecting system (Fig. 2-36). These should be differentiated from a hydrocalyx, which develops from infundibular stricturing with focal hydronephrosis. A hydrocalyx tends to have a squared-off contour distinctly different from that seen with a calyceal diverticulum.

Mesoblastic nephroma

Mesoblastic nephroma is a benign neoplasm. It is the most commonly diagnosed neonatal renal neoplasm; however, its incidence is still rare. Mesoblastic nephroma is a hamartoma of the kidney. The mesoblastic nephroma also has been described by other names, including fetal renal hamartoma, stromal hamartoma, and leiomyomatous hamartoma. The etiology of these tumors is unknown, but one hypothesis suggests that they develop from a line of metanephric cells that have lost their potential for divergent differentiation. One report describes a

small series of mesoblastic nephromas that contained mature nephrons and demonstrated minimal excretion of iodinated contrast material. However, this is the exception rather than the rule for mesoblastic nephroma imaging, because most of these are nonfunctioning masses. These tumors are almost always diagnosed in children aged less than 2 years. Demographics aside, these lesions have an appearance similar to that of most solid renal masses. They grow by expansion into ball-shaped, exophytic lesions. Excision usually is performed for diagnosis rather than cure because radiographically these tumors can mimic malignant renal neoplasms, such as Wilms' tumors.

Nephroblastomatosis

Nephroblastomatosis is a disease in which multiple foci of primitive renal tissue are intermingled with normal renal parenchyma. Primitive metanephric blastema tissue can be present normally until 36 weeks of gestation. After this period, the presence of this tissue is abnormal. Severe forms of congenital nephroblastomatosis lead to marked renal enlargement, with multifocal areas of nonfunctioning renal tissue, which may be detected with urography, contrast-enhanced CT (Fig. 2-37), or MR imaging. The foci of primitive renal tissue also can cause mass effect

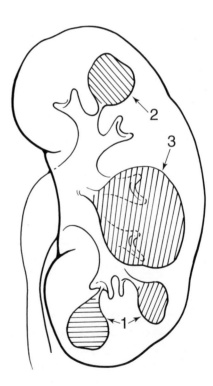

Fig. 2-34   Classification of calyceal diverticula. Diagram illustrates the three types of calyceal diverticula. Type I (1) originates directly from a minor calyx. Type II (2) originates from an infundibulum draining a calyx. Type III (3) originates directly from the renal pelvis.

Box 2-9	Classification of Calyceal Diverticulum

Type I originates from minor calyx
Type II originates from calyceal infundibulum
Type III originates from renal pelvis

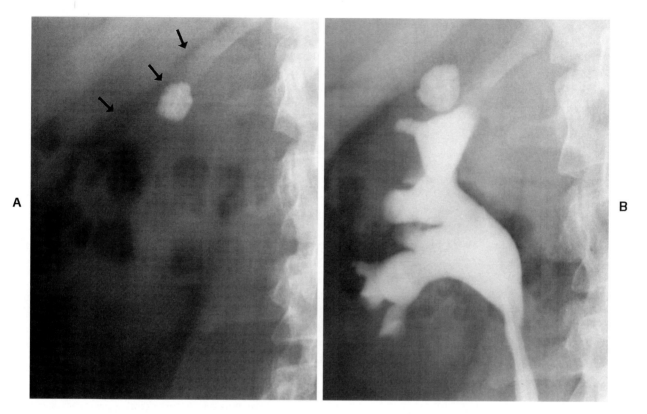

Fig. 2-35 Type I calyceal diverticulum containing stones. **A,** A cone-down radiograph of the right upper quadrant demonstrates a large round kidney stone, which is located very near the edge of the renal parenchyma (arrows), unusual for a calyceal stone. **B,** A retrograde pyelogram demonstrates that this stone is outside the confines of the calyces. The stone is obscured by contrast material, apparently enlarging its radiographic shadow, which indicates that this stone is within a cavity communicating with the upper pole calyx, typical of a Type I calyceal diverticulum.

with calyceal distortion. The major significance of neph-roblastomatosis lies in its association with an increased risk for developing Wilms' tumors. Wilms' tumors often contain primitive blastema elements. Multiple foci of these nephrogenic rests are found in up to 25% of kidneys harboring Wilms' tumors. Patients with nephroblas-tomatosis also have a considerably increased risk of for-mation of multiple and bilateral Wilms' tumors. The de-posits of primitive renal tissue usually are dispersed in predominantly subcapsular locations within the kidney. These rare lesions should be suspected in young patients with renal enlargement and evidence of multiple renal masses.

URETEROPELVIC JUNCTION OBSTRUCTION

The UPJ is the most common site of congenital ob-struction of the urinary tract. Its cause is unclear, and the stricture has been attributed to inherent abnormalities in ureteral bud development, in utero ischemia, aberrant crossing vessels, and fibrous bands compressing the ure-

teric bud. In all patients, there is excessive collagen tissue in the affected segment of the ureter, leading to an ady-namic segment of ureter and resulting in hydronephrosis and renal pelvic distension. In patients with severe cases, function of the kidney is profoundly impaired, and there is minimal renal cortex. In all patients, early diagnosis is important for preserving functional renal mass and detecting significant associated anomalies. UPJ obstruc-tion occurs bilaterally in 20% of patients. In addition, other congenital urinary tract anomalies may be associ-ated, most notably contralateral MDK, contralateral renal agenesis, ureteral duplication, and vesicoureteral reflex.

Ureteropelvic junction obstruction can be diagnosed with a variety of imaging techniques, including urogra-phy, sonography, CT, MR imaging, and scintigraphy. Im-aging studies demonstrate hydronephrosis (Fig. 2-38). The focal narrowing at the UPJ usually can be demon-strated with intravenous urography or with retrograde pyelography (Fig. 2-38). With longstanding disease, the renal pelvis is markedly redundant, and the upper ureter often develops a corkscrew contour. When abrupt angu-lation at the UPJ is noted with urography or pyelography, the presence of an aberrant crossing vessel in association

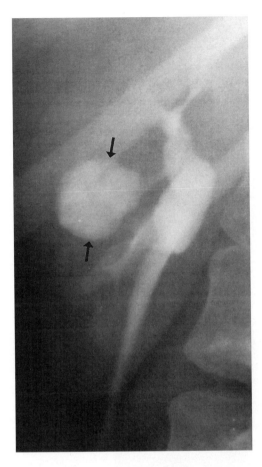

Fig. 2-36   Calyceal diverticulum. This Type I calyceal diverticulum demonstrates typical radiographic features. The contrast-containing diverticulum (arrows) is spherical and smooth. The draining infundibulum, not visible on this radiograph, usually is difficult to demonstrate because of its short and narrow course from the adjacent calyx.

with the obstruction should be suspected. If endoscopic surgery is contemplated for management of the obstruction, preoperative vascular imaging may be necessary and can be performed with CT angiography or MR angiography. Both of these techniques appear to be acceptable for demonstrating crossing arteries of significant size.

NORMAL ANATOMY OF THE RETROPERITONEUM

The anatomy of the retroperitoneum is complex; however, a basic knowledge of retroperitoneal anatomy is important for understanding pathways of disease spread, which often involve the urinary tract. The retroperitoneal space is bounded anteriorly by the posterior parietal peritoneum (Fig. 2-39). The posterior border of the retroperitoneal space is the transversalis fascia. The superior extent of the retroperitoneum is the diaphragm, and the space extends inferiorly to the pelvis. Three discrete retroperitoneal compartments make up the retroperitoneal space (Box 2-10). These compartments include the perirenal space, the anterior pararenal space, and the posterior pararenal space. Some authorities include a distinct fourth compartment encompassing the aorta, the inferior vena cava, and the tissues immediately surrounding these vessels, which is called the retroperitoneal vascular compartment.

The term *Gerota's fascia,* frequently used to describe the anterior and the posterior segments of renal fascia,

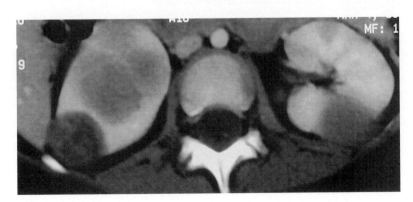

Fig. 2-37   Nephroblastomatosis. This contrast-infused computed tomography demonstrates multifocal subcapsular areas of low attenuation in this child. Open biopsy of these lesions demonstrated nephroblastomatosis. This radiographic pattern in a young child is very suggestive of nephroblastomatosis. In adults, this pattern would be more typical of renal metastases.

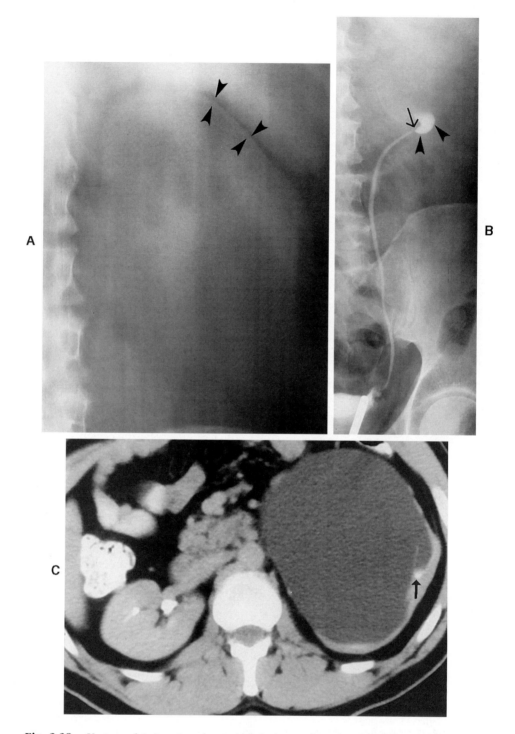

Fig. 2-38   Ureteropelvic junction obstruction. **A,** A cone-down view of the left renal bed from an intravenous urogram demonstrates reniform enlargement of the left kidney. A thin rim of residual cortex (arrowheads) surrounds this markedly hydronephrotic kidney. **B,** A retrograde pyelogram demonstrates a normal left ureter with focal obstruction (arrow). Cephalad to the obstruction, the renal pelvis is dilated and tortuous (arrowheads). **C,** Computed tomography scan of a different patient with findings typical of long-standing ureteropelvic obstruction. There is severe hydronephrosis with marked parenchymal atrophy. Minimal contrast excretion is noted (arrow). Lower scans demonstrated absence of ureteral dilatation.

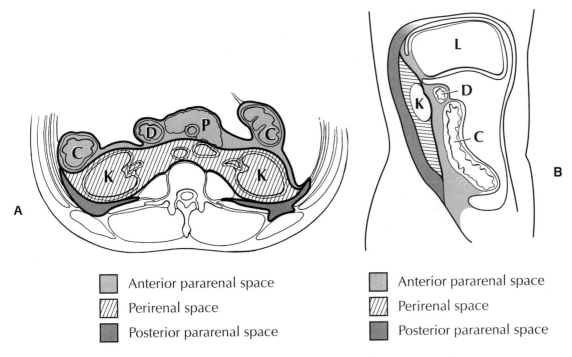

Anterior pararenal space

Perirenal space

Posterior pararenal space

Anterior pararenal space

Perirenal space

Posterior pararenal space

Fig. 2-39   **A,** Diagram illustrating retroperitoneal anatomy from an axial orientation. **B,** Sagittal view. The kidneys (RK, LK) are within the perinephric space, which communicates across the midline adjacent to the vena cava (V) and the aorta (A). The anterior pararenal space contains the pancreas (P) and the retroperitoneal portions of the colon (C) and the duodenum (D). The posterior pararenal space is a potential space containing no organs.

refers to the connective tissue that surrounds the perinephric fat (Box 2-11). Gerota's fascia sometimes is subdivided into the posterior layer, also known as Zuckerkandl's fascia, and the anterior layer. With this terminology, the anterior layer of perirenal fascia is also known as Gerota's fascia or the fascia of Toldt. Where the anterior and posterior layers of the renal fascia fuse laterally, the perirenal space takes on a triangular shape as seen on cross-sectional imaging studies. The fascia in this area is described as the lateroconal fascia, and it continues anterolaterally behind the colon to blend with the parietal peritoneum. We will use Gerota's fascia to describe the entirety of the surrounding renal fascia. The perinephric space is surrounded by Gerota's fascia. Gerota's fascia is a dense collection of connective tissue, normally less than 2 mm thick. It surrounds the kidney, the

adrenal gland, the renal hilum including the renal vessels and the proximal collecting system, and the perinephric fat. Throughout the perinephric fat, bridging septa subdivide the space into multiple compartments. These perinephric septa, also known as Kunin's septa in recognition of the first researcher to describe their appearance on CT, normally are visible with high-resolution CT in patients with adequate perinephric fat. The septa appear as fibrous bands within the perinephric fat. Perinephric septa may become thickened in association with pathologic processes, including renal infection, renal vein thrombosis, renal tumors, and retroperitoneal fluid collections. Thickened perinephric septa have been described as perinephric cobwebs or perinephric stranding.

The simplest of these three compartments is the posterior pararenal space, which is situated between the posterior renal fascia and its extension, the lateroconal fascia, anteriorly and the transversalis fascia posteriorly. It contains no organs and only a moderate amount of fat.

The anterior pararenal space is bordered posteriorly by Gerota's fascia and anteriorly by the posterior parietal peritoneum. This space contains most of the pancreas and the retroperitoneal portions of the duodenum and the colon.

The retroperitoneal spaces extend superiorly and inferiorly. The superior extent of the perirenal space is con-

---

Box 2-11   Divisions of the Perirenal Fascia

Anterior layer—Gerota's fascia, fascia of Toldt
Posterior layer—Zuckerkandl's fascia
Lateral junction—lateroconal fascia

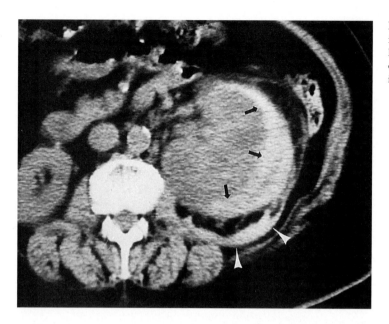

Fig. 2-40   Perirenal fluid. High-density acute hemorrhage is seen in the left perinephric space. This blood is subcapsular (arrows) and extracapsular (arrowheads). Hemorrhage occurred spontaneously from an occult renal cell carcinoma in this kidney.

tiguous with the bare areas of the liver and spleen. The perirenal space also may communicate with the mediastinum via diaphragmatic perforations, lymphatics, or splanchnic foramina. The perirenal space extends inferomedially and forms a cone shape. Inferiorly, the perirenal space melds and communicates with the periureteric connective tissues. In some patients, the perirenal fascia is patent inferiorly and communicates with the extraperitoneal pelvic compartments. Fluids can spread between these compartments in some patients. In most patients,

the perirenal spaces appear to have the potential for intercommunication across the midline, which has been cited as the reason for demonstration of blood in the perirenal space when there is bleeding from the abdominal aorta. In some patients, such bleeding is limited to the periaortic region, and there appears to be a lack of communication between the vascular compartment and the perirenal space. This remains an area of controversy in descriptions of the retroperitoneal spaces.

Inferiorly, the anterior and posterior pararenal spaces

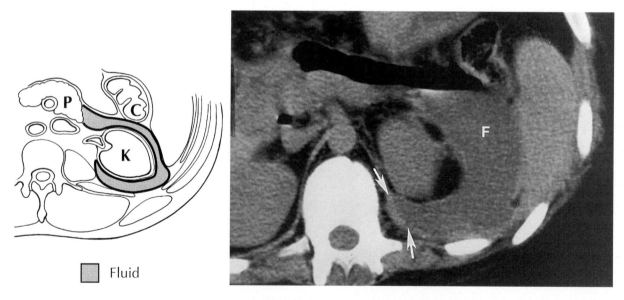

Fluid

Fig. 2-41   Diagram and computed tomography illustration of fluid in the left anterior pararenal space. Fluid (F) from acute pancreatitis is localized in the anterior pararenal space. As sometimes occurs, this fluid has dissected between the leaves of Gerota's fascia and extends behind the kidney to mimic fluid in the posterior pararenal space. The wedge shape of this posterior fluid (arrows) is typical of fluid in the anterior pararenal space.

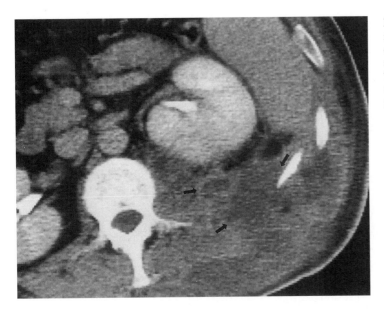

Fig. 2-42 Inflammatory fluid in the left posterior pararenal space extending cephalad from a pelvic abscess. Axial computed tomography scan demonstrates fluid infiltrating and expanding the left posterior pararenal space (arrows). The shape of this fluid collection is distinctly different from that seen with posterior extension of fluid in the anterior pararenal space.

intercommunicate caudally with the lower aspect of the perirenal fascia, which allows free communication of the pararenal spaces with the prevesical space and other pelvic extraperitoneal compartments.

Knowledge of the retroperitoneal spaces and their contents can help in analyzing retroperitoneal pathology and fluid collections. Perirenal fluid collections (Fig. 2-40) usually result from renal bleeding, extravasation of urine, or extension of bleeding from the aorta. Urine extravasation causes lipolysis and induces encapsulation of the urinoma. Thus, with chronicity, urinomas assume a saccular configuration. The shape of the urinoma usually parallels the shape of the perirenal space. Some urinomas circumferentially surround the kidney.

Key features of perirenal space pathologic processes include perirenal infections usually originate from the kidney; chronic urinomas usually are conically shaped within the perirenal space; renal cell carcinoma, lymphoma, and melanoma are the most common causes of solid masses; amyloid and fibrosis tend to form a rind enveloping the kidney; a diaphragmatic "pseudotumor" can occur, and it is the only cause of a solid, linear lesion in the perirenal space.

Fluid in the anterior pararenal space usually results from pancreatitis. When present in the left anterior pararenal space, it usually results from pancreatitis of the pancreatic tail. Fluid in the right anterior pararenal space usually results from pancreatitis involving the head of the pancreas or from leakage of fluid from the duodenum. When extensive, particularly when associated with the proteolytic enzymes seen with pancreatitis, fluid in the anterior pararenal space can dissect into the potential space formed between the two major layers of Gerota's fascia. This potential space extends dorsally to the kidney

and may simulate fluid in the posterior pararenal space. The fact that this actually represents fluid in the anterior pararenal space can be recognized by the characteristic wedge shape of the fluid dorsal to the kidney (Fig 2-41).

Pathologic processes involving the posterior pararenal space are uncommon. Most commonly, fluid collections in this space result from extraperitoneal hemorrhage and usually are seen in patients who have received excessive anticoagulation therapy. Fluid collections also can extend from pelvic extraperitoneal spaces into the posterior pararenal space (Fig. 2-42).

SUGGESTED READINGS

Barakat AJ, Drougas JG: Occurrence of congenital abnormalities of kidney and urinary tract in 13,775 autopsies, *Urology* 38:347-350, 1991.

Bosniak MA, Ambos MA: Polycystic kidney disease, *Semin Roentgenol* 10:133-143, 1975.

Castillo OA, Boyle ET Jr, Kramer SA: Multilocular cysts of kidney: a study of 29 patients and review of literature, *Urology* 37:156-162, 1991.

Chapman AB, Rubinstein D, Hughes R, et al: Intracranial aneurysms in autosomal dominant polycystic kidney disease, *N Engl J Med* 327:916-920, 1992.

Daneman A, Alton DJ: Radiographic manifestations of renal anomalies, *Radiol Clin North Am* 29:351-363, 1991.

Donaldson JS, Shkolnik A: Pediatric renal masses, *Semin Roentgenol* 23:194-204, 1988.

Dretler SP, Olsson C, Pfister RC: The anatomic, radiologic and clinical characteristics of the pelvic kidney: an analysis of 86 cases, *J Urol* 105:623-627, 1971.

Hartman DS, Davis CJ, Sanders RC, et al: The multiloculated renal mass: considerations and differential features, *Radiographics* 7:29-52, 1987.

Hayden CK Jr, Swischuk LE, Smith TH, et al: Renal cystic disease in childhood, *Radiographics* 6:97-116, 1986.

Herman TE, McAlister WH: Radiographic manifestations of congenital anomalies of the lower urinary tract, *Radiol Clin North Am* 29:365-382, 1991.

Kääriäinen H, Jääskeläinen J, Kivisaari L, et al: Dominant and recessive polycystic kidney disease in children: classification by intravenous pyelography, ultrasound, and computed tomography, *Pediatr Radiol* 18:45-50, 1988.

Kleiner B, Filly RA, Mack L, et al: Multicystic dysplastic kidney: observations of contralateral disease in the fetal population, *Radiology* 161:27-29, 1986.

Kneeland JB, Auh YH, Rubenstein WA, et al: Perirenal spaces: CT evidence for communication across the midline, *Radiology* 164:657-664, 1987.

Kunin M: Bridging septa of the perinephric space: anatomic, pathologic, and diagnostic considerations, *Radiology* 158:361-365, 1986.

Mall JC, Ghahremani GG, Boyer JL: Caroli's disease associated with congenital hepatic fibrosis and renal tubular ectasia, *Gastroenterology* 66:1029-1035, 1974.

Meyers MA: *Dynamic radiology of the abdomen: normal and pathologic anatomy*, ed 4, New York, 1994, Springer-Verlag.

Mindell HJ, Mastromatteo JF, Dickey KW, et al: Anatomic communications between the three retroperitoneal spaces: determination by CT-guided injections of contrast material in cadavers, *AJR Am J Roentgenol* 164:1173-1178, 1995.

Olsen A, Højhus JH, Steffensen G: Renal medullary cystic disease: findings at urography and ultrasonography, *Acta Radiol* 29:527-529, 1988.

O'Toole KM, Brown M, Hoffmann P: Pathology of benign and malignant kidney tumors, *Urol Clin North Am* 20:193-205, 1993.

Papanicolaou N, Pfister RC, Yoder IC: Spontaneous and traumatic rupture of renal cysts: diagnosis and outcome, *Radiology* 160:99-103, 1986.

Parfrey PS, Bear JC, Morgan J, et al: The diagnosis and prognosis of autosomal dominant polycystic kidney disease, *N Engl J Med* 323:1085-1090, 1990.

Rosenberg HK, Sherman NH, Tarry WF, et al: Mayer-Rokitansky-Kuster-Hauser syndrome: US aid to diagnosis, *Radiology* 161:815-819, 1986.

Silva JM, Jafri SZH, Cacciarelli AA, et al: Abnormalities of the kidney: embryogenesis and radiologic appearance, *Appl Radiol* 24:19-24, 27-28, 1995.

Sirinelli D, Silberman B, Baudon JJ, et al: Beckwith-Wiedemann syndrome and neural crest tumors: a report of two cases, *Pediatr Radiol* 19:242-245, 1989.

Uhlenhuth E, Amin M, Harty JI, et al: Infundibulopelvic dysgenesis: a spectrum of obstructive renal disease, *Urology* 35:334-337, 1990.

Veréb J, Tischler V, Pavkoveková O: Differential x-ray diagnosis of renal dystopias and ectopias in children, *Pediatr Radiol* 7:205-210, 1978.

Young DW, Lebowitz RL: Congenital abnormalities of the ureter, *Semin Roentgenol* 21:172-187, 1986.

Renal Masses

Detection of renal masses is a high-priority task for radiologists examining the abdomen. Renal masses may be detected, often incidentally, with a variety of modalities. This chapter describes the radiographic clues that are useful in the diagnosis of renal masses. Additionally, once detected, renal masses should be characterized and, if necessary, staged for proper management. Although this task may seem daunting at first, a few basic principles can be used to assist in the diagnosis of renal masses in a majority of patients.

BALLS *VERSUS* BEANS

One concept that is very helpful in detecting and classifying renal masses is the basic shape of the mass (Boxes 3-1, 3-2). Most renal masses grow by expansion. These masses are shaped similarly to spheres or balls, and they displace and compress rather than invade normal structures (Fig. 3-1). As these masses enlarge, they expand from the normal parenchymal margins either peripherally to the kidney or into the renal sinus, depending on the primary direction of growth. Alternatively, some renal lesions grow by a second pattern—infiltration. These lesions grow along the lattice work of the normal renal parenchyma. Infiltrating lesions may swell the area of involved parenchyma, but they do not greatly deform the shape of the kidney (Fig. 3-2). The kidney retains its bean shape, and these reniform lesions often are referred to as "beans," in distinction to the previously described "balls." Beans often are more difficult to detect radiologically than balls because little mass effect is associated with them.

In addition, ball- and bean-shaped lesions may be solitary or multiple, and the number of lesions often is helpful in determining the correct diagnosis. Boxes 3-3 and 3-4 list lesions in each of these two categories. The ball category includes most of the common renal masses, such as simple cysts, renal cell carcinoma (RCC), angiomyolipoma, most metastases, oncocytoma, and abscesses. Alternatively, with geographic infiltrating lesions, one should also consider the three *I*'s: *i*nfiltrating neoplasms, *i*nflammatory lesions, and *i*nfarction. Infiltrating neoplasms include transitional cell carcinoma (TCC) and squamous cell carcinoma (SCC), which spread

Box 3-1   Expansile Renal Masses—Radiographic Characteristics
Ball shaped Exophytic Displace normal structures Well-demarcated margins

Box 3-2   Infiltrative Renal Masses—Radiographic Characteristics
Maintain "bean" shape of kidney Infiltrate normal structures Poorly demarcated margins

from the urothelium to the renal parenchyma, the uncommon infiltrating RCC, the recently described renal medullary carcinoma, some metastases, leukemia, and lymphoma. All of these lesions are described in greater detail in this chapter.

DETECTION

Plain Films

Commonly, the first hint of a renal mass may be found on an abdominal radiograph. Renal masses may be visible on a radiograph or a tomogram of the abdomen, usually as exophytic ball-shaped masses extending from the kidney. Uncommonly, fat within the mass may increase the mass's conspicuity. This finding is virtually diagnostic of an angiomyolipoma. Confirmation of intratumoral fat should be obtained with computed tomography (CT) or magnetic resonance (MR) imaging before making a diagnosis of angiomyolipoma, which is a benign tumor. More commonly, calcifications are detected within a

mass originating from the kidney (Fig. 3-3). Calcification within a renal mass is worrisome. Before the refinement of cross-sectional imaging, a urology rule of thumb was "a calcified renal mass is a surgical renal mass." This tenet remains true for many calcified renal masses today. Although cross-sectional imaging is required to better characterize and guide management of a calcified renal mass, plain film findings often give significant information regarding the etiology of these masses.

When calcification is detected, its pattern should be scrutinized (Box 3-5). A thin, peripheral rim calcification most commonly occurs within the wall of a benign cyst (Fig. 3-4). Although only 1% of cysts contain calcium, renal cysts are ubiquitous. Unfortunately, peripheral rim calcifications also can develop in renal neoplasms, particularly cystic RCCs. Eighty percent of isolated rim calcifications that are identified with radiography in renal masses are benign cysts, and 20% are malignancies. On the opposite end of the spectrum are renal masses that contain central, irregular calcifications (Fig. 3-3). Eighty-seven percent of these lesions are RCCs, and the re-

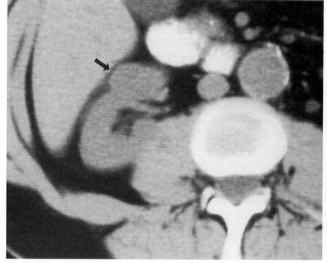
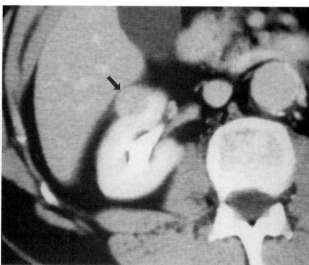

A

B

Fig. 3-1   The typical computed tomography appearance of an exophytic renal mass. This small renal cell carcinoma (arrow) is well seen before intravenous contrast material injection **(A).** This ball-shaped renal mass (arrow) is even more easily identified after the intravenous injection of contrast material **(B).**

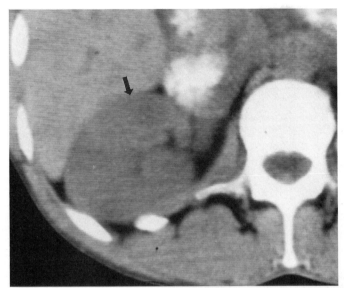

A

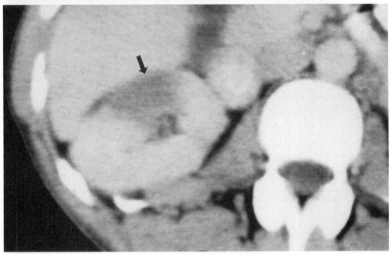

B

Fig. 3-2   Typical computed tomography appearance of an infiltrating renal mass. Before contrast material infusion **(A)**, this infiltrating mass in the right kidney (arrow) barely is discernible as an area of subtle low density. After the intravenous injection of contrast material **(B)**, this geographic area of decreased enhancement (arrow) is readily identifiable. Typical of an infiltrating lesion, this infiltrating renal cell carcinoma does not grossly affect the bean shape of the kidney.

Box 3-3   Solitary Expansile Renal Masses (Balls)

Common
  Cyst
  Renal cell carcinoma
Uncommon
  Angiomyolipoma
  Abscess
  Metastases
Rare
  Oncocytoma
  Multilocular cystic nephroma
  Localized renal cystic disease
  Focal xanthogranulomatous pyelonephritis

Box 3-4   Infiltrating Renal Masses (Beans)

Common
  Transitional cell carcinoma
  Pyelonephritis
Uncommon
  Squamous cell carcinoma
  Infiltrating renal cell carcinoma
  Lymphoma
  Metastases
  Renal infarct
Rare
  Renal medullary carcinoma
  Collecting duct carcinoma

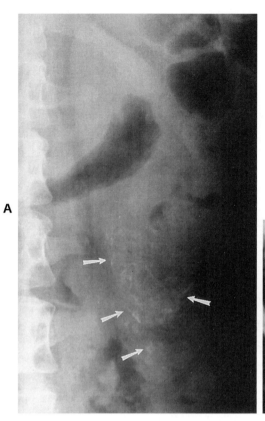

A

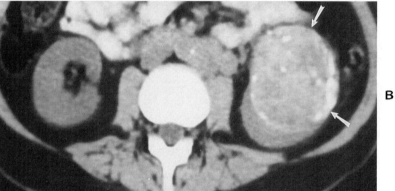

Fig. 3-3   Calcifications in a renal cell carcinoma. **A,** This cone-down view of the left upper quadrant demonstrates irregular calcifications (arrows) extending from, and projecting over, the lower pole of the left kidney. This pattern is worrisome for a renal cell carcinoma. **B,** Uninfused computed tomography of the same patient demonstrates a large, solid renal cell carcinoma (arrows) of the left kidney. This mass contains numerous calcifications corresponding to those seen on the abdominal radiograph.

B

maining 13% are cysts complicated by previous infection or hemorrhage. Some renal masses contain thin, peripheral calcifications and focal, central calcifications. Half of these renal masses are RCCs, and the other half are simple cysts. Approximately 15% of RCCs contain calcifications that are visible on abdominal radiographs. Taking all of these variables into account, 60% of renal masses that contain calcium that is visible on an abdominal radiograph, regardless of the calcification pattern, are RCCs. Cross-sectional imaging allows distinction between benign and malignant calcified renal masses in most patients.

Other plain film findings of importance are skeletal abnormalities. RCC often spreads hematogenously to the skeleton, causing lytic skeletal lesions. These lesions

sometimes grow slowly and lead to bubbly lesions that focally expand the bone. The lesions can mimic numerous types of bone lesions, including other metastases, primary bone neoplasms, and myeloma. Multiple osteo-

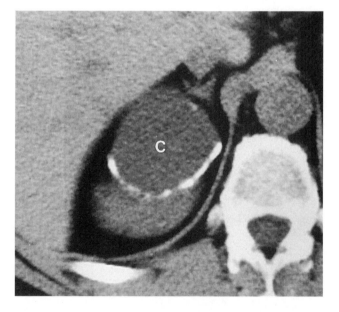

Fig. 3-4   Calcification in the rim of a simple cyst. This uninfused computed tomography scan demonstrates a thin rim of calcification in the wall of a simple cyst (C).

Box 3-5   Renal Mass Calcifications—Imaging Statistics

Renal cell carcinoma—up to 31% contain calcium
Cysts—1%–2% contain calcium
Peripheral rim only—80% are cysts
Central, irregular—87% are renal cell carcinomas
Mixed central and peripheral—50% renal cell carcinomas, 50% cysts

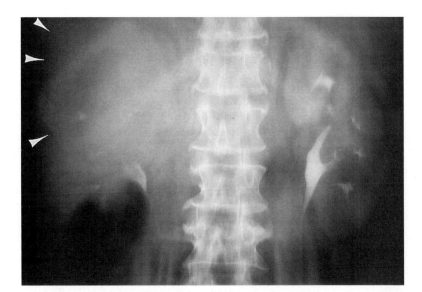

Fig. 3-5 Intravenous urography of an exophytic renal mass. This cone-down view of the kidneys demonstrates a large solid mass extending from the upper pole of the right kidney. This mass compresses and displaces calyces, and its margins (arrowheads) extend beyond the expected margins of the kidney. This mass was a renal cell carcinoma.

mas, or bone islands, are another interesting type of skeletal abnormality sometimes seen in association with renal masses. Patients with tuberous sclerosis can have multiple osteomas, which are predominant particularly in the skull and spine. Angiomyolipoma of the kidney develops in 80% of these patients, and multiple renal cysts develop in a smaller percentage.

Intravenous Urography

Renal masses often are detected with intravenous urography (IVU). Exophytic renal masses (Box 3-3) lead to a focal bulge extending from the kidney and displacing normal renal structures (Figs. 3-5, 3-6). Contour abnormalities are best detected during the nephrogram phase, and detection of masses may be improved with nephrotomography during this phase of IVU. Large masses lead

to calyceal splaying, stretching, and draping, whereas infiltrating renal lesions usually produce little, if any, parenchymal mass effect. However, within infiltrated parenchyma, function is absent or greatly diminished, and therefore, opacification in the involved region is diminished during the nephrogram phase. In addition, infundibular stricture with resulting hydrocalyx and calyceal amputation (Fig. 3-7) is a typical urographic finding associated with infiltrating renal masses. Because many of these masses originate or invade the calyces, calyceal filling defects also may be evident on IVU.

Ultrasonography

Ultrasonography is very useful in the detection of exophytic renal masses and in characterizing renal masses, a use that is described later in this chapter. Ultrasonogra-

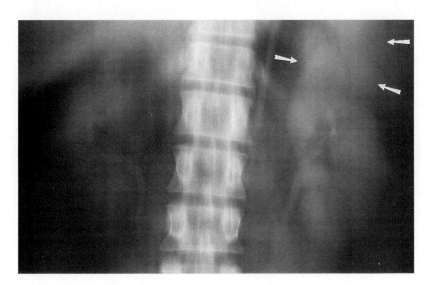

Fig. 3-6 Nephrotomogram demonstrating a left upper pole renal cell carcinoma. A bilobed mass (arrows) extends from the upper pole of the left kidney. This mass is solid and enhances similar to the density of the normal renal parenchyma.

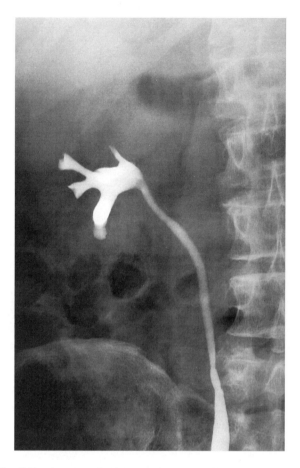

Fig. 3-7 Amputated calyx. A transitional cell carcinoma is present in the upper pole of this right kidney, causing stricturing of the upper pole infundibulum and calyceal amputation. These features are typical of an infiltrating process.

phy, unfortunately, is of little value in the detection of infiltrating renal lesions because these lesions often cause only subtle sonographic abnormalities or none at all. Extensive infiltrating lesions often lead to secondary abnormalities, including hydronephrosis and vascular encasement with diminished flow to the area of involvement. These abnormalities may be detectable with ultrasound and suggest the presence of an infiltrating process.

Cross-sectional Imaging

Cross-sectional imaging, i.e., CT and MR imaging, is the most useful imaging modality for the detection and characterization of renal masses. Exophytic renal masses are found routinely with CT scanning. Additionally, CT with contrast material infusion or MR imaging is extremely accurate in renal mass diagnosis and staging of renal neoplasms. Exophytic renal masses 5 mm or larger are detected routinely with these two imaging modalities. Detection of infiltrating lesions can be somewhat more difficult. Contrast material infusion with CT is essential for the detection of infiltrating lesions because they cause little or no contour abnormality (Fig. 3-2). With contrast infusion, these lesions are detectable usually with CT examination. With MR imaging, intravenous contrast infusion usually is not necessary for lesion detection. Unfortunately, neither CT nor MR imaging is completely reliable for characterization of infiltrating renal lesions, once detected, because of the considerable amount of overlap of the CT and MR imaging findings of various infiltrating lesions.

Angiography

Renal angiography, once a basic element in the diagnosis of renal masses, is of little value in the evaluation of most renal masses. Angiography is reserved for mapping vascular supply to the kidney harboring a renal mass when a partial nephrectomy is contemplated, although noninvasive techniques, such as CT or MR angiography, can be used to derive similar information regarding renal vasculature. Renal arteriography also is useful as part of a procedure for embolization of renal masses. This technique can be useful to devascularize a tumor before excision or to diminish symptoms from an inoperable renal malignancy. Rarely, angiography may be useful in distinguishing various renal masses. In particular, angiography may be an alternative to open biopsy in the diagnosis of infiltrating renal neoplasms. Urothelial neoplasms, inflammatory lesions, and infarcts are nearly always hypovascular or avascular. An uncommon subtype of RCC is the infiltrating variety. The fact that this tumor is usually very vascular distinguishes it from other infiltrating lesions. Therefore, an infiltrating renal mass that is hypervascular strongly suggests an infiltrating RCC. This finding is important because RCC traditionally is managed with nephrectomy, whereas TCC is managed with nephroureterorectomy, and many other infiltrating lesions are managed medically.

CLASSIFICATION OF RENAL MASSES

For ease of understanding, renal masses can be separated into categories according to their growth pattern. The categories are solitary exophytic masses, multiple exophytic masses, and geographic infiltrating lesions.

Ball-Shaped Masses

Box 3-3 lists lesions that form exophytic masses on the kidney. Of these, the simple renal cyst is the most common lesion. With cross-sectional imaging, these are seen in 50% or more of patients aged more than 50 years. Simple renal cysts are not uncommon in younger patients, although the presence of a simple renal cyst in

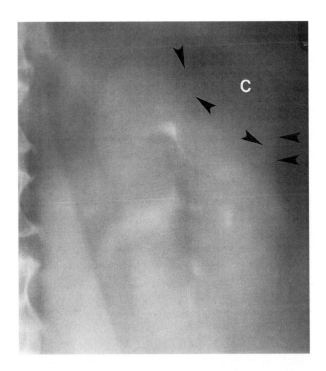

Fig. 3-8 The "beak" sign of a simple renal cyst on urography. A 3-cm simple cyst (C) is present in the upper pole of the left kidney on this nephrotomogram. The edges of the renal parenchyma (arrowheads) are draped around this mass, forming the shape of a bird's beak. This typifies the appearance of a slow-growing, exophytic renal mass, usually a simple cyst.

a child should raise the possibility of underlying renal disease, such as polycystic kidney disease, medullary cystic disease, or another hereditary disorder. Simple cysts may be visible on plain films of the abdomen as large, round, water-dense masses extending from the kidney. These cysts usually are perfectly round with smooth margins. On IVU, simple cysts do not enhance, they have an

imperceptible outer margin, and because of their slow growth, renal parenchyma drapes around the edge of the mass (Fig. 3-8) where the cyst meets the kidney. Renal parenchyma draped around the edges of the cyst often is referred to as the "beak" sign. Although these findings are typical of a simple cyst, the accuracy of diagnosing a simple cyst solely on the basis of IVU results is about 90%, a level of accuracy that is unacceptably low in today's environment. These lesions can be confirmed easily as simple cysts with renal ultrasonography. On ultrasound examination, simple renal cysts are anechoic with enhancement of through sound transmission and a well-demarcated back wall (Fig. 3-9). Simple cysts may have one or two delicate septations. Any variance from these criteria suggests that the lesion is a renal neoplasm and that additional imaging may be necessary. Simple cysts are completely benign. They occasionally cause symptoms because of mass effect, but usually simple cysts are an incidental finding of no clinical significance.

Cystic lesions

Cystic renal masses with more complex imaging features have been studied extensively with CT. The Bosniak classification system is useful for categorizing these lesions as to their etiology and for management guidelines. Box 3-6 summarizes the Bosniak classification system for cystic renal masses seen on CT examination. Class I is a simple cyst. Findings that are diagnostic of a simple renal cyst include a water-dense mass that does not enhance and has an imperceptible or barely perceptible peripheral margin. Class II lesions have multiple septations and thin peripheral calcifications (Fig. 3-4), are typical high-density cysts (Fig. 3-10), or have features typical of infected cysts. On CT examination, one can be reasonably confident that these Class II lesions are benign. However, Class II lesions do merit follow-up CT scanning in 6 to

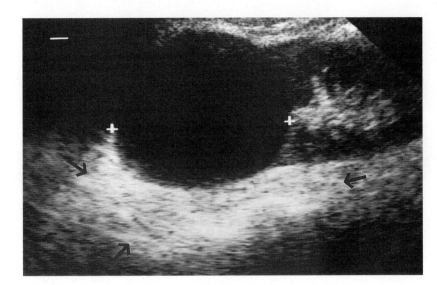

Fig. 3-9 Sonogram of a simple renal cyst. This upper pole simple renal cyst demonstrates typical sonographic features. It is anechoic, spherical, and has enhancement of through sound transmission (arrows).

Box 3-6 Cystic Masses—Bosniak Computed Tomography Classification

*   I   Simple cysts
*   II   Septated, minimal calcium, nonenhancing high-density cysts, infected cysts
† III Multiloculated, hemorrhagic, dense calcification, nonenhancing solid component
‡ IV   Marginal irregularity and enhancing solid component

*Nonoperative management.
†Renal-sparing surgery.
‡Radical nephrectomy.

12 months to exclude progression. Septations and high-density internal material are thought to develop after cyst infection or hemorrhage, which leads to the development of fibrinous internal septa, dystrophic calcifications in the wall of the cyst, or internal proteinaceous material reflected by high density on uninfused CT scans. The high-density cysts are the most problematic for radiologists. These lesions appear to be of higher density than the kidney on uninfused CT scanning. With contrast infusion, they appear hypodense to the kidney, and there is no internal enhancement of these lesions with contrast material injection. Management of these lesions is controversial. Although the lack of enhancement seems to indicate that these are benign lesions, some researchers believe that ultrasound examination of these lesions is helpful in confirming that they are benign, albeit complicated, cysts. Unfortunately, these lesions often contain internal echoes when imaged ultrasonographically, and follow-up imaging or surgical extirpation is necessary for additional evaluation. Because the overwhelming majority of these lesions are benign, follow-up CT examination seems to be the more prudent approach. If these lesions contain enhancing components, they are not Class II lesions but rather Class IV lesions, and surgical removal is indicated.

Class III lesions have more complex imaging characteristics, including dense, thick calcifications, numerous septa, or solid components that do not enhance (Fig. 3-11). Approximately 50% of these lesions are cystic RCCs. The remainder are benign lesions, such as cysts complicated by infection or hemorrhage, or a benign tumor known as multilocular cystic nephroma. There is no reliable way to distinguish these lesions without surgery. Because many of them are benign, renal-sparing surgery can be considered for these patients, but surgical excision generally is indicated for complex cystic masses. Class IV lesions always are considered malignant. The major criterion of a Class IV lesion is an area of enhancing solid tissue. With cystic neoplasms, this tissue often is at

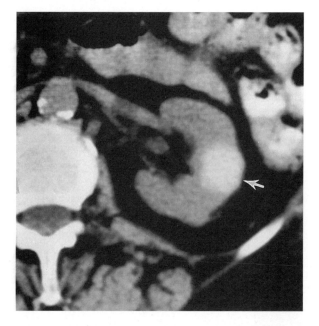

Fig. 3-10   High-density cyst. This uninfused computed tomography scan demonstrates a homogeneously high-density lesion (arrow) in the left kidney, which did not enhance with contrast infusion and with sonography-demonstrated features of a simple cyst. These cysts usually contain hemorrhage or highly concentrated proteinaceous material.

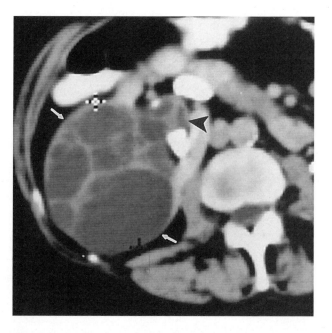

Fig. 3-11   Bosniak Class III renal mass. This multilocular right renal mass (arrows) has numerous septations, and it did not enhance with contrast infusion. Note there is extension centrally, or herniation (arrowhead), of this mass into the renal sinus. This was a benign multilocular cystic nephroma.

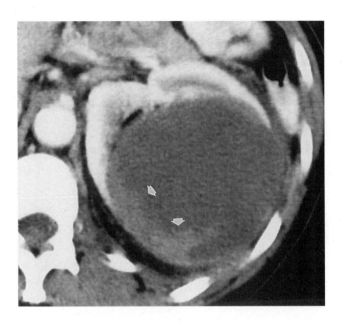

Fig. 3-12 Bosniak Class IV renal mass. This papillary renal cell carcinoma demonstrates solid tissue with subtle peripheral enhancement (arrowheads). Enhancing tissue in a cystic renal mass strongly suggests a malignant tumor.

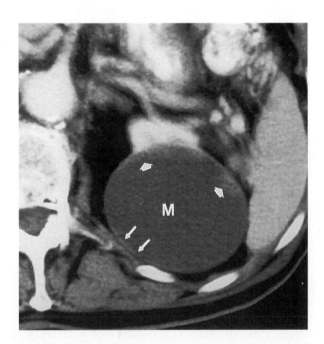

Fig. 3-13 Bosniak Class IV cystic renal cell carcinoma. This contrast-infused computed tomography demonstrates a predominantly cystic left renal mass (M). Areas of peripheral enhancement (arrowheads) and an enhancing rim (arrows) make this a Bosniak Class IV tumor.

the periphery, and enhancement may be subtle (Figs. 3-12, 3-13). Careful evaluation of the margins of the cystic mass on the infused CT scan may reveal an area of enhancement. If so, the lesion should be presumed to be RCC, and surgery is indicated.

In our experience, 20% of RCCs appear predominantly cystic on CT examination or MR imaging. Seventy-five percent of these are solid RCCs that have undergone central liquefaction necrosis. With growth, these lesions tend to outstrip their blood supply, and central areas become ischemic and necrotic. The remaining lesions are truly cystic RCCs. This subgroup usually has a papillary cellular growth pattern, which has been associated with a decreased rate of metastases and has better prognosis than other forms of RCC. Papillary RCCs also are often multifocal. These tumors tend to be slow-growing masses with fronds of tissue protruding centrally from the margins. Fluid may be a large component of these masses. The masses usually are hypovascular, even after attaining a large size. Although these lesions may have subtle features on CT examination, indicating their true nature, ultrasound examination often demonstrates the complex internal architecture (Fig. 3-14) typical of a papillary RCC.

In addition, cysts may be associated with renal malignancies in other ways. Because renal cysts are common, cysts and tumors in the same kidney usually are not causally related. A renal tumor may occur adjacent to a solitary or dominant cyst. This pattern of abnormalities is likely related and occurs because of the neoplasm obstructing renal tubules and causing dilatation and cyst formation. Because recognition of these cysts may lead to detection of the nearby renal tumor, these focal, solitary cysts sometimes are referred to as "sentinel" cysts. Some conditions cause formation of renal cysts and renal neoplasms. This category includes von Hippel-Lindau disease, tuberous sclerosis, and long-term dialysis. These entities are discussed later in this chapter. Finally, the rarest cyst–renal neoplasm association is the formation of an RCC in the wall of a preexisting simple renal cyst. Once sizable, these neoplasms can be detected with ultrasound or CT examination or MR imaging as a solid nodule originating in the wall of the cyst. The solid component of these masses usually enhances with contrast material injection, and these tumors are managed identically to other RCCs.

Renal cell carcinoma

Renal cell carcinoma is commonly referred to as renal adenocarcinoma, Grawitz's tumor, hypernephroma, and renal clear cell carcinoma. It is the most common primary renal malignancy. Twenty thousand new cases of RCC occur in the United States annually. Because of its protean and often nonspecific clinical manifestations, it is sometimes referred to as the "great imitator" by clinicians. The classic clinical triad associated with the diagnosis of RCC is a combination of flank pain, hematuria, and a palpable flank mass. Although often cited, this triad is seen in only 10% of patients with RCC and usually indicates the presence of advanced disease with a poor prognosis. Early detection is crucial for cure; management of

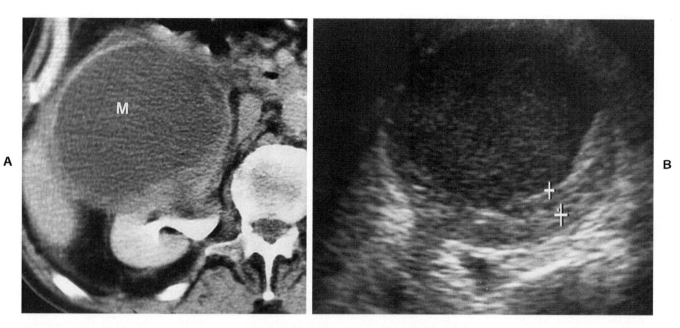

Fig. 3-14 Papillary renal cell carcinoma, computed tomography, and sonographic features. **A,** Contrast-infused computed tomography demonstrates a Bosniak Class IV renal mass (M). Most of this mass appears cystic. **B,** Transverse sonogram through the right kidney in this patient demonstrates a thick rind of solid tissue. The cystic component contains many low level echoes and this component of the mass is not simply cystic.

advanced disease is largely ineffective. The cure rate is high for patients with early stage RCC, whereas the prognosis for patients with advanced disease is abysmal.

Renal cell carcinoma originates from renal tubular epithelium and usually develops in the cortex of the kidney. Recognized risk factors include male gender, with a twofold to threefold increase in the risk of developing RCC, and advancing age (median age at diagnosis, 55 years).

Once the main imaging tool in the diagnosis of RCC, IVU has been superseded by the more sensitive and specific cross-sectional imaging modalities: ultrasound or CT examination and MR imaging. However, because IVU remains a common screening test for patients with suspected urinary tract disease, careful interpretation of these studies for signs of RCC is essential for diagnosis at an early stage. Unfortunately, some small RCCs are undetectable with IVU; one third of RCCs less than 3 cm in diameter cannot be detected with IVU. Therefore, normal IVU results in patients who have clinical evidence of RCC should be supplemented with either CT or ultrasound examination or MR imaging or additional clinical evaluation.

An RCC detected with IVU usually appears as an exophytic contour bulge (Box 3-7; Figs. 3-5, 3-6). Because RCC typically grows by expansion rather than infiltration, the tumor usually displaces calyces. Occasionally, an RCC grows predominantly outward, and no detectable mass effect is exerted on the calyceal system. RCCs that extend either exclusively anteriorly or exclusively posteriorly from the kidney are very difficult to detect with IVU

because the mass contour is obscured by superimposed normal kidney. The detection of a mass with IVU is rather nonspecific diagnostically. A second imaging study should always be obtained to characterize any renal mass detected with IVU. When IVU findings suggest a simple renal cyst (e.g., water density; sharp, distinct interface with kidney; and imperceptible or barely perceptible outer capsule; Fig. 3-8), renal ultrasonography should be performed to confirm this diagnosis and to exclude a cystic neoplasm. If the mass does not meet these IVU criteria, it is more likely a neoplasm, and MR imaging or CT examination should be performed to characterize and, if necessary, stage the tumor.

Calcifications can be detected with standard radiographs in 13% of RCCs. Patterns of calcifications are helpful in determining whether a mass is benign or malignant, but unfortunately there is a substantial degree of pattern overlap. Pure rim-like calcification in a renal mass is caused by benign renal cysts in 80% of patients and by

---

Box 3-7   Renal Cell Carcinoma— Intravenous Urography Features

Exophytic mass
Calyceal displacement, compression
Ureteral notching
Diminished function, if vein occluded

RCCs in 20% of patients. Conversely, 87% of masses with central, diffuse, amorphous, or dense calcifications are RCCs, and 13% are benign tumors. Overall, the majority of all renal masses with associated calcifications are RCCs, therefore, the presence of calcification in a renal mass strongly suggests RCC.

Other IVU signs of RCC are secondary to mass effect and need for increased perfusion. These signs include notching of the renal pelvis or the ureter, obstruction or invasion of the collecting system, and diminished or absent renal function. Notching results from enlargement of ureteric and renal pelvic vessels, which are recruited to feed or drain a hypervascular RCC. Overall, 78% of RCCs are hypervascular compared with normal renal parenchyma. Focal or diffuse hydronephrosis usually occurs with a large RCC and results from compression of major calyces, the renal pelvis, or the upper ureter. Less commonly, an RCC grows by infiltration rather than by expansion. In these cases, malignant stricturing of the collecting system occurs and is secondary to encasement and invasion of the urothelium.

Decreased or absent renal function requires additional renal imaging to exclude RCC, unless another etiology is suggested by IVU results. The finding of globally decreased function in a kidney with a renal mass is nearly diagnostic of RCC. RCC has a predilection for venous extension. Tumor thrombus in the renal vein is the most common cause of absent renal function in a kidney harboring an RCC. Less commonly, diminished or absent renal function can result from RCC-induced hydronephrosis, as described previously.

With CT or MR imaging, RCC can be diagnosed with better than 95% accuracy. This high degree of accuracy reflects the fact that nearly all RCCs conform to a standard profile on CT and MR imaging: RCCs are exophytic, with solid components (Box 3-8). Some RCCs are predominantly cystic, but they exhibit evidence of neoplasia on CT or MR imaging. In addition, because RCCs do not contain discernible fat, the presence of fat in a renal mass suggests an angiomyolipoma and excludes an RCC, unless the tumor has grown to engulf normal perirenal fat. This pattern usually is distinguishable from that of true intrinsic tumor fat.

Older reports suggested the following CT characteristics as typical of RCC: (1) soft-tissue renal mass, (2) isodensity compared with the kidney before contrast enhancement, (3) hypodensity compared with the kidney after contrast enhancement, (4) inhomogeneous internal density, (5) indistinct mass–kidney interface, (6) lobulated and irregular margins, and frequently, (7) calcification. Many RCCs do not meet all of these CT criteria. We have found that the CT features of RCC change considerably as the tumor enlarges. Most small RCCs (5 cm in diameter or less) have a less aggressive appearance than the previously mentioned criteria would suggest.

The radiographic appearance of RCCs varies greatly. In our own experience with CT, 94% of RCCs are detected as exophytic masses, whereas the remaining 6% grow by infiltration without significant disruption of the reniform shape of the involved kidney. The precontrast enhancement density of RCCs compared with the background renal parenchyma can be hypodense, isodense, or hyperdense. Hyperdensity presumably results from acute hemorrhage, calcium, or proteinaceous debris within the tumor. Almost half of RCCs display a transient hyperdense blush during bolus contrast material injection (Fig. 3-15), but all are hypodense to kidney during

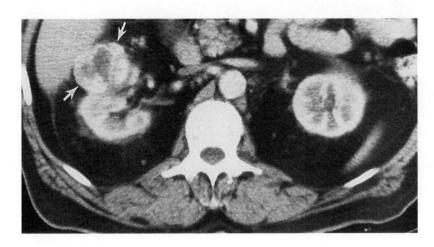

Fig. 3-15 Computed tomography of the transient hyperdense blush seen in some renal cell carcinomas. This computed tomography scan taken during a bolus injection of intravenous contrast material demonstrates an exophytic right renal mass (arrows). This mass enhances to a slightly greater density than does normal renal parenchyma. This feature commonly is seen with hypervascular renal cell carcinomas.

the infusion phase of contrast enhancement. Tumor homogeneity, distinctness of the RCC–kidney interface, and the shape and sharpness of the tumor margins largely depend on tumor size. RCCs less than 5 cm in diameter usually are homogeneous masses with a distinct mass–

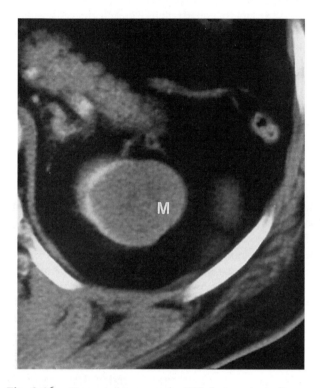

Fig. 3-16 Computed tomography (CT) features typically seen with small renal cell carcinomas. This contrast-infused CT demonstrates a homogeneous, well marginated renal mass (M) that has a distinct interface with normal enhancing renal parenchyma. This 4-cm mass was proven to be a renal cell carcinoma.

kidney interface and smooth, sharp margins (Fig. 3-16). These features are rare in large RCCs. Calcifications are visible with CT in 31% of RCCs, a larger percentage than with plain radiography studies.

Renal cell carcinomas sometimes appear cystic, and about 22% of proven RCCs are predominantly cystic. However, the CT appearance of a cystic RCC is different from the CT criteria of a simple cyst. In cystic RCCs, areas of wall thickening and contrast material enhancement are present, therefore, simple renal cysts are excluded.

Large RCCs usually display features typical of malignant growth, including central necrosis resulting from inadequate vascular supply, marginal lobulation reflecting differential growth rates within the tumor (Fig. 3-17), infiltration of surrounding tissues, and production of an indistinct mass–kidney interface.

Size is not a valid CT criterion for differentiating malignant from benign renal masses (Fig. 3-18). Small RCCs are more likely to be contained within Gerota's fascia and have a less aggressive imaging appearance. However, extirpation of these tumors is mandatory for cure and to prevent progression to a more advanced disease stage. Surgical therapy generally offers patients with small RCCs a good prognosis. In one of our own RCC series, two of eight patients with RCCs 30 mm or smaller had advanced stage disease at the time of diagnosis (Fig. 3-19), highlighting the fact that tumor size alone may underestimate tumor stage. Tumor size is, at best, a rough indicator of prognosis but is not an indicator of diagnosis.

Other differential diagnoses to be considered when a solitary renal mass is demonstrated with CT or MR imaging include metastatic disease, invasive urothelial neoplasm, inflammatory lesions of the kidney, and benign renal neoplasms. Although CT or MR imaging, especially

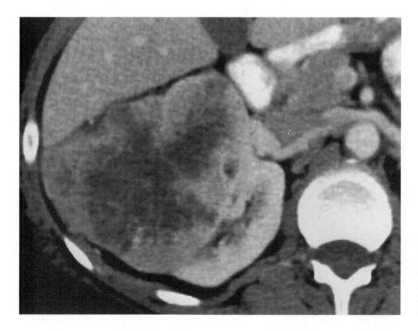

Fig. 3-17 Computed tomography of a large renal cell carcinoma. This large right renal cell carcinoma demonstrates features typical of larger renal cell carcinomas. Heterogeneity with central necrosis, irregular margins, and an indistinct interface with normal kidney are demonstrated in this renal mass.

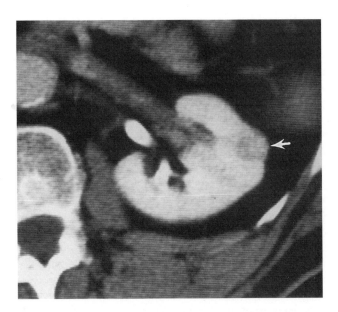

Fig. 3-18 A 1.5-cm renal cell carcinoma. This 1.5-cm left renal mass (arrow) was detected incidentally during an abdominal computed tomography scan for another reason. This mass clearly is solid, and no fat was detected within it. Renal-sparing surgery confirmed it was a renal malignancy.

in conjunction with the patient's clinical data, may permit differentiation of RCC from these other entities, imaging features often exhibit considerable overlap. Some of the pertinent benign entities to be considered and the radiographic features that assist in their diagnosis are discussed later in this chapter. In patients with known extrarenal malignancies, guided needle biopsy of a solitary renal mass may help to differentiate between primary renal malignancy and metastasis. This distinction may be important if the metastasis would be managed nonsurgically. It is one of the few indications for percutaneous

renal mass biopsy because the imaging appearances of an RCC and a metastasis can overlap, although their clinical management often differs.

For some RCCs, appearance strongly suggests the diagnosis, but in other cases appearance is not conclusive. Infiltrating RCCs, an uncommon subtype, do not substantially alter the reniform shape of the kidney, and these lesions often have homogeneous internal architecture (Fig. 3-2). They are detectable mainly because of their hypodensity compared with surrounding parenchyma on contrast-enhanced CT or gadolinium-enhanced MR imaging. Without the use of other diagnostic modalities, such as angiography or biopsy, these tumors are indistinguishable from invasive urothelial malignancies.

The clinical presentation also may confound the correct diagnosis of RCC. Rarely, patients present with a renal abscess when RCC underlies the process. In these cases, the necrotic tumor center becomes infected secondarily. Follow-up renal imaging studies of patients with renal abscess after resolution of their symptoms are necessary to exclude an occult RCC.

Finally, nontraumatic spontaneous renal hemorrhage, subcapsular hemorrhage, or spontaneous perirenal hemorrhage (SPH; Fig. 3-20) may be an unusual presentation of patients with RCC. Of all SPHs, up to 55% result from underlying RCCs. Unfortunately, extensive hemorrhage often obscures the underlying tumor, making it undetectable with CT or MR imaging. In these cases, if a renal mass is not detected initially when SPH is diagnosed, a renal arteriogram should be acquired to detect evidence of a vasculitis or other vascular lesion. If none is detected, CT or MR imaging should be repeated after 1 month to search again for a renal mass while the hemorrhage is resolving. Follow-up CT or MR imaging should be repeated if no lesion is detected. If a benign mass like angiomyolipoma is detected (Fig. 3-21), which is com-

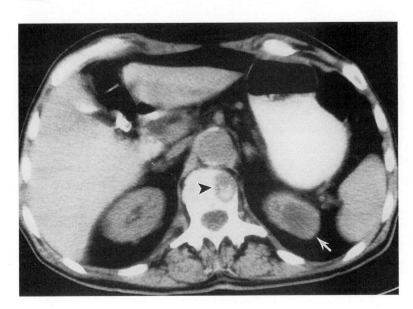

Fig. 3-19 Small renal cell carcinoma with metastatic disease. This contrast-infused computed tomography scan demonstrates a 2.5-cm mass (arrow) in the upper pole of the left kidney. Although this mass does not appear particularly aggressive, this patient already had distant metastases. A lytic metastasis (arrowhead) from this renal cell carcinoma is present in an adjacent vertebra.

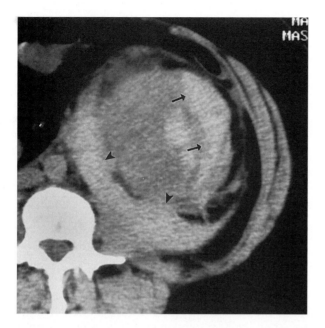

Fig. 3-20 Spontaneous perirenal hemorrhage in a patient with renal cell carcinoma. This uninfused computed tomography scan demonstrates subcapsular (arrows) and perirenal (arrowheads) high attenuation fluid, which is typical of acute hemorrhage and suggests underlying abnormality in that kidney. Additional scanning demonstrated a solid renal mass with features typical of a renal cell carcinoma in this kidney.

monly associated with SPH, it may be managed nonsurgically or with renal-sparing surgery. Detection of an RCC usually leads to nephrectomy. This approach to SPH minimizes nephrectomy for benign diseases.

Because sonography of the kidneys is performed often either in the evaluation of the urinary tract or as part of a larger upper abdominal examination, RCCs often are detected on ultrasound examination. The sonographic

features of RCC are typical of this lesion, but they are not diagnostic. Most RCCs appear as exophytic, solitary renal masses. They may be hypoechoic, isoechoic, or hyperechoic compared with the renal parenchyma. As RCCs enlarge, they often develop heterogeneous echo patterns with internal cystic areas (Fig. 3-22). Several sonographic features of RCC are of interest. In particular, the sonographic appearance of small (less than 5 cm in diameter) RCCs can mimic that of angiomyolipoma. With renal sonography, most small RCCs appear as masses that are only slightly hyperechoic compared with the normal kidney. However, approximately 15% of small RCCs appear as markedly hyperechoic renal masses (Fig. 3-23), and these lesions may be indistinguishable on ultrasound examination from the benign tumor angiomyolipoma. Although CT or MR imaging is required to further categorize these hyperechoic lesions, some sonographic features strongly suggest a diagnosis of RCC. An anechoic perimeter, or the presence of cystic areas within the hyperechoic mass, typifies RCC and should not be seen with an angiomyolipoma. However, there is substantial overlap in the sonographic appearance of RCC and other renal masses. For this reason, detection of a renal mass with sonography always should be complemented with CT or MR imaging to further categorize the renal mass for tumor staging if the lesion is malignant. Both modalities are exquisitely sensitive for the detection of intratumoral fat, the presence of which confirms the diagnosis of angiomyolipoma.

Another interesting sonographic feature in the evaluation of renal masses is the capacity to show the internal architecture of renal tumors better than other imaging techniques. Some renal masses appear cystic or homogeneous with CT and MR imaging. Ultrasound examination of these lesions may demonstrate complex internal components (Fig. 3-14) with septations, fronds of solid tissue

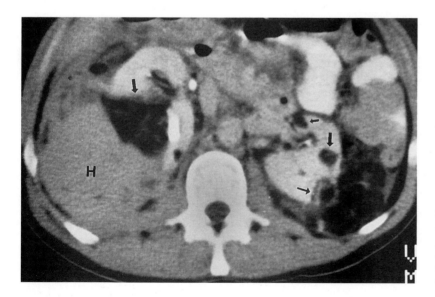

Fig. 3-21 Bilateral renal angiomyolipoma with right spontaneous perinephric hemorrhage. This patient with tuberous sclerosis has bilateral angiomyolipomas (arrows). In addition, there is high-density liquid in the right perirenal space (H), typical of acute hemorrhage.

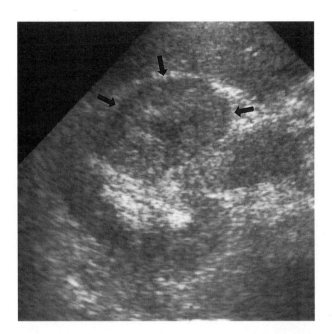

Fig. 3-22 Sonogram of a renal cell carcinoma. This transverse sonogram demonstrates an exophytic right renal mass (arrows). This mass is slightly hyperechoic and heterogeneous compared with normal renal parenchyma. These features are typical of most renal cell carcinomas.

lining the periphery of the mass, or other evidence of malignancy. Therefore, sonography may be used as an adjunctive test when CT findings are equivocal, particularly when CT findings suggest the presence of a cystic lesion that lacks features typical of a simple cyst but is not obviously malignant.

Once RCC is suspected, staging is critical for appropriate disease management. Table 3-1 summarizes the commonly used staging algorithms for RCC. Stage I and II RCCs are managed surgically with either a partial or radical nephrectomy. Stage III lesions usually are managed with radical nephrectomy and extirpation of tumor-filled veins, tumor thrombectomy, local lymph node excision, or a combination of these. Patients with Stage IV disease generally are spared surgery and are treated palliatively unless nephrectomy is used to relieve intractable symptoms.

By using meticulous CT or MR imaging technique, accurate RCC staging can be achieved in more than 90% of patients (Box 3-9). Often, the most difficult imaging task with CT is accurate evaluation of tumor extension to the renal vein. Once a renal mass is identified, the level of the appropriate renal vein should be determined before injection of contrast material. After power-injected contrast material administration, thin CT slices made at the level of the renal vein will yield 95% accuracy in detecting renal vein thrombus with RCC. Secondary signs of renal vein involvement are unreliable. Renal vein enlargement and displacement are not accurate signs of venous invasion because the renal vein often is enlarged simply because of the high flow of blood from a hypervascular RCC. Venous displacement reflects distortion of its normal course from a bulky renal tumor or displacement from extrinsic nodal disease. The normal left renal vein may have an abrupt caliber change where it crosses between the superior mesenteric artery and aorta; elsewhere, such changes usually indicate the presence of tumor thrombus. However, the most reliable sign of tumor invasion is direct visualization of the low-attenuation thrombus in an otherwise opacified vein (Fig. 3-24). These criteria also apply to the diagnosis of tumor thrombus in the inferior vena cava. Bland thrombus may propagate in veins adjacent to tumor thrombus and may mimic more extensive tumor thrombus than actually is present. CT can be used to differentiate bland thrombus from tumor thrombus only in unusual instances when neovascularity or substantial contrast enhancement is detectable within the tumor thrombus.

Computed tomography and MR imaging are very effective in detecting retroperitoneal lymphadenopathy. Nodes 1.5 cm or larger are abnormally enlarged and therefore suggestive of lymphatic metastases. This criterion assures accurate detection of most nodal metastases. Unfortunately, malignant lymphadenopathy cannot be differentiated from lymph node enlargement with CT because of benign hyperplasia. Benign hyperplasia of regional nodes is more commonly seen with RCCs complicated by tumor necrosis and venous extension. Also, nodes in the 1- to 1.5-cm range, particularly if they are more numerous than expected, are considered indeterminate but suspicious for spread of malignant disease. Rarely, normal-sized nodes (less than 1 cm) harbor microscopic tumor foci. These nodes are not identifiable with CT size criteria.

Distant metastases within the abdomen to organs such as the liver and bone generally are easy to identify with CT or MR imaging. Organ-appropriate window settings of scans should be done in all patients to maximize the CT visualization of metastatic deposits. Because RCC metastases are often hypervascular, making them difficult to detect in the enhanced liver, CT examination of the liver before injection of contrast material is helpful in identifying many of these lesions. Detection of metastases in organs such as the liver, skeleton, and lung bases may obviate the need for additional diagnostic studies of these areas and negate indications for surgery.

It is often impossible to differentiate between Stage I and Stage II RCCs with CT and MR imaging. In most settings, this drawback is of no clinical significance other than for prognostication because radical nephrectomy is the treatment of choice in either case. However, a growing number of surgeons are treating patients with early-stage RCC with partial nephrectomy or tumorectomy. Results suggest that partial nephrectomy is effective man-

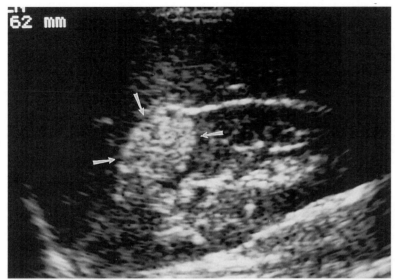

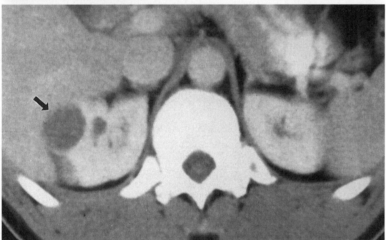

Fig. 3-23   Sonogram demonstrating a hyperechoic renal cell carcinoma. **A,** This longitudinal sonogram of the right kidney demonstrates a well-circumscribed hyperechoic right renal mass (arrows). **B,** Contrast-infused computed tomography scan in the same patient demonstrates that this mass is solid (arrow) without visible internal fat. This mass was resected and proven to be a renal cell carcinoma.

Table 3-1   Staging Systems of Renal Cell Carcinoma

Robson stage		TNM stage
I	Tumor within renal capsule	
	Small tumor	T1
	Large tumor	T2
II	Tumor spread to perinephric fat	T3a
IIIA	Venous tumor extension	
	Limited to renal vein	T3b
	Infradiaphragmatic inferior vena cava	T3c
	Supradiaphragmatic	T4b
IIIB	Regional lymph node metastasis	N1–N3
IIIC	Venous tumor extension *and* regional node metastasis	
IVA	Direct invasion beyond Gerota's fascia	T4a
IVB	Distant metastasis	M1a–d, N4

Box 3-9   Abdominal Imaging in Patients with Renal Cell Carcinoma: Areas of Particular Interest

Contralateral kidney
Renal vein
Vena cava
Regional lymph nodes
Adjacent organs
Liver
Skeleton

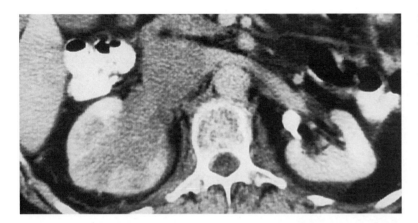

Fig. 3-24   Renal cell carcinoma extending into the right renal vein and the inferior vena cava. This contrast-infused computed tomography demonstrates solid tissue extending into and enlarging the right renal vein and the inferior vena cava. The portion in the inferior cava is outlined by a meniscus of opaque contrast material entering the cava from the normal left renal vein.

agement for Stage I and Stage II RCCs. When partial nephrectomy is being considered, it is important to scrutinize the ipsilateral adrenal gland for evidence of tumor involvement. When present, this form of Stage II RCC will necessitate adrenalectomy in conjunction with tumor removal. Otherwise, the adrenal gland is spared.

Some signs have been considered suggestive of extracapsular (Stage II) tumor spread; these signs include visualization of the following features in the perinephric space: stranding or cobwebbing, collateral vessels, fat obliteration, discrete soft-tissue masses, and fascial thickening. Obliteration of perinephric fat and visualization of perinephric collateral vessels are not reliable signs of Stage II disease, and their significance for staging is minimal. Fat obliteration indicates only mass effect, not invasion, in the perinephric space, and collateral vessels form in response to a vascular lesion but do not indicate extension of tumor. Likewise, perinephric stranding should not be considered a sign of extracapsular tumor spread. Perinephric stranding results from thickening of perinephric septa by edema, inflammation, or vascular congestion. Although fascial thickening often results from direct tumor spread, it can on occasion result from reactive edema or hyperemia. The most reliable imaging sign of RCC spread to the perinephric space is the presence of a discrete perinephric soft-tissue mass. The presence of a focal perinephric mass larger than 1 cm in diameter is strongly indicative of Stage II RCC. This finding is seen in less than 50% of patients with Stage II disease. To date, the reliable differentiation between Stage I and Stage II disease remains in the domain of the pathologist.

Other staging quandaries encountered when using CT or MR imaging include bulky right renal masses that obscure the right renal vein and adjacent inferior vena cava, vena cava wall invasion *versus* intraluminal tumor thrombus, and differentiation of RCCs abutting adjacent organs from those invading adjacent organs.

Although MR imaging is very accurate in staging RCC, its cost, length of examination time, and somewhat limited accessibility have led most physicians to use CT as the major staging technique for RCC. Thus far, the major role of MR imaging in RCC evaluation lies primarily in staging of RCC left indeterminate after CT evaluation or in imaging of patients for whom obtaining optimal CT scans is impossible. The MR imaging characteristics of RCC (Fig. 3-25) are similar to those seen on CT examination. RCC signal characteristics vary greatly from patient

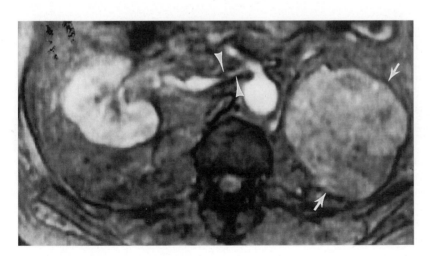

Fig. 3-25   Magnetic resonance (MR) image demonstrating a left renal cell carcinoma. This axial gradient–echo MR image demonstrates a solid, heterogeneous mass (arrows) in the left kidney. With gradient–echo techniques, flowing blood has high signal. The left renal vein (arrowheads) is normal without extension of tumor as it crosses under the superior mesenteric artery.

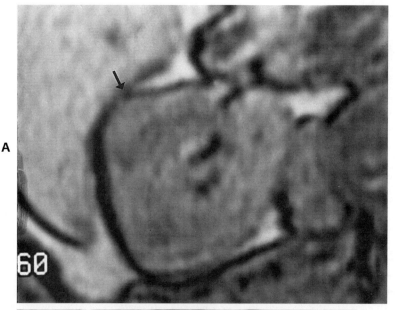

A

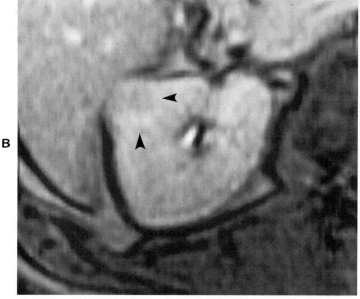

B

Fig. 3-26 Magnetic resonance (MR) image of a small renal cell carcinoma that demonstrates enhancement with gadolinium infusion. **A,** This axial T_1-weighted MR imaging of the right kidney demonstrates a subtle contour abnormality (arrow). This bulge has similar signal characteristics as the remainder of the kidney. **B,** After gadolinium infusion, a T_1-weighted axial image demonstrates peripheral enhancement (arrowheads) of this small renal cell carcinoma.

to patient. RCCs may be similar to surrounding kidney in signal characteristics, depending on scanner field strength and imaging parameters, and some RCCs are isointense with surrounding parenchyma on T_1 and T_2 pulse sequences. Therefore, the diagnosis of RCC depends on visualization of a contour-disrupting mass, and small RCCs could be undetectable. Gadolinium contrast enhancement overcomes this limitation (Fig. 3-26). With gadolinium injection, as with injection of contrast material for CT, RCCs enhance and become conspicuous within renal parenchyma. The diagnosis of RCC with MR imaging particularly is useful in patients for whom iodinated intravascular contrast media present a significant health risk because gadolinium injection is safe in these patients. Additionally, multiplanar MR images can

be helpful in determining the organ of origin of tumors when this remains unclear after CT and US examination.

With MR imaging, as with CT, no reliable criteria have been established for differentiating Stage I and Stage II RCC. Multiplanar imaging of the abdomen and the ability to enhance the signal of flowing blood make MR imaging helpful for staging RCC. Sagittal and coronal MR images usually are definitive in excluding the presence of direct adjacent organ invasion when a fat plane exists between the RCC and that organ. Altered signal characteristics within adjacent organs must be interpreted with care when they are the sole abnormality, because signal changes in compressed segments of liver resulting from congestion and edema may mimic changes of direct invasion. The degree of venous tumor extension also is accu-

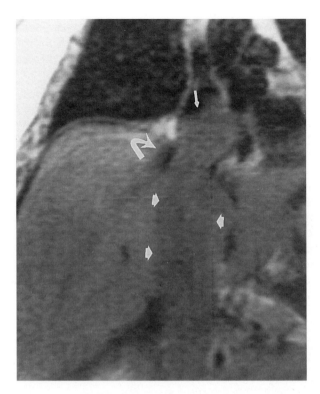

Fig. 3-27   Coronal magnetic resonance (MR) image demonstrating the extent of tumor thrombus. This coronal MR imaging scan demonstrates extensive renal cell carcinoma in the inferior vena cava (arrowheads). The upper extent of this tumor (arrow) is in the right atrium, well above the hepatic vein entry (curved arrow) into the inferior vena cava.

rately depicted with multiplanar MR imaging (Fig. 3-27). Coronal scans usually show the level of hepatic vein entry into the inferior vena cava. Tumor extension at or above the level of the hepatic veins dictates the surgical approach. If the tumor does not extend beyond hepatic inflow, an abdominal approach may be used for tumor excision and thrombectomy. Extension above this level necessitates an intrathoracic approach, which requires intraoperative cardiopulmonary bypass.

Although venous extension of tumor thrombus is well demonstrated with standard spin–echo T_1-weighted images, on which flowing blood appears black because of signal void, low flip-angle gradient–echo scans enhance the signal of flowing blood (Fig. 3-25). The resulting "bright blood" images are similar in appearance to inferior vena cavograms and renal vein phlebography; thrombus appears as a low-signal filling defect surrounded by the high signal of flowing blood.

With MR imaging metastatic deposits in the liver can be detected readily and distinguished from benign hemangiomas. Metastases to the spleen can be very difficult to identify because of the MR imaging characteristics of the spleen, which can mask focal tumors.

The accuracy of MR imaging in detecting lymphadenopathy is similar to that of CT. However, as with CT,

size is the only reliable MR imaging criterion for detecting abnormal lymph nodes. MR imaging has no advantage over CT in evaluating RCC involvement of lymph nodes that are normal or equivocal in size.

Distant metastases can be detected by MR imaging, but with no proven advantage over CT imaging. MR imaging may be more sensitive than CT in the detection of unsuspected bony metastases because of its exquisite bone marrow imaging capability.

Sonography is less accurate than either CT or MR imaging for staging of RCC. Sonography should not be used as the sole modality for staging RCC. Ultrasound examination may be a helpful adjunct to other imaging techniques in staging problematic RCCs. The major limitations of sonography in staging RCC are the inability to image the renal vein and the subhepatic inferior vena cava reliably and the limited detection of abdominal lymphadenopathy. For staging, it mainly is used as an adjunct examination when tumor extension into the inferior vena cava is detected with CT scanning but the exact superior extent of the tumor thrombus cannot be determined by CT. In these patients, ultrasound examination is completely accurate in determining whether tumor thrombus extends into the intrahepatic inferior vena cava (Fig. 3-28). This portion of the vena cava can be visualized by ultrasound examination in 100% of patients. Likewise, tumor thrombus in this segment of the IVC is identifiable whenever present. Because the level of extension of tumor thrombus within the inferior vena cava affects management planning, this is an important indication for ultrasound evaluation of these enigmatic RCCs. Although this area also can be evaluated with either MR imaging or venography, sonography is the most cost-effective technique to resolve this isolated staging problem.

Oncocytoma

Oncocytomas are benign renal tumors with no metastatic potential. Unfortunately, preoperative diagnosis often is impossible because imaging characteristics of these lesions overlap substantially with those of RCC. In addition, biopsy is of little value because some RCCs contain benign-appearing oncocytic elements that are indistinguishable from an oncocytoma. In imaging renal masses, one goal is to look for findings that suggest histology other than RCC (Boxes 3-10 to 3-16). If such findings are present, they suggest the possibility of a benign entity preoperatively. The surgeon then can consider renal-sparing surgery if open biopsy confirms a benign lesion. Some imaging features are suggestive of oncocytoma. On IVU, oncocytomas often are large at initial detection and have very smooth margins. Ultrasound findings are nonspecific. Oncocytomas usually are isoechoic to the kidney, with well-demarcated margins. Masses that exceed 6 cm in diameter may have areas of central necrosis. A central scar, typical of oncocytoma, may be visible on ultrasound examination. With CT or MR imaging, these lesions appear well circumscribed and have homogeneous enhancement patterns. Often, the appearance of a pseudocapsule is seen at the periphery of the mass. The pseudocapsule is formed from renal parenchyma

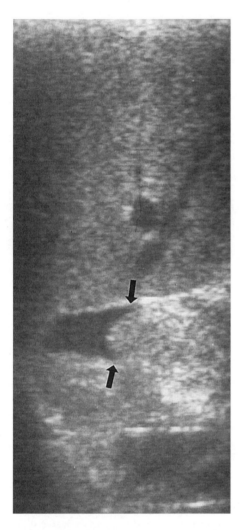

Fig. 3-28 Sonogram demonstrating tumor extension into the inferior vena cava. A longitudinal transabdominal sonogram demonstrates the upper extent of this renal cell carcinoma (arrows) within the intrahepatic inferior vena cava.

Box 3-10 Features of Oncocytoma

Typically, 50- to 70-year-old men
Solid exophytic renal mass
Isoechoic or heterogeneous on ultrasound examination
Homogeneous enhancement with computed tomography
Pseudocapsule
Central scar typical
"Spoke wheel" arteriographic pattern

---

compressed around the edge of the mass. As these lesions enlarge, a central, stellate scar may be detectable with CT (Fig. 3-29) or MR imaging. Although this scar is typical of oncocytoma, it is not diagnostic, and RCC may have an identical appearance. Angiography may be obtained before attempting renal-sparing surgery. The typical angiographic pattern of an oncocytoma is one of a "spoke wheel" with circumferential vessels at the periphery of the lesions and feeding vessels penetrating to the avascular central scar (Fig. 3-30). These tumors lack the bizarre tumor vascularity often seen with RCC. At best, the presence of some of these imaging features may suggest the possibility of an oncocytoma and may prompt an attempted renal-sparing approach to the tumor. At surgery, histologic assessment of the specimen can confirm the diagnosis of oncocytoma. If malignant elements indicating an RCC are found, partial or radical nephrectomy can be completed.

Multilocular cystic nephroma

Multilocular cystic nephroma (MLCN) is an interesting benign renal mass that occurs uncommonly. Epidemiologically, these lesions have a biphasic peak of occur-

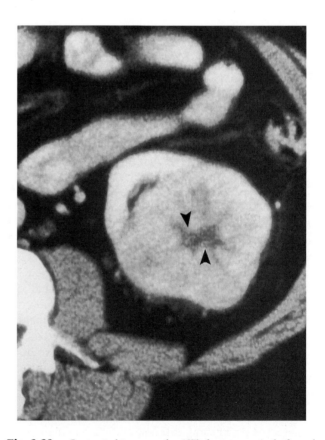

Fig. 3-29 Computed tomography (CT) features typical of renal oncocytoma. This contrast-infused CT scan demonstrates a homogeneous renal mass with a central stellate scar (arrowheads). Although this mass was an oncocytoma, there is considerable overlap of these imaging features with renal cell carcinomas.

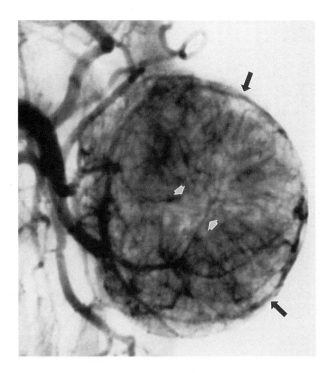

Fig. 3-30 Typical angiographic features of an oncocytoma. This oncocytoma demonstrates the typical "spoke wheel" angiographic pattern. A rim of blood vessels (arrows) outlines the mass, and radially arrayed vessels penetrate the mass centrally. A relatively avascular stellate scar is located centrally (arrowheads).

Box 3-11 Features of Multilocular Cystic Nephroma
50% occur in boys aged less than 3 years 50% occur in women aged more than 40 years Exophytic cystic renal mass Herniation into collecting system commonly Enhancing septa with computed tomography Hemorrhage absent Hypo- or avascular with arteriography

rence; half of these lesions occur in boys aged less than 3 years, and the other half occur mostly in middle-aged women (Box 3-11). These tumors, which originate from primitive metanephric blastema, are smooth masses with innumerable septations. The septa within an MLCN may be visible with IVU. MLCNs have a predilection to herniate into the renal pelvis from the renal parenchyma. This herniation is very characteristic of MLCN. On ultrasound examination, these masses appear multiloculated with numerous sonolucent areas with interspersed echogenic septations (Fig. 3-31). With CT or MR imaging, MLCNs are well-defined masses with visible septations (Fig. 3-31). Internal hemorrhage characteristically is absent in these benign tumors. MLCNs are hypovascular or avascular. Like oncocytomas, these tumors have characteristic fea-

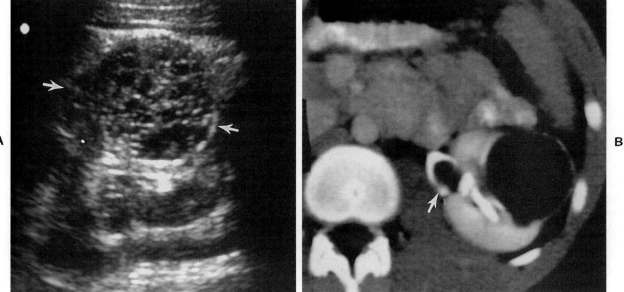

Fig. 3-31 Sonogram and computed tomogram (CT) of a multilocular cystic nephroma. **A,** Sonography of this renal mass (arrows) demonstrates numerous cystic locules with interposed septa. **B,** CT of this same mass demonstrates features typical of a multilocular cystic nephroma. This cystic mass is well circumscribed with thin septations. Centrally, it is seen to herniate (arrow) into the renal pelvis.

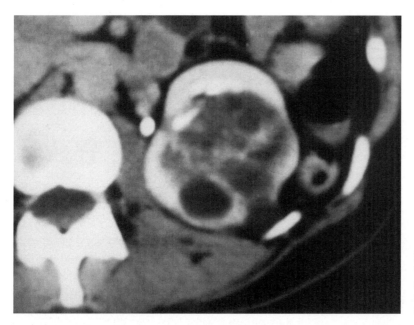

Fig. 3-32 Multilocular cystic renal cell carcinoma. This contrast-infused computed tomography demonstrates a multilocular cystic renal mass with thick septa. This mass surgically was proven to be a renal cell carcinoma.

tures, none of which, however, distinguish them reliably from RCC. Therefore, at best, one can suggest the diagnosis preoperatively, so that renal-sparing surgery may be attempted in some patients.

When a multiloculated cystic renal mass is detected, MLCN should come to mind. Other diagnoses should be considered as well (Box 3-12), including cystic RCC (Fig. 3-32), segmental multicystic dysplastic kidney (MDK), localized renal cystic disease (LRCD), and renal abscess. Of these, RCC is the most common. Multilocular cystic RCC often is indistinguishable from benign diseases before surgery. RCC usually occurs in later life and more commonly in men than in women. A cystic RCC often contains solid areas of contrast-enhancing tissue. Cystic RCCs may show other evidence of malignancy, including

---

Box 3-12 Causes of Multilocular Cystic Renal Masses

Common
    Renal cell carcinoma
    Septated renal cyst
    Renal abscess
Uncommon
    Segmental multicystic dysplastic kidney
    Wilms' tumor
    Multilocular cystic nephroma
Rare
    Focal xanthogranulomatous pyelonephritis
    Malacoplakia
    Localized renal cystic disease
    Echinococcus

---

intratumoral hemorrhage, extensive neovascularity, and marginal irregularity. RCC grows by expansion and characteristically does not extend into the lumen of the renal pelvis, as does MLCN. Segmental MDK is a rare, localized form of MDK. It is seen segmentally only when renal duplication is present. As with other forms of MDK, the involved area is nonfunctional or minimally functional. The normal renal parenchyma is replaced with cystic areas because of failure of induction of maturation of the primitive metanephric blastema. The cysts usually are of varying size and are spread randomly throughout the involved area. The presence of a duplication anomaly and absence of hemorrhage, function, and contrast-enhancing solid components help to distinguish MDK from cystic RCC. LRCD is a rare cause of a multiloculated renal mass mimicking MLCN. It is caused by the development of numerous simple renal cysts in a focal area of one kidney. This condition is idiopathic and nonfamilial. The collection of cysts appears tumefactive because it is localized, but close scrutiny of CT or MR images reveals a nonencapsulated cluster of cysts with interspersed functioning renal parenchyma. The remainder of the affected kidney and the entire contralateral kidney are normal. The imaging key to the diagnosis of this nonprogressive, benign entity is recognition that it is a cluster of cysts rather than a multiloculated cystic tumor. Usually, at least one cyst is separated from the cluster by normal renal tissue. This finding, in addition to the lack of abnormalities in the remainder of the kidneys, strongly suggests a diagnosis of LRCD.

Renal abscess

Renal abscesses usually result from inadequate management of pyelonephritis, which leads to central lique-

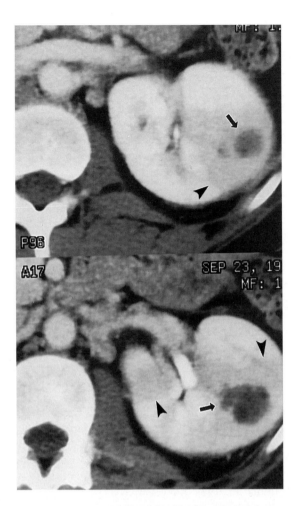

Fig. 3-33 Computed tomography (CT) scan of a renal abscess. Two contiguous CT slices through a left renal abscess (arrows). This cystic mass is very irregular, and the kidney demonstrates numerous heterogeneous areas of enhancement (arrowheads), typical of pyelonephritis in association with this renal abscess.

faction and formation of a discrete intrarenal abscess. The majority of patients with renal abscess have clinical symptoms that are resistant to standard antibiotic therapy, suggesting pyelonephritis. Although imaging typically is not used in the evaluation of routine pyelonephritis, renal infections with clinical symptoms that continue beyond 72 hours despite appropriate antibiotic manage-

ment suggest the possibility of renal abscess. CT is the best imaging modality for diagnosis of renal abscesses, because some small abscesses are undetectable by ultrasound examination and IVU. Abscesses, when visible, appear as thick-walled cystic masses on IVU or US evaluation (Box 3-13). On ultrasound examination, lesions usually have mixed echogenicity and less through sound transmission than simple cysts of comparable size. On CT examination, abscesses appear as rounded, well-defined, low-density masses with central liquefaction (Fig. 3-33). These lesions usually have a thick peripheral wall if they extend beyond the confines of the renal capsule and perinephric signs of inflammation, including septal thickening and perinephric fluid. With injection of contrast material, there is substantial rim enhancement around the abscess. Occasionally, gas is evident within an abscess. This finding is diagnostic of abscess. The presence of a renal abscess generally indicates the need for percutaneous drainage in conjunction with systemic antibiotic management. It is imperative that ureteral obstruction, if coexistent, also be managed to improve renal blood flow and antibiotic delivery to the renal parenchyma.

Focal xanthogranulomatous pyelonephritis

Tumefactive or focal xanthogranulomatous pyelonephritis (XGP) results from a focal area of renal inflammation. Typically, XGP occurs with chronic infection-based stone disease and urinary infection (Box 3-14). All forms of XGP occur in women more often than in men. In some patients, lipid-laden histocytes focally infiltrate and replace the involved renal parenchyma. As a result, focal renal masses may form and mimic malignancy. Ipsilateral renal stones are evident in at least 80% of these patients. The inflammatory masses formed by tumefactive XGP are nonfunctional, although some enhancement may occur with contrast injection. A history of chronic urinary tract infection is typical and may suggest the etiology of these masses. No imaging characteristics are diagnostic of focal XGP. With IVU, a hypofunctioning focal mass is evident. On ultrasound examination, this mass may have increased echogenicity resulting from the innumerable lipid-laden macrophages that make up the mass. On CT examination, focal XGP appears as a nonspecific solid or cystic renal mass, often in association with a renal calculus (Fig. 3-34).

Box 3-13 Features of Renal Abscess

Clinical evidence of infection
Hypoechoic with less through sound transmission than cyst
Thick wall rim enhancement on computed tomography
Neovascularity in wall on arteriogram

Box 3-14 Features of Focal Xanthogranulomatous Pyelonephritis

Middle-aged women with recurrent urinary infections
Focal hypofunctioning renal mass
Infection-based stones common

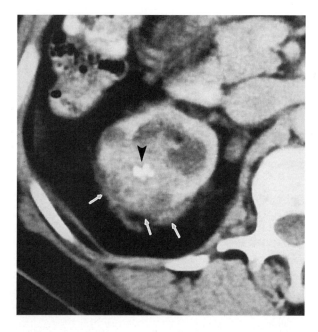

Fig. 3-34 Focal xanthogranulomatous pyelonephritis. This contrast-infused computed tomography scan of an elderly woman with chronic urinary tract infections demonstrates an inhomogeneous mass (arrows) in the upper pole of the right kidney. A stone (arrowhead) is centered in this renal mass, and there is adjacent thickening of perinephric septa.

Perinephric inflammatory changes often coexist with XGP. Typical history and these imaging features may suggest the diagnosis of focal XGP before surgery. These lesions are irreversible and are best managed with renal-sparing surgery.

Renal metastases

Rarely, a solitary renal metastasis or solitary focus of renal lymphoma may occur. In a patient with known extrarenal malignancy, percutaneous biopsy or surgical biopsy usually is necessary to distinguish RCC from a

Box 3-15 Features of Renal Lymphoma
Usually with systemic lymphoma
Usually bilateral
Multifocal, diffuse, or focal pattern
Hypoechoic without through sound transmission
Often with massive lymphadenopathy

solitary metastasis. Lesions that account for most renal metastases include carcinoma of the breast, lung, or gastrointestinal tract or malignant melanoma. Also, lymphoma commonly spreads to the kidneys, but true primary renal lymphoma is extremely rare. Most patients in whom lymphoma spreads to the kidney have extensive lymphoma elsewhere (Box 3-15). Probably as a result of its spread along lymphatics, lymphoma has a predilection for spread directly from the retroperitoneum into the renal sinus (Fig. 3-35) and perinephric space (Fig. 3-36) concurrently with parenchymal invasion. A solitary renal lymphoma metastasis in a patient with lymphoma is very uncommon. When present, renal lymphoma usually appears as a homogeneous solid mass. IVU, CT, and MR imaging features of focal renal lymphoma are nonspecific. Sonographic features often are typical of renal lymphoma, regardless of its distribution in the kidney. More common than a solitary focal mass in patients with renal lymphoma are two other patterns. In the majority of patients, multiple homogeneous parenchymal implants (Fig. 3-37), typical of a hematogenous spread pattern, are detectable with CT or MR imaging. The second most common appearance with renal lymphoma is that of diffuse infiltration of the kidney, which usually is a bilateral process that leads to reniform enlargement (Fig. 3-38) and diminished function of the kidney. This pattern also can be seen in renal involvement with leukemia and

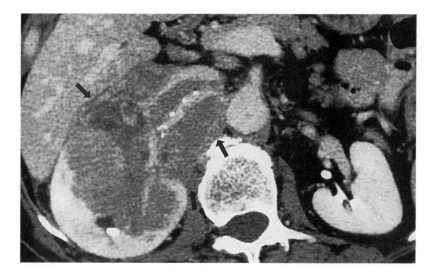

Fig. 3-35 Retroperitoneal lymphoma spreading into the perinephric space. This contrast-infused computed tomography scan from a patient with non-Hodgkin's lymphoma demonstrates a retroperitoneal mass (arrows) originating adjacent to the aorta, encasing the renal vessels, and spreading into the renal sinus and the renal parenchyma. This pattern is very suggestive of lymphoma.

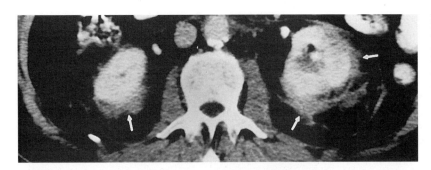

Fig. 3-36 Perinephric involvement from lymphoma. This contrast-infused computed tomography scan demonstrates irregular soft-tissue masses (arrows) encasing both kidneys. The perinephric space is a favorite area of spread for lymphoma.

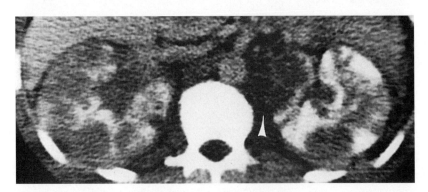

Fig. 3-37 Renal lymphomas with multiple parenchymal masses. This contrast-infused computed tomography scan demonstrates innumerable focal low attenuation masses in the parenchyma of both kidneys. Typical of lymphoma, these masses are homogeneous with little mass effect and no contour deformity. The normally enhancing renal parenchyma is displaced minimally by these infiltrating metastases. Associated retroperitoneal lymphadenopathy (arrowhead) also is present.

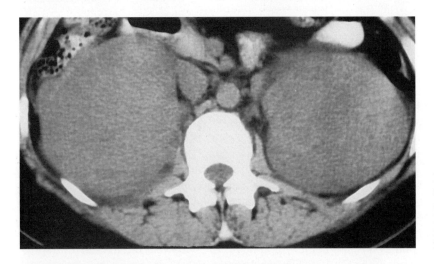

Fig. 3-38 Diffuse infiltration of the kidneys from lymphoma. This uninfused computed tomography scan demonstrates massive reniform enlargement of both kidneys secondary to lymphoma infiltration. The kidneys are homogeneous, with loss of normal architectural patterns.

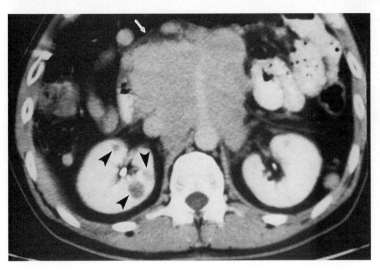

Fig. 3-39 Massive retroperitoneal lymphadenopathy with associated renal metastases. This contrast-infused computed tomography scan demonstrates multiple homogeneous renal masses (arrowheads) resulting from lymphoma. In addition, there is massive retroperitoneal lymphadenopathy (arrow). This degree of lymphadenopathy is very typical of lymphoma, and its presence implies the etiology of the renal masses.

is more commonly seen with leukemia than with lymphoma. On ultrasound examination, renal lymphoma often has a typical appearance because lymphoma masses are formed from a proliferation of a monoclonal line of cells that form a densely packed homogeneous mass. On ultrasound examination, the masses are homogeneously hypoechoic or anechoic, with no through sound transmission. This appearance should not be confused with the similar, yet distinctive, appearance seen with simple cysts, which exhibit considerable through sound transmission. Renal lymphoma often is associated with coexistent retroperitoneal adenopathy. The adenopathy may be massive (Fig. 3-39 on p. 105) and suggests lymphoma rather than RCC in a patient with a solitary renal mass. Massive adenopathy uncommonly is associated with RCC. Otherwise, in the rare case of a solitary renal mass attributable to lymphoma, preoperative diagnosis will be impossible based on the imaging characteristics alone.

Angiomyolipoma

Angiomyolipoma is one of the most important of the renal masses described. It is one of the few masses that usually can be diagnosed definitively on the basis of imaging features (Box 3-16) alone without the need for surgery or biopsy. Angiomyolipomas are not rare renal masses, but most angiomyolipomas are found incidentally and do not cause symptoms. Approximately 80% of angiomyolipomas occur in middle-aged adults and most frequently in women. These lesions usually are small, solitary, and asymptomatic. The remaining 20% of patients with angiomyolipomas have tuberous sclerosis, a syndrome that is described more fully later in this chapter. Among patients with tuberous sclerosis, angiomyolipomas are common, developing in approximately 80%. These patients usually have multiple bilateral angiomyolipomas, which commonly attain a large size and often cause symptoms (Fig. 3-21). Angiomyolipomas associated with tuberous sclerosis usually are detectable before the fourth decade of life, earlier than angiomyolipomas unassociated with tuberous sclerosis. Although angiomyolipomas may become symptomatic, they are benign hamartomas. Angiomyolipomas are made up of varying

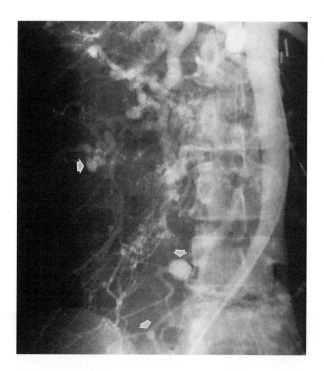

Fig. 3-40 Hypervascular angiomyolipoma with aneurysms on feeding vessels. This patient with tuberous sclerosis had a massive right-sided angiomyolipoma. This arteriogram demonstrates diffuse neovascularity with aneurysms (arrowheads) on several of the feeding vessels. This angiographic pattern is typical of angiomyolipomas.

proportions of angioid, myoid, and lipoid components. Some angiomyolipomas contain a large angioid component, i.e., they are hypervascular. Typically, small aneurysms develop on some of the arteries feeding an angiomyolipoma (Fig. 3-40). This angiographic finding suggests the diagnosis angiomyolipoma, but it can occur with other tumors, including RCC. These vascular lesions may hemorrhage spontaneously, and the hemorrhage may be massive and life threatening. When angiomyolipomas become symptomatic, the symptoms often result from spontaneous hemorrhage. Other symptoms may be caused purely by mass effect when an angiomyolipoma compresses adjacent structures. Because most angiomyolipomas are detected incidentally, protocols have been developed to determine which of these lesions require prophylactic excision. A general rule states that angiomyolipomas smaller than 4 cm in diameter rarely become symptomatic and should be followed with sonographic evaluation every 6 to 12 months. Angiomyolipomas larger than 4 cm in diameter are more likely to hemorrhage and therefore often are excised surgically with renal-sparing partial nephrectomy. If larger angiomyolipomas are not amenable to renal-sparing surgery, sonographic monitoring may be used to detect angiomyolipoma enlargement or development of complicating features that would necessitate nephrectomy.

Box 3-16   Features of Angiomyolipoma

80% in adults (usually women), aged 30 to 50 years
20% in patients with tuberous sclerosis
Well-defined hyperechoic mass
Fat, even small amounts, diagnostic with computed
   tomography
Neovascularity with aneurysms on arteriography
Unlikely to bleed if <4 cm

In the diagnosis of angiomyolipoma with imaging techniques, intratumoral fat is the key component. At least 90% of angiomyolipomas contain fat that is detectable with thin-section CT or MR imaging. The detection of fat within a renal mass (Fig. 3-41) is considered diagnostic of angiomyolipoma. Isolated cases of RCC and oncocytoma with intratumoral fat have been reported. These cases are rare, and most authorities agree that renal tumors containing fat should be diagnosed as angiomyolipomas based on the imaging features alone. The detection of intratumoral fat in a renal lesion is the only radiologic finding that can differentiate an angiomyolipoma from an RCC. Therefore, efforts must be made to detect small foci of fat in renal tumors with otherwise nonspecific imaging features, thereby avoiding unnecessary surgery in patients with small, asymptomatic angiomyolipomas. Thin-section (5 mm or thinner) CT scanning optimizes the detection of intratumoral fat. In difficult cases, CT pixel mapping over a region of interest within the tumor may be useful to detect small quantities of fat. With pixel mapping, three to six continuous pixels with negative Hounsfield units averaging below −10 HU indicates intratumoral fat and a diagnosis of angiomyolipoma.

Finally, it is important to recognize that angiomyolipomas may grow with time. Therefore, once intratumoral fat has been confirmed with CT or MR imaging and the angiomyolipoma is not excised, sonographic follow-up evaluation should be performed. Approximately 25% of angiomyolipomas smaller than 4 cm will grow during an observation period of 4 years or less. Up to 50% of larger

A

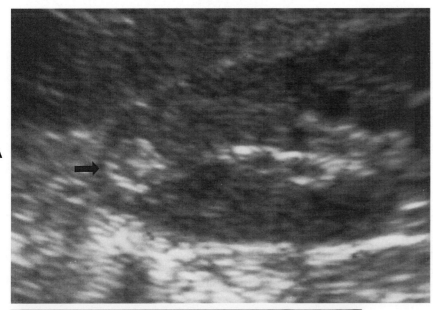

B

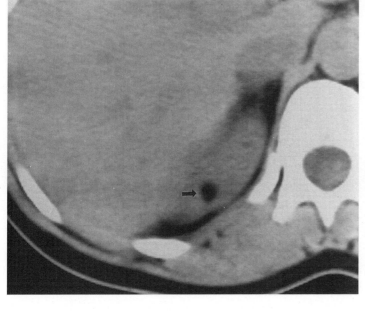

Fig. 3-41 Sonogram and computed tomography (CT) scan of a small angiomyolipoma. **A,** A well-circumscribed, hyperechoic lesion (arrow) is present in the upper pole of the right kidney. **B,** An uninfused CT scan through this region demonstrates that this mass (arrow) contains low attenuation fat, which is diagnostic of angiomyolipoma.

angiomyolipomas will demonstrate growth during a similar observation period. Angiomyolipoma enlargement progresses more rapidly in patients who also have tuberous sclerosis than in patients without tuberous sclerosis. Although angiomyolipoma usually grows slowly, growth rates cannot be predicted on the basis of initial imaging features. Continued growth of an angiomyolipoma may prompt prophylactic excision, even in asymptomatic patients.

Multiple Expansile Renal Masses

Multiple primary renal masses (Box 3-17) have the same appearance as their solitary counterparts. Other clinical features, such as the presence of a coexistent syndrome, often lead to the correct diagnosis.

Cysts

Multiple simple renal cysts are seen commonly in elderly patients. Usually detected incidentally, these cysts are of no clinical significance and usually are not associated with detectable renal insufficiency. The imaging features of each of these lesions are identical to those described previously for solitary simple cysts. Detection of a large number of simple cysts in a younger patient suggests an underlying disease state, most commonly autosomal dominant polycystic kidney disease (ADPKD). Patients with ADPKD usually present when aged 20 to 39 years with clinical symptoms such as flank pain, pyelonephritis, hematuria, urolithiasis, hypertension, or renal insufficiency. The diagnosis of ADPKD can be made with ultrasound examination or other imaging techniques, such as CT (Fig. 3-42) or MR imaging. IVU often is bypassed because these patients usually have renal insufficiency at presentation. CT may be more sensitive than sonography for detecting cysts early in the course of ADPKD. Because ADPKD is inherited in an autosomal dominant pattern, approximately 50% of the children of an afflicted parent will develop the disease. This disease has a high penetrance rate; that is, the disease develops clinically in nearly all people who inherit the gene for ADPKD. Criteria have been developed for diagnosis of ADPKD in persons genetically at risk before clinical symptoms develop. For persons at risk, ADPKD should be diagnosed if renal ultrasound examination demonstrates two or more cysts in both kidneys combined in a person aged less than 30 years. Two or more renal cysts in each kidney are indicative of ADPKD in patients who are aged between 30 and 60 years. Patients aged more than 60 years with ADPKD will have at least four detectable renal cysts in each kidney. The risk of renal malignancy does not appear to be increased in these patients. However, extrarenal abnormalities are common. Cysts of other abdominal viscera are most frequent; up to 50% of these patients have coexistent simple cysts in the liver (Fig. 3-43). Less common sites of cysts include the pancreas, adnexa, spleen, or lung parenchyma. Up to 15% of these patients have berry aneurysms in their central nervous system (CNS) circulation. In addition, the incidence of

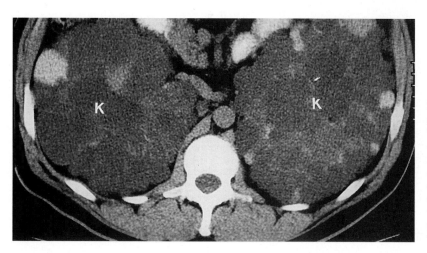

Fig. 3-42 Computed tomography (CT) scan of autosomal dominant polycystic kidney disease. This unenhanced CT scan through the kidneys demonstrates massive enlargement of both kidneys (K). The normal renal parenchyma is replaced completely with renal cysts. Some of these cysts demonstrate high attenuation, indicating previous complications with internal hemorrhage or proteinaceous contents. This radiographic pattern is typical of advanced autosomal dominant polycystic kidney disease.

Box 3-18   Syndromes Associated with Multiple Renal Cysts*

Acrorenal-mandibular syndrome
Apert's syndrome
Beckwith-Wiedemann syndrome
Brachmann-de Lange syndrome
Caroli's syndrome
Cerebrocostomandibular
Chondrodysplasia punctata
Congenital rubella
Cutis laxa
Deletion of long arm of chromosome 13
DiGeorge's syndrome
Duplication of long arm of chromosome 10
Duplication of short arm of chromosome 10
Ectromelia-ichthyosis syndrome
Ehlers-Danlos syndrome
Elajalde syndrome
Goldenhar's syndrome
Goldson's syndrome
Hajdu-Cheney syndrome
Jeune's asphyxiating thoracic dystrophy
Kaufman-McKusick syndrome
Laurence-Moon or Bardet-Biedl syndrome
Lissencephaly syndrome
Maizer-Saldino syndrome
Marden-Walker syndrome
Meckel-Gruber syndrome
Miranda's syndrome
Myotonic dystrophy
Nail–patella syndrome
Noonan's syndrome
Oculo-renal syndrome
Oral-facial-digital syndrome, type no. 1 (Gorlin's syndrome)
Passage
Robert's syndrome (pseudothalidomide syndrome)
Schwartz-Jampel syndrome
Senior-Loken syndrome
Simopoulos' short rib–polydactyl syndrome
Spherocytosis
Translocation syndrome
Triploidy
Trisomy 13-15 (trisomy D)–Patau's syndrome
Trisomy 16-18 (trisomy E)–Edward's syndrome
Trisomy 21–Down syndrome
Tuberous sclerosis
Turner's syndrome
von Hippel-Lindau syndrome
Zellweger's syndrome (cerebrohepatorenal syndrome)

*Adapted from Hartman DS: An overview of renal cystic disease, In Hartman DS, ed: *Renal cystic disease*, Philadelphia, 1989, WB Saunders.

valvular heart disease and coarctation of the aorta appears to be increased in patients with ADPKD.

Cysts detected predominantly in the medulla of the kidney suggest a different entity: medullary cystic disease, which is characterized by progressive salt-wasting nephropathy with renal insufficiency. Another variety of this entity is juvenile nephronophthisis, which usually develops during childhood or early adolescence. These related diseases inevitably lead to irreversible renal failure, resulting from progressive tubular atrophy.

Multiple simple renal cysts have been described in association with numerous syndromes of multiple malformations. Some of these are listed in Box 3-18.

von Hippel-Lindau disease

Several diseases are associated with the development of renal neoplasms and renal cysts. These include von Hippel-Lindau disease (VHL), acquired cystic disease of dialysis, and tuberous sclerosis. RCC develops in 40% of patients with VHL. In 75% of these patients, multifocal RCC develops. In addition, up to 75% of patients with VHL have simple renal cysts. Characteristically, these patients also develop hemangioblastomas of the CNS (Fig. 3-44). These are benign, slow-growing tumors of the cerebellum or the spinal cord. Retinal angiomas are another component of VHL. The coexistence of multiple RCCs and simple renal cysts (Fig. 3-45) strongly suggests the diagnosis of VHL. In addition, multiple pancreatic cysts occur in up to 50% of patients with VHL. These pancreatic cysts may be extensive, replacing most of the pancreas. In some patients, pancreatic insufficiency and diabetes mellitus result. Pancreatic cysts are uncommon in other diseases affecting the kidneys. In patients with VHL, simple cysts may develop in other abdominal viscera, including the liver and spleen. Other neoplasms that may develop in patients with VHL include pheochromocytomas, hepatic adenomas, pancreatic adenocarcinomas, islet cell tumors, and pancreatic microcystic adenomas. Of these, pheochromocytomas are the most common. They occur in up to 15% of these patients. Fifty to eighty percent of patients with VHL who have a pheochromocytoma will have multiple, often bilateral, and extraadrenal pheochromocytomas.

Acquired cystic disease of dialysis

Up to 7% of patients undergoing long-term dialysis will develop RCC. The development of RCC usually follows the development of cystic disease of the kidneys (Fig. 3-46) seen in association with renal insufficiency and long-term dialysis. Dysplastic cells are believed to line the margins of many of these acquired cysts and lead to a predilection for the development of RCC. The radiographic features of RCC (Fig. 3-47) in patients undergoing dialysis are identical to those seen elsewhere. Most RCCs that develop in these patients have a low metastatic

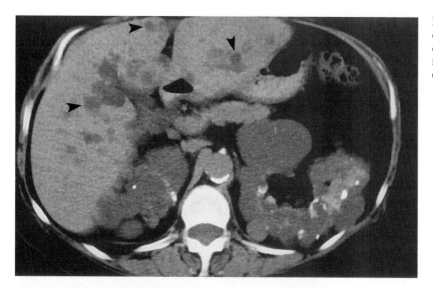

Fig. 3-43 Autosomal dominant polycystic disease with hepatic involvement. Extensive bilateral cysts are noted. Some of these cysts contain calcifications. As is common, numerous simple cysts (arrowheads) of the liver also are present.

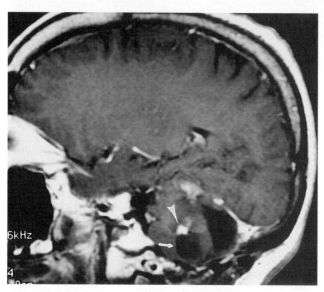

Fig. 3-44 Hemangioblastoma of the cerebellum in a patient with von Hippel-Lindau disease. This sagittal MR imaging scan demonstrates a cystic mass (arrow) in the cerebellum. There is a brightly enhancing mural nodule (arrowhead) in this mass. These features are typical of hemangioblastoma.

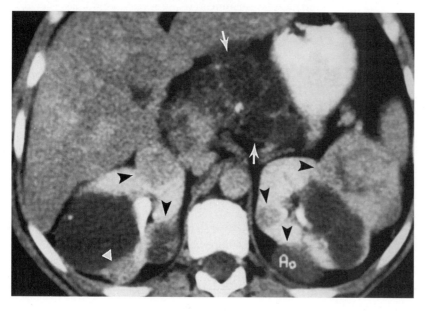

Fig. 3-45 Renal cell carcinomas, cysts, and pancreatic cysts in a patient with von Hippel-Lindau disease (VHL). This contrast-infused computed tomography scan demonstrates numerous pancreatic cysts (arrows). Cystic renal lesions are noted in association with multiple renal cell carcinomas (arrowheads). This constellation of abnormalities is typical of VHL.

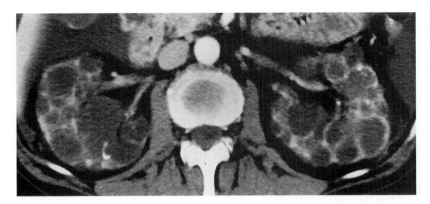

Fig. 3-46 Acquired cystic disease of dialysis. This contrast-infused computed tomography scan demonstrates innumerable simple cysts spread throughout both kidneys. This patient developed these cysts after the initiation of hemodialysis.

potential. Because of the less aggressive behavior of these RCCs and the limited life expectancy of patients undergoing dialysis, the clinical significance of the need for removal of these RCCs has been the subject of some controversy. In our opinions, because the clinical course of these tumors is unpredictable, nephrectomy should be undertaken unless the patient's life expectancy is very limited.

Tuberous sclerosis

Renal abnormalities that are seen with tuberous sclerosis have been described previously. Eighty percent of these patients develop renal angiomyolipomas, and simple renal cysts often coexist with angiomyolipomas in patients with tuberous sclerosis. In a subset of these patients, usually those in whom tuberous sclerosis is diagnosed during childhood, innumerable renal cysts develop (Fig. 3-48) without associated renal angiomyolipomas. The radiographic appearance of these kidneys mimics that seen with ADPKD, but that disease is not a part of the family history, and other signs of tuberous sclerosis usually are present. Tuberous sclerosis is an autosomal recessive disorder, and patients usually have adenoma sebaceum, seizures, and mental retardation. However, one or more of these abnormalities may be absent. Ade-

noma sebaceum is a multifocal, wart-like lesion that occurs in a malar distribution on the face. Seizures and mental retardation in patients with tuberous sclerosis usually result from CNS damage caused by cerebral hamartomas. These appear as periventricular calcifications (Fig. 3-49) on CNS imaging studies. Rarely, these hamartomas undergo malignant transformation into giant cell astrocytomas, lesions characteristically associated with tuberous sclerosis. Other manifestations include a discolored skin lesion known as a shagreen patch, cardiac rhabdomyomas and rhabdomyosarcomas, multiple skeletal osteomas, and pulmonary lymphangioleiomyomatosis. This particular pulmonary abnormality results in increased interstitial lung markings, recurrent chylous pleural effusions, and recurrent pneumothoraces. Although tuberous sclerosis is rare, its numerous manifestations increase the likelihood of encountering some of these patients.

Other multifocal renal masses

Other causes of multiple ball-shaped renal masses include multiple RCCs, metastases, lymphoma, multiple abscesses, and multiple oncocytomas. All of these are somewhat uncommon. A second RCC can be found in 2% of patients with RCC unless VHL or acquired cystic

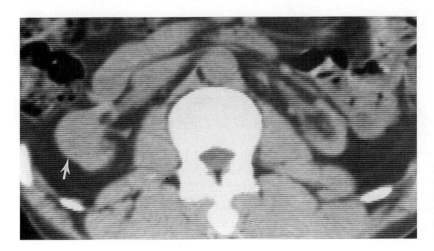

Fig. 3-47 Renal cell carcinoma in a long-term dialysis patient. This unenhanced computed tomography scan through the kidneys demonstrates renal atrophy resulting from chronic renal insufficiency. In addition, there is a 3-cm solid renal cell carcinoma (arrow) originating in the right kidney.

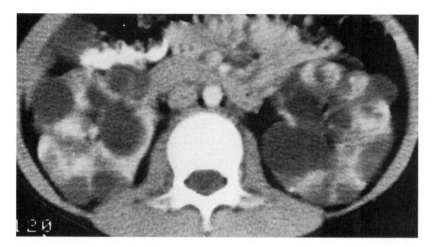

Fig. 3-48 Renal cystic disease in an 8-year-old child with tuberous sclerosis. A contrast-infused computed tomography scan through the kidneys of this child demonstrates innumerable bilateral simple renal cysts. No angiomyolipomas were detected. In a subset of patients with tuberous sclerosis, renal abnormalities similar to those seen with polycystic kidney disease develop.

disease of dialysis is present. In these subgroups, the risk of multiple RCCs is higher. The risk of multiple RCCs also appears to be higher in patients with RCCs of papillary histology. Multiple abscesses typically are seen in immunosuppressed patients, intravenous drug abusers, or patients with bacterial endocarditis who develop multiple septic emboli. Multiple oncocytomas have been reported in the literature numerous times. These lesions are virtually indistinguishable from multiple RCCs and have no apparent association with any known syndrome. The presence of a central stellate scar in these renal tumors

may suggest this diagnosis preoperatively. Most renal metastases, excluding lymphoma and SCC, lead to multiple ball-shaped masses. The multiplicity of these lesions in conjunction with the usual history of a known primary malignancy should confirm a diagnosis of secondary renal neoplasms. Percutaneous fine-needle biopsy can be performed safely if histologic confirmation is required before treatment. Renal metastases usually occur in patients with advanced malignant disease, and management of the renal lesions generally is unnecessary. Multiple masses from renal lymphoma or metastatic SCCs usually lead to multiple infiltrating renal masses, which are discussed in the next section of this chapter.

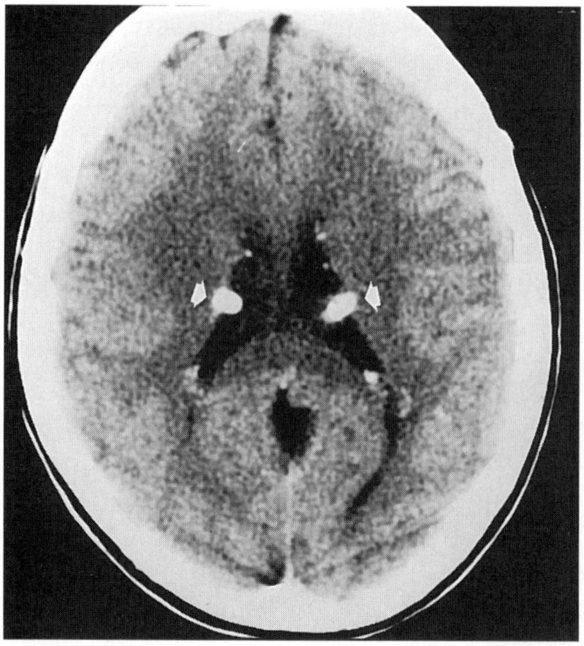

Geographic Infiltrating Renal Masses

Although the detection and characterization of exophytic renal masses are relatively straightforward tasks, geographic lesions usually are more problematic. Early in the growth of exophytic masses, renal contour deformity occurs, but the fact that infiltrating lesions lead to little or no contour deformity makes their detection more difficult. In addition, the considerable amount of overlap in the radiographic appearance among various infiltrating lesions makes their classification more challenging.

Geographic infiltrating renal masses may be unifocal or multifocal. These masses are difficult or impossible to detect with standard radiography, urography, or sonography. They often are undetectable unless intravenous contrast material is used with CT scanning. By whichever modality they are detected, these lesions, by definition, maintain the reniform shape of the kidney and have an ill-defined interface between the lesion and normal renal parenchyma. These imaging characteristics have been shown to correlate with histologic findings of infiltration of the renal parenchyma. This pattern is distinctly different from an expansile growth pattern. Therefore, a lesion that appears to be infiltrative with CT or MR imaging

Fig. 3-49 Calcified periventricular hamartomas in a patient with tuberous sclerosis. This unenhanced computed tomography scan demonstrates periventricular calcifications (arrowheads) typical of the calcified cerebral hamartomas seen in patients with tuberous sclerosis.

generally is confirmed as such on histologic examination. Not all of these lesions are neoplasms, and infiltration may result from edema, hemorrhage, or inflammation. Although imaging features of these lesions may imply or even strongly indicate a particular diagnosis, many cases remain enigmatic. Percutaneous biopsy should be used cautiously in these patients for two major reasons. First, a substantial number of these lesions result from urothelial neoplasms, such as TCC. These tumors have a tendency to seed biopsy tracts, leading to extrarenal spread of the neoplasm. Second, fine-needle biopsy of nonneoplastic infiltrating geographic lesions may yield nondiagnostic samples that do not contribute to a final diagnosis. Renal infarction, inflammation, and some renal neoplasms, such as lymphoma, may be difficult or impossible to diagnose with fine-needle aspiration or percutaneous core biopsy. Imaging features and their implications for the diagnosis may be crucial for treatment of these patients.

Geographic infiltrating renal masses are grouped into three major categories of lesions: infiltrating neoplasms, inflammatory lesions, and renal infarction. When these lesions are detected, additional clinical information may be crucial to determine the correct diagnosis.

Infiltrating neoplasms

Neoplasms that infiltrate the renal parenchyma include TCC, SCC, infiltrative RCC, renal medullary carcinoma, renal lymphoma, and some renal metastases. Except for lymphoma and metastases, these tumors are nearly always solitary and unilateral. Urothelial neoplasms, including TCC and SCC, that originate in the intrarenal collecting system spread into the kidney parenchyma in 25% of patients. Although most TCCs in the collecting system have a papillary, exophytic growth pattern, once these lesions invade the renal parenchyma, they universally spread by infiltration. Ninety percent of urothelial neoplasms result from TCC, and the remaining 10% result from SCC. Renal medullary carcinoma and infiltrative RCC are uncommon or rare. Although only TCC and SCC originate in the renal collecting system, all four of these neoplasms tend to invade calyces and lead to overlapping features when imaged with urography or retrograde pyelography. Urographic findings typical of infiltrating neoplasms include intraluminal filling defects attributable to tumor (Fig. 3-50) or blood and amputated (Figs. 3-7, 3-50) or obliterated calyces resulting from malignant infundibular stricturing. With cross-sectional imaging, TCC and SCC usually are ill-defined, soft-tissue masses (Fig. 3-50) centered within the renal sinus, sometimes with a prominent component infiltrating the parenchyma. These centrally located neoplasms usually are heterogeneous but contain calcifications in less than 2% of patients. The soft-tissue component in the renal sinus obliterates and displaces intervening fat to blend imperceptibly with the adjacent renal parenchyma. This appearance has been described as the "faceless kidney"

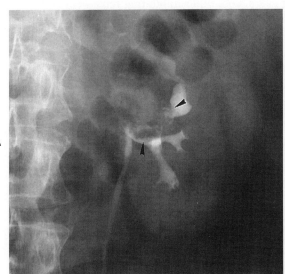 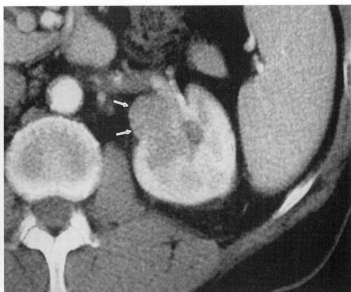

Fig. 3-50 Transitional cell carcinoma causing calyceal amputation and renal pelvic filling defects. **A,** A coned-down view of the left kidney from an intravenous urogram demonstrates a polypoid mass (arrowheads) extending into the renal pelvis. The upper pole calyces are amputated. **B,** A computed tomography scan in the same patient demonstrates a soft-tissue mass (arrows) centered in the renal sinus. At this level, the renal sinus is obliterated, and there is infiltration of the adjacent renal parenchyma.

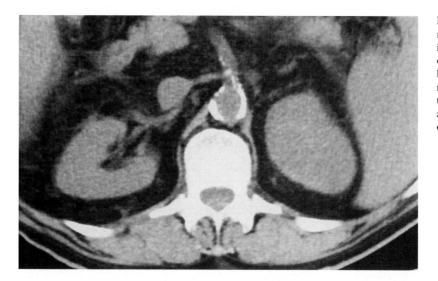

Fig. 3-51   Extensive infiltration of the left kidney from transitional cell carcinoma. This contrast-infused computed tomography scan demonstrates extensive infiltration of the lower pole of the left kidney from an infiltrating transitional cell carcinoma. There is reniform enlargement of this portion of the kidney. The kidney has a "faceless" appearance, with loss of normal architecture and obliteration of the renal sinus fat.

(Fig. 3-51). This pattern of growth is very unusual for RCC. This distinction is important because the recommended therapeutic approaches for renal TCC and RCC are different. Standard therapy for RCC is nephrectomy, whereas renal TCC is managed with nephroureterectomy with resection of a bladder cuff adjacent to the involved ureterovesical junction.

Radiographically, SCC mimics TCC, and the two usually are indistinguishable. Clues that may suggest SCC preoperatively include the fact that SCC tends to be a very aggressive, fast-growing tumor, therefore, rapid progression on sequential imaging studies favors a diagnosis of SCC. In addition, SCC develops after metaplasia of the urothelium from transitional epithelium to squamous epithelium, which usually results from chronic inflam-

mation often caused by nephrolithiasis. In up to 50% of patients with renal SCC, a coexistent renal calculus is evident on imaging studies. Therefore, the presence of a renal stone in association with a geographic infiltrating renal lesion with a large renal sinus component implies the diagnosis of SCC.

Infiltrating RCC is an unusual form of RCC. Unlike TCC, infiltrating RCC originates and is centered in the renal parenchyma (Fig. 3-52). Unfortunately, these tumors often extend into the renal sinus, making them indistinguishable from invasive TCC or SCC. Like SCC, these tumors tend to be very aggressive and have a poor prognosis. One feature can help to distinguish these infiltrating RCCs from other infiltrating renal neoplasms. Infiltrative RCCs usually are very vascular, whereas uro-

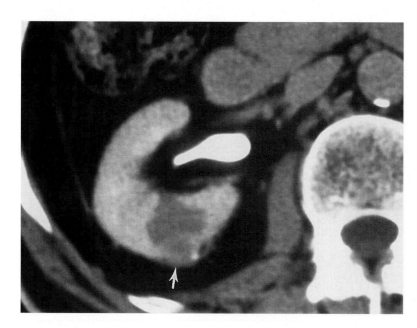

Fig. 3-52   Infiltrating renal cell carcinoma. A contrast-infused computed tomography scan through the right kidney demonstrates an infiltrating mass (arrow). The epicenter is within the renal parenchyma, and the adjacent renal sinus is normal. These features suggest an infiltrating renal cell carcinoma.

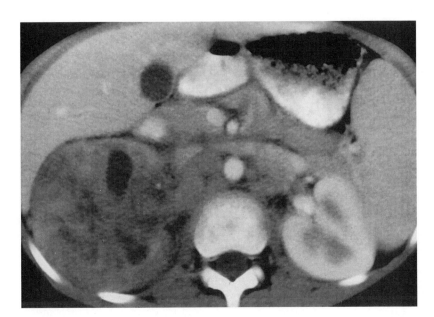

Fig. 3-53 Renal medullary carcinoma. This 10-year-old boy with sickle cell disease was found to have a right renal medullary carcinoma. At the time of diagnosis, extensive bony and pulmonary metastases were present. Radiographically, this mass is heterogeneous, is centered near the junction of the renal sinus and renal parenchyma, and grows mainly by infiltration with a prominent renal sinus component.

thelial neoplasms, metastases, and other geographic infiltrating lesions are hypovascular or avascular. Therefore, if a solitary infiltrating renal lesion is shown to be hypervascular with arteriography, it is almost certainly an infiltrative RCC, and appropriate surgery can be planned. Unfortunately, infiltrating RCC is associated with a high incidence of metastases and a very poor prognosis.

An interesting infiltrating renal neoplasm is the renal medullary carcinoma. This neoplasm only recently has been described, and it appears to represent a new class of renal neoplasm. This tumor originates from the collecting tubules of the renal medulla. Like TCC, SCC, and the rare collecting duct carcinoma, renal medullary carcinoma appears to originate from elements of the kidney originally derived from the ureteric bud. However, these tumors have several distinct pathologic and clinical features. Clinically, these tumors are found in young patients, aged less than 40 years. They are highly associated with sickle cell trait and less commonly with sickle cell disease. They also tend to present at an advanced stage with metastatic disease and, therefore, have an extremely poor prognosis; the mean survival time after diagnosis is less than 4 months. Radiographically, these lesions are indistinguishable from other infiltrating renal neoplasms. These are centrally located; they demonstrate an infiltrative growth pattern in the renal parenchyma; and they often spread into the renal sinus, causing encasement or obliteration of the collecting system (Fig. 3-53). However, urothelial tumors are rare in patients aged less than 40 years. Therefore, when an infiltrating renal mass is detected in a young patient, the patient's race should be established because virtually all patients with renal medullary carcinoma are black, and evidence of sickle cell trait or sickle cell disease should be sought. If present, these clinical features strongly indicate a diagnosis of renal medullary carcinoma.

Renal lymphoma and renal metastases are not uncommon in autopsy series of patients with malignancies. However, they are much less commonly detected in life. Unlike other infiltrating renal neoplasms, these tumors usually are multifocal and usually are accompanied by evidence of extrarenal metastases. The history usually includes diagnosis of a primary malignancy. In 5% of patients with lymphoma, renal metastases are seen during autopsy. These patients usually have advanced disease, and renal metastases are a late finding. On imaging studies, renal lymphoma typically appears as multiple infiltrative nodules (Fig. 3-37) that appear to have spread to the kidneys via a hematogenous route. Unlike primary RCC, these nodules often cause little mass effect, are homogeneous radiographically, and rarely contain calcification. Less commonly, renal lymphoma can appear as diffuse infiltration of the kidney (Fig. 3-38) without a focal lesion. The involved kidney is enlarged but maintains its reniform shape. Involvement of the renal sinus and perinephric space (Figs. 3-35, 3-36), favored sites of lymphoma spread, often is extensive. Regardless of the pattern, renal lymphoma is bilateral in at least 50% of patients. Massive lymphadenopathy of the retroperitoneum (Fig. 3-39) often coexists with renal lymphoma. This constellation is nearly diagnostic of renal lymphoma because massive lymphadenopathy is rare with other renal neoplasms. Although retroperitoneal lymphadenopathy often is present with primary RCC, massive lymphadenopathy in this situation is uncommon. One other characteristic feature of renal lymphoma is its sonographic pattern. These tumors tend to be formed by a large number of uniform lymphoma cells. The result can be a homogeneous, nearly anechoic, appearance on renal ultrasound examination. At first glance, these lesions can mimic simple cysts. However, there is little, if any, through transmission of sound, and subtle low-level internal echoes may be detectable. This sonographic pattern is virtually unique for renal lymphoma.

Most other renal metastases lead to exophytic masses. Other tumors that commonly metastasize to the kidney include malignancies originating in the lung, breast, and gastrointestinal tract and malignant melanoma. Of these, renal metastases of squamous cell origin usually cause infiltrative rather than exophytic renal masses. These tumors usually originate from a squamous cell bronchogenic carcinoma and spread to the kidney hematogenously. SCCs originating from other organ systems and spreading to the kidney also may grow by infiltration of the renal parenchyma.

Inflammatory lesions

Lesions in this group that may lead to infiltrative abnormalities include pyelonephritis, renal tuberculosis, and xanthogranulomatous pyelonephritis. History and clinical findings often are diagnostic in these patients.

Pyelonephritis, a bacterial infection of the renal parenchyma and collecting system, is a common abnormality. It is diagnosed clinically, and imaging rarely is required in these patients. However, imaging may be helpful if a more complicated infection, such as renal abscess, is suspected. Pyelonephritis usually is suspected in patients whose symptoms are refractory to standard antibiotic treatment. As with other infiltrating renal lesions, pyelonephritis is difficult to diagnose with urography or sonog-

raphy. However, contrast-infused CT is highly sensitive in this diagnosis. With CT, renal enlargement with wedge-shaped heterogeneous areas is seen in the kidney, usually with associated parenchymal striations (Fig. 3-54). In conjunction with appropriate clinical symptoms, this CT appearance is virtually diagnostic of acute pyelonephritis and is distinctly different from that of other infiltrating renal lesions.

Renal tuberculosis often is difficult to diagnose because of the subtle or nonspecific clinical abnormalities and absence of distinctive imaging features. Renal tuberculosis results from secondary reactivation of the tuberculous infection. The reactivation occurs near the corticomedullary junction and enlarges by infiltration of surrounding parenchyma. Eventually, papillary necrosis occurs and extends into the renal collecting system. Antegrade spread of infection can occur. Spread into the renal collecting system usually corresponds to the onset of clinical symptoms of renal tuberculosis. Unfortunately, no imaging features are specific for renal tuberculosis; diagnosis depends on bacteriologic studies of the urine. However, radiologic findings can be suggestive of tuberculosis, and the extent of infection can be well delineated with imaging studies. Once the collecting system is involved, stricturing may be evident. Radiographically, this infection mimics TCC with calyceal stricturing and obliteration. If results of a nephrogram appear normal but large areas of the kidney lack visualization of subtending calyces, calyceal amputation is likely to be present. This finding strongly suggests a diagnosis of renal tuberculosis or an invasive urothelial neoplasm. If multiple small ulcerations also are seen along the involved urothelium (Fig. 3-55; also described as "moth-eaten"), the diagnosis of tuberculosis is very likely. Other imaging studies often

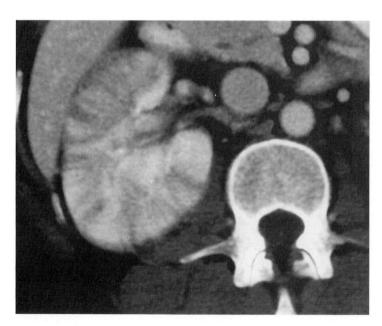

Fig. 3-54 Computed tomography (CT) scan of acute pyelonephritis. This contrast-infused CT scan demonstrates reniform enlargement of the right kidney with numerous striations resulting from parenchymal edema and stasis of urine in the renal tubules. With the appropriate clinical history, these radiologic features are diagnostic of acute pyelonephritis.

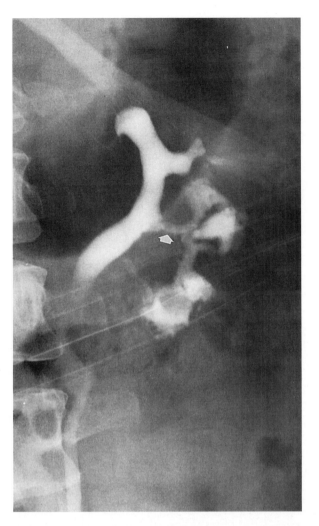

Fig. 3-55 "Moth-eaten" pattern of calyceal renal tuberculosis. The urogram demonstrated amputated lower pole calyces. This retrograde pyelogram demonstrates narrowing of the major calyx (arrowhead), draining the lower pole. The involved calyces are irregular and ulcerated, typical of renal tuberculosis.

Box 3-19	Features of Xanthogranulomatous Pyelonephritis

Marked female predominance
History of urinary infections
Nephrolithiasis
Renal enlargement
Ipsilateral renal hypofunction
Fractured calculus sign
Cystic parenchymal areas
Extrarenal extension common

are nonspecific in the diagnosis of renal tuberculosis. The parenchymal disease is infiltrative, and there may be a large renal sinus component as the disease spreads to the collecting system. Radiographically, this will be indistinguishable from an infiltrating renal neoplasm. Some other radiographic findings are suggestive of urinary tuberculosis. As fibrosis ensues from tuberculosis, calcification commonly occurs, and its presence is more suggestive of tuberculosis than of other infiltrating renal processes. In addition, extensive ureteral wall thickening and periureteral fibrosis in association with renal parenchymal abnormalities strongly suggest advanced renal tuberculosis.

Diffuse XGP also can lead to reniform enlargement of the kidney and marked diminution or absence of renal function (Box 3-19). A renal stone coexists in at least

80% of patients with xanthogranulomatous pyelonephritis (XGP). XGP appears to result from a chronic, low-grade form of pyonephrosis. Pyonephrosis implies ureteral obstruction and coexistent urinary infection. Typically, pyonephrosis is an aggressive, fulminant infection, whereas XGP almost always develops in patients with chronic urinary tract infections and infection-based nephrolithiasis. Infection-based stones usually are branched or laminated, and this finding is a major clue to their etiology. Although infectious stones rarely cause high-grade obstruction, their presence undoubtedly leads to some degree of mild obstruction from mass effect and surrounding inflammation. In some patients, these chronic abnormalities lead to XGP.

XGP describes infiltration of the renal parenchyma with lipid-laden histiocytes. These histiocytes enlarge the renal contour and replace the kidney's functional elements. Although a focal, tumefactive form of XGP sometimes occurs, at least 80% of XGP occurrences lead to diffuse involvement of the kidney. XGP usually is a unilateral process. Involvement of the renal parenchyma often spreads to adjacent structures. In the collecting system, diffuse inflammation is common, and perirenal structures also are commonly involved. Like other granulomatous processes, XGP does not respect normal tissue barriers. It commonly spreads into the perinephric fat and through Gerota's fascia. Inflammation of the psoas commonly is associated with XGP, and renal cutaneous or renal enteric fistulas also may develop.

Imaging features of XGP are very typical. The classic urographic triad of XGP is rather specific and includes an enlarged kidney, nephrolithiasis, and markedly diminished or absent renal function. Ultrasound examination usually demonstrates the renal pelvic stone, reniform enlargement of the kidney, and diffusely abnormal parenchymal echogenicity with absence of the normal corticomedullary distinction. The CT features of XGP also are very characteristic. The involved kidney is enlarged and contains multiple low-attenuation cystic areas and a cen-

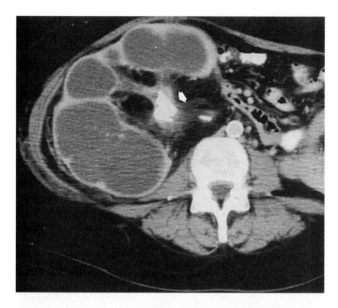

Fig. 3-56 Computed tomography (CT) features of diffuse xanthogranulomatous pyelonephritis. This contrast-infused CT scan demonstrates a renal pelvic stone (arrowhead) with a contracted and irregular collecting system. The renal parenchyma is replaced by multiple cystic areas representing necrosis and histiocyte infiltration. Minimal enhancing renal parenchyma surrounds the cystic areas.

Box 3-20 Features of Renal Infarcts

Wedge-shaped
Cortical rim sign
Usually multifocal
Progressive atrophy with chronicity

tral stone (Fig. 3-56). A thin rim of renal parenchyma may persist in this area and will enhance after intravenous contrast material injection. These cystic areas correspond to necrotic regions within the parenchyma, although radiographically they suggest the presence of hydronephrosis. Retrograde pyelographic studies usually demonstrate a contracted, markedly irregular collecting system rather than hydronephrosis. Because of the central stone and the peripheral cystic areas within the kidney, the CT appearance of XGP has been likened to the print of a bear paw. Another radiographic clue to the diagnosis of XGP that is seen in some patients is the "fractured calculus" sign. In most patients with infectious stones, the stones enlarge contiguously. However, renal complications such as XGP may lead to rapid parenchymal enlargement, which may cause the stone to fracture and the fragments to become displaced. Therefore, the radiographic finding of a fractured and displaced infection-based kidney stone should suggest stone disease complicated by another abnormality such as XGP.

Renal infarction

Renal infarction may be caused by emboli, renal artery dissection, thrombosis, or vasculitis. Regardless of their etiology, renal infarcts usually are demonstrated on contrast-infused CT scans (Box 3-20) as multiple wedge-shaped defects with the base of the wedge extending to the renal cortex (Fig. 3-57). A characteristic sign of infarcts is the cortical rim sign seen with contrast-infused CT. Because the renal capsular artery is an early branch from the renal artery, capsular flow often is preserved

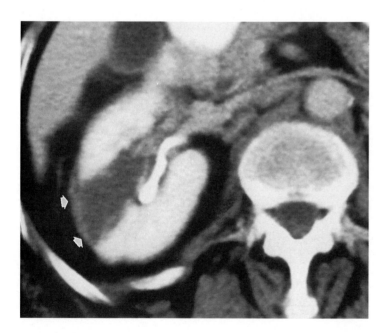

Fig. 3-57 Computed tomography (CT) features of renal infarction. A contrast-infused CT scan demonstrates a wedge-shaped area of decreased attenuation in the right kidney. This wedge extends to the edge of the renal cortex. There is a thin rim of enhancing cortex (arrowheads) overlying this infarction. This cortical rim sign is characteristic of renal infarcts.

in patients with segmental renal infarcts. The capsular arteries then provide collateral blood flow to a thin rim of cortex overlying the infarction. This rim of enhancement adjacent to a wedge-shaped hypofusion defect is characteristic of renal infarction, as it is not seen with other infiltrating renal lesions. Unfortunately, the cortical rim sign is seen in only half of renal infarcts. In addition, patients with vasculitis or emboli usually have multiorgan involvement, and infarcts will be visible in abdominal viscera.

DIAGNOSTIC APPROACH FOR INFILTRATING RENAL LESIONS

Infiltrating renal lesions can be difficult to detect, but they usually are visible with contrast-infused CT scanning. The correct diagnosis of these lesions is important for proper therapeutic planning. Radiographic features often can be helpful in determining the exact diagnosis. If multiple geographic infiltrating lesions are present, either renal metastatic disease, pyelonephritis, or renal infarction is the most likely diagnosis. Presence of the cortical rim sign associated with wedge-shaped defects is virtually diagnostic of infarction and should prompt a search for a history of vascular disease. With pyelonephritis, clinical signs of infection usually will be evident, and contrast-infused CT scanning usually demonstrates striations in the parenchyma. Alternatively, in patients with renal metastases, a known primary neoplasm usually is present. If not, the presence of massive retroperitoneal lymphadenopathy or extensive tumor involvement of the renal sinus and perinephric space strongly suggests a diagnosis of renal lymphoma.

The presence of a solitary infiltrating renal lesion suggests other diagnoses. Involvement of the entire kidney with reniform enlargement suggests either XGP or renal lymphoma. With XGP, a stone usually coexists and it has features typical of infection-based calculi. XGP is rarely bilateral. On the contrary, renal lymphoma often is bilateral, and extensive disease usually is evident elsewhere in the body.

Focal infiltrating renal lesions suggest a primary neoplasm or tuberculosis. Distinguishing among these entities is challenging. Lesions centered in the renal sinus with apparent secondary invasion of the renal parenchyma usually are TCCs. The coexistence of a renal stone with a solitary geographic infiltrating renal lesion should suggest that this tumor may be an uncommon SCC. The appearance of a solitary geographic infiltrating renal lesion in a young patient should raise the possibility of a renal medullary carcinoma. This diagnosis can be confirmed by determining the patient's race and by searching for evidence of sickle cell trait or another sickle cell hemoglobinopathy. Thus far, this lesion has been reported only in patients aged less than 40 years. The epicenter of these lesions is in the renal medulla, but a large renal sinus component also may be present. Infiltrative RCC tends to have a more prominent parenchymal component, with minimal renal sinus invasion. A suspected RCC can be confirmed with arteriography because RCCs are uniquely vascular, unlike other infiltrating renal tumors. Finally, early renal tuberculosis usually is associated with subtle imaging abnormalities. A small area of parenchymal infiltration may be associated with renal papillary necrosis, a major clue suggesting tuberculosis. As the infection spreads, calcification and fibrosis become prominent. With fibrosis, hydronephrosis and parenchymal dysfunction ensue. Findings of calyceal amputation, obliteration, or ulceration may be the first imaging indication of urinary tract tuberculosis. Clinical symptoms may be absent or may include hematuria, flank pain, and sterile pyuria. Bacteriologic confirmation of tuberculosis is essential for the diagnosis. Incidentally, chest radiography is of little help in establishing a diagnosis of renal tuberculosis, although the organism originally spread to the kidney from a pulmonary source. In at least 50% of patients with renal tuberculosis, results of chest radiography are normal. In the remaining 50%, findings of previous pulmonary tuberculosis do not necessarily indicate renal involvement because these abnormalities are commonly seen on chest radiographs of patients with unrelated renal abnormalities.

INDETERMINATE MASSES

The overwhelming majority of significant renal masses easily can be classified and management planned on the basis of radiographic guidelines outlined previously in this chapter. However, some masses remain indeterminate on the basis of imaging features. Small renal masses commonly are seen on CT or MR imaging studies of the kidney. Their small size often makes classification difficult. Nearly all of these tiny lesions are small simple renal cysts. Our policy is to assume that lesions smaller than 5 mm are simple cysts, unless obvious atypical features are evident, such as solid components, nodularity, marginal irregularity, calcification, or intrinsic fat. For other indeterminate renal lesions, numerous options are available for additional evaluation. The two most effective approaches include follow-up imaging or exploratory surgery with excision of the lesion. Obviously, in most patients, noninvasive imaging is preferred. However, some lesions, such as Bosniak Class III cystic masses, are best approached with surgical exploration and excision because half or more of these lesions are malignant. Imaging surveillance is another viable option in the evaluation of some indeterminate renal masses because malignant lesions and some benign tumors, such as angiomyolipoma, demonstrate growth over an extended period of time. It is uncommon for RCC to spread beyond the kidney when the primary tumor is smaller than 3 cm in diameter. Follow-up studies of RCCs have shown variable growth rates for small lesions. On average, RCCs less than 3 cm in diameter grow about 0.5 cm in diameter per year; therefore, it is safe for a solitary small, indeterminate renal mass to be followed with renal CT to check for progression or for the development of detectable intratumoral fat. Enlargement of the mass, in the absence of observable intrinsic fat, indicates that the lesion is an RCC, and surgical extirpation should be considered. Enlarging lesions with intratumoral fat can be diagnosed as angiomyolipomas and managed appropriately. In general, small, indeterminate renal masses, other than infiltrating lesions, should be followed with a CT scan 6 months after initial detection and then yearly afterward to detect enlargement. Lesions that reach 2 cm in diameter or that show definite enlargement should be managed surgically, preferably with renal-sparing techniques.

Sequential imaging of infiltrating lesions also can be of use in some patients. In patients with abnormalities suggesting renal infarction but with some atypical imaging features, CT scanning can be repeated in 1 to 2 months. Unlike neoplasms, infarcts show progressive atrophy over this time period, confirming the diagnosis.

Cyst puncture and percutaneous needle biopsy rarely are indicated in the evaluation of renal masses. Most renal masses easily are classified as surgical or nonsurgical lesions with cross-sectional imaging techniques. Percutaneous needle biopsy usually is reserved for two situations. Patients who have a known extrarenal malignancy and a solitary renal mass may require percutaneous biopsy to distinguish between a solitary metastasis that could be managed nonsurgically and an RCC. Also, patients with multiple bilateral renal masses without a known coexisting disease, such as VHL, may undergo percutaneous needle biopsy for diagnosis. In these patients, diagnosis is essential before therapy because surgery may require bilateral nephrectomy. Multiple solid renal masses may be caused by metastatic disease, RCCs, lymphoma, angiomyolipomas, or oncocytomas. In these patients, observation or nonsurgical therapy may be an option once the histologic diagnosis is established. One caveat regarding the percutaneous biopsy of a suspected oncocytoma is that biopsy results suggesting an oncocytoma should be viewed with some skepticism because some RCCs contain oncocytic components that are indistinguishable from those seen in benign oncocytomas. For this reason, percutaneous biopsy of a solitary renal mass thought to be an oncocytoma is not recommended. The results will be inconclusive, at best, in excluding RCC. However, in the patient with multiple solid renal masses, multiple oncocytomas could be considered. If percutaneous biopsy of several lesions reveals histologic evidence of an oncocytoma without evidence of malignancy, conservative management with follow-up imaging, rather than bilateral renal surgery, can be recommended.

Finally, MR imaging essentially is equivalent to contrast-infused CT in the evaluation of renal masses. The use of MR imaging in the evaluation of patients with an indeterminate renal mass is rarely beneficial if a high-quality CT scan already has been obtained. Conversely, CT rarely adds valuable information in patients with an indeterminate renal mass detected with MR imaging. MR imaging is most useful in the evaluation of renal masses in patients who cannot tolerate intravenous contrast material for a standard renal CT scan. In these patients, the improved contrast resolution of MR imaging and the ability to administer intravenous gadolinium make it a very useful test, affording a high likelihood of successful renal mass characterization.

SUGGESTED READINGS

Afsar H, Yagci F, Meto S, et al: Hydatid disease of the kidney: evaluation and features of diagnostic procedures, *J Urol* 151:567–570, 1994.

Birnbaum BA, Bosniak MA, Megibow AJ, et al: Observations on the growth of renal neoplasms, *Radiology* 176:695–701, 1990.

Bosniak MA: Angiomyolipoma (hamartoma) of the kidney: a preoperative diagnosis is possible in virtually every case, *Urologic Radiology* 3:135–142, 1981.

Bosniak MA: Problems in the radiologic diagnosis of renal parenchymal tumors, *Urol Clin North Am* 20:217–230, 1993.

Bosniak MA: The current radiological approach to renal cysts, *Radiology* 158:1–10, 1986.

Bosniak MA: The small (#3.0 cm) renal parenchymal tumor: detection, diagnosis, and controversies, *Radiology* 179:307–317, 1991.

Bosniak MA, Megibow AJ, Hulnick DH, et al: CT diagnosis of renal angiomyolipoma: the importance of detecting small amounts of fat, *AJR Am J Roentgenol* 151:497–501, 1988.

Carter MD, Tha S, McLoughlin MG, et al: Collecting duct carcinoma of the kidney: a case report and review of the literature, *J Urol* 147:1096–1098, 1992.

Charnsangavej C: Lymphoma of the genitourinary tract, *Radiol Clin North Am* 28:865–877, 1990.

Choyke PL, Filling-Katz MR, Shawker TH, et al: von Hippel-Lindau disease: radiologic screening for visceral manifestations, *Radiology* 174:815–820, 1990.

Coulam CM, Brown LR, Reese DF: Hippel-Lindau syndrome, *Semin Roentgenol* 11:61–66, 1976.

Daniel WW Jr, Hartman GW, Witten DM, et al: Calcified renal masses: a review of ten years experience at the Mayo Clinic, *Radiology* 103:503–508, 1972.

Didier D, Racle A, Etievent JP, et al: Tumor thrombus of the inferior vena cava secondary to malignant abdominal neoplasms: US and CT evaluation, *Radiology* 162:83–89, 1987.

Dimopoulos MA, Logothetis J, Markowitz A, et al: Collecting duct carcinoma of the kidney, *Br J Urol* 71:388-391, 1993.

Gash JR, Zagoria RJ, Dyer RB: Imaging features of infiltrating renal lesions, *Crit Rev Diagn Imaging* 33:293-310, 1992.

Harrison RB, Dyer R: Benign space-occupying conditions of the kidneys, *Semin Roentgenol* 22:275-283, 1987.

Hartman DS: An overview of renal cystic disease. In Hartman DS, ed: *Renal cystic disease,* Philadelphia, 1989, WB Saunders.

Hartman DS, Davidson AJ, Davis CJ Jr, et al: Infiltrative renal lesions: CT-sonographic-pathologic correlation, *AJR Am J Roentgenol* 150:1061-1064, 1988.

Honda H, Coffman CE, Berbaum KS, et al: CT analysis of metastatic neoplasms of the kidney: comparison with primary renal cell carcinoma, *Acta Radiol* 33:39-44, 1992.

Ikeda AK, Korobkin M, Platt JF, et al: Small echogenic renal masses: how often is computed tomography used to confirm the sonographic suspicion of angiomyolipoma? *Urology* 46:311-315, 1995.

Jennings CM, Gaines PA: The abdominal manifestation of von Hippel-Lindau disease and a radiological screening protocol for an affected family, *Clin Radiol* 39:363-367, 1988.

Johnson CD, Dunnick NR, Cohan RH, et al: Renal adenocarcinoma: CT staging of 100 tumors, *AJR Am J Roentgenol* 148:59-63, 1987.

Kandel LB, McCullough DL, Harrison LH, et al: Primary renal lymphoma: does it exist? *Cancer* 60:386-391, 1987.

Leder RA, Dunnick NR: Transitional cell carcinoma of the pelvicalices and ureter, *AJR Am J Roentgenol* 155:713-722, 1990.

Lieber MM: Renal oncocytoma, *Urol Clin North Am* 20:355-359, 1993.

Mead GO, Thomas LR Jr, Jackson JG: Renal oncocytoma: report of a case with bilateral multifocal oncocytomas, *Clin Imaging* 14:231-234, 1990.

Mooring FJ, Kaude JV, Wajsman Z: Bilateral renal oncocytomas, *Journal of Medical Imaging* 3:27-30, 1989.

Narla LD, Slovis TL, Watts FB, et al: The renal lesions of tuberosclerosis (cysts and angiomyolipoma)—screening with sonography and computerized tomography, *Pediatr Radiol* 18:205-209, 1988.

Oesterling JE, Fishman EK, Goldman SM, et al: The management of renal angiomyolipoma, *J Urol* 135:1121-1124, 1986.

Parienty RA, Pradel J, Parienty I: Cystic renal cancers: CT characteristics, *Radiology* 157:741-744, 1985.

Ruchman RB, Yeh H-C, Mitty HA, et al: Ultrasonographic and computed tomographic features of renal sinus lymphoma, *J Clin Ultrasound* 16:35-40, 1988.

Schwartz DT, Mascatello VJ, David-Nelson MA: Malacoplakia of the kidney, *South Med J* 76:1427-1429, 1983.

Seidenwurm DJ, Barkovich AJ: Understanding tuberous sclerosis, *Radiology* 183:23-24, 1992.

Semelka RC, Hricak H, Stevens SK, et al: Combined gadolinium-enhanced and fat-saturation MR imaging of renal masses, *Radiology* 178:803-809, 1991.

Siegel SC, Sandler MA, Alpern MB, et al: CT of renal cell carcinoma in patients on chronic hemodialysis, *AJR Am J Roentgenol* 150:583-585, 1988.

Steiner MS, Goldman SM, Fishman EK, et al: The natural history of renal angiomyolipoma, *J Urol* 150:1782-1786, 1993.

Takahashi K, Honda M, Okubo RS, et al: CT pixel mapping in the diagnosis of small angiomyolipomas of the kidneys, *J Comput Assist Tomogr* 17:98-101, 1993.

Wallace S, Charnsangavej C, Carrasco CH, et al: Interventional radiology in renal neoplasms, *Semin Roentgenol* 22:303-315, 1987.

Watson RC, Fleming RJ, Evans JA: Arteriography in the diagnosis of renal carcinoma: review of 100 cases, *Radiology* 91:888-897, 1968.

Weiss LM, Gelb AB, Medeiros LJ: Adult renal epithelial neoplasms, *Am J Clin Pathol* 103:624-635, 1995.

Yamashita Y, Ueno S, Makita O, et al: Hyperechoic renal tumors: anechoic rim and intratumoral cysts in US differentiation of renal cell carcinoma from angiomyolipoma, *Radiology* 188:179-182, 1993.

Zagoria RJ, Bechtold RE, Dyer RB: Staging of renal adenocarcinoma: role of various imaging procedures, *AJR Am J Roentgenol* 164:363-370, 1995.

Zagoria RJ, Dyer RB: Computed tomography of primary renal osteosarcoma, *J Comput Assist Tomogr* 15:146-148, 1991.

Zagoria RJ, Dyer RB, Wolfman NT, et al: Radiology in the diagnosis and staging of renal cell carcinoma, *Crit Rev Diagn Imaging* 31:81-115, 1990.

Zagoria RJ, Wolfman NT, Karstaedt N, et al: CT features of renal cell carcinoma with emphasis on relation to tumor size, *Invest Radiol* 25:261-266, 1990.

Zbar B, Glenn G, Lubensky I, et al: Hereditary papillary renal cell carcinoma: clinical studies in 10 families, *J Urol* 153:907-912, 1995.

CHAPTER 4

The Kidney: The Diffuse Parenchymal Abnormality

Diffuse parenchymal abnormalities of one or both kidneys often are recognized during renal imaging. These diseases usually result in abnormalities of renal size, of renal shape, or of the collecting system. Diagnosis of the underlying abnormality often is possible on the basis of the pattern of abnormalities. In this chapter, various patterns are discussed, and suggestions are given for determining the most likely diagnosis for each patient. Often, additional imaging studies or percutaneous biopsy may be needed to confirm the diagnostic findings. However, in many patients, the radiologic findings are diagnostic, and additional evaluation is unnecessary. Depending on the imaging modality—radiography, sonography, computed tomography (CT), and magnetic resonance (MR) imaging—some variables of pattern classification may be undetectable, although other variables are apparent. Findings such as calyceal shape, mass effect on the intrarenal collecting system, and parenchymal echo texture may be detectable with only one of these modalities.

In evaluating the diffusely abnormal kidney, a few general guidelines are in order. These include kidney size, kidney contour, calyceal anatomy, renal function, echo texture, and pattern of calcifications. In healthy individuals, both kidneys are similar in length. A discrepancy of more than 2 cm between the kidneys suggests underlying disease. To determine which kidney is abnormal, other findings, such as absolute renal size and additional abnormalities of either kidney, are important. With radiography, kidney length should exceed the length from the top of L1 to the bottom of L3, including the intervening disc spaces, but be no longer than L1–L4. Because the kidneys lie adjacent to the vertebral column, this method takes into account magnification factors and variability in body habitus that may affect kidney and vertebra size. That is, large patients tend to have large spines and large kidneys, whereas small patients have smaller spines and kidneys. In most men, the absolute length of the kidneys measured on abdominal radiographs ranges from 10 to 14 cm and in women from 9 to 13 cm. With sonography, magnification is less of a factor, and normal renal lengths measure less by 1 to 2 cm. In addition, it often is stated that the left kidney in many patients is somewhat longer than the right kidney. More recent studies with ultrasound examination have shown little variability in the length of the right and left kidneys. Differences in kidney length should be less than 2 cm in healthy persons. Sometimes, differences in length result from tilting of either kidney with resulting foreshortening of the renal axis on radiographic studies. This limitation may be avoided with sonography because the transducer easily is reoriented in a plane along the true longitudinal axis of the kidney being examined.

SMALL SCARRED KIDNEY

Abnormalities of small kidneys fall into several groupings. Is the kidney smooth or scarred? If the kidney is scarred or if both kidneys are small and scarred, several other factors must be considered. Where are the scars

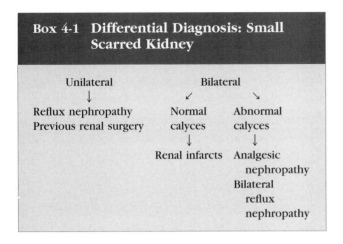

Box 4-1 Differential Diagnosis: Small Scarred Kidney

Unilateral   Bilateral
↓   ↙   ↘
Reflux nephropathy   Normal   Abnormal
Previous renal surgery calyces   calyces
                          ↓   ↓
                     Renal infarcts Analgesic
                                     nephropathy
                                     Bilateral
                                     reflux
                                     nephropathy

located in relationship to the calyces, and are the calyces normal? Small scarred kidneys usually result from ischemic disease caused by small-vessel occlusions in the kidney, from reflux nephropathy, or from analgesic nephropathy (Box 4-1). Renal scarring resulting from reflux usually is unilateral. Scarring caused by small-vessel disease and analgesic nephropathy is bilateral. Occlusion of interlobar arteries usually results from advanced atherosclerosis, and small-vessel involvement typically is seen in patients with diabetes, hemoglobinopathy, or collagen-vascular diseases. Interlobar arteries are radially arrayed vessels extending between renal lobules. Each of these lobules has one or more calyces in its center. Parenchymal scarring caused by occlusion of these interlobar arteries results in thinning of the parenchyma in areas of the kidney between calyces. The parenchyma directly adjacent to the calyx is of normal thickness. In addition, the calyces get their arterial supply from a separate network of vessels derived from the main renal artery and the ureteric arteries. Therefore, occlusion of interlobar arteries does not lead to structural changes in the calyces, and small scarred kidneys with scars centered between calyces and normal calyces indicate renal atrophy resulting from remote interlobar artery occlusions.

Alternatively, bilateral small kidneys with scars centered over calyces or with medullary calcifications indicate a diagnosis of analgesic nephropathy. Findings of papillary necrosis often are present.

Reflux nephropathy, sometimes referred to as chronic atrophic pyelonephritis, is a major cause of renal atrophy with an irregular contour. Parenchymal scarring can be caused by reflux of either sterile or bacteria-infested urine. For scarring to develop, reflux must be chronic and usually massive. The occurrence of this combination of factors almost always is limited to children. However, the kidney's structural changes often are detected during adulthood. Reflux confined to the calyces leads to calyceal blunting without overlying parenchymal atrophy. Atrophic parenchymal changes occur when reflux ex-

tends through the ducts of Bellini into the renal medulla. This process tends to follow a typical pattern. Previous work has demonstrated that the ducts of Bellini vary in their antireflux characteristics. Most ducts of Bellini are slit-like and effective in preventing parenchymal spread of urinary reflux. Atrophy of the kidney overlying these areas occurs only after long-standing, massive reflux. Alternatively, some ducts of Bellini are circular and, therefore, less effective at inhibiting intraparenchymal reflux. Circular ducts occur most commonly in compound calyces. In addition, compound calyces usually are present in the poles (upper and lower) of the kidney as described in Chapter 2, which leads to an interesting radiographic pattern, typical of reflux nephropathy. In most patients, the first, and often the only, signs of reflux nephropathy occur in the upper and lower poles of the kidney (Fig. 4-1), sparing the midportion of the kidney. The parenchymal scars are broad-based and centered over the subtending calyx. In addition, the underlying calyx is abnormal. As a result of parenchymal atrophy and chronic reflux, the calyx loses its normal concave shape and becomes

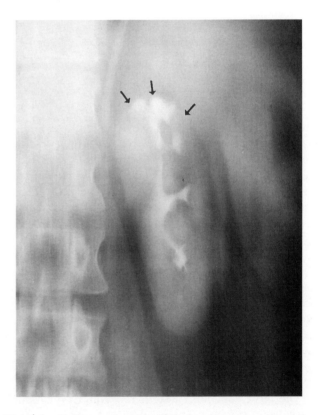

Fig. 4-1 Reflux nephropathy limited to the upper pole of the left kidney. This film from an intravenous urogram demonstrates a clubbed compound calyx in the upper pole of the left kidney. This calyx has convex margins. There is marked atrophy of the upper pole renal parenchyma adjacent to this calyx (arrows). The remainder of the kidney is normal without evidence of calyceal clubbing or parenchymal scarring. These features are typical of reflux nephropathy.

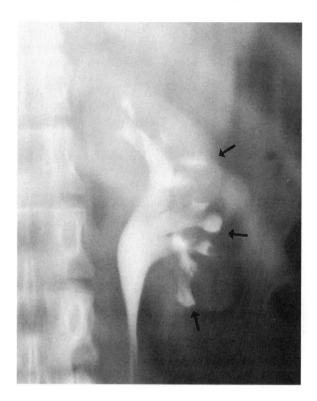

Fig. 4-2   Severe reflux nephropathy of the left kidney. A film from a urogram demonstrates severe changes of reflux nephropathy with multiple broad-based parenchymal scars (arrows) overlying clubbed calyces.

club-shaped with convex margins (Fig. 4-2). Additional parenchymal contour irregularity may originate from compensatory hypertrophy in the unaffected areas of the kidney, which can lead to exaggeration of the contour irregularities induced by reflux nephropathy. Although reflux nephropathy usually is unilateral, bilateral changes are not rare. Severe reflux nephropathy is not an uncommon cause of irreversible renal insufficiency.

Typical changes of reflux nephropathy include a small scarred kidney with the scars centered over an abnormal calyx. Scars develop first in, and may be limited to, the renal poles, but advanced cases involve the kidney globally.

UNILATERAL SMALL SMOOTH KIDNEY

The most common cause of this pattern is chronic renal artery stenosis. Other causes of a unilateral small smooth kidney include chronic renal vein thrombosis, postobstructive atrophy, renal hypoplasia, previous renal trauma with subcapsular hematoma, and previous radiation therapy to the renal bed (Box 4-2). Secondary radiographic features are helpful in distinguishing this group of abnormalities. On intravenous contrast studies (intra-

---

Box 4-2   Differential Diagnosis: Unilateral Small Smooth Kidney

Smooth, reniform

Normal calyces	Abnormal calyces
↓	↓
Renal artery stenosis	Postobstructive atrophy
Chronic renal vein thrombosis	
Renal hypoplasia	
Subcapsular hematoma	
Radiation therapy	

---

venous urography [IVU], CT, or MR imaging with gadolinium), findings suggestive of renal artery stenosis include a small, smooth kidney with delayed nephrogram, delayed pyelogram, and late development of a hyperdense pyelogram (Fig. 4-3; Box 4-3). The calyces and ureter are normal. The calyces may appear very delicate because of decreased urine output by the ischemic kidney. Because the contrast material is delivered with the blood stream, there usually is a delay in nephrographic opacification. Unfortunately, this delay may not be detectable with standard urographic techniques because films are not obtained quickly enough after contrast material injection. However, delayed pyelogram (Fig. 4-3), i.e., the opacification of the calyces and renal pelvis, usually is evident and is a key finding to suggest renal artery stenosis. Delay of pyelographic opacification results from slowed blood flow through the kidney with decreased pressure propelling contrast material through the nephrons and collecting ducts. This delay and inability to reabsorb contrast material through the tubular epithelium leads to development of the hyperdense pyelogram. When the time required for passage of contrast media in the tubules is prolonged, reabsorption of water increases and leads to higher concentration of contrast media in the tubules of the affected kidney than in the normally perfused kidney. Radiographically, this leads to a higher density of contrast media in the ischemic kidney than in the normal kidney in the pyelographic phase. Another sign, sometimes iden-

---

Box 4-3   Urographic Signs of Renal Artery Stenosis

Small smooth kidney
Delayed nephrogram
Delayed pyelogram
Hyperdense pyelogram
Ureteral "notching"

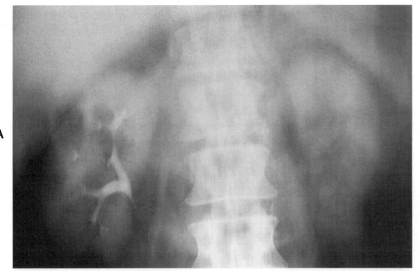

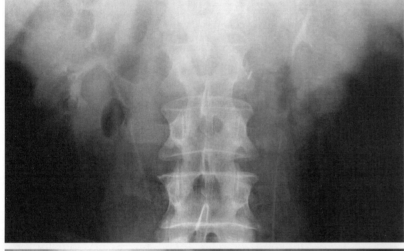

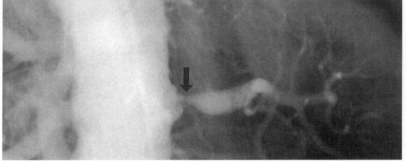

Fig. 4-3   Urographic findings of severe renal artery stenosis. **A,** A 1-minute nephrotomogram demonstrates a normal right kidney with normal temporal progression of contrast enhancement. The left kidney is small but has smooth margins and retains a reniform shape. There is delay in opacification of the calyces on the left. **B,** A 20-minute film from the same urogram demonstrates opacification of a nondilated left collecting system and ureter. The left pyelogram is slightly hyperdense compared with the normal right pyelogram. **C,** A single film from an aortogram in the same patient demonstrates a tight ostial stenosis (arrow) with poststenotic dilatation of the left renal artery. This stenosis accounts for the urographic abnormalities seen in this patient.

tified urographically in association with renal artery stenosis, is notching of the ureter and renal pelvis (Fig. 4-4) caused by enlarged collateral ureteric arteries. These arteries are recruited and enlarged to give additional blood supply to the ischemic kidney. Ureteric vessels originate from lumbar arteries and branches of the iliac artery. These vessels form a network of anastomoses, with ureteric branches originating from the main renal artery. The connection of the ureteric vessel network with the main renal artery often is distal to the stenosis.

Thus, ureteric vessels can enlarge to help supply more blood to the ischemic kidney. Notching caused by enlarged ureteric arteries appears as persistent, eccentric, and extrinsic indentations on the ureter and renal pelvis (Fig. 4-4).

Intravenous urography is not a good screening test for renovascular hypertension. The IVU has low specificity and sensitivity for renal artery stenosis, although the abnormalities described previously sometimes are seen in these patients. For patients with suspected renovascular hypertension, the best screening examination, after thorough history and physical examination, is the radionuclide renogram augmented with captopril. Another test that has been used for screening is renal sonography augmented with Doppler analysis of the renal arteries.

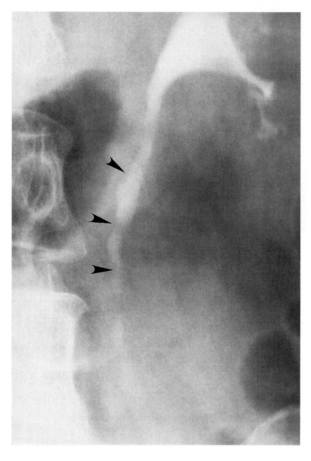

Fig. 4-4   Left ureteral notching resulting from enlarged ureteric collaterals in a patient with renal artery stenosis. Multiple eccentric indentations (arrowheads) of the upper left ureter were noted consistently throughout this urogram. An arteriogram confirmed left renal artery stenosis in this patient with hypertension.

Results for this technique have been variable. Some institutions have a high detection rate of renal artery stenosis with this technique, whereas other reports indicate that this test is unreliable. It appears that in some centers, Doppler sonography may allow a fairly high degree of accuracy in the detection of renal artery stenosis. Confirmation of renal artery stenosis is best obtained using arteriography with either standard filming or digital subtraction technique. Digital subtraction technique has the advantage of requiring lower volumes of contrast material while still retaining a high degree of resolution. For patients with contraindications to the administration of intravascular contrast material, magnetic resonance angiography appears to be a promising technique for evaluation of the proximal renal arteries for stenotic lesions.

It also is important to differentiate between renal artery stenosis and ureteral obstruction because they share some radiographic features. Acute ureteral obstruction also leads to delayed nephrogram and pyelogram. However, hydroureteronephrosis and a dilute pyelogram and symptoms of ureteral colic usually accompany ureteral obstruction.

Chronic renal vein thrombosis is another vascular cause of renal ischemia. If inadequate venous collaterals develop, a small ischemic kidney will result from chronic renal vein thrombosis. Chronic renal vein thrombosis also can lead to other radiographic features mimicking renal artery stenosis, including delayed pyelogram (Fig. 4-5), hyperdense pyelogram, and nondilated normal-appearing calyces and ureter. Sonography with Doppler evaluation of the renal artery and vein often leads to the correct diagnosis. Definitive diagnosis of renal vein thrombosis or renal artery stenosis may require renal angiography or other noninvasive angiographic techniques, such as magnetic resonance angiography or CT angiography. These last two techniques are in various stages of development, and their accuracy compared with that of conventional angiography is not known.

Renal hypoplasia appears radiographically as a small, smooth kidney with a small number of calyces (Fig. 4-6).

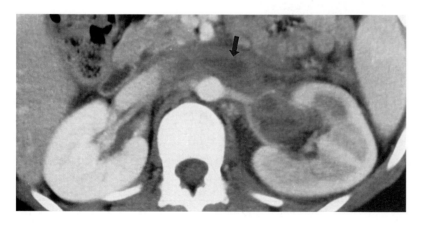

Fig. 4-5   Subacute left renal vein thrombosis. This CT scan demonstrates thrombus in the left renal vein (arrow). Although the left kidney is not atrophic, there is delay in opacification in the left kidney compared with the right. The right kidney is diffusely opacified, whereas the left kidney demonstrates delayed opacification of the medullary portion of the kidney.

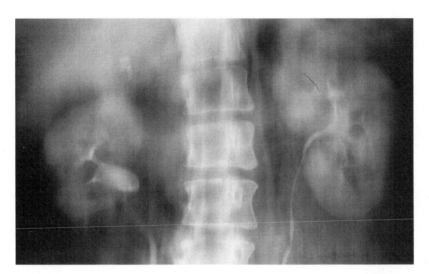

Fig. 4-6   Hypoplasia of the right kidney. This patient was asymptomatic and was being evaluated for pelvic surgery. A film from the urogram demonstrates a small smooth kidney with three calyces. Other than its small size and low number of calyces, this kidney appears essentially normal. These features are typical of renal hypoplasia.

This entity is thought to result from underperfusion of the fetal kidney. The small kidney functions normally and has normal parenchymal thickness, however, by definition, there will be five or fewer calyces in the intrarenal collecting system. Although there are few calyces, they appear completely normal. No additional signs of abnormality, such as those seen with renal artery stenosis, are present with the hypoplastic kidney. Renal arteriography demonstrates a diminutive, but widely patent, renal artery. The artery is small because of a small volume of renal parenchyma requiring arterial supply.

The ''Page kidney'' is another name for renal atrophy resulting from subcapsular hematoma. Because the renal capsule is rigid, an arterial subcapsular hematoma exerts hydraulic pressure throughout the renal parenchyma. If unmanaged, this eventually leads to parenchymal ischemia and atrophy (Fig. 4-7). The kidney usually maintains a near reniform shape, and the calyces appear normal. As with renal artery stenosis, hypertension often results from overstimulation of the renin–angiotensin system by parenchymal ischemia. The key to this diagnosis is a clinical history of flank trauma, which can occur in deceleration injuries but more often is identified in young patients with sports-related injuries. These subcapsular hematomas may go unrecognized at the time of acute injury and may be identified incidentally during imaging at a later time for another reason. In some patients, the remnant of the subcapsular hematoma is visible with cross-sectional imaging. This result confirms the diagnosis of Page kidney.

Radiation therapy that includes the renal bed can lead to parenchymal ischemia because of small-vessel arteritis

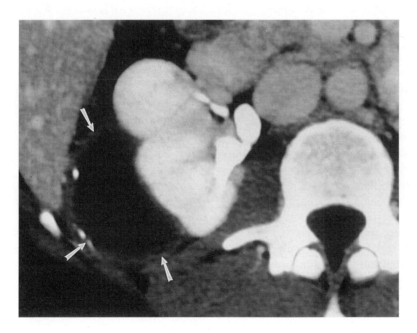

Fig. 4-7   Page kidney. This patient has a chronic right subcapsular hematoma (arrows). Dystrophic calcifications are noted in the wall of this hematoma. The chronic subcapsular hematoma has led to renal atrophy with some deformity of the kidney shape. The calyces are delicate and nondilated.

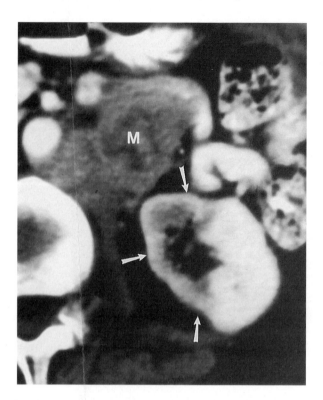

Fig. 4-8 Atrophy of the kidney after radiation therapy. This patient has a retroperitoneal mass (M) adjacent to the left kidney. The radiation port used in management of this mass included the medial segment of the left kidney. Atrophy of the exposed segment of the kidney (arrows) occurred after treatment.

induced by the radiation therapy. This arteritis results in parenchymal atrophy (Fig. 4-8) and mimics other vascular causes of renal ischemia, including chronic renal vein thrombosis and renal artery stenosis. This arteritis is rarely seen with modern radiation therapy techniques but should be considered in patients who have undergone radiation treatment for tumors in the region of the kidney. Other radiographic clues suggesting previous radiation therapy sometimes can be identified in the adjacent spine. These clues include osteonecrosis and resulting scoliosis.

Finally, an uncommon cause of a unilateral small, smooth kidney is postobstructive atrophy. This condition can be seen in patients who have experienced long-standing ureteral obstruction for any of a variety of causes. High-grade ureteral obstruction with sterile urine must persist for at least 1 week to lead to irreversible parenchymal atrophy. During the acute obstructive phase, the kidney usually is edematous, swollen, and distended (Fig. 4-9), rather than atrophic. However, when long-standing obstruction is relieved, parenchymal atrophy becomes evident (Fig. 4-9). Unlike reflux nephropathy, ureteral obstruction leads to increased pres-

sure spread throughout the renal parenchyma. Once the obstruction is relieved, some renal function returns, but global atrophy and residual ectasia of the collecting system (Fig. 4-9) will be evident. Collecting-system ectasia, with dilatation and residual clubbing of the calyces, distinguishes this entity from other causes of a unilateral small, smooth kidney. In many patients there will be a history of previous intervention to relieve the ureteral obstruction. In particular, postobstructive atrophy often is seen in patients with pelvic malignancies, including bladder and ureteral neoplasms. If these are surgically resected or if the urinary stream is diverted after a significant period of ureteral obstruction, postobstructive atrophy will be evident.

A unilateral small smooth kidney with normal calyces most likely results from renal artery stenosis. Additional radiographic signs of renal artery stenosis should be sought. A small smooth kidney with associated calyceal ectasia suggests postobstructive atrophy. A small, smooth kidney that is normal except that it contains a complement of five or fewer calyces is likely a congenital hypoplastic kidney. Other entities with this pattern that should be considered include chronic renal vein thrombosis, Page kidney, and previous radiation therapy affecting the renal bed.

SHOCK NEPHROGRAM

One urographic pattern of bilateral abnormality that must be recognized is the shock nephrogram. Although hypotension from any cause occurring during the course of radiographic contrast material excretion can cause this pattern, it almost always is seen in association with a severe adverse reaction to the administered contrast material. Prompt recognition of this pattern is necessary and should lead to assessment of the patient and initiation of appropriate therapy when indicated. When arterial perfusion pressure to the kidneys drops below the minimum level required for glomerular filtration, tubular stasis occurs. Any contrast material that has been excreted into the kidney stagnates. Some salt and water resorption continues, but additional excretion of contrast material subsides. With urography, this sequence of events usually is demonstrated over a short time span. Initially, contrast excretion usually is normal. There is normal nephrographic opacity and development of a pyelogram in a prompt fashion (Fig. 4-10). However, once hypotension develops, the overall kidney size will decrease slightly, caused by diminished arterial inflow. Nephrographic density will persist and become progressively denser resulting from hyperconcentration of the stagnant contrast material in the tubules. The most dramatic finding is regression or disappearance of the pyelogram phase (Fig.

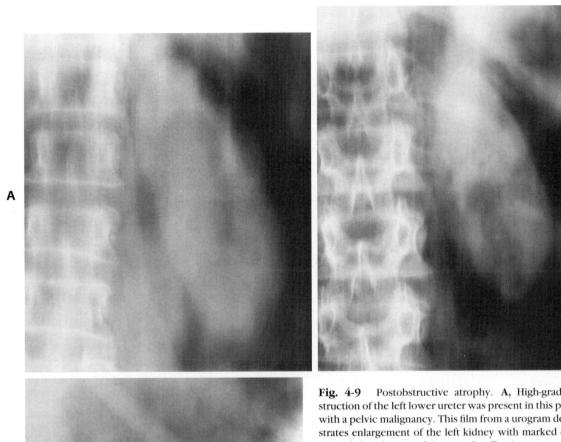

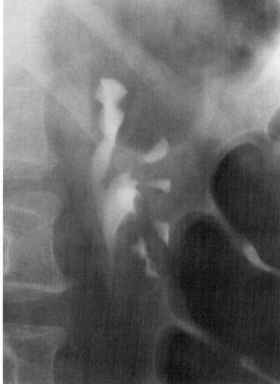

Fig. 4-9 Postobstructive atrophy. **A,** High-grade obstruction of the left lower ureter was present in this patient with a pelvic malignancy. This film from a urogram demonstrates enlargement of the left kidney with marked dilatation of the obstructed intrarenal collecting system. The dilated collecting system causes a "negative pyelogram," resulting from nonopacification of the urine against the well-opacified renal parenchyma. **B,** A urogram obtained several months after decompression of the obstructed ureter demonstrates atrophy of the left kidney. The kidney now spans less than three lumbar vertebral bodies. Its shape is reniform, and its contours are smooth. **C,** A later film from this urogram demonstrates abnormal calyces in this patient with postobstructive renal atrophy. The calyces are blunted and clubbed, typical of residual ectasia from remote obstruction in this patient.

4-10). After hypotension develops, contrast material that has been excreted into the calyces or ureter will progress to the bladder. However, further excretion will be interrupted, leading to disappearance of pyelographic opaci-

fication. This constellation of findings, delayed recurrence of dense nephrogram and disappearance of pyelogram opacification often seen in conjunction with decreased size of the kidneys, is an alarming development

A

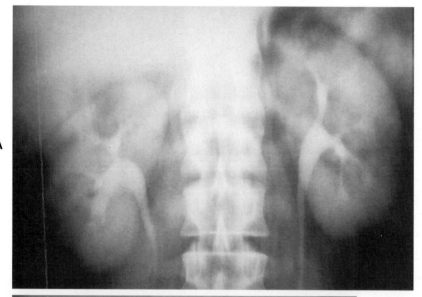

B

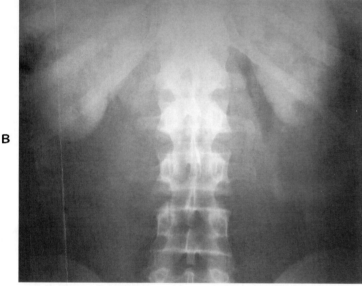

Fig. 4-10   Shock nephrogram. **A,** A 1-minute film from this intravenous urogram demonstrates normal kidneys with good opacification of the calyces and ureter. **B,** A 10-minute film demonstrates persistently dense nephrograms with regression and disappearance of the pyelogram phase. Contrast material that had been in the calyces and ureter has progressed into the bladder, whereas the underperfused kidneys are no longer excreting contrast material. This patient was suffering from severe hypotension as a result of an adverse response to the contrast material.

and usually indicates the onset of life-threatening hypotension as a result of an adverse reaction to the administered contrast material.

BILATERAL SMALL SMOOTH KIDNEYS

Significant bilateral renal atrophy usually is associated with renal insufficiency. Patients generally are imaged with nonenhanced CT, sonography, or MR imaging. Renal insufficiency usually results from chronic medical renal disease of various etiologies, including chronic glomerulonephritis, nephrosclerosis resulting from hypertension, bilateral renal artery stenosis, analgesic nephropathy, hereditary nephropathy, or remote acute tubular necrosis. Evidence of renal artery stenosis may be ob-

tained with noninvasive techniques such as Doppler sonography or magnetic resonance angiography and can be confirmed with conventional angiography if treatment is contemplated. Other entities may require biopsy for a tissue diagnosis. The atrophy is likely to be irreversible, and, at best, renal function could be stabilized rather than improved.

One unique entity that may lead to this pattern is medullary cystic disease of the kidney. It usually is seen in children who develop a salt-wasting nephropathy, but a subtype occurs in adults in whom renal insufficiency and salt-wasting develop insidiously. The kidneys usually are small and contain numerous medullary cysts. There is no known management for this disease, which usually occurs sporadically, although some cases appear to be inherited. CT or sonographic demonstration of numerous

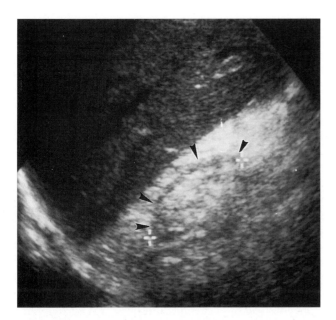

Fig. 4-11 Chronic medical renal disease. A longitudinal sonogram of the right kidney in this patient with chronic glomerulonephritis demonstrates a small, diffusely atrophied right kidney (arrowheads). The kidney maintains its reniform shape with smooth margins and no focal scarring. The renal parenchyma is hyperechoic compared with the adjacent liver. These features are typical of chronic medical renal disease of various etiologies.

medullary cysts in small kidneys and an appropriate clinical history should suggest this diagnosis. Other entities in this category lead to small, hyperechoic kidneys (Fig. 4-11) without increased cyst formation.

UNILATERAL SMOOTH RENAL ENLARGEMENT

In patients with unilateral smooth renal enlargement, one kidney is abnormally large without focal mass effect. The renal contour should be smooth or minimally lobulated in a manner consistent with persistent fetal lobation. Also, there should be no evidence of focal renal masses affecting the renal collecting system. Renal function may be impaired; if so, this finding is helpful in classifying these cases. Underlying abnormalities resulting in this pattern fit into one of five categories: ureteral obstruction, renal duplication anomalies, acute vascular abnormalities, parenchymal infiltration, and glomerular hypertrophy (Box 4-4).

The most common underlying abnormality in this group is ureteral obstruction. In the acute obstructive phase, the kidney is engorged and edematous because of urinary outflow obstruction. Contrast-material injection demonstrates the swollen kidney with delayed opacification of the collection system and a dense persistent nephrogram. Varying degrees of hydronephrosis are evi-

Box 4-4 Causes of Unilateral Reniform Enlargement

Ureteral obstruction
Duplication anomalies and hypertrophy
Parenchymal infiltration
    Cellular infiltrates
        Pyelonephritis
        Xanthogranulomatous pyelonephritis
        Contusion
        Infiltrating neoplasm
    Edema
        Acute renal vein occlusion
        Acute arterial occlusion and arteritis

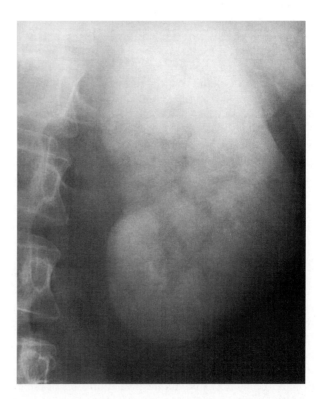

Fig. 4-12 High-grade ureteral obstruction with a striated nephrogram. This film taken 45 minutes after contrast injection in this patient with an obstructing distal ureteral stone demonstrates reniform enlargement of the left kidney. Lucent striations are noted extending from the renal sinus to the cortex. Unilateral smooth reniform enlargement with delayed and persistent nephrogram and striations most commonly is found in patients with acute ureteral obstruction.

dent on delayed films, depending on the severity and duration of obstruction. In many patients, high-grade ureteral obstruction leads to a striated nephrogram (Fig. 4-12). The term *striated nephrogram* implies linear lucencies extending from the renal medulla into the renal cortex on a contrast-infused study of the kidney, which

Box 4-5   Causes of Striated Nephrogram

Common
   Acute ureteral obstruction
   Pyelonephritis
Uncommon
   Autosomal recessive polycystic kidney disease
   Acute renal vein thrombosis
   Renal contusion
Rare
   Radiation nephritis

is most commonly seen with high-grade ureteral obstruction and is thought to result from a combination of interstitial edema and stasis of unopacified urine in renal tubules adjacent to contrast-filled tubules.

The striated nephrogram can be seen with a number of other entities, including autosomal recessive polycystic kidney disease, pyelonephritis, acute renal vein thrombosis, renal contusion, and, acutely, after radiation therapy to the kidney (Box 4-5).

Whether a striated nephrogram is present, delayed films should be obtained when acute obstruction is suspected to confirm the presence of hydronephrosis because other nephrographic findings of obstruction can be identical to the findings associated with other entities, such as renal vein thrombosis. When evidence of ureteral dilatation also is detected, it indicates ureteral obstruction. Diagnosis of obstruction usually is not difficult with IVU, CT, or sonography.

Duplication anomalies generally lead to enlargement of the kidney as a result of the overall increase in renal mass. These easily can be diagnosed with most imaging modalities because separate collecting systems with separate surrounding renal sinus fat and intervening renal parenchyma invaginating and separating the two moieties of the kidney will be demonstrated. Rarely, triplication, tetraplication, and duplication anomalies of greater number are detected, although they are of little or no clinical significance.

Infiltration of the kidney parenchyma can lead to reniform enlargement, which usually results from inflammatory processes such as acute pyelonephritis, chronic xanthogranulomatous pyelonephritis (XGP), or infiltration secondary to trauma and renal contusion. We routinely do not image the kidneys of patients with acute pyelonephritis because this is a clinical diagnosis, and imaging usually adds nothing to treatment planning. However, on occasion, pyelonephritis is detected in patients being imaged for other reasons, or we may evaluate a patient who has not responded to appropriate antibiotic treatment for pyelonephritis. Results of IVU in a patient with acute pyelonephritis most often appear normal. In 30%

of patients with pyelonephritis, results of the IVU are abnormal, but findings usually are nonspecific. Various abnormalities may be detected, including kidney enlargement, delayed or decreased function of the involved kidney (Fig. 4-13), and a striated nephrogram. On occasion, the causative bacteria release an endotoxin, which leads to diminished muscle tone and results in hydroureteronephrosis. This finding is of particular concern because it can lead to an erroneous diagnosis of ureteral obstruction. One should be aware of this enigmatic urographic finding and be cautious in diagnosing ureteral obstruction in patients with suspected pyelonephritis. Contrast-infused CT is sensitive in detecting abnormalities of pyelonephritis. With CT, a heterogeneous nephrogram is typical. The kidney is swollen and contains areas of striation. There are wedge-shaped regions of hypofunction (Fig. 4-14), and perinephric inflammatory changes often are present. Pyelonephritis can affect segments of the kidney instead of occurring diffusely. Focal pyelonephritis is less common than the diffuse form. When pyelonephritis is focal, findings are similar as those seen with diffuse pyelonephritis. The affected area will demonstrate hypofunction, swelling, and heterogeneous nephrogram. Because swelling is focal, the infected segment of the kidney may mimic an infiltrating tumor. However, striations and wedge-shaped areas of decreased opacification on CT usually suggest the correct diagnosis. In the proper clinical setting, these findings are indicative of pyelonephritis. Although these findings are of interest, the major thrust of renal imaging in parenchymal infections should be the exclusion of parenchymal abscesses. The presence of liquefaction usually implies the need for additional or prolonged treatment of infected patients. Antibiotic therapy often is coupled with percutaneous or surgical drainage of parenchymal abscesses.

Emphysematous pyelonephritis, an uncommon form of acute pyelonephritis, is characterized by renal infection with a gas-producing organism. Emphysematous pyelonephritis usually is seen in people with diabetes and is a particularly severe infection. Unmanaged emphysematous pyelonephritis has been associated with a mortality rate up to 90%. Although emergency nephrectomy is the therapy generally accepted for emphysematous pyelonephritis, some patients can be treated with percutaneous drainage and systemic antibiotics. Gas in the renal bed usually is visualized on plain abdominal radiographs (Fig. 4-15). Once gas in the renal bed is suggested, CT should be obtained to confirm its presence and exactly localize the gas collection (Fig. 4-15). The management algorithms somewhat depend on the location and distribution of gas around the kidney. With CT, the location of the gas can be identified accurately. Additionally, gas within the kidney should be characterized as localized or diffuse. If gas is diffusely spread throughout the renal parenchyma (Fig. 4-15), surgical nephrectomy is indi-

A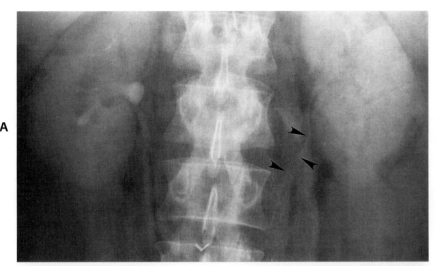

B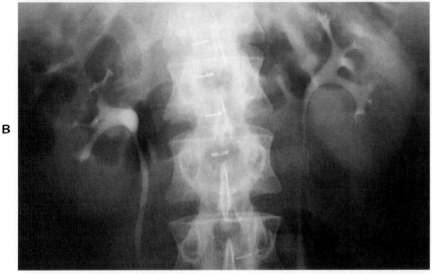

Fig. 4-13 Acute pyelonephritis. **A,** This film from a urogram in a patient with left-sided pyelonephritis demonstrates poor opacification of the left calyces and ureter. There is minimal contrast excretion from the left kidney with only a thread of contrast within the left ureteral lumen (arrowheads). **B,** A urogram 1 week later, after successful antibiotic management of pyelonephritis demonstrates a completely normal left kidney and collecting system.

cated in most patients. Nephrectomy is indicated to remove the source of infection and because the kidney likely is irreversibly damaged and unsalvageable. However, if gas is localized within one area of the renal parenchyma (Fig. 4-16) and if preservation of functioning renal tissue is a high priority, percutaneous drainage of this focal infection can be attempted. This drainage usually is performed under CT guidance. When percutaneous management is contemplated, it is essential to evaluate the involved kidney for possible ureteral obstruction, which often coexists with emphysematous pyelonephritis and must be managed simultaneously. If present, obstruction should be managed with stenting or percutaneous nephrostomy placement and drainage of the emphysematous pyelonephritis. Finally, systemic antibiotics must be administered. This nonsurgical approach to the management of localized emphysematous pyelonephritis usually is successful and results in resolution of infection and preservation of function in the involved kidney. If

the infection continues to progress after adequate percutaneous drainage and if urinary tract decompression has been obtained, surgical nephrectomy may still be required.

Gas collections elsewhere in the renal bed also can be treated nonsurgically in many patients. Perinephric gas-containing abscesses usually are managed successfully with percutaneous drainage and systemic antibiotic therapy. Gas that is localized within the intrarenal collecting system or ureter (Fig. 4-17 on p. 136), which is the result of a gas-producing infection, also is treated nonsurgically in most patients. A gas-producing infection in this area also is known as emphysematous pyelitis, which usually is seen with obstruction of the ureter and coexistent infection. It is really a subtype of pyonephrosis and is managed in a similar fashion. Systemic antibiotics coupled with urinary tract decompression usually result in prompt resolution of the infection. Urinary tract decompression can be obtained with either ureteral stenting or percutaneous nephrostomy drainage. In most patients, nephrostomy drainage is preferred because a large-bore catheter may be necessary to drain the viscus, infectious debris mixed with the urine.

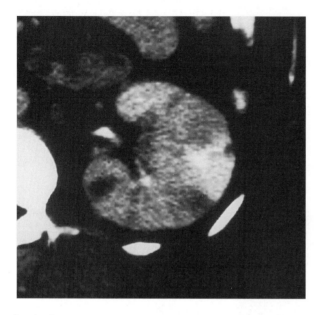

Fig. 4-14 Contrast-infused CT of a kidney with acute pyelonephritis. This CT scan demonstrates reniform enlargement of the left kidney with wedge-shaped areas of hypofunction and linear striations. These features are typical of diffuse pyelonephritis.

Infiltration of the kidney also can be caused by cellular infiltrates from chronic inflammation, as is seen with XGP. These patients typically have a history of chronic or recurrent urinary tract infections, usually with *Proteus* or *Escherichia coli* bacteria. In 80% of patients, nephrolithiasis coexists and is the likely cause of XGP. XGP most likely results from chronic, low-grade obstruction coupled with chronic bacteriuria. A minority of patients with this combination will develop XGP. Histologically, XGP results from replacement of renal parenchyma with lipid-laden histiocytes, which leads to reniform enlargement of the kidney, with diminished or absent function. The classic urographic triad associated with XGP includes nephrolithiasis associated with renal enlargement (Fig. 4-18) and diminished or absent renal function (Box 4-6). One radiographic clue that aids in the diagnosis of XGP is the "fractured stone" sign. When XGP develops, it may lead to rapid infiltration and expansion of the renal parenchyma, which may cause fracture and dispersion of the associated renal calculus. Many infection-based calculi are branched, but fragments usually are contiguous or at least closely related. Identification of a fractured branched stone suggests the development of XGP, and additional imaging is indicated. XGP may be diagnosed with other imaging techniques. Although ultrasound examination will demonstrate reniform enlargement, intraparenchymal debris-filled cystic spaces, loss of the cortical medullary junction, and the renal calculus, often

Fig. 4-15 Emphysematous pyelonephritis. **A,** A coned-down view of the left renal bed demonstrates striated gas spread throughout the left kidney. Several crescentic collections of gas are noted in a subcapsular location. **B,** A CT scan in the same patient demonstrates diffuse emphysematous pyelonephritis.

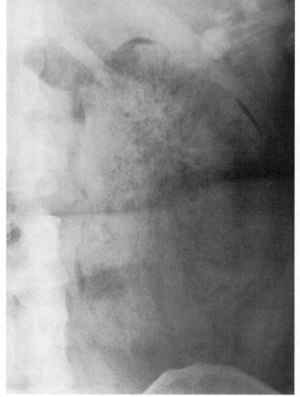

A

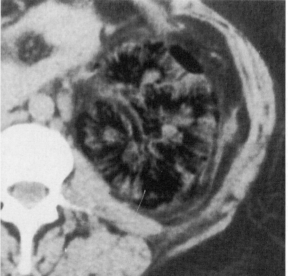

B

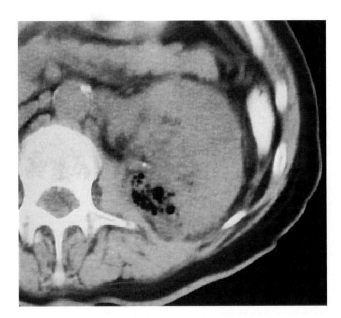

Fig. 4-16   Localized emphysematous pyelonephritis. A computed tomography scan in this patient demonstrates a focal collection of gas in the dorsal aspect of the left kidney. This patient successfully was treated with percutaneous drainage of this area of infection in conjunction with systemic antibiotic treatment.

sonography is less diagnostic than urography or CT. On CT scans, the central renal stone usually is visualized on uninfused studies. Extrarenal inflammatory changes often are evident. With contrast infusion, some residual parenchymal enhancement is demonstrated in most patients. This parenchyma surrounds radially oriented cystic spaces representing necrotic debris within the parenchyma. This appearance may radiographically mimic hydronephrosis. The cystic spaces represent parenchymal cavities rather than obstructed calyces. Retrograde pyelograms usually demonstrate a very contracted and irregular pyelocalyceal system. Flow into extraurinary fistulas may be demonstrated with contrast studies. There is a marked female predominance with XGP, probably because of the higher prevalence of pyelonephritis in the female population. Ten percent of patients with XGP have diabetes mellitus, and this probably reflects the propensity of patients with diabetes for urinary tract infections. Although XGP is a benign condition, it often spreads beyond the kidney. Inflammatory changes often are seen in contiguous structures, including the perinephric space, the psoas muscle, and other retroperitoneal structures. Cutaneous or enteric fistulas may develop. In some patients, an elevation in liver enzymes occurs and suggests associated liver disease. After nephrectomy, liver enzymes will return to normal. It is likely that liver enzymes are elevated because of massive tissue necrosis associated with the renal parenchymal replacement seen with XGP. Unlike people with typical acute renal infections, these patients usually present with chronic systemic symptoms with a background of chronic urinary infections. Anorexia, malaise, weight loss, and fever typically are associated with XGP. Because the kidney is damaged irrevocably with the diffuse form of XGP, nephrectomy is the only appropriate therapy.

Renal contusion in the acute phase can lead to diffuse enlargement of the kidney (Fig. 4-19). Obviously, this is seen in the trauma setting, and the diagnosis is not in doubt. Associated with parenchymal swelling is the heterogeneous nephrogram, particularly well demonstrated on CT scans. Parenchymal striations and renal hypofunction often are associated with contusion.

Acute ischemia or vascular engorgement also can lead to smooth enlargement of the involved kidney. This pattern is most typical of acute renal vein thrombosis (RVT). With acute RVT, the kidney is swollen and hypofunctioning (Fig. 4-20 on p. 138). Excretion of contrast material will be delayed or even absent in severe cases. Hydronephrosis is not present because the ureter is unaffected in RVT. The thrombosis may be demonstrated with sonography, MR imaging, or contrast-infused CT. RVT in adults most commonly is associated with coagulopathy as associated with diffuse intravascular coagulopathy, collagen-vascular diseases, and some hemoglobinopathies. RVT also is seen in patients with acute glomerulonephritis of the membranoproliferative subtype. In many patients, RVT is idiopathic. Because symptoms and some imaging features (reniform enlargement, delayed opacification, flank pain, and hematuria) mimic those of ureteral obstruction, imaging of the collecting system is crucial in patients with possible RVT. Absence of collecting-system dilatation suggests a vascular etiology, such as RVT.

Another vascular abnormality that leads to reniform enlargement of the kidney in the acute phase is arterial occlusion, which usually is seen in patients with acute renal artery dissection or thromboembolic disease. When renal infarction is global, the kidney swells acutely and is nonfunctional. The diagnosis can be confirmed with Doppler ultrasound examination or contrast-infused CT scan. With contrast infusion, a rim nephrogram usually is present and is indicative of parenchymal ischemia associated with minimal residual perfusion of the outer cortex, which is supplied by capsular collateral arteries. This finding is typical for acute arterial obstruction. Segmental infarcts rarely lead to significant reniform enlargement of the kidney but otherwise have similar imaging features in the involved segments of the kidney.

Some renal neoplasms grow by infiltration of the kidney, that is, they grow along and replace normal renal parenchyma. These neoplasms can lead to unilateral reniform enlargement and are discussed in detail in Chapter 3. However, because these neoplasms may cause unilateral smooth renal enlargement, they must be considered in this category of patterns. The most common of these neoplasms is the transitional cell carcinoma (TCC). TCC

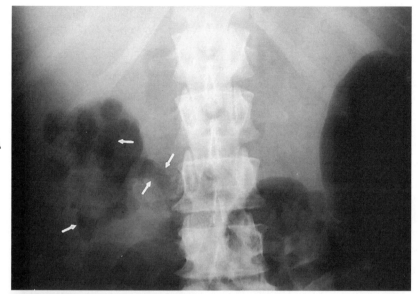

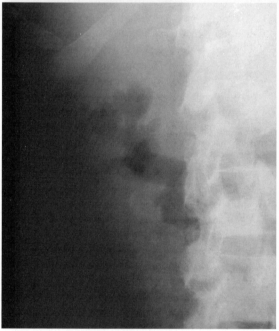

Fig. 4-17 Emphysematous pyelitis. **A,** This abdominal radiograph was obtained in a patient with diabetes with sepsis and abdominal pain. Gas in the right collecting system and right ureter (arrows) is obscured partially by overlying colon. **B,** An oblique view of the right renal bed confirms gas in the calyces and upper ureter, which was managed successfully with percutaneous nephrostomy drainage and systemic antibiotic administration.

patients usually present with gross hematuria. Radiographic features that support a diagnosis of TCC include nonvisualization of calyces, polypoid filling defects in the calyces or renal pelvis, soft tissue mass in the renal sinus, and associated retroperitoneal lymphadenopathy. Another neoplasm with similar appearance is the squamous cell carcinoma (SCC), an uncommon urothelial neoplasm. Radiographically, this appears identical to the TCC with the same features as those mentioned previously. However, some clues may suggest the diagnosis of SCC rather than TCC. For primary SCC to develop, there must be preexisting metaplasia of the normal transitional epithelium of the collecting system, which occurs as a result of chronic irritation, often caused by renal stone disease. Therefore, the presence of a renal stone in association

with an infiltrating renal neoplasm is strongly suggestive of SCC. A renal stone can be detected in approximately 50% of patients with renal SCC. Other primary infiltrating renal neoplasms are rare. Some secondary neoplasms may involve the kidney, causing renal enlargement. Neoplasms that typically cause this pattern of renal involvement include leukemia, lymphoma, and metastatic SCC. With these patients, lesions usually are multiple and typically bilateral, another radiographic pattern that is discussed later in this chapter.

Finally, acute arteritis induced by radiation therapy leads to swelling of the kidney and hypofunction. The appearance is similar to that of other vascular causes of renal enlargement. In ensuing months, renal atrophy develops in the affected kidney.

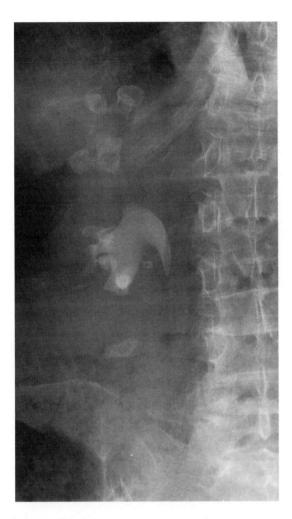

Fig. 4-18   Xanthogranulomatous pyelonephritis (XGP). This scout film for a urogram demonstrates a staghorn calculus in the right kidney. The renal outline is not well demonstrated, but based on the size of the renal stone, the kidney is definitely enlarged. After contrast material injection, there was no perceptible function in this right kidney. This triad of findings is typical of XGP.

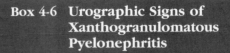

Box 4-6   Urographic Signs of Xanthogranulomatous Pyelonephritis

Unilateral reniform enlargement
Unilateral renal hypofunction
Renal stone
"Fractured stone" sign

The final category leading to unilateral smooth enlargement of the kidney is hypertrophy. Unilateral renal hypertrophy usually is the result of an abnormality of the contralateral kidney, which may result from renal absence or functional impairment. Hypertrophy implies enlargement of existing glomeruli rather than generation of new glomeruli (impossible in mature kidneys). Renal hypertrophy is possible in patients of all ages, but it seldom occurs in patients aged more than 60 years. Renal hypertrophy usually presents little diagnostic difficulty because the kidney will be enlarged but appears normal otherwise. In addition, the contralateral renal absence or abnormality will be evident. On occasion, compensatory hypertrophy occurs focally in the kidney and leads to the formation of a pseudotumor. Renal pseudotumor implies focal enlargement of normal renal parenchyma, which in some ways mimics a neoplasm and usually occurs when part of a kidney is atrophic or diseased so that hypertrophy of these segments is limited or impossible. Normal segments undergo hypertrophy when needed, which can lead to development of a pseudotumor. In all other regards, this area of kidney appears normal, with normal subtending calyces and echo texture.

In rare cases, renal hypertrophy is caused by underly-

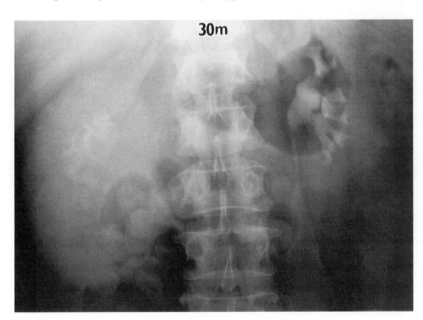

30m

Fig. 4-19   Renal contusion causing unilateral renal enlargement. This 30-minute film from a urogram in a trauma patient demonstrates reniform enlargement of the right kidney with a dense, persistent nephrogram and delay in pyelographic opacification. These findings are typical of diffuse renal contusion in a trauma patient. Computed tomography scanning was performed and confirmed the absence of more severe renal injury.

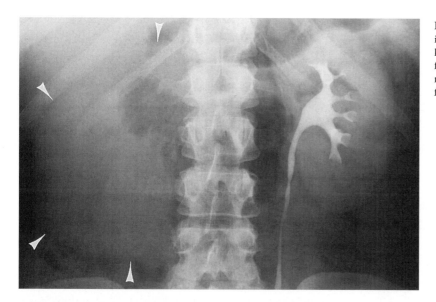

Fig. 4-20   Acute renal vein thrombosis. There is no excretion of contrast material from the right kidney on this urogram. The right kidney is diffusely and smoothly enlarged (arrowheads). Sonography of this patient with systemic lupus confirmed right renal vein thrombosis.

ing congenital abnormality. When patients suffer hemihypertrophy, the kidney on the involved side may enlarge. Although this disease is rare, it is of interest to the uroradiologist, because hemihypertrophy is associated with other genitourinary pathology. In a small number of patients with medullary sponge kidney, a common urographic abnormality, hemihypertrophy is an associated abnormality (Fig. 4-21). In these patients, medullary sponge kidney is evident, and careful scrutiny of the radiographs also yields evidence of unilateral reniform enlargement and musculoskeletal asymmetry, often associated with scoliosis. Other abnormalities associated with hemihypertrophy include Wilms' tumors, pheochromo-

cytoma, and syndromes such as the Beckwith-Wiedemann syndrome.

The cause of unilateral smooth enlargement of the kidney often can be determined with imaging studies, which lead to a diagnosis of acute ureteral obstruction, duplication anomaly, or compensatory hypertrophy. Clinical evidence of pyelonephritis should be sought in patients with this radiographic abnormality. If patients do not readily fit into one of these categories, vascular etiologies or infiltrating neoplasms are strongly suggested, and these are usually well evaluated with sonography or contrast-infused CT. The coexistence of an infection-based stone and markedly diminished renal function

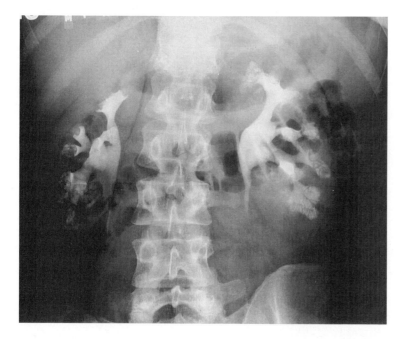

Fig. 4-21   Renal enlargement resulting from hemihypertrophy. A urogram in this patient demonstrates diffuse changes of medullary sponge kidney. In addition, unilateral enlargement of the left kidney is noted. There also is enlargement of the left iliac wing and associated scoliosis. This patient had hemihypertrophy, which is sometimes found in association with medullary sponge kidney.

is virtually diagnostic of XGP. If none of these entities appropriately fit the radiographic findings, additional or follow-up imaging may be needed. On occasion, a focal renal mass located in one pole of the kidney may mimic reniform enlargement of the kidney. Once detected, renal tumors become the major diagnostic consideration. Rarely, unilateral enlargement may represent the early presentation of bilateral renal disease, and later imaging will demonstrate more symmetric involvement of both kidneys.

BILATERAL RENAL ENLARGEMENT

In seeking a diagnosis for patients who have bilateral renal enlargement, the first major task is to distinguish between patients with multiple renal masses causing enlargement from those with diffuse renal enlargement in the absence of focal renal masses. Renal masses usually are evident with imaging studies because they cause focal contour abnormalities and substantial calyceal splaying and displacement. If these features are present, multiple renal masses must be considered as the cause of kidney enlargement, and the diagnostic paradigm is completely different than for bilateral smooth renal enlargement.

Reniform Enlargement

The list of diseases causing bilateral smooth renal enlargement is extensive (Box 4-7). Many of the entities are obscure. However, it is useful to be aware of many of these entities to plan further imaging for clinical evaluation and management. The most common cause of bilateral smooth renal enlargement is diabetic nephropathy, which accounts for at least 50% of cases. Diabetes can affect the kidney in a number of ways and often eventually leads to renal insufficiency. Parenchymal hypertrophy can occur in this nephropathy spectrum. In some patients, bilateral renal enlargement precedes definitive chemical evidence of diabetes by 1 year or more. In patients with diabetes and adequate renal function, the kidneys may be enlarged but otherwise appear normal with good contrast excretion on radiographic studies (Fig. 4-22). On ultrasound examination, echogenicity of the kidneys is normal. Therefore, confirmation of diabetic nephropathy depends on clinical parameters indicating coexistent diabetes mellitus or on biopsy.

The second most common cause of this radiographic pattern is acute glomerulonephritis. This disease encompasses a spectrum of histologic abnormalities, and any of these processes, during its acute phase, can lead to renal enlargement. The renal enlargement is thought to result from edema incited by diffuse parenchymal inflammation initiated by glomerulonephritis. Because these patients often present with renal insufficiency, con-

Box 4-7   Causes of Bilateral Smooth Renal Enlargement

Common
    Diabetic nephropathy
Uncommon
    Acute glomerulonephritis
    Collagen-vascular diseases
    Vasculitis
    AIDS nephropathy
    Leukemia
    Lymphoma
    Autosomal recessive polycystic kidney disease
    Acute interstitial nephritis
Rare
    Hemoglobinopathy (sickle cell, thalassemia)
    Acromegaly
    Acute urate nephropathy
    Amyloidosis
    Myeloma
    Fabry's disease
    Bartter's syndrome
    Von Gierke's disease

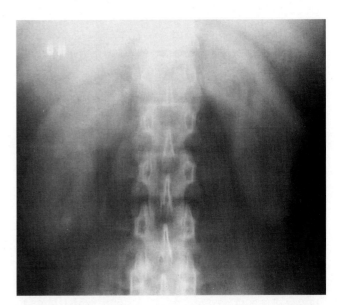

Fig. 4-22 Bilateral renal enlargement resulting from diabetes. This nephrotomogram demonstrates smooth reniform enlargement of both kidneys in this patient with early diabetic nephropathy. Other than enlargement, the kidneys appear healthy, and on later films, there was excretion of contrast material into normal calyces and ureters.

trast studies usually are bypassed. Other imaging studies are nonspecific and demonstrate only smooth bilateral renal enlargement. Definitive diagnosis usually depends on percutaneous biopsy. The major role of imaging in these patients is to exclude postrenal causes of renal

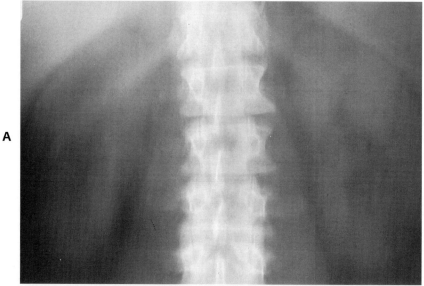

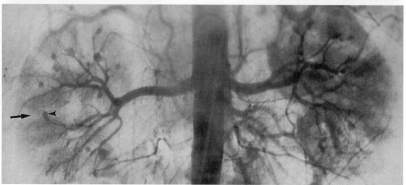

Fig. 4-23   Renal enlargement from polyarteritis nodosa. **A,** A nephrotomogram demonstrates diffuse reniform enlargement of both kidneys in this patient with intermittent gross hematuria. **B,** A renal arteriogram in this patient demonstrates multiple renal artery branch aneurysms (arrowhead) with adjacent infarctions (arrow). These angiographic findings are suggestive of polyarteritis nodosa, although they uncommonly are seen with other forms of arteritis.

insufficiency because these may be reversible with urinary tract decompression.

Collagen-vascular diseases, autoimmune disorders, and vasculitides also can cause bilateral smooth renal enlargement. Entities in this group include systemic lupus erythematosus, Goodpasture's syndrome, Wegener's granulomatosis, Henoch-Schönlein purpura syndrome, and polyarteritis nodosa. Associated clinical symptoms often suggest the correct diagnosis. Pulmonary hemorrhage is usually associated with Goodpasture's syndrome. Diffuse purpura is seen in association with Henoch-Schönlein purpura syndrome. Wegener's granulomatosis usually is associated with sinusitis and hemoptysis. Polyarteritis nodosa is a multiorgan disease process, although hematuria and renal disease often are the dominant problems. Polyarteritis nodosa is a strong possibility when numerous aneurysms are detected by angiography (Fig. 4-23) and when there is laboratory evidence of an ongoing inflammatory process. Renal biopsy may be required to confirm the etiology of the renal disease.

Other causes of smooth bilateral renal enlargement are included in Box 4-7. Many of the other entities in this list are uncommon or they uncommonly involve the kidneys. Clinical information is crucial, although biopsy often is required for exact diagnosis of entities in this category.

Bilateral Renal Enlargement with Multiple Masses

Parenchymal enlargement may result from displacement of normal parenchyma by multiple renal masses, leading to overall enlargement of the renal shadow (Box 4-8). Contour bulges and collecting-system displacement are associated. A number of these entities are described in detail in chapter 3; others deserve additional discussion here. The most common cause of marked renal enlargement with multiple renal masses is autosomal dominant polycystic kidney disease (ADPKD). This autosomal dominant hereditary disorder is characterized by the development of innumerable simple renal cysts. Commonly, these cysts lead to massive enlargement of the renal shadows. Sometimes, in addition, a feature somewhat unique to ADPKD is massive enlargement of the collecting system (Fig. 4-24) in association with the parenchymal enlargement. Unlike other mass lesions in the kidney that

Box 4-8   Bilateral Renal Enlargement with Masses

Common
  Autosomal dominant polycystic kidney disease
Uncommon
  Acquired renal cystic disease
  Multiple simple cysts
  Lymphoma
  Metastases
  Wilms' tumors
Rare
  Tuberous sclerosis
  von Hippel-Lindau disease
  Multiple oncocytomas
  Nephroblastomatosis

compress the collecting system, in some patients, ADPKD leads to dilatation unrelated to obstruction. This appearance is akin to enlargement of the uterine cavity, as is seen in association with multiple uterine fibroids. Other cystic diseases of the kidneys are not known to cause this pattern.

Clinical features of ADPKD are typical, although there is a spectrum of disease. This disease does have a high degree of penetrance, which means that those who inherit the gene are very likely to manifest typical abnormalities. Patients often first present when aged 20 to 40 years with a variety of symptoms, including hypertension, flank pain, pyelonephritis, urolithiasis, hematuria, or renal insufficiency. Imaging studies usually demonstrate a large number of simple cysts spread throughout both kidneys in a disorganized fashion. The cysts usually vary in size, and with time, they progress to replace virtually all normal renal parenchyma. Because so many cysts are present, complicated cysts often are seen coexisting with simple cysts. Complicated cysts include those that contain hemorrhage, with evidence of infection, septations, or peripheral calcifications. Clinical symptoms in patients with complicated cysts often are related to infection or hemorrhage into preexisting simple renal cysts. There does not appear to be greater risk of renal malignancy in these patients, however, incidence of renal malignancy in this group appears no lower than that of a cohort of patients without ADPKD. In up to 50% of patients, simple hepatic cysts also are demonstrated. Cysts also occur in other solid organs but at considerably lower incidence rates. Cysts may be detected in the spleen, the pancreas, the pelvic organs, and the lung. Important associations include a 10% to 15% rate of intracranial berry aneurysm formation and a high rate of mild valvular heart disease. In addition, patients with ADPKD may have an increased

risk of coarctation of the thoracic aorta. Although the diagnosis of ADPKD with imaging studies usually is straightforward, some cases are atypical. In approximately 10% of patients, renal cystic disease is markedly asymmetric. Usually, the less affected kidney develops innumerable cysts typical of ADPKD, but at presentation, this kidney may appear nearly normal. Usually some cysts are present in both kidneys, even in markedly asymmetric cases. Age at presentation, family history, and other clinical factors usually suggest the correct diagnosis. If in doubt, surveillance sonography or computed tomography will demonstrate progression of disease bilaterally with time. In other patients, the presentation of ADPKD may be delayed or may progress slowly; some patients survive until aged 60 to 80 years without significant renal insufficiency. Such long survival is uncommon, but it is one extreme of the spectrum of ADPKD.

Other causes of multiple renal masses that can lead to bilateral renal enlargement are listed in Box 4-8. Numerous syndromes that are associated with cystic dis-

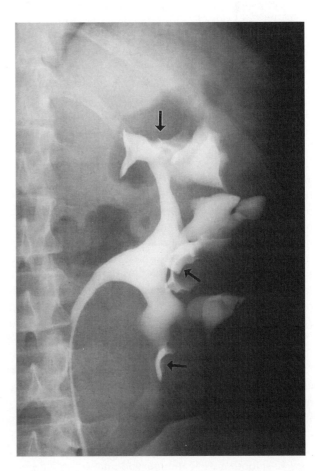

Fig. 4-24   Renal enlargement with associated collecting system enlargement. A retrograde pyelogram in this patient with known autosomal dominant polycystic kidney disease demonstrates massive enlargement of the left collecting system. Several areas of calyceal splaying (arrows) are caused by the parenchymal cysts.

eases of the kidney are similar radiographically to ADPKD. In addition, multifocal primary renal tumors or renal metastasis may lead to multiple solid renal masses that enlarge the renal contours.

Finally, three clinical entities are known to be associated with the development of simple renal cysts and solid renal masses. These are von Hippel-Lindau (VHL) disease, tuberous sclerosis, and acquired cystic disease of dialysis (ACD). In patients with VHL disease, 75% or more develop simple renal cysts. Renal cell carcinoma (RCC) develops in 40% of patients with VHL, and 75% of these patients have multiple, and often bilateral, RCCs. In addition, these patients have hemangioblastomas of the central nervous system (CNS) and retinal angiomas. Other associated abnormalities include cysts of other solid abdominal organs (particularly the pancreas), pheochromocytomas, pancreatic and hepatic adenomas, and cysts of pelvic organs.

Eighty percent of patients with tuberous sclerosis will develop renal angiomyolipomas. Although angiomyolipomas are described more thoroughly in Chapter 3, these benign hamartomas contain variable components of vascular, fat, and muscle tissue. In patients with tuberous sclerosis, angiomyolipomas usually are multifocal and often grow large. Although they are benign, the mass effect caused by these tumors may lead to pain and urinary outflow obstruction. In addition, angiomyolipomas are known for their predilection to hemorrhage, but hemorrhage is rare in those masses smaller than 4 cm in diameter. Larger angiomyolipomas can hemorrhage massively and cause acute symptoms and, in some patients, life-threatening blood loss. Patients with tuberous sclerosis also have an increased incidence of simple renal cyst formation. These cysts are less common than angiomyolipomas in these patients, but cysts and angiomyolipomas often coexist. The coexistence of multiple angiomyolipomas with one or more simple renal cysts is said to be diagnostic of tuberous sclerosis. In one subgroup of patients with tuberous sclerosis, primarily in young children, numerous simple renal cysts develop in the absence of angiomyolipoma formation. The radiographic appearance of these kidneys closely resembles that of ADPKD. However, other clinical parameters usually point to tuberous sclerosis. Associated findings include a facial skin lesion known as adenoma sebaceum, mental retardation, and seizure disorder. The central nervous system abnormalities are related to periventricular hamartomas, which usually calcify and are evident on CNS imaging studies. Other known associations include CNS giant-cell astrocytomas; truncal shagreen patch of rough, discolored skin; cardiac smooth muscle tumors; and pulmonary lymphangioleiomyomatosis, which causes interstitial lung disease, and recurrent chylous effusions and pneumothorax. Also commonly seen are multiple bone islands or osteomas. Although this entity is rare, tuberous sclerosis and VHL disease include many radiographically important abnormalities whose manifestations should be well known by radiologists.

Last in this category is ACD. Patients with preserved native kidneys who undergo dialysis, either hemodialysis or peritoneal dialysis, usually develop cystic disease of the kidneys. After 3 years of dialysis, at least 50% of patients have ACD. Usually ACD is manifested radiographically as innumerable small parenchymal simple cysts spread throughout the kidneys. In some patients, these cysts attain a large size, and the appearance of the kidneys is identical to that of ADPKD. Seven percent of patients with ACD also will develop solid renal tumors. Although most of these tend to progress very slowly, most are classified as malignant RCCs. Therefore, imaging of the native kidneys is recommended in these patients if any symptoms of renal disease, such as hematuria or flank pain, develop. Demonstration of a solid renal mass on imaging studies indicates renal adenocarcinoma. Because these tumors often do not metastasize, nephrectomy usually is curative.

NEPHROCALCINOSIS

The term *nephrocalcinosis* has been used to describe various patterns of renal parenchymal calcification. However, the term is most appropriate when multifocal renal parenchymal calcifications exist so that focal dystrophic calcifications in solitary renal masses and focal areas of remote renal inflammation are excluded. Nephrocalcinosis easily is identified on imaging studies. Sonography and CT are more sensitive for the detection of small quantities of parenchymal calcification than standard radiography. However detected, nephrocalcinosis should be classified to generate a reasonable list of possible underlying abnormalities. Nephrocalcinosis is a classic radiographic finding, and a differential diagnosis should be committed to every radiologist's memory. Nephrocalcinosis can be divided into two distinct subtypes: medullary and cortical. It is very uncommon for cortical and medullary nephrocalcinosis to coexist in the same patient. Nephrocalcinosis can be classified on the basis of its radiographic appearance. In patients with cortical nephrocalcinosis, the calcifications are limited to the peripheral 1 to 2 cm of renal parenchyma (Fig. 4-25). The calcification often appears as an "eggshell" around the periphery of the kidney. Because the cortex also is seen *en face*, some calcifications project over the medullary portion of the kidney. The cortical position of these calcifications is best demonstrated by looking at the segment of the kidney in profile, at its periphery. Medullary nephrocalcinosis does not involve the extreme periphery of the kidney. In medullary nephrocalcinosis, the cortex is spared from the calcifying process; calcifications are

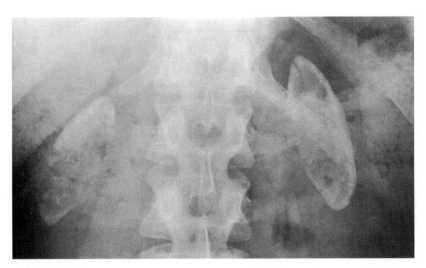

Fig. 4-25   Cortical nephrocalcinosis. This abdominal radiograph demonstrates eggshell calcification of both kidneys. This patient had chronic glomerulonephritis and demonstrates a calcification pattern typical of cortical nephrocalcinosis.

limited to the renal pyramids, which are arrayed in triangular orientation away from the calyces (Fig. 4-26). The base of these triangles is situated at the cortical–medullary junction of the renal parenchyma. These calcified renal pyramids are separated by unaffected renal parenchyma representing columns of renal cortex. With cortical nephrocalcinosis, the entire cortex of both kidneys usually is diffusely involved. Calcifications usually are evenly dispersed, forming a shell-like lining. With medullary nephrocalcinosis, the pattern of calcification somewhat depends on the underlying disease process. However, the calcifications usually are irregular and chunky in appearance. Calcifications may involve all pyramids, or there may be patchy, asymmetric involvement of the renal medulla. In addition, patients with cortical nephrocalcinosis usually have chronic renal insufficiency, and the kidneys are markedly atrophic. In a minority of patients with medullary nephrocalcinosis, the kidneys also are diminutive. In a smaller minority of these patients, there is smooth enlargement of the kidneys associated with the underlying disease process.

Once the classification is determined according to the pattern of calcification, an appropriate list of differential diagnoses can be considered.

Medullary Nephrocalcinosis

Medullary nephrocalcinosis is considerably more common than the cortical variety. The major causes of medullary calcinosis are listed in Box 4-9. The majority of cases result from hypercalcemic states, renal tubular acidosis, and medullary sponge kidney.

Hypercalcemic states may result from a number of underlying diseases, including hyperparathyroidism, sarcoidosis, vitamin D intoxication, milk–alkali syndrome, neoplastic states, and a myriad of other diseases. Regardless of the underlying cause, hypercalcemia can lead to the deposition of metastatic calcifications in otherwise normal tissues. This metabolic imbalance can lead to medullary nephrocalcinosis. As a result of hypercalciuria, these patients also have higher incidence of urolithiasis, which may require them to undergo radiographic studies. Severe long-standing hypercalcemia also is a well-known cause of irreversible renal insufficiency resulting from tubulointerstitial damage. Although hypercalcemia is a clinical and laboratory diagnosis, the pattern of medullary nephrocalcinosis present in these patients usually suggests this damage as the underlying abnormality. Because this is a systemic disease, the calcification pattern is sym-

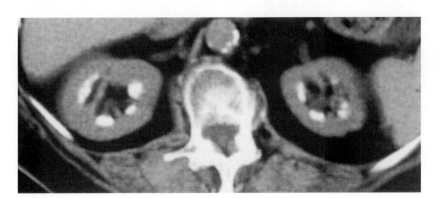

Fig. 4-26   Medullary nephrocalcinosis. Unenhanced computed tomography scan in this patient with renal tubular acidosis demonstrates bilateral medullary calcifications typical of medullary nephrocalcinosis.

Box 4-9 Causes of Medullary Nephrocalcinosis

Common
  Medullary sponge kidney
  Hypercalcemia
  Renal tubular acidosis
Uncommon
  Papillary necrosis
  Tuberculosis
  Hyperoxaluria
Rare
  Chronic furosemide use

metric and diffuse, involving all of the renal pyramids of both kidneys. In addition, because the nephrocalcinosis often is associated with chronic medical renal disease, the kidneys often are smaller than normal but smooth. Therefore, a possible diagnosis in a patient with diffuse symmetric medullary nephrocalcinosis with small smooth kidneys is chronic hypercalcemia.

Renal tubular acidosis (RTA) has a number of subtypes. Medullary nephrocalcinosis develops only in patients with type I, distal RTA. These patients generally develop progressive renal insufficiency. These patients, like those with other common varieties of medullary nephrocalcinosis, are more likely to have urolithiasis. RTA is associated with abnormally low levels of citrate in the urine. Citrate is an inhibitor of urolithiasis, and this deficiency may explain the development of uroliths and medullary nephrocalcinosis in these patients. With RTA, the distal tubule is unable to secrete adequate amounts of the hy-

drogen ion. These patients have inadequately acidified urine, even when a substantial degree of metabolic acidosis is present. Hypercalciuria develops to compensate for the hydrogen cation secretion deficiency. Presumably, medullary nephrocalcinosis is caused by chronic hypercalciuria combined with citrate deficiency. In this disease, the medullary calcifications are diffuse and symmetric (Fig. 4-27), involving all renal pyramids of both kidneys. In addition, the kidneys are normal in size and maintain a normal contour. Therefore, patients with diffuse symmetric medullary nephrocalcinosis and normal-sized kidneys are most likely to have distal RTA.

The most common cause of medullary nephrocalcinosis is medullary sponge kidney (MSK). This disorder is thought to be congenital. Although it is found in approximately one of every 200 intravenous urograms performed, in most patients, it is only an incidental finding of little clinical significance. However, MSK is associated with a markedly increased risk of urolithiasis, and there may be a slightly increased risk of pyelonephritis because of urinary stasis in the ectatic tubules. MSK, also known as benign renal tubular ectasia, often involves a limited number of renal pyramids. Although it is possible for all pyramids to be involved, MSK more commonly spares some of the renal pyramids from visible tubular ectasia. In patients with MSK, there is idiopathic ectasia of some of the distal collecting tubules in the renal medulla. The ectasia leads to urine stasis and precipitation of calcium and related minerals. When calcifications occur, they usually are rounded and multiple, arrayed radially, emanating from the renal papilla. Because these calcifications actually are contained within the ectatic tubules, they are obscured by excreted contrast material during urography. Their density blends imperceptibly with that of the surrounding contrast material, therefore, their shadow

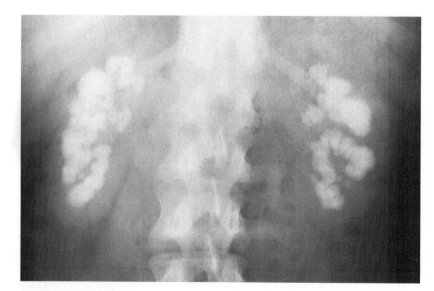

Fig. 4-27 Medullary nephrocalcinosis in a patient with renal tubular acidosis. A plain abdominal radiograph demonstrates diffuse and symmetric medullary nephrocalcinosis in normal-size kidneys. These features are suggestive of renal tubular acidosis.

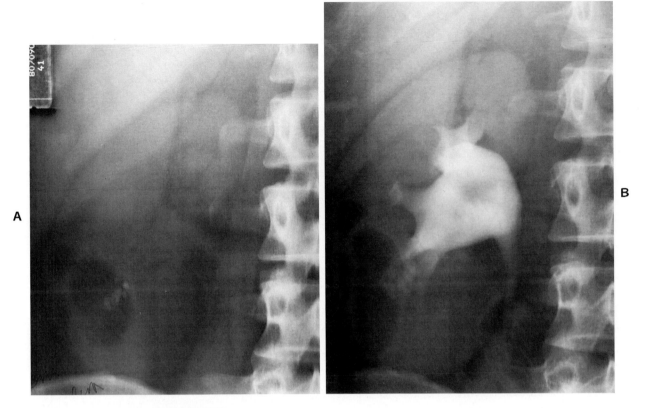

Fig. 4-28   The growing calculus sign with focal medullary sponge kidney. **A,** A preliminary radiograph demonstrates focal medullary calcification in the lower pole of the right kidney. **B,** After contrast material injection, the shadows of these calcifications apparently enlarge as they blend imperceptibly with the surrounding contrast material. These calcifications are contained within cystically dilated tubules in the renal medulla typical of medullary sponge kidney.

often appears to increase (Fig. 4-28) on radiographs after injection of contrast material. This "growing calculus" sign is classic, and when it occurs with other typical abnormalities, it is diagnostic of MSK. In many patients, discrete ectatic tubules are visualized as linear or cystic opacifications on a contrast-enhanced study. They are seen in the absence of medullary calcifications. Although this condition is undoubtedly a form of MSK, it often is described as benign renal tubular ectasia, which sounds less ominous and avoids labeling patients with a worrisome disease process. Most patients with MSK and benign tubular ectasia have normal-sized kidneys. In some patients, idiopathic enlargement of both kidneys is associated with MSK. A small subgroup of patients with MSK have associated hemihypertrophy (Fig. 4-21). With hemihypertrophy, one side of the body, including the kidney, is enlarged. Hemihypertrophy also is associated with more serious conditions, including Wilms' tumors, pheochromocytomas, and various congenital syndromes.

Analgesic nephropathy can cause medullary nephrocalcinosis, which most often is caused by chronic ingestion of large doses of nonsteroidal antiinflammatory drugs, such as phenacetin, aspirin, and acetaminophen.

Diffuse papillary necrosis may coexist. Analgesic nephropathy appears to be more common outside the United States, with high rates in Australia and Europe. This geographic distribution may result from the increased availability of combination analgesics in these areas. Analgesic nephropathy causes chronic renal insufficiency. Radiographically, analgesic nephropathy causes small kidneys, which often are irregularly scarred and occasionally smooth. Medullary nephrocalcinosis combined with bilateral small scarred kidneys (Fig. 4-29) strongly suggests analgesic nephropathy.

Rarely, other conditions are associated with medullary nephrocalcinosis, including hyperoxaluria, either primary or acquired, renal tuberculosis, and chronic furosemide usage in infants. Hyperoxaluria results from disruption of the normal enterohepatic metabolic pathways. The primary form is rare, and hyperoxaluria more commonly results from extensive disease or surgical resection of the distal small bowel. This form causes increased urinary secretion of oxalates, leading to formation of calcium oxalate stones and medullary nephrocalcinosis. Rarely, hyperoxaluria also can lead to cortical nephrocalcinosis. Primary hyperoxaluria generally is irreversible

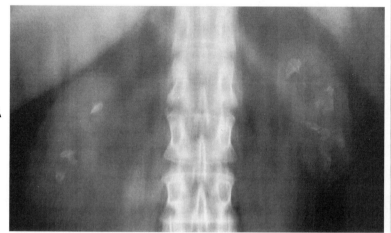

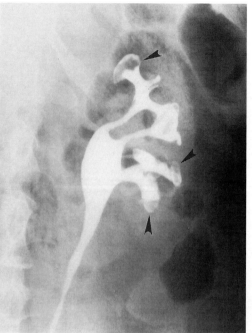

Fig. 4-29 Medullary nephrocalcinosis resulting from analgesic nephropathy. **A,** An abdominal radiograph in this patient with chronic renal failure demonstrates multiple medullary calcifications with smooth atrophy of both kidneys. **B,** A retrograde pyelogram demonstrates papillary necrosis (arrowheads), which often is seen in association with analgesic nephropathy.

and leads to death at a young age. Secondary hyperoxaluria is caused by extensive disease of the distal small bowel or small bowel resection and may be treatable. Hyperoxaluria is one of the few causes of calcium urolithiasis and nephrocalcinosis in children. Another is administration of furosemide, usually as a treatment for cardiovascular diseases in premature infants.

Finally, renal tuberculosis causes urinary tract calcifications in approximately 10% of patients. This form of secondary tuberculosis almost always originates in one kidney, focally involving a single renal papilla. As the infection grows, there is spread into the renal calyx with associated papillary necrosis. Infection then can extend along the urothelium and lead to inflammation and later fibrosis. Hydronephrosis and, eventually, autonephrectomy may develop. Parenchymal calcifications occur in a minority of patients with renal tuberculosis. These calcifications usually are focal and unilateral (Fig. 4-30), and they occur at sites of pyelitis acutely or fibrotic changes later in the disease course. This pattern of focal, unilateral calcification associated with cicatrization is less typical of other causes of medullary nephrocalcinosis. However, in some patients with renal tuberculosis, medullary calcifications may be extensive and may mimic other forms of medullary nephrocalcinosis. Contrast studies demonstrating inflammatory and fibrotic changes (Fig. 4-30) can be used to exclude other causes of nephrocalcinosis and to determine the underlying infectious etiology.

Cortical Nephrocalcinosis

Cortical nephrocalcinosis is an uncommon radiographic finding. Box 4-10 lists the major causes of this radiographic pattern. The most common cause of cortical nephrocalcinosis is chronic glomerulonephritis, in which chronic renal failure is associated with marked renal atrophy with smooth renal contours. Shell-like calcifications develop in the renal cortex in a small number of these patients and persist after successful renal transplantation and normalization of renal function. These calcifications are likely dystrophic and related to chronic renal cortical ischemia.

Box 4-10 Causes of Cortical Nephrocalcinosis

Common
    Chronic glomerulonephritis
    Acute cortical necrosis
Uncommon
    Hyperoxaluria
Rare
    Alport's syndrome
    Chronic transplant rejection

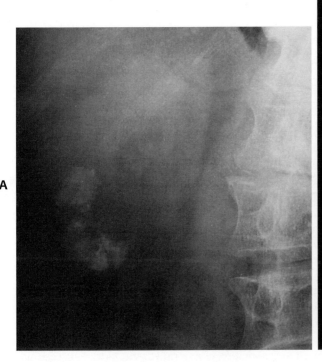
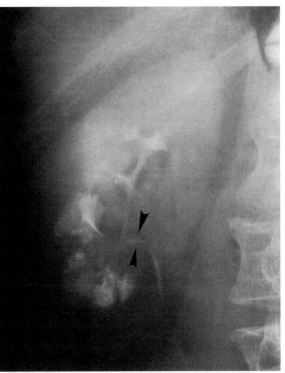

Fig. 4-30 Medullary nephrocalcinosis resulting from renal tuberculosis. **A,** A scout view of the right kidney demonstrates medullary nephrocalcinosis localized to the lower portion of the right kidney. **B,** A urogram in this patient with a remote history of renal tuberculosis demonstrates stricturing of the renal pelvis (arrowheads) and of the calyx adjacent to the parenchymal calcifications.

The other major cause of cortical nephrocalcinosis is calcification resulting from acute cortical necrosis. Among several possible causes, the most common is severe hypotension, which can occur as a complication of childbirth, sepsis, or severe hemorrhage. Acute cortical necrosis also can result from ingested nephrotoxins, such as ethylene glycol, a chemical commonly used in automobile antifreeze. In such patients, chronic renal failure is inevitable, and again, these cortical calcifications are dystrophic because of cortical necrosis. The radiographic pattern of calcification is identical to that seen with chronic glomerulonephritis.

Other, less common causes of cortical nephrocalcinosis are hyperoxaluria, Alport's syndrome, and chronic renal transplant rejection. Hyperoxaluria has been described previously, and it is unique because it may lead to the development of either medullary or cortical nephrocalcinosis. Alport's syndrome is a rare hereditary disorder consisting of congenital nephritis and sensorineural deafness. Patients with this condition may develop cortical nephrocalcinosis associated with chronic renal failure. Also, patients who have received renal transplants and suffer from chronic transplant rejection may develop cortical nephrocalcinosis, which occurs in the transplant kidney only and results from cortical necrosis with sec-

ondary formation of dystrophic calcifications in the necrotic areas.

Unlike medullary nephrocalcinosis, cortical nephrocalcinosis is uncommon, and radiographic findings usually are not useful in distinguishing the underlying causes. Fortunately, the patient's medical history usually readily indicates the underlying disease process leading to cortical calcifications.

IMAGING OF RENAL FAILURE

Causes of renal failure fall into several broad categories, including prerenal, renal, and postrenal diseases (Box 4-11). Prerenal processes include underperfusion of the kidneys as a result of severe cardiac disease or extensive renal atherosclerosis. Renal diseases causing renal failure include all of the chronic glomerulonephritides, which often are broadly categorized as medical renal disease; parenchymal replacement processes, such as severe polycystic kidney disease, either autosomal dominant or recessive, and uncommon infiltrative disorders. Although these diseases are chronic, patients may present with previously undiagnosed renal insufficiency, and the chronicity of the finding initially will be uncertain. Postre-

Box 4-11   Causes of Renal Failure

Prerenal
    Underperfusion
Renal
    Diffuse parenchymal disease
Postrenal
    Bladder outlet obstruction
    Bilateral ureteral obstruction

nal causes of acute renal failure include processes that obstruct urine outflow, such as bilateral ureteral obstruction or bladder outlet obstruction. Initial imaging evaluation of patients with newly diagnosed renal failure should begin with ultrasound evaluation. With sonography, postrenal obstructive causes of renal failure usually can be distinguished from the other two categories. This distinction is important, because urinary tract decompression often can reverse renal failure in this group of patients. Alternatively, prerenal and renal causes of renal failure are managed noninvasively. Ultrasound evaluation of patients with renal failure usually is straightforward. Because renal insufficiency induced by obstruction indicates longstanding blockage, hydronephrosis will be present. In the majority of patients with obstructive renal failure, hydronephrosis is bilateral. On occasion, unilateral obstruction associated with severe contralateral renal disease of a different etiology, such as reflux nephropathy or renal artery stenosis, can account for renal insufficiency. Because one healthy kidney is adequate for normal renal function, both kidneys must be diseased before a patient develops renal insufficiency. If bilateral hydro-

nephrosis is present, patients should be triaged to receive urinary tract decompression. Decompression may be successful with bladder catherization alone in patients with bladder outlet obstruction. Alternatively, ureteral stenting or percutaneous nephrostomy may be required.

Although varying degrees of parenchymal atrophy often are associated with longstanding ureteral obstruction, the reversibility of renal insufficiency cannot be predicted accurately from the quantity of residual renal parenchyma demonstrated with imaging studies before urinary tract decompression. Once urinary decompression is achieved, renal function gradually returns to a new baseline level, and the level of function of the renal mass can be assessed with a radionuclide renogram. Kidneys that appear severely atrophied on occasion regain surprisingly high levels of renal function when decompressed.

Renal sonography also is useful in identifying chronic medical renal disease. Patients with this disease have marked parenchymal atrophy with smooth reniform contour of the kidneys (Fig. 4-11). These kidneys appear small and hyperechoic. In patients with ADPKD, innumerable simple cysts replace the normal parenchyma. Patients with autosomal recessive polycystic kidney disease will develop reniform enlargement of both kidneys. In addition, the innumerable cystically dilated tubules present in ARPKD increase the echogenicity of the renal parenchyma so that the kidneys are equal to, or greater than, adjacent liver or spleen in echogencity. Nephropathy caused by HIV infection also causes increased echogenicity of the kidneys with reniform renal enlargement (Fig. 4-31).

Finally, newer sonographic techniques can be useful in identifying some patients with prerenal disease-

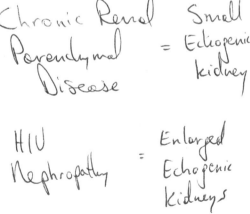

Chronic Renal Parenchymal Disease = Small Echogenic kidneys

HIV Nephropathy = Enlarged Echogenic Kidneys

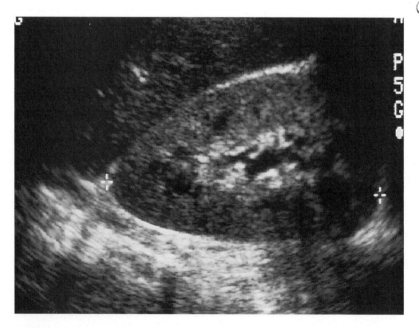

Fig. 4-31   HIV nephropathy. A longitudinal sonogram of the right kidney in this patient with AIDS demonstrates smooth reniform enlargement of the right kidney. Typical of HIV nephropathy, the renal parenchyma is hyperechoic compared with the adjacent liver. This pattern is very unusual in other disease entities.

induced renal insufficiency. Underperfusion of the kidneys can be caused by bilateral renal artery stenosis, which may be identified with duplex ultrasound evaluation of the renal arteries. Newer techniques, such as CT angiography and MR angiography, are in the developmental phase and also may be useful in diagnosing renal artery stenosis. Although vascular sonography appears to be a useful screening test at some institutions for patients in whom renal artery stenosis is suspected, angiography remains the standard for diagnosis and management planning of this disease. In patients with renal insufficiency, digital angiography should be used to minimize the nephrotoxicity of the administered intravascular contrast media. Revascularization procedures, either surgery or angioplasty, can stabilize or even reverse renal failure in some patients with renal artery stenosis.

Patients with renal failure of undiagnosed cause should be evaluated first with ultrasound examination. Bilateral renal disease with hydronephrosis suggests a remediable cause of renal failure, and urinary tract decompression should be undertaken. Patients with chronic medical renal disease usually have typical findings, including small atrophic kidneys indicative of longstanding parenchymal disease. Finally, duplex examination of the renal arteries may be useful in evaluating patients for possibly remediable renal artery stenosis.

RENAL TRAUMA

Urinary tract injury occurs in 10% of trauma patients. The kidney is the area of the urinary tract that most commonly is injured, and blunt trauma is the cause of 90% of traumatic renal injuries. Blunt injuries usually occur during motor vehicle accidents or athletic injuries and can damage the kidney because of compression or shearing forces. Blunt injury also can lead to laceration of the kidney by adjacent fractured bones. A minority of renal injuries result from penetrating trauma. The other sites of urinary tract injury in order of descending frequency are the bladder, the urethra, and the ureters. Radiologic evaluation of these areas of the urinary tract often precedes renal evaluation.

Various systems for classifying renal injuries have been used. One such system classifies traumatic renal injuries into five categories: renal contusion, renal laceration, renal fracture, shattered kidney, and vascular pedicle injury. The choice of the initial imaging examination to evaluate the kidneys should be governed by knowledge of the mechanism of injury, condition of the patient, and the degree of suspicion of underlying renal trauma. The kidneys should be evaluated radiologically in all blunt trauma patients who have either gross hematuria or microscopic hematuria with clinical evidence of ongoing hemorrhage, such as hypotension. Although the absence

of gross hematuria can be used to avoid unnecessary radiologic evaluation of the kidneys in blunt trauma patients, this is not true in patients with penetrating injuries involving either kidney. With penetrating trauma to the kidneys, not only does the severity of hematuria fail to correlate with the severity of renal trauma, but hematuria can be absent with major renal injury. Hematuria is absent in up to 14% of patients with renal lacerations and renal vascular injuries from penetrating trauma.

Contrast-infused CT and IVU are the two radiologic examinations used to evaluate the kidneys of trauma patients. IVU should be used for patients who have experienced penetrating trauma and whose condition requires immediate surgery. In these patients, IVU is useful to evaluate the contralateral kidney for unsuspected abnormalities. An IVU examination can yield false-negative results for the kidney injured by penetrating trauma. Because penetrating injuries cause damage in a focal, defined area of the abdomen, unstable patients are best treated with exploratory surgery focused on the area of injury. IVU for trauma patients can be performed in the emergency department or intraoperatively with portable radiographic equipment. IVU is a good test to exclude major renal injuries caused by blunt trauma if gross hematuria is present in patients whose condition is unstable. Normal IVU results in a blunt trauma patient virtually exclude any serious renal trauma. However, urograms of trauma patients must be scrutinized for subtle abnormalities, including contrast extravasation, diminished nephrogram, or mass effects. An abdominal CT should be obtained for additional evaluation whenever IVU results for a trauma patient are abnormal. CT is useful in definitively classifying the type of renal injury involved, information that is helpful for guiding treatment decisions. CT should be used as the first radiologic examination to evaluate the kidneys and the other abdominal viscera in stable victims of blunt trauma. In addition to allowing accurate classification of renal injuries, CT offers the potential to detect damage to other organs. The condition of a trauma patient must be reasonably stable to undergo CT scanning.

Overall, clinically significant renal injuries are uncommon. Of diagnosed renal injuries, 65% are classified as contusion, and 30% are classified as laceration. Both of these types of injuries are generally managed conservatively, without surgery, in the patient whose condition is stable. The remaining 5% of renal injuries comprise renal fractures, shattered kidneys, and vascular pedicle injuries.

Renal contusion is a parenchymal bruise with interstitial edema and hemorrhage. On imaging studies, the affected kidney generally is enlarged because of swelling (Fig. 4-19). The contused kidney demonstrates hypofunction, which may be visualized radiographically as delay in the pyelographic phase, persistence of the nephro-

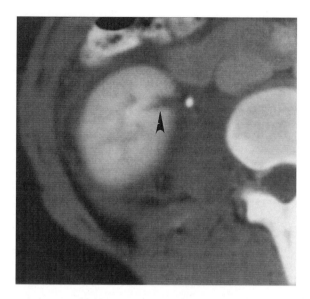

Fig. 4-32 Renal laceration. A contrast-infused computed tomography scan in this adolescent who was injured in a motor vehicle accident demonstrates a focal renal laceration (arrowhead). There is extensive perirenal blood from the laceration.

gram, and diminished density of the contrast material in the calyces and ureter. This decreased density results from impaired concentration capacity of the contused kidney. The kidney has been "stunned" by the trauma, and its function has not yet returned to normal. With CT, a heterogeneous nephrogram usually is demonstrated in the contused kidney. Some degree of renal contusion commonly coexists with more severe renal injuries, including renal laceration. With pure contusion, extravasation of urine or blood does not occur. Renal contusion is a self-limited abnormality.

Renal laceration refers to a rent in the renal parenchyma, which inevitably leads to formation of a perirenal urinoma, hematoma, or both. On imaging studies, the hallmark of renal laceration is extravasation of contrast material or perinephric fluid collections. With CT, the actual renal laceration usually is visualized (Fig. 4-32). Renal lacerations usually are managed nonsurgically if the trauma patient's condition is hemodynamically stable. On occasion, active arterial bleeding may be demonstrated on contrast-infused CT scans. This finding usually prompts intervention, either renal arteriography with embolization or surgical exploration.

A renal fracture is a severe form of renal laceration. In this situation, the laceration extends completely through the full thickness of the renal parenchyma, which divides the kidney into two or three separate segments. Fractures are more severe than limited lacerations, and patients with renal fractures tend to be hemodynamically unstable. The choice of treatment for these patients depends on patient condition, particularly the integrity

of the renal vasculature. With imaging techniques, a renal fracture appears similar to a renal laceration but with more numerous defects. Prominent areas of contrast extravasation and perirenal hemorrhage are present. In the patient whose condition is stable, selective renal arteriography may be useful to evaluate the integrity of the renal vasculature, with the possibility of embolizing small arteries that are actively bleeding, which may preclude the need for emergency surgery.

The most severe form of renal laceration is the shattered kidney. In this situation, the kidney is fractured into three or more separate segments. Patients with this severe type of injury usually are hemodynamically unstable, and the kidney damage is extensive and irreversible. Nephrectomy generally is indicated to prevent critical bleeding from the injured renal arterial branches. Because of the severity of this injury, the involved kidney rarely functions well enough to visualize the fractured segments with IVU. However, the shattered kidney can be well evaluated by CT scanning. As with other renal injuries, evaluating other abdominal organs in patients with shattered kidneys is crucial. The force to the retroperitoneum that is necessary to shatter a kidney usually results in injuries to other abdominal organs. Particularly susceptible are the spleen, liver, and pancreas because they are located in the same region.

Renal vascular pedicle injury can occur as a result of renal trauma. This injury usually is associated with deceleration-related blunt injuries that result in transection or dissection of the main renal artery or the renal vein. In addition, penetrating injuries can lacerate or transect the renal vessels. Patients with these injuries usually present with hypotension and evidence of massive hemorrhage. If the diagnosis is made rapidly, within 3 to 6 hours of the injury, surgical revascularization of the affected kidney may be attempted. Often, the kidney is damaged irreparably, and revascularization is not an option. Nephrectomy generally is the required treatment for these patients. These patients' conditions usually are hemodynamically unstable. Any evidence of diminished nephrogram on IVU in a trauma patient should raise the possibility of decreased blood flow to the kidney, possibly the result of a renal vascular pedicle injury. With CT scanning, extensive perirenal hemorrhage will be noted along the course of the renal artery. Other findings associated with renal pedicle injury are the delayed and diminished nephrogram, diminished opacification of the lateral segments of the main renal artery, and a rim nephrogram. The rim nephrogram results from persistent perfusion of the outermost rim of renal cortex via the renal capsular artery. The capsular artery branches off very early from the renal artery and rarely is affected by renal artery transection. The result is greater opacification of the outer rim of cortex than the remainder of the kidney because most of the kidney will be underperfused. Finally, renal arteriography is useful in the diagnosis of renal vascular pedicle injury. Aortography usually demonstrates active renal artery bleeding or renal artery occlusion resulting from transection and thrombosis. Thrombosis of the transected renal artery should not indicate that this injury has spontaneously reached a point of stability. Renal artery transection requires surgical repair. If not treated, renal artery bleeding will recur and may result in severe hemorrhage.

SUGGESTED READINGS

Becker JA: Renal tuberculosis, *Urologic Radiology* 10:25–30, 1988.

Bourgoignie JJ, Pardo V: HIV-associated nephropathies, *N Engl J Med* 327:729–730, 1992.

Campos A, Figueroa ET, Gunasekaran S, et al: Early presentation of tuberous sclerosis as bilateral renal cysts, *J Urol* 149:1077–1079, 1993.

Carlin BI, Resnick MI: Indications and techniques for urologic evaluation of the trauma patient with suspected urologic injury, *Semin Urol* 13:9–24, 1995.

Chen Y-T, Coleman RA, Scheinman JI, et al: Renal disease in type I glycogen storage disease, *N Engl J Med* 318:7–11, 1988.

Dyer RB, Munitz HA, Bechtold R, et al: The abnormal nephrogram, *Radiographics* 6:1039–1063, 1986.

Elseviers MM, De Schepper A, Corthouts R, et al: High diagnostic performance of CT scan for analgesic nephropathy in patients with incipient to severe renal failure, *Kidney Int* 48:1316–1323, 1995.

Fanney DR, Casillas J, Murphy BJ: CT in the diagnosis of renal trauma, *Radiographics* 10:29–40, 1990.

Gedroyc WMW, Chaudhuri R, Saxton HM: Normal and near normal caliceal patterns in reflux nephropathy, *Clin Radiol* 39:615–619, 1988.

Gedroyc WMW, Saxton HM: More medullary sponge variants, *Clin Radiol* 39:423–425, 1988.

Gold RP, McClennan BL, Rottenberg RR: CT appearance of acute inflammatory disease of the renal interstitium, *AJR Am J Roentgenol* 141:343–349, 1983.

Hamper UM, Goldblum LE, Hutchins GM, et al: Renal involvement in AIDS: sonographic-pathologic correlation, *AJR Am J Roentgenol* 150:1321–1325, 1988.

Hayes WS, Hartman DS, Sesterhenn IA: Xanthogranulomatous pyelonephritis, *Radiographics* 11:485–498, 1991.

Herschorn S, Radomski SB, Shoskes DA, et al: Evaluation and treatment of blunt renal trauma, *J Urol* 146:274–277, 1991.

Jabour BA, Ralls PW, Tang WW, et al: Acquired cystic disease of the kidneys: computed tomography and ultrasonography appraisal in patients on peritoneal and hemodialysis, *Invest Radiol* 22:728–732, 1987.

Kenney IJ, Aiken CG, Lenney W: Frusemide-induced nephrocalcinosis in very low birth weight infants, *Pediatr Radiol* 18:323–325, 1988.

Kuhlman JE, Browne D, Shermak M, et al: Retroperitoneal and pelvic CT of patients with AIDS: primary and secondary involvement of the genitourinary tract, *Radiographics* 11:473–483, 1991.

Levine E, Grantham JJ: High-density renal cysts in autosomal dominant polycystic kidney disease demonstrated by CT, *Radiology* 154:477–482, 1985.

Levine E, Slusher SL, Grantham JJ, et al: Natural history of acquired renal cystic disease in dialysis patients: a prospective longitudinal CT study, *AJR Am J Roentgenol* 156:501–506, 1991.

Morehouse HT, Weiner SN, Hoffman JC: Imaging in inflammatory disease of the kidney, *AJR Am J Roentgenol* 143:135–141, 1984.

Novick AC: Evaluation and management of atherosclerotic renal vascular disease to prevent end-stage renal failure, *Semin Urol* 12:67–73, 1994.

Penter G, Arkell DG: The fragmented staghorn calculus: a radiological sign of pyonephrosis, *Clin Radiol* 40:61–63, 1989.

Pollack HM, Wein AJ: Imaging of renal trauma, *Radiology* 172:297–308, 1989.

Premkumar A, Lattimer J, Newhouse JH: CT and sonography of advanced urinary tract tuberculosis, *AJR Am J Roentgenol* 148:65–69, 1987.

Sandler DP, Smith JC, Weinberg CR, et al: Analgesic use and chronic renal disease, *N Engl J Med* 320:1238–1243, 1989.

Saunders HS, Dyer RB, Shifrin RY, et al: The CT nephrogram: implications for evaluation of urinary tract disease, *Radiographics* 15:1069–1085, 1995.

Sclafani SJA, Becker JA: Radiologic diagnosis of renal trauma, *Urologic Radiology* 7:192–200, 1985.

Segel MC, Lecky JW, Slasky BS: Diabetes mellitus: the predominant cause of bilateral renal enlargement, *Radiology* 153:341–342, 1984.

Soulen MC, Fishman EK, Goldman SM, et al: Bacterial renal infection: role of CT, *Radiology* 171:703–707, 1989.

CHAPTER 5

The Renal Sinus, Pelvocalyceal System, and Ureter

EMBRYOLOGY AND ANATOMY

Although embryology of the urinary tract is complex and often baffling, its important features actually are rather simple. The ureteral bud originates from the mesonephric duct early in gestation and forms the ureter, pelvocalyceal system, and renal collecting tubules. A physical association between the ureteral bud and the metanephric blastema, the primordium of renal parenchyma, is necessary for development of the kidney and the calyces. Differentiation of the metanephric blastema into renal parenchyma depends on induction by the ure-

teral bud; ureteral bud branching depends on induction by the metanephric blastema. If all goes well, the pelvocalyceal system and ureter develop into tubular conduits for urine with approximately 10 to 25 calyces per kidney. The ureters are lined by transitional epithelium. The transitional epithelium and the supporting connective tissue constitute the mucosa of the ureter. The mucosa is surrounded by the muscularis layer, which is made up of smooth muscle with longitudinal and circular fibers. The outermost lining of the normal ureter is the adventitia, which is composed of connective tissue.

RENAL SINUS

The renal sinus is surrounded laterally by and abuts the renal parenchyma. Medially, it communicates with the perinephric space. The normal constituents of the renal sinus include the intrarenal collecting system, renal blood vessels, lymphatics, nerve fibers, fat, and varying quantities of fibrous tissue. Aside from lesions contained within the intrarenal collecting system, such as stones, and lesions originating from the collecting system, such as urothelial tumors, significant disease of the renal sinus is unusual. Most abnormalities of the renal sinus are asymptomatic and are of interest primarily so they will not be confused with more serious abnormalities. Lesions of the intrarenal collecting system are discussed later in this chapter.

Fat is the largest single constituent of the renal sinus, and it is readily visible with ultrasound, computed tomography (CT), and magnetic resonance (MR) imaging examinations of the kidney. Normally, the quantity of fat in the renal sinus gradually increases with age. Very little, if any, renal sinus fat is present at birth, whereas approximately 20% of total renal volume is a result of renal sinus fat in the adult. With aging, fat proliferates in the renal sinus to compensate for atrophy of the renal parenchyma.

Box 5-1   Renal Sinus Fat Proliferation

Renal sinus lipomatosis—increased fat with little mass effect
Replacement lipomatosis—renal atrophy, massive fat

Box 5-2   Renal Sinus Cysts

Peripelvic—multiple, small, insinuating cysts
Parapelvic—typical simple renal cyst
Uriniferous—urine extravasation

Fatty proliferation that leads to mass effect on the intrarenal collecting system usually is referred to as renal sinus lipomatosis (Box 5-1). This mass effect manifests radiographically as attenuation and stretching of the infundibula, the resulting appearance being described as a "spidery" collecting system. Mass effect from renal sinus lipomatosis rarely leads to symptoms because calyceal obstruction does not result from simple sinus lipomatosis. Whereas renal sinus lipomatosis generally is seen in the aged, fatty proliferation can be accelerated in patients with increased exogenous or endogenous steroids, but it is seen more commonly in patients who are experiencing renal parenchyma atrophy. In these patients, the volume of atrophied renal parenchyma is replaced with a similar volume of renal sinus fat. In patients with extreme cases, replacement lipomatosis occurs (Box 5-1). This term describes massive renal sinus lipomatosis with severe parenchymal atrophy, usually the result of severe renal infection or vascular ischemia. Radiographically, replacement lipomatosis appears as massive overgrowth of the renal sinus with marked thinning of the renal parenchyma. The proliferation of renal sinus fat, which is diffused throughout the renal sinus, leads to attenuation and stretching of the collecting system without a dominant area of mass effect. This appearance is typical of replacement lipomatosis or extensive renal sinus lipomatosis and should not be confused with focal fat-containing neoplasms originating in the renal sinus.

Renal Sinus Cysts

Renal sinus cysts also are common (Box 5-2). True renal sinus cysts, also known as peripelvic cysts, usually are small and multiple, and they grow to insinuate themselves throughout the renal sinus in a distribution similar to that seen with renal sinus lipomatosis (Fig. 5-1). These fluid-containing cysts are thought to be congenital and of lymphatic origin, and they rarely are symptomatic. On occasion, these cysts can lead to focal hydronephrosis, which necessitates cyst drainage and ablation. On ultrasound examination, these water-containing structures may mimic hydronephrosis (Fig. 5-2) because they often parallel the normal calyces and renal pelvis. With urography or contrast-enhanced CT, the extraluminal position of these cysts is readily apparent (Fig. 5-2). Rather than hydronephrosis, an attenuated, "spidery" collecting system is demonstrated. Renal sinus lipomatosis and renal sinus cysts often are indistinguishable with urography unless the renal sinus fat lucency is identifiable on precontrast radiographs. Simple renal cysts originating in the medial renal parenchyma can protrude into the renal sinus. These also are known as parapelvic cysts, and despite their location, their origin appears to be different from that of peripelvic cysts. Parapelvic cysts, like other simple cysts of the renal parenchyma, usually are discrete, spherical, water-density masses (Fig. 5-3). They usually are solitary or few in number, unlike peripelvic

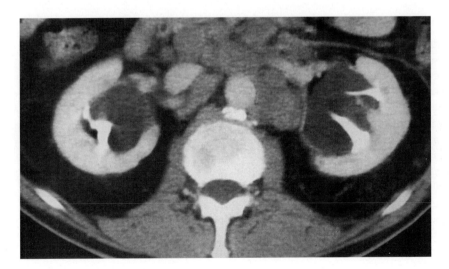

Fig. 5-1   Renal sinus cysts. This contrast-infused CT scan demonstrates multiple peripelvic cysts infiltrating the renal sinus bilaterally. The calyces are stretched and attenuated but not obstructed by these cysts. In addition, there is extensive retroperitoneal lymphadenopathy in this patient with lymphoma.

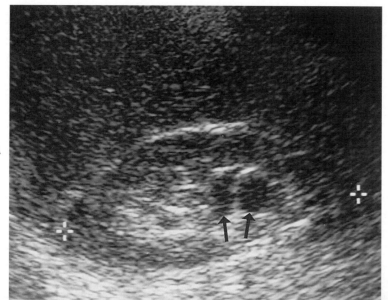

A

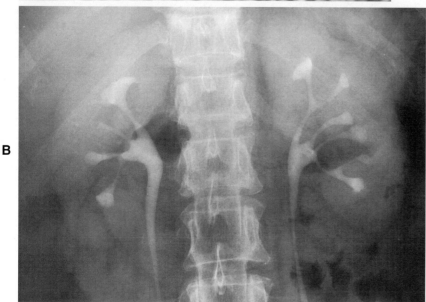

B

Fig. 5-2 Renal sinus cysts. **A,** Longitudinal sonogram of the right kidney in this patient demonstrates normal renal parenchyma. Several cystic areas are seen in the lower pole of the kidney (arrows), and other cystic areas are seen elsewhere in the renal sinus. The sonographic appearance suggests hydronephrosis. **B,** A urogram of the same patient demonstrates stretched and attenuated calyces bilaterally with an appearance described as a "spidery" collecting system. No hydronephrosis is present. Taken in conjunction with the sonogram, these studies are diagnostic of peripelvic cysts.

cysts. Diagnostically, parapelvic cysts should meet all the radiologic criteria for simple cysts elsewhere in the kidney. Unfortunately, because of their central location, it often is difficult to demonstrate the complete absence of internal echoes on ultrasound examination. On occasion, CT or MR imaging may be necessary to confirm the benign nature of these lesions and to exclude a parenchyma neoplasm.

Less commonly, a urinoma may originate in the renal sinus. Urinomas usually are associated with ureteral obstruction secondary to stone disease with resulting collecting system rupture. Occasionally, renal sinus urinomas may result from traumatic laceration of the collecting system. Extravasated urine usually diffuses throughout the renal sinus and into the perinephric space without causing a dominant uriniferous cyst. On occasion, a focal urinoma can develop, but spontaneous resolution usually occurs with adequate decompression of the urinary tract, and additional management rarely is required.

Renal Sinus Masses

Vasculopathic processes that can involve the renal sinus include focal lesions such as a large renal artery aneurysm or arteriovenous malformation. These lesions often originate in or protrude into the renal sinus, leading to mass effect. They are readily identifiable with modern sonography or with angiography. Management may be

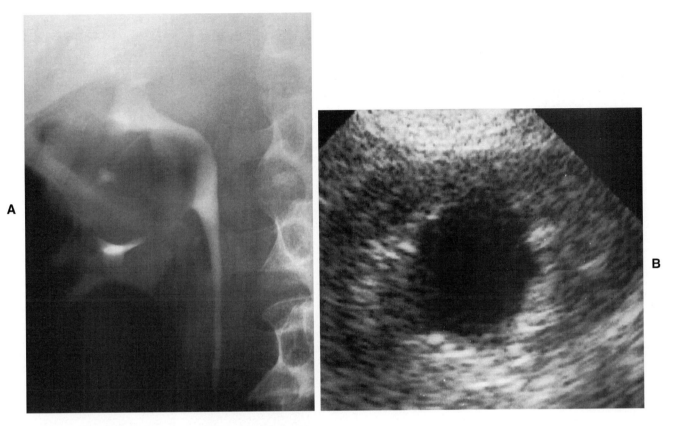

Fig. 5-3   Parapelvic cysts. **A,** A cone-down view of the right kidney from a urogram demonstrates splaying of calyces and compression of the renal pelvis, suggestive of a mass. **B,** A longitudinal sonogram of the right kidney in this patient confirms a simple cyst protruding into the renal sinus. This is the typical appearance of a parapelvic cyst.

Box 5-3   Renal Sinus Neoplasms

Renal parenchymal neoplasms
    Adenocarcinoma, angiomyolipoma, multilocular
       cystic nephroma
Primary renal sinus neoplasm
    Angiomyolipoma
    Teratoma
    Lipoma and liposarcoma
    Fibroma and fibrosarcoma
    Neuroma and neurosarcoma
    Leiomyoma and leiomyosarcoma
    Malignant fibrous histiocytoma

---

undertaken with catheter-introduced embolic materials to ablate aneurysms or vascular malformations.

Neoplasms may involve the renal sinus (Box 5-3), but most neoplasms do so secondarily. Renal parenchyma neoplasms, such as renal cell carcinoma (RCC), commonly extend into the renal sinus and lead to focal hydronephrosis or calyceal displacement. These lesions can be readily diagnosed with cross-sectional imaging, and their true site of origin usually is not in doubt. One tumor of interest is the multilocular cystic nephroma (MLCN). This tumor has a bimodal peak of incidence as it occurs predominantly in boys and middle-aged women. This cystic lesion has numerous thick septa, and it originates from the renal parenchyma. MLCN has a predilection to protrude and to herniate into the renal sinus. Herniation can lead to an intraluminal filling defect within the intrarenal collecting system. This feature is characteristic of MLCN, although not truly diagnostic because the more common RCC occasionally mimics this appearance.

Renal sinus lymphoma is one of the more common renal manifestations of lymphoma. It usually spreads directly and contiguously from retroperitoneal lymph nodes. This solid neoplastic tissue infiltrates and replaces the normal constituents of the renal sinus (Fig. 5-4), often with contiguous spread into the perinephric space. This situation is most common in patients with advanced non-Hodgkin's lymphoma.

Finally, neoplasms originating primarily in the renal sinus are rare but include benign tumors such as angiomyolipoma and teratoma and tumors, both benign and

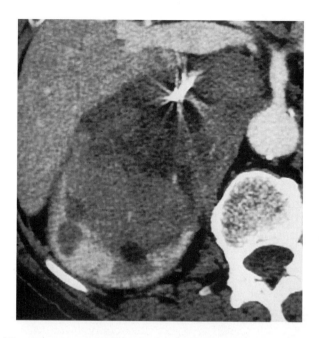

Fig. 5-4   Renal sinus lymphoma. A contrast-infused CT scan in this patient with known non-Hodgkin's lymphoma demonstrates a retroperitoneal mass originating adjacent to the aorta and spreading into the right perinephric space. The mass has insinuated itself into the renal sinus and has replaced or obliterated normal renal sinus components. This pattern is very suggestive of lymphoma.

malignant, originating from mesenchymal tissue. These mesenchymal tumors may originate from smooth muscle, fat, fibrous tissue, or nerve fiber. Radiographically, the characteristics of these tumors often are nonspecific. Mesenchymal tumors originating in the renal sinus appear identical to those originating elsewhere.

PELVOCALYCEAL SYSTEM AND URETER

Normally, approximately 8 to 15 minor calyces subtend each kidney. A single, or simple, calyx is a concave structure applied to the papilla of the renal medulla. When seen *en face,* a simple calyx appears circular. When viewed in profile, the simple calyx is concave and has two well-defined, sharp forniceal angles. Single or multiple simple calyces are drained by an infundibulum, also known as a major calyx, which empties into the renal pelvis. Frequently, calyces fail to divide completely, and they form a larger compound calyx. This normal variant most commonly is seen in the upper and lower poles of the kidney. The shape of the compound calyx becomes distorted, and the circular shape of the simple calyx often is lost. Familiarity with the typical appearance of a compound calyx will prevent confusing it with changes resulting from obstruction or scarring. Compound calyces do have an association with the development of adjacent parenchymal scarring caused by urinary reflux.

The renal pelvis generally is triangular, and it tapers smoothly to its junction with the ureter. The ureteropelvic junction (UPJ) is an ill-defined area where the renal pelvis joins the ureter (Fig. 5-5). The ureter also is somewhat narrowed where it crosses the iliac vessels (Fig. 5-5) and enters the pelvis and at the ureterovesical junction (Fig. 5-5) where the ureter tunnels through the bladder wall. The ureter is a dynamic organ, and frequent constrictions result in transient areas of narrowing as urine is transmitted toward the bladder. A focal dilation of the ureter just above the iliac vessel crossover point frequently is seen. This dilation has been described as the ureteral spindle. This normal phenomenon again reflects a peristaltic wave that stalls transiently as it crosses the iliac vessels.

The ureter normally extends along the ventral surface of the psoas muscle (Box 5-4). It lies just anterior to the transverse processes of the lumbar spine. There often is a focal segment coursing horizontally, usually at L3, as the ureter crosses over the lateral psoas edge. The ureter

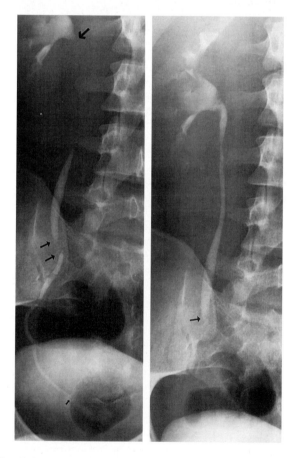

Fig. 5-5   Areas where relative narrowing of the ureter is expected. Two films from an intravenous urogram demonstrate expected locations of relative narrowing of the ureter (arrows). These areas of narrowing occur at the ureteropelvic junction, where the ureter crosses the iliac vessels, and at the ureterovesical junction. These also are sites where ureteral stones commonly impact.

Box 5-4   Ureter—Normal Course

Less than 1 cm lateral to the transverse process
Not medial to the pedicle
The two are separated by 5 cm or more

should not be more than 1 cm lateral to the tip of the nearest transverse process. The ureter should not course medially to the ipsilateral vertebral pedicle. Sometimes the ureter does course just anterior to the pedicle, and this variant usually is normal. This variant is particularly common as the ureter nears the lower lumbar spine. Nearly 20% of urograms will demonstrate the ureter medial to a lower lumbar or upper sacral pedicle. This is particularly common on the right, usually is unilateral, and usually occurs in patients aged 20 to 40 years. However, if this course is associated with any other signs of abnormality, it must be investigated further. In addition, the abdominal ureters should be separated by 5 cm or more. Ureters in closer proximity than 5 cm suggest medial deviation of one or both ureters. As the ureters enter the pelvis, they follow a slightly medial course as they cross the common iliac vessels. In the pelvis, the ureters course laterally to parallel the inner margin of the bony pelvis. Finally, the ureters enter the posterior lateral surface of the bladder.

Congenital Anomalies

Congenital variants of the pelvocalyceal system and ureter are common. Duplication anomalies are represented by a spectrum of findings. Mild anomalies include bifid renal pelvis and incomplete ureteral duplications. These anomalies are seen in up to 4% of the general population and develop when two or more ureteral buds form from the mesonephric duct. Incomplete ureteral duplication usually represents a clinically unimportant finding, but on occasion, "yo-yo" reflux can occur. Urine descending one ureter refluxes up the second ureter during its relaxation phase of peristalsis. Yo-yo reflux can cause urinary infections and flank pain.

Complete ureteral duplications, when two separate ureters drain a single kidney, are substantially less common than incomplete duplications. However, the clinical significance of complete duplication anomalies is considerably greater than that of incomplete duplications. It is important to be familiar with the Weigert-Meyer rule, which states that the upper pole of the kidney drains via the ureter, which inserts inferior and medial to the normal, expected ureteral insertion point. This is the truly ectopic ureter in a complete duplication. This ectopic ureter is prone to development of ectopic ureteroceles

(Fig. 5-6) and extravesical insertions. Less commonly, the ectopic ureter is susceptible to reflux. Ectopic ureteroceles occur in one third of patients with duplicated ectopic ureters. It has been hypothesized that ureteroceles form as a result of a failure of the normal epithelial membrane to recanalize between the bladder and the ureter (Chwalla's membrane). The ectopic ureterocele represents marked submucosal dilatation of the intramural ureter at the ureterovesical junction. This dilated ureteral segment often projects into the lumen of the bladder. The ureterocele may cause distortion and obstruction of the other ipsilateral ureteral orifice, causing obstruction. In addition, large ureteroceles may prolapse and obstruct the urethral orifice, leading to bilateral ureteral dilation. Ectopic ureteroceles are seen predominantly in the female population; the female-to-male ratio is 4 to 1. Ectopic ureteroceles rarely are found in blacks. Ectopic ureteroceles generally cause obstruction of the ureter above the ureterocele. An ectopic ureterocele unassociated with a duplicated ureter is rare. A second cause of obstruction of an ectopic ureter is extravesical insertion of its caudal end. In female patients, the ectopic ureter often inserts into the bladder neck, the urethra, or directly into the vagina (Fig. 5-7). Because these areas are exposed chronically to infection, fibrosis and stenosis often develop in the lower ureter and lead to hydronephrosis of the upper moiety. In male patients, the ureter never inserts inferior to the external sphincter, so it is protected from infection, and incontinence is rarely a symptom. On the contrary, extravesical insertion of the ureter in female patients frequently is associated with

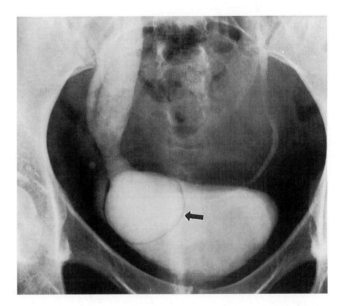

Fig. 5-6   Ectopic ureterocele. A large ectopic ureterocele (arrow) protrudes into the right side of the bladder and obstructs the ureter draining the upper moiety of the right kidney in this patient with a complete duplication of the right collecting system and ureter.

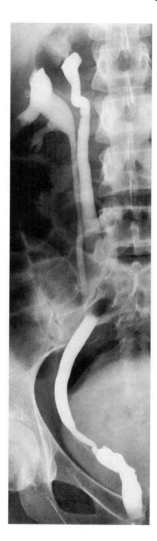

Fig. 5-7   Obstruction of the upper moiety resulting from extravesical insertion of the ureter. A right retrograde pyelogram in this adult with incontinence demonstrates complete duplication of the right collecting system and ureter. The lower moiety was opacified separately. The ureter draining the upper moiety empties into the vagina and is obstructed partially. There is dilatation and irregularity of its lowermost segment resulting from chronic infection and fibrosis.

chronic incontinence. Classically, extravesical ureter insertion in a female patient causes the triad of continuous urine leakage, normal voiding, and some degree of functional renal impairment.

The lower moiety of the completely duplicated system generally is normal. However, an increased incidence of vesicoureteral reflux is seen with the lower moiety (Fig. 5-8).

Another form of ureterocele is the orthotopic ureterocele, which also is known as a simple, or adult-type, ureterocele. Although thought to be a congenital anomaly, orthotopic ureterocele usually is identified only in adults. Usually, this is an incidental radiologic finding

unrelated to symptoms. An orthotopic ureterocele is a cystic dilatation and invagination of the intramural segment of the ureter where it joins the bladder. The cause of orthotopic ureteroceles is unknown, but it may be related to partial persistence of Chwalla's membrane, an embryologic vestige. These focal ureteral dilatations usually are asymptomatic. As ureteroceles grow they more commonly are associated with complications. Ureteroceles more than 2 cm in greatest diameter are more likely to be associated with ureteral obstruction and stone formation within the ureterocele (Fig. 5-9). Radiographically, orthotopic ureteroceles usually are demonstrated with intravenous urography. They have a bulbous appearance as they prolapse into the bladder lumen. The focally dilated lumen of the ureter fills with opaque contrast material, which is circumscribed by the radiolucent ureteral wall and bladder mucosa. Typically, this is described as a "cobra-head," or "spring onion" appearance (Fig. 5-10). This anomaly appears similar to a prolapsing hemorrhoid seen in the colon. The focally dilated lumen is surrounded by a thin membrane, representing the wall of the normal structure. Radiographically, it is important to distinguish orthotopic ureteroceles from pseudoureteroceles. Pseudoureteroceles suggest underlying abnor-

Pseudoureteroceles!

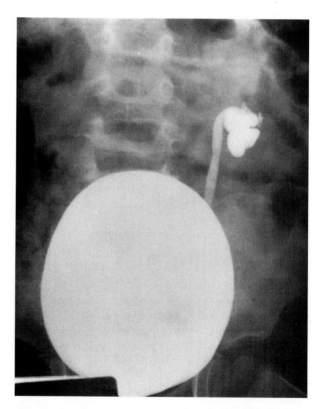

Fig. 5-8   Refluxing lower moiety in a duplicated system. A cystogram in this patient with chronic pyelonephritis demonstrates reflux into a left ureter. The upper calyces are not visualized and drain via a separate ureter, typical of a complete duplication.

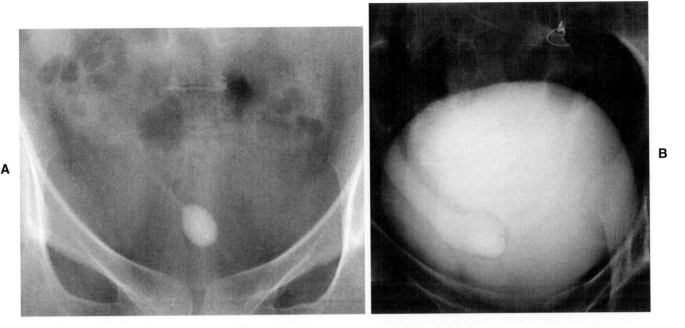

Fig. 5-9   Large simple ureterocele containing a stone. **A,** A view of the pelvis demonstrates a large oval calcification near the midline in this patient with chronic right flank pain. **B,** An intravenous urogram demonstrates bilateral simple ureteroceles. The large stone exists within the right simple ureterocele. Stones can form in ureteroceles resulting from chronic stasis of urine.

mality such as infiltrating transitional cell carcinoma (TCC) or ureteral stone impaction. With an orthotopic ureterocele, the radiolucent line surrounding the ureterocele will be no thicker than 2 mm and will be uniform throughout. Irregularity or focal thickening of this radiolucent margin (Figs. 5-11, 5-12) suggests abnormality and indicates a pseudoureterocele.

When evaluating congenital anomalies of the urinary tract, such as duplications, remember that up to one third of patients have a second coexisting significant congenital abnormality of the urinary tract. Duplication anomalies frequently are associated with strictures of the UPJ, in addition to the previously described ureteroceles and refluxing ureterovesical junctions.

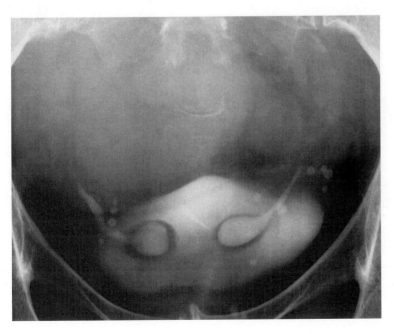

Fig. 5-10   Bilateral orthotopic ureteroceles. A pelvic film from an intravenous urogram demonstrates bilateral orthotopic ureteroceles. The bulbous end of each ureter is surrounded by a thin, smooth lucent line.

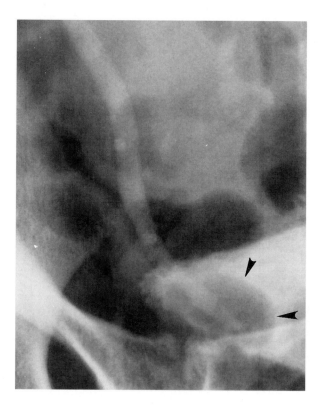

Fig. 5-11   Pseudoureterocele caused by an impacted ureteral stone. This oblique view of the pelvis from an intravenous urogram demonstrates a thick lucent rind (arrowheads) surrounding the right ureterovesical junction. A small stone was impacted at the ureterovesical junction, causing edema and the appearance of a pseudoureterocele.

Although duplication anomalies of some degree are seen commonly in everyday practice, other supernumerary anomalies of the ureter and pelvocalyceal system are distinctly uncommon. Triplication, tetrafication, and pentafication anomalies have been described. Because of the rarity of these anomalies, little is known regarding their association with reflux, ureteroceles, and other urinary tract abnormalities. It is known that the Weigert-Meyer rule is violated in at least 50% of the patients with triplication and greater supernumerary anomalies.

Another uncommon form of ureteral duplication occurs when incomplete development results in a congenital ureteral diverticulum, which most likely develops from a duplicated ureteric bud when one moiety fails to connect with the metanephric blastema, and as a result, a blind-ending segment of ureter is connected to the otherwise normal ureter. Radiographically, the blind-ending ureter appears either saccular or cylindrical, and it usually communicates with the normal ureter (Fig. 5-13). Although this anomaly is of little clinical significance, the ureteral diverticulum can reservoir relatively static urine, increasing the risk of infection and stone disease.

Congenital abnormalities of the ureter, which typically result in hydronephrosis or ureteral dilatation, include congenital strictures, retrocaval ureter, primary megaureter, prune belly syndrome, and vesicoureteral reflux. When hydroureteronephrosis is detected, attention should be directed to defining the cause of dilatation. A search should be made to define the transition point from dilated ureter to normal ureter. Congenital strictures of the ureter are the most common congenital anomalies

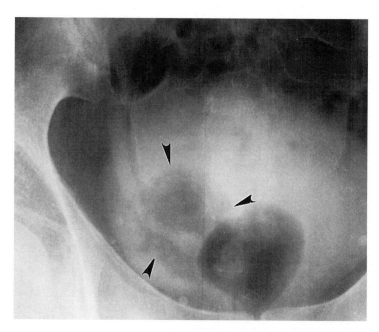

Fig. 5-12   Pseudoureterocele from a transitional cell carcinoma. A view of the pelvis from a urogram demonstrates a markedly irregular lucent rind (arrowheads) surrounding the focally dilated right ureterovesical junction. This irregularity seen with a pseudoureterocele is typical of neoplasm.

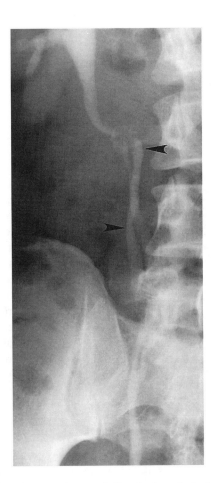

Fig. 5-13   Congenital ureteral diverticulum. A single film from a urogram demonstrates a blind-ending ureteral diverticulum (arrowheads) originating from the right ureter.

of the ureter. These fibrotic strictures may develop at any site along the course of the ureter (Fig. 5-14), but the majority develop near the ureteropelvic junction (UPJ) and at the ureterovesical junction. UPJ obstruction is the most common cause of fetal hydronephrosis. The etiology of these strictures is unclear, however, it has been postulated that in utero ureteral ischemia leads to the formation of a focal stricture. The degree of hydroureteronephrosis varies, as does the clinical significance of these strictures. The most extreme form of UPJ stricture results in a nonfunctioning, hydronephrotic form of multicystic dysplastic kidney. Milder forms of UPJ stricture often go unnoticed until adulthood. Typical symptoms of a UPJ stricture are flank pain, hematuria, infection, or stone disease. The delayed presentation of UPJ stricture in an adult is common and is believed to result from gradual worsening of UPJ scarring caused by intermittent subclinical inflammation or increased urine production with growth. Approximately 5% of UPJ strictures are caused by anomalous accessory renal arteries crossing

and compressing the UPJ. The diagnosis of UPJ stricture caused by a crossing artery is of clinical significance, because surgeons generally select open pyeloplasty repair over percutaneous endopyelotomy in these situations. Although most UPJ strictures, regardless of the cause, have the same appearance; if the narrowed segment of ureter at the UPJ curves smoothly laterally with a concave medial margin (Fig. 5-15), an associated crossing artery should be suspected. An anomalous vessel can be confirmed with arteriography (Fig. 5-15) or with noninvasive techniques, such as helical CT scanning with bolus contrast infusion or MR angiography. The diagnosis of nephrolithiasis associated with a UPJ stricture also is clinically significant. The combination of these two abnormal-

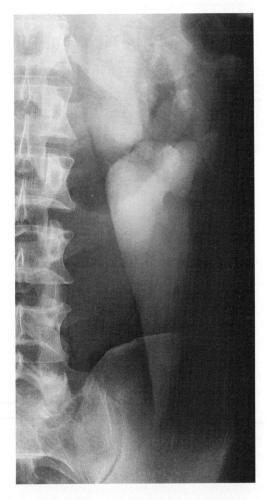

Fig. 5-14   Congenital midureteral stricture. A film from an intravenous urogram demonstrates massive hydroureteronephrosis down to the level of the left sacroiliac joint. Complete evaluation of this ureter demonstrated no underlying pathology, and this was attributed to a congenital midureteral stricture. Most congenital ureteral strictures occur at the ureteropelvic junction or ureterovesical junction, but they can occur anywhere along the course of the ureter.

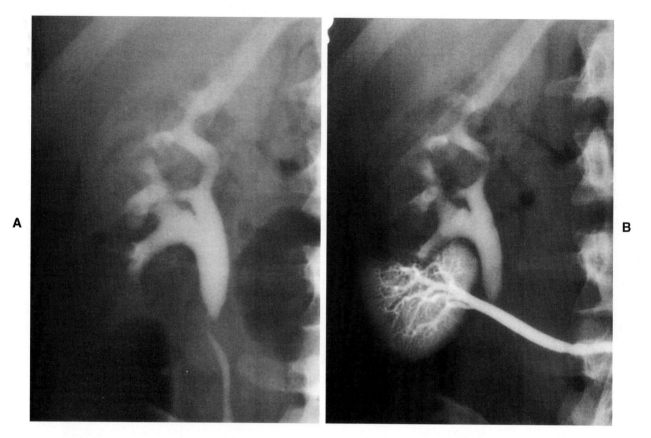

Fig. 5-15 Ureteropelvic junction stricture caused by a crossing vessel. **A,** This young patient complained of intermittent right flank pain. An intravenous urogram demonstrates mild ureteropelvic junction stricture. The ureteropelvic junction has a smooth concave medial curvature. **B,** A selective arteriogram in this patient demonstrated an anomalous lower pole renal artery causing the ureteropelvic junction stricture.

ities encourages clinicians to choose percutaneous neph-rolithotomy and endopyelotomy for management. In these patients, renal calculi can be removed and endopyelotomy can be performed percutaneously during the same procedure.

The frequency of multiple coexistent urinary tract anomalies is an important concept when a UPJ stricture is detected. Up to 25% of patients with congenital UPJ obstruction will have a contralateral congenital urinary tract anomaly. Frequently associated anomalies include contralateral multicystic dysplastic kidney and contralateral UPJ obstruction. Detection of these contralateral anomalies may be greatly significant and may affect management. For example, detection of a multicystic dysplastic kidney opposite a UPJ stricture may lead to more aggressive management of the UPJ stricture.

Other abnormalities of the ureter can be classified into several groups according to radiologic pattern. These are abnormalities of ureteral course or caliber and filling defects. Similar abnormalities can be seen in the renal pelvis and calyces.

Deviations of the Ureter

The ureter may be deviated medially or laterally, and deviation can occur along its entire course or segmentally. Abnormalities of ureteral course rarely result from primary ureteral disease but rather from abnormalities extrinsic to the ureter. Causes of ureteral deviation are listed in Boxes 5-5 and 5-6. In most patients, a definitive diagnosis of the underlying pathology cannot be made without cross-sectional imaging techniques. When ureteral deviation is visualized by urography or retrograde pyelography, CT or MR imaging usually is indicated to further evaluate the adjacent retroperitoneal structures. Some patterns of ureteral deviation are characteristic and indicative of a single diagnosis and therefore negate the need for additional evaluation. For example, abrupt medial deviation of the upper segment of the right ureter with a course resembling a fish hook and with the medial portion located within the adjacent vertebral pedicle is diagnostic of a retrocaval ureter (Fig. 5-16; Box 5-7). No additional imaging is required to confirm this diagnosis.

Box 5-5 Medial Deviation of the Ureter

Upper ureter
  Lower pole renal mass
  Lateral retroperitoneal mass
  Psoas enlargement
  Retroperitoneal fibrosis
  Retrocaval ureter
Lower ureter
  Lymphadenopathy
  Pelvic lipomatosis
  Iliopsoas enlargement
  Pelvic mass or fluid collection
  Iliac vessel ectasia
  Abdominoperineal resection
  Cystocele

Box 5-7 Retrocaval Ureter—Urographic Findings

Right ureter
Abrupt medial deviation
Courses medial to pedicle
Fish hook shape
Hydronephrosis

and recurrent urinary tract infections. Cystitis glandularis is a premalignant bladder lesion that is associated with pelvic lipomatosis.

Unilateral deviation of the upper two thirds of the left ureter often results from abdominal aortic aneurysm (Fig. 5-19 on p. 167). Atherosclerotic calcifications of the aorta often are seen in association with this type of deviation. Focal lateral deviation of the upper left ureter in a young man suggests lymph node metastases from a testicular carcinoma (Fig. 5-20 on p. 167). These neoplasms typically spread via the lymphatic system. A primary path of lymphatic drainage of the left testicle parallels the left testicular vein and empties into nodes near the left renal vein. Bilateral deviation of the upper ureters most commonly results from hypertrophy of the psoas muscles (Fig. 5-21 on p. 168) and usually occurs in muscular young men. The enlarged muscles often are visible on an abdominal radiograph. This form of deviation is asymptomatic and incidentally detected. If the psoas muscle is wider than 8 cm from the edge of a vertebral body to its lateral edge at the upper edge of the iliac bone, psoas hypertrophy is likely the cause of ureteral deviation. Often, the pelvic ureters also are medially deviated in these muscular individuals because of large iliacus and obturator internus muscles, with resulting displacement of the ureters. An alternative cause of this pattern of ureteral deviation is massive lymphadenopathy. Massive retroperitoneal and pelvic lymphadenopathy causes lateral deviation of the upper ureters and medial deviation of the lower ureters (Fig. 5-22 on p. 168). It typically is seen in patients with lymphoma or chronic leukemia. Another typical pattern of ureteral deviation is seen after mobilization and peritonealization of the ureters as treatment for retroperitoneal fibrosis. In these patients, the ureters exhibit marked lateral deviation (Fig. 5-23 on p. 169) with other postsurgical findings, i.e., surgical clips or wire sutures. In this surgery, the ureters are dissected away from the retroperitoneal fibrotic process, mobilized laterally, and wrapped in peritoneum or omentum to protect them from additional involvement with the retroperitoneal disease.

Several other conditions are associated with deviations that have a typical radiographic pattern. Focal lateral

In another typical pattern, both ureters are deviated medially in their midsegments, usually at L3 to L5, with associated hydronephrosis and ureteral narrowing (Fig. 5-17). This pattern is typical of retroperitoneal fibrosis. Unfortunately, medial deviation of the ureter occurs in only about 50% of patients with retroperitoneal fibrosis, and it alone is not diagnostic of this disease. Additionally, retroperitoneal fibrosis can involve one ureter and spare the contralateral ureter. Cross-sectional imaging often is helpful to confirm the abnormality or to guide biopsy in these patients. Symmetric medial deviation of the pelvic ureters with associated lucency in the pelvis is typical of pelvic lipomatosis (Fig. 5-18 on p. 166), which is an idiopathic process in most patients. It more commonly is seen in young black men, and it can lead to bilateral hydroureteronephrosis. It usually causes extrinsic compression of the bladder, resulting in the characteristic pear-shaped or teardrop-shaped bladder (Fig. 5-18). Often, the rectum also is involved, and concentric narrowing and straightening of the rectosigmoid colon may occur. These patients often have difficulties with voiding

Box 5-6 Lateral Deviation of the Ureter

Upper ureter
  Malrotated or horseshoe kidney
  Lymphadenopathy
  Psoas hypertrophy
  Aortic aneurysm
  Retroperitoneal mass or fluid
  Ureter mobilization surgery
Lower ureter
  Central pelvic mass or fluid collection
  Sciatic ureteral hernia

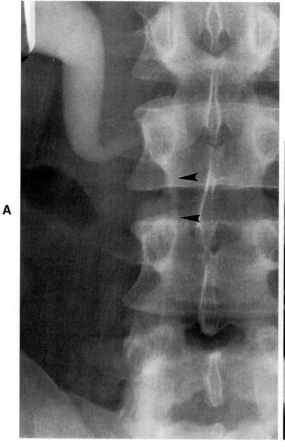

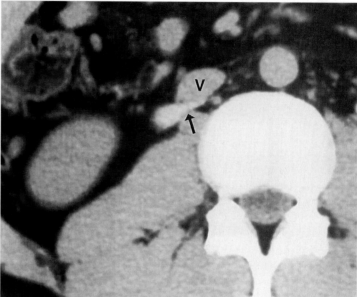

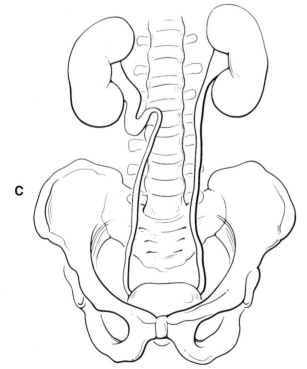

Fig. 5-16   Retrocaval ureter. **A,** An intravenous urogram demonstrates the typical appearance of a retrocaval or circumcaval ureter with abrupt medial deviation of the right ureter. The ureter takes on an appearance analogous to a fish hook. The medial portion of the ureter (arrowheads) is within the ipsilateral vertebral pedicle. **B,** A CT scan in this same patient demonstrates the right ureter (arrow) as it courses behind the vena cava (V). The ureter then will course medially to the vena cava and pass back laterally over the ventral surface of the cava. **C,** A diagram of the expected course of a retrocaval ureter.

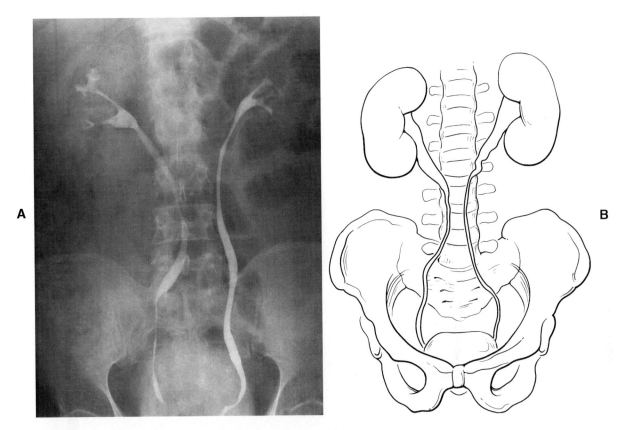

Fig. 5-17   Medial deviation of the ureters caused by retroperitoneal fibrosis. **A,** A single film from a urogram demonstrates marked medial deviation of the right ureter and mild medial deviation of the left ureter at L4. There is no significant ureteral narrowing associated with this case of retroperitoneal fibrosis. **B,** Diagram of the typical medial deviation of the ureters sometimes seen with retroperitoneal fibrosis.

deviation of the ureter at the level of the upper sacrum (Fig. 5-24 on p. 169) usually results from an aneurysm of the iliac artery. Because other abnormalities, including focal lymphadenopathy, can cause a similar appearance, confirmation with other imaging usually is indicated. After abdominoperineal resection, the pelvic ureters will lie more medially than normal (Fig. 5-25 on p. 170). There is loss of the normal lateral curvature of the ureteral course in patients after this form of surgery. Typically, on entering the pelvis, the ureters course directly inferior to the bladder. A history or radiographic evidence of substantial previous abdominal surgery usually is evident. A common site of bladder diverticulum is just inferior to the ureterovesical junction. A diverticulum in this specific location often is referred to as a Hutch diverticulum. When large, these diverticuli will deviate the ureter. Typically, this leads to focal medial deviation of the ureter (Fig. 5-26 on p. 170) as it nears the ureterovesical junction. This usually is a unilateral process. Segments of the ureter may herniate, leading to typical deviation patterns. Ureteral hernias in general are more common in middle-aged men and usually are unilateral, involving the right ureter only. With ureterosciatic herniation, the ureter

deviates laterally into the greater sciatic foramen (Fig. 5-27 on p. 171), which leads to a focal lateral deviation of the ureter in the pelvis. Inguinal and femoral herniation of the ureter also occurs. With inguinal herniation, the ureter in the pelvis focally deviates inferiorly (Fig. 5-28 on p. 171) into the inguinal canal. Femoral hernias have a similar appearance (Fig. 5-28), but the herniation occurs in a more lateral location. Ureteral herniation may be asymptomatic, and these hernias often go unrecognized unless surgical repair is undertaken. In some patients, ureteral hernias cause ureteral obstruction.

The other causes of ureteral deviation have nonspecific findings radiographically. The presence of one of these nonspecific forms of deviation should prompt a CT scan of the abdomen and pelvis to establish a definitive diagnosis or to exclude significant retroperitoneal disease.

Abnormalities of Ureteral Caliber

Caliber abnormalities of the ureter encompass dilatation and narrowing. Causes of ureteral dilatation and narrowing are summarized in Boxes 5-8 and 5-9 on p. 172.

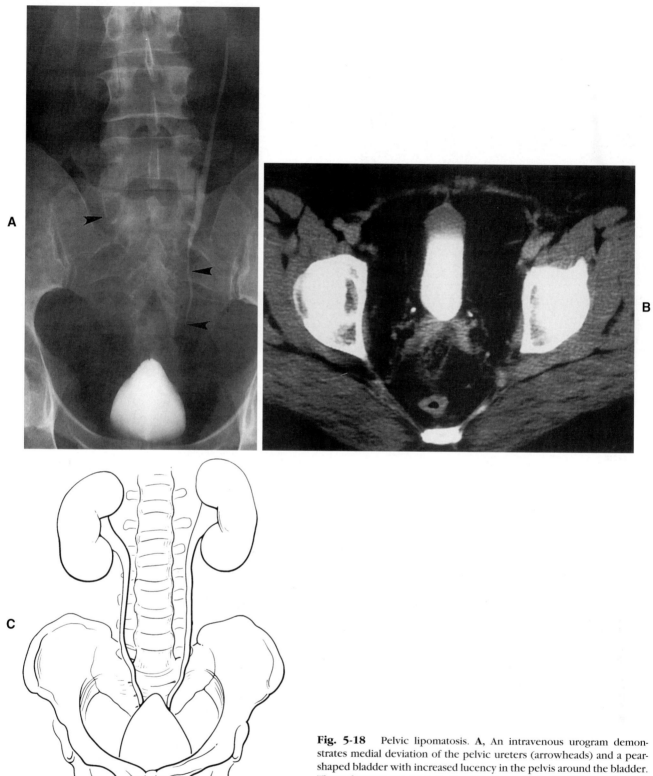

Fig. 5-18   Pelvic lipomatosis. **A,** An intravenous urogram demonstrates medial deviation of the pelvic ureters (arrowheads) and a pear-shaped bladder with increased lucency in the pelvis around the bladder. These features are typical of pelvic lipomatosis. **B,** CT scan through the pelvis in this same patient demonstrates marked proliferation of perivesical and perirectal fat, diagnostic of pelvic lipomatosis. **C,** Diagram of lower ureteral deviation seen with pelvic lipomatosis.

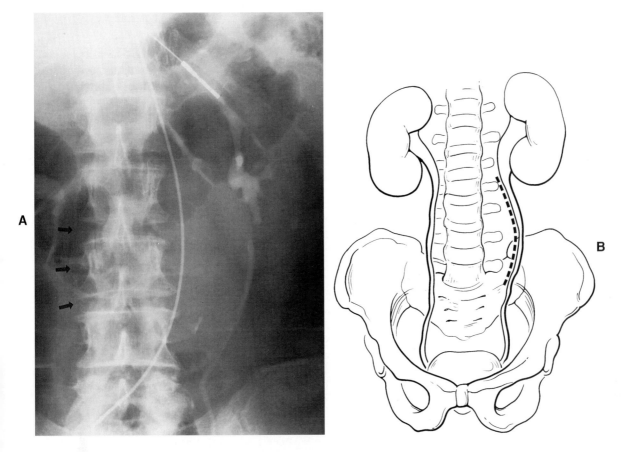

Fig. 5-19 Lateral deviation of the left ureter resulting from an abdominal aortic aneurysm. **A,** The upper left ureter is deviated laterally. Atherosclerotic calcifications are seen within the wall (arrows) of this aneurysm. **B,** Diagram of the ureteral deviation typically seen with a large abdominal aortic aneurysm.

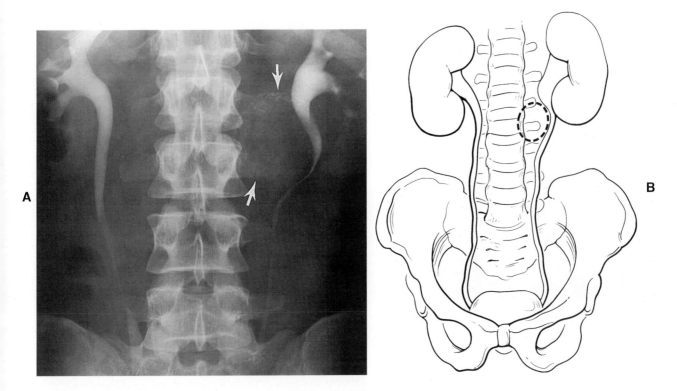

Fig. 5-20 Focal deviation of the upper left ureter caused by lymphadenopathy. **A,** The intravenous urogram in this patient with treated carcinoma of the testicle demonstrates partially calcified lymphadenopathy (arrows) near the renal hilum, which is causing focal lateral deviation of the upper left ureter. This pattern is typical for lymphadenopathy from testicular neoplasms. **B,** Diagram of the typical ureteral deviation seen with perirenal lymph node metastasis from a left testicular neoplasm.

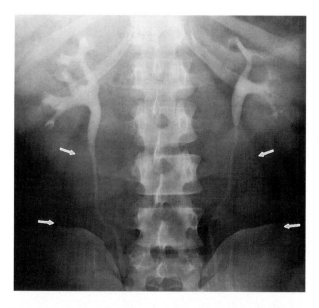

Fig. 5-21   Ureteral deviation from psoas hypertrophy. An intravenous urogram in a young man demonstrates large psoas muscles (arrows) causing mild lateral deviation of the upper ureter bilaterally.

Obviously, some overlap occurs between these two classes of abnormalities, because ureteral narrowing often leads to obstruction with dilatation. However, ureteral dilatation can be seen without associated ureteral obstruction (Box 5-10 on p. 172), in which case it may result from mechanical distention from intraluminal mass, diminished tone of the ureteral musculature, or increased intraluminal volume in the ureter. The ureter may be universally or segmentally dilated.

Ureteral dilatation

One of the most important causes of ureteral dilatation is focal distention from an intraluminal mass. This finding is characteristic of a mucosal neoplasm. Although the neoplasm is nearly always a TCC, other tumors such as metastases or squamous cell carcinoma (SCC) rarely appear identical. Obviously, this focal dilatation of the ureter will be associated with an intraluminal filling defect on contrast studies. Typically, ureteral dilatation involves the entire ureter cephalad and a short segment caudal to the mass (Fig. 5-29 on p. 173). This appearance

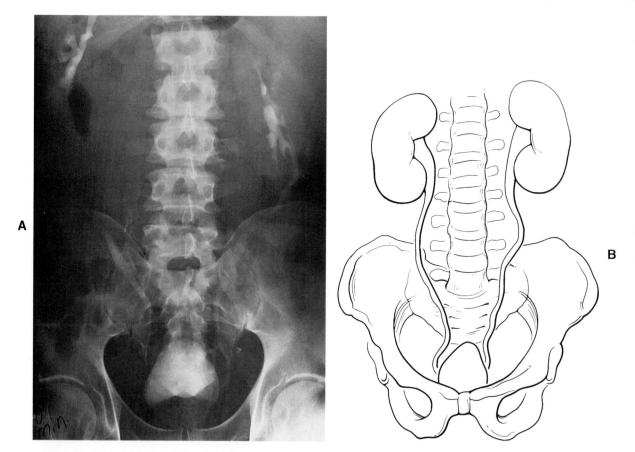

Fig. 5-22   Ureteral deviation from massive retroperitoneal lymphadenopathy. **A,** An intravenous urogram in a patient with chronic lymphocytic leukemia demonstrates lateral deviation of the upper ureters, medial deviation of the lower ureters, and uplifting of the bladder base, all resulting from diffuse lymphadenopathy. **B,** Diagram demonstrating typical ureteral deviation seen with extensive lymphadenopathy.

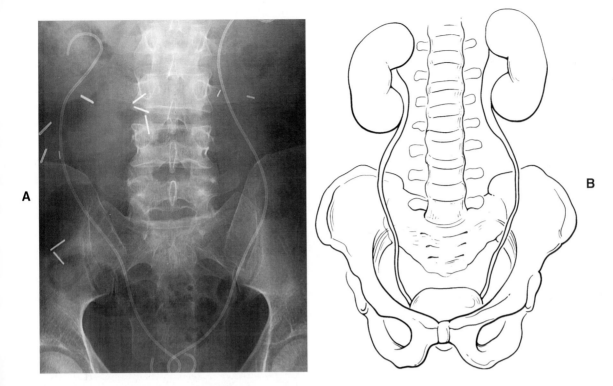

Fig. 5-23   Deviation of the ureters after mobilization and peritonealization of the ureters. **A,** Bilateral ureteral stents demonstrate the marked lateral course of the ureters in this patient who has been treated surgically for retroperitoneal fibrosis. The ureters are mobilized, moved laterally, and wrapped in mesentery or peritoneum. **B,** Diagram of the expected course of the ureters after this surgical procedure.

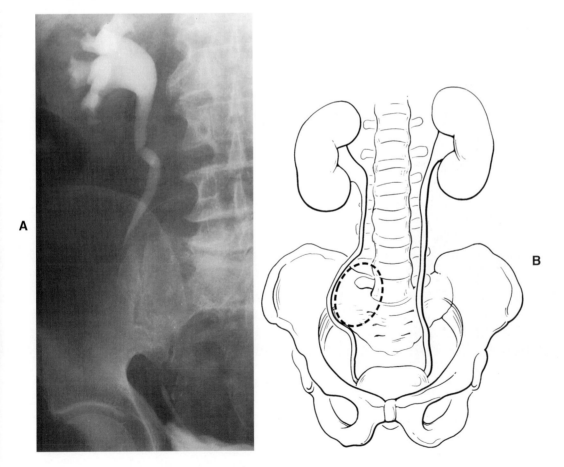

Fig. 5-24   Focal ureteral deviation caused by a large iliac artery aneurysm. **A,** An intravenous urogram demonstrates marked lateral deviation of the right ureter overlying the sacrum. A calcified iliac artery aneurysm is the cause of this deviation. **B,** Diagram of the typical course of the ureter when it is deviated by an iliac artery aneurysm.

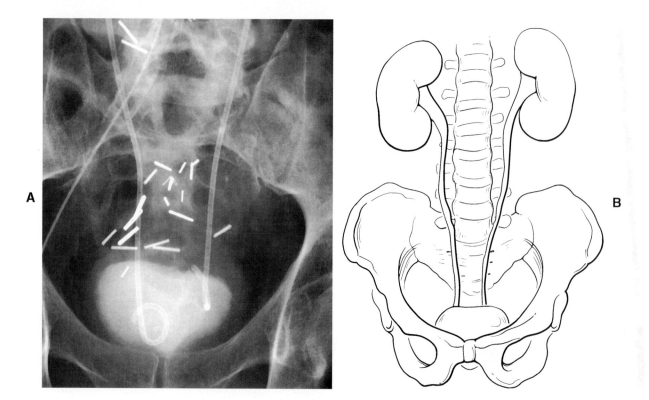

Fig. 5-25 Deviation of the ureters after abdominoperineal resection. **A,** The pelvic ureters, containing ureteral stents, are deviated medially with loss of the normal lateral curvature of the pelvic ureters. This pattern is typical after this surgical procedure. **B,** Diagram of the typical course of the ureters after abdominoperineal resection.

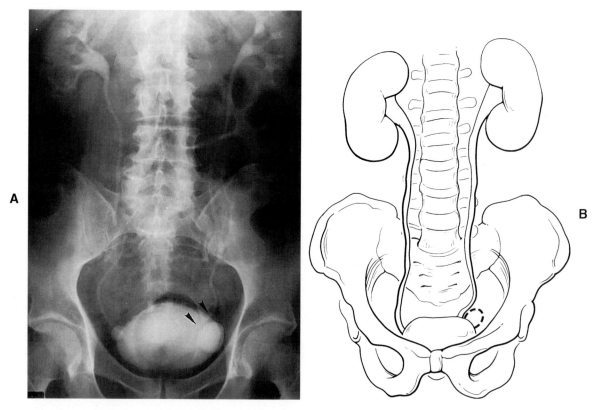

Fig. 5-26 Focal ureteral deviation resulting from a bladder diverticulum. **A,** There are bilateral bladder diverticula. The left-sided diverticulum is larger and occurs at the ureterovesical junction. There is typical medial deviation of the ureter (arrowheads) as it crosses over the top of this left-sided diverticulum. **B,** Diagram of the typical medial deviation of the lower ureter caused by a Hutch diverticulum.

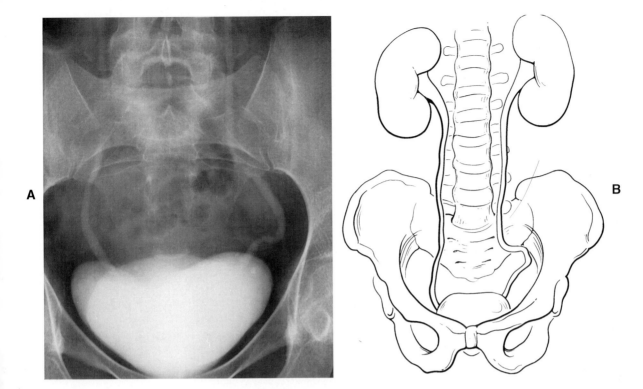

Fig. 5-27 Ureterosciatic herniation. **A,** Intravenous urography demonstrates focal deviation of the left ureter at the sciatic notch, typical of this type of hernia. **B,** Diagram of a ureterosciatic hernia on the left.

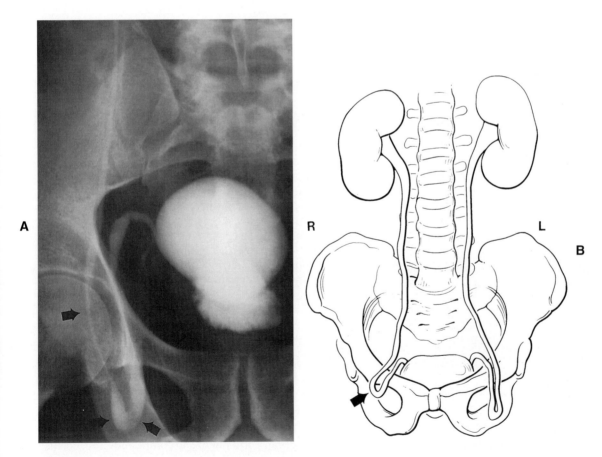

Fig. 5-28 Inguinal and femoral hernias of the ureter. **A,** An intravenous urogram demonstrates herniation of the right ureter (arrows) into the right inguinal canal. **B,** Diagram of a left-sided inguinal hernia and a less common femoral hernia (arrow) of the right ureter.

Box 5-8   Location and Extent of Ureteral Dilatation in Absence of Intrinsic Ureteral Obstruction

Entire ureter
  Bilateral
    Bladder outlet obstruction (mechanical and functional)
    Extensive bladder neoplasm
    Bladder inflammation
    Prune belly (Eagle-Barrett) syndrome
    Diabetes insipidus
    Polydipsia
    Primary megaureter
  Unilateral
    Vesicoureteral reflux (Grades II–IV)
    Primary megaureter
    Ectopic ureter inserting below bladder
    Bacterial infection
Lower ureter only
  Primary megaureter
  Vesicoureteral reflux (Grade I)
Upper ureter only
  Retrocaval or retroiliac ureter
  Enlarged uterus
  Postpartum ectasia

Box 5-9   Ureteral Narrowing

Malignancy
  Urothelial
  Local extension of extrinsic tumor
  Distant metastasis
  Lymphoma
Congenital
  Congenital strictures
Infectious conditions
  Tuberculosis
  Schistosomiasis
Inflammatory bowel disease
  Regional enteritis
  Diverticulitis
  Appendicitis
Gynecologic
  Endometriosis
Trauma
  Stone passage
  Iatrogenic
    Mechanical stone extraction
    Ureterolithotomy
    Radiation therapy
Miscellaneous conditions
  Retroperitoneal fibrosis
  Pelvic lipomatosis
  Amyloidosis

Box 5-10   Nonobstructive Causes of Ureteral Dilatation

Mechanical distention from intraluminal mass
  Mucosal neoplasm (goblet sign)
Decreased or flaccid ureteral musculature
  Prune belly (Eagle-Barrett) syndrome
  Bacterial infection with endotoxin release
  Residual dilatation from remote obstruction
Increased intraluminal volume
  Vesicoureteral reflux (primary and acquired)
  Primary megaureter
  Diabetes insipidus
  Polydipsia

---

has been described as the goblet sign because the tumor causes a meniscus-shaped filling defect (Fig. 5-29) in the dilated, contrast-filled ureter, much like the appearance of fluid in a goblet. Dilatation below an intraluminal filling defect never is seen with nonneoplastic processes. The dilatation inferior to the tumor is believed to be caused by normal peristalsis, leading to continual intussusception of the tumor into the immediately adjacent ureter. Over time, focal dilatation of the ureter occurs below the neoplasm. Less chronic, nongrowing intraluminal lesions cause contraction of the ureter caudal to the lesion because of spasm and accommodation to the diminished urine volume. The goblet sign is not seen with all TCCs of the ureter. It is seen with a minority of papillary neoplasms. Two thirds of TCCs are papillary, and the remainder are nonpapillary, or infiltrating. TCC is the most common type of urothelial neoplasm; it accounts for approximately 85% of these tumors. Five percent of urothelial neoplasms result from SCC, 1% from adenocarcinoma, and 10% from benign tumors. These tumors usually are indistinguishable by radiologic techniques. One important feature of TCCs is their propensity for multifocal disease (Box 5-11). When the ureter is involved, up to 40% of patients have or will develop other sites of TCC (Fig. 5-30). Typically, these sites are located on the same side in the collecting system, elsewhere in the same

ureter, or anywhere in the bladder lumen. The entire length of urothelium should be examined for other foci of TCC. TCCs rarely are seen in children and typically appear in middle-aged or older adults. Numerous carcinogens are known to increase the risk of TCC. These include aniline dyes and other benzene compounds, tobacco use, analgesic abuse, bone marrow transplantation, some chemotherapeutic agents (such as cyclophosphamide) that

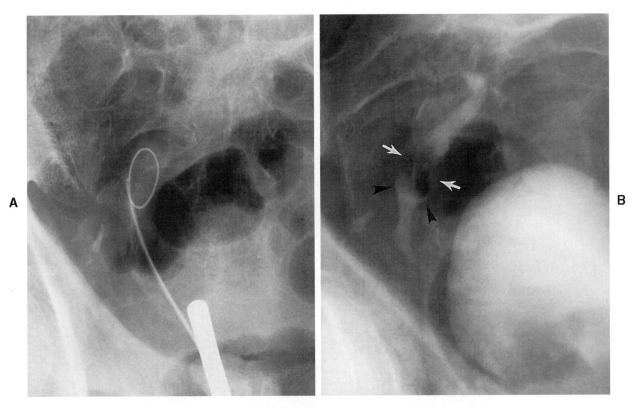

Fig. 5-29   Ureteral dilatation resulting from a papillary transitional cell carcinoma (TCC). **A,** Cystoscopy followed by cannulation of the right ureter with a catheter and guidewire demonstrates coiling of the guidewire in the lower right ureter. Coiling of the guidewire or catheter in this dilated segment of ureter is suggestive of ureteral TCC. This finding has been referred to as Bergman's coiled catheter sign and is analogous to the urographic goblet sign. **B,** An intravenous urogram in this same patient demonstrates the papillary TCC (arrows). There is a meniscus shape of the contrast material in the short dilated segment of ureter (arrowheads) just below the mass.

are used to manage malignant neoplasms outside the urinary tract, and in rare cases, Balkan nephropathy.

Prune belly syndrome

Dilatation of the ureter without obstruction often results from diminished tone in the ureteral musculature. Patients with prune belly syndrome often have inadequate ureteral musculature, which leads to massive diffuse, bilateral ureteral dilatation and hydroureteronephrosis (Fig. 5-31). There is no mechanical obstruction of the ureters, but the dilatation results from flaccidity

of the ureters. Because these patients have inadequate abdominal musculature with characteristic clinical findings, the diagnosis generally is obvious before ureteral imaging. Prune belly syndrome, also known as Eagle-Barrett syndrome, is seen almost exclusively in male patients, and cryptorchidism is common. Prostate and urethral anomalies often coexist.

Endotoxins

Pyelonephritis also can be associated with ureteral dilatation without mechanical obstruction. This enigmatic finding results from bacterial release of an endotoxin that paralyzes the ureteral musculature and inhibits ureteral peristalsis. If infection is suspected, exclusion of ureteral obstruction is crucial because its presence will inhibit entry of antibiotics into the infected urinary system. Obstruction also promotes rapid propagation of bacteria, destruction of renal parenchyma, and development of septicemia. Uncomplicated pyelonephritis resolves within 72 hours with appropriate antibiotic management. Radiographic abnormalities or symptoms of infection that continue longer than 3 days suggest compli-

---

Box 5-11   Transitional Cell Carcinoma Facts

Two-thirds papillary
85% of urothelial neoplasms
20% multifocal
Associations include aniline dyes, tobacco, analgesics, and Balkan nephropathy

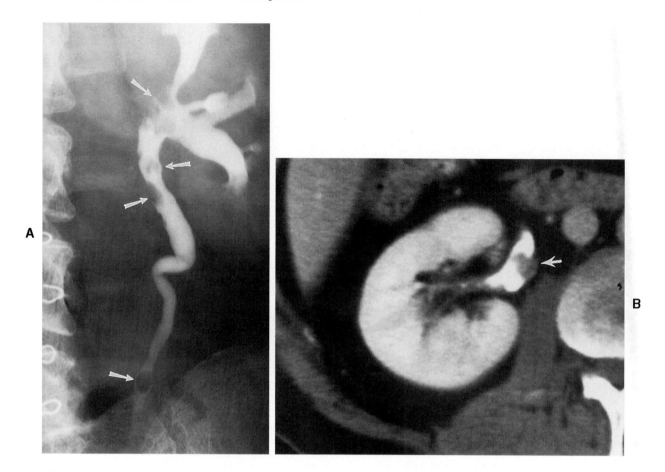

Fig. 5-30   Multifocal transitional cell carcinomas (TCC). **A,** Intravenous urography in a patient with gross hematuria demonstrates multiple radiolucent filling defects (arrows). These were biopsied and found to be papillary TCC. **B,** Contrast-infused CT of a different patient demonstrates the CT appearance of a papillary TCC (arrow).

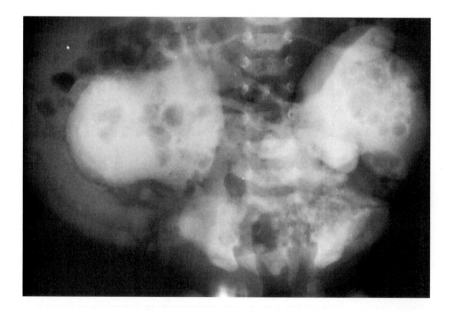

Fig. 5-31   Massive nonobstructive hydroureteronephrosis resulting from prune belly syndrome. A delayed film from an intravenous urogram in this child with prune belly syndrome demonstrates massive dilatation and redundancy of the ureters and renal pelvis resulting from deficient ureteral muscles.

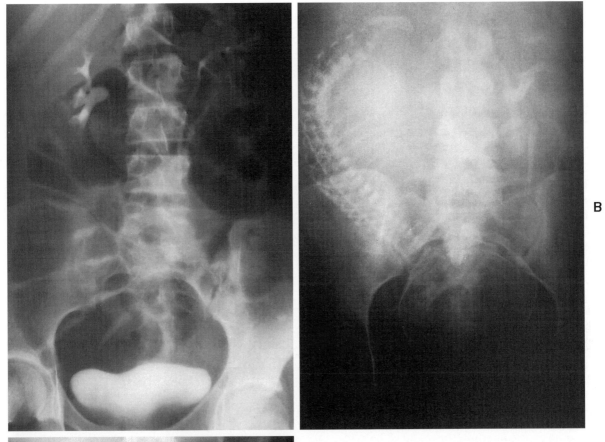

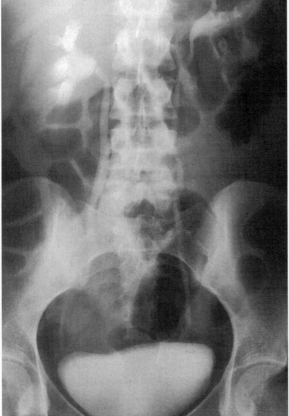

Fig. 5-32   Postpartum ureteral dilatation. **A,** An intravenous urogram in this patient obtained before pregnancy demonstrates normal caliber ureters and calyces. **B,** An abdominal radiograph taken during third trimester of pregnancy in this same patient demonstrates the position of the fetus overlying the right ureter as it crosses the iliac vessels. Mechanical compression of the right ureter is thought to be the major cause of postpartum ureteral dilatation. **C,** A urogram taken 6 months after delivery of a healthy infant demonstrates mild residual ectasia of the upper two-thirds of the right ureter and the right calyces. This nonobstructive dilatation can persist for months or years after childbirth.

cated pyelonephritis. Complicated pyelonephritis can result from ureteral obstruction, stone disease, unusual pathogens, or renal abscess.

Residual ectasia

The most common cause of ureteral dilatation associated with decreased muscle tone is residual ectasia related to remote obstruction. In these patients, ureteral imaging will demonstrate dilatation of a ureteral segment without any other signs of obstruction. For example, there will be no temporal delay in opacification of the collecting system or ureter. The normal caliber ureter below the dilated segment will opacify normally. Administration of a diuretic will lead to rapid and symmetric contrast material washout from the affected and the unaffected kidney. Permanent ureteral ectasia requires a long-standing obstruction, i.e., one that lasts months or years. Once this obstruction has been relieved, the kidney regains function, but the ureter remains dilated, albeit unobstructed. One common form of this abnormality is postpartum dilatation of the ureter (Fig. 5-32 on p. 175), which is a unilateral abnormality that involves the right ureter only. Mild dilatation of the upper two thirds of the right ureter in women after childbirth often results from compression of the ureter between the enlarged uterus and the iliac vessels. The left ureter is protected from compression by the interposed sigmoid colon. This segmental, right-sided ureteral dilatation can be marked during pregnancy because of ongoing compression, and it may be enhanced by hormonal inhibition of smooth muscle contraction during pregnancy. In most patients, the caliber of the ureter returns to normal after childbirth, however, in some patients, this dilatation persists (Fig. 5-32). It has been hypothesized that these patients experienced more severe compression during pregnancy or that they had a subclinical urinary tract infection coexisting with the partial obstruction during pregnancy. Postpartum ureteral ectasia is not uncommon. However, this is a diagnosis of exclusion, and one must ensure that the transition from dilated to normal ureter is not associated with an ongoing obstruction. An intravenous urogram augmented with diuretic administration is usually adequate for this exclusion. Typically, the transition from dilated to normal ureter occurs as the ureter crosses the iliac vessels. The ureter in this transitional segment is gently tapered and smooth, and filling defects are absent.

Increased urine volume

The final class of nonobstructive causes of ureteral dilatation includes increased intraluminal volume. Chronic excessive urine output resulting from diabetes insipidus or polydipsia can lead to diffuse, bilateral dilatation of the ureters. Vesicoureteral reflux also can lead

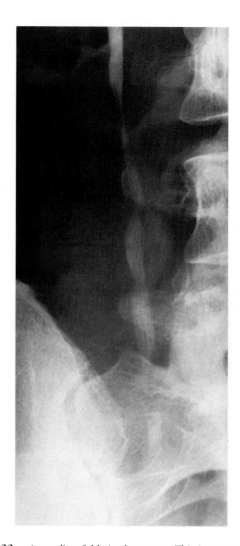

Fig. 5-33 Accordion folds in the ureter. This intravenous urogram demonstrates linear lucencies extending within the lumen of the lower right ureter. The right ureter also is mildly dilatated. This patient had chronic reflux leading to dilatation and ectasia of the ureter. These lucencies are thought to represent infolding of the ureteral mucosa, much like an accordion. Some inflammatory processes can cause linear lucent filling defects within the ureter, and if symptoms suggest an acute abnormality, endoscopy may be necessary for diagnosis.

to ureteral dilatation because the ureter must dilate to accommodate the increased volume of urine in the segment affected by reflux. In Grade 1 reflux, only the lower third of the ureter is involved and dilated to accommodate the normal antegrade flow of excreted urine and the volume of refluxed urine. If reflux is minor, the ureter may contract to a normal caliber between episodes. Often, this ureteral segment has visible longitudinal linear lucencies indenting the contrast column (Fig. 5-33). This appearance is caused by infolding of redundant mucosa, analogous to the folds of an accordion. These folds are effaced during distention.

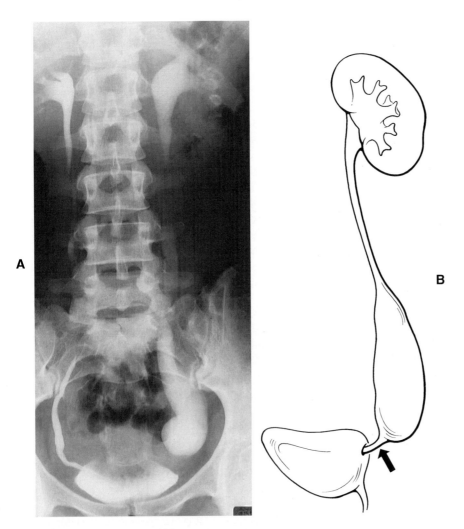

Fig. 5-34   Primary megaureter. **A,** An intravenous urogram in this patient with recurrent urinary tract infections demonstrates massive dilatation of the lower third of the left ureter. The left calyces are delicate and nondilated. This pattern is incompatible with ureteral obstruction and is typical of primary megaureter. A cystogram done 1 week later demonstrated no evidence of ureteral reflux. **B,** Diagram of the typical appearance of a primary megaureter. The primary abnormal segment is normal in caliber (arrow) at the ureterovesical junction.

Primary megaureter

One interesting form of ureteral dilatation caused by increased volume is primary megaureter, an idiopathic congenital abnormality. Primary megaureter results from inadequate musculature inhibiting peristalsis along a short segment of ureter near the ureterovesical junction. This segment of ureter appears normal radiographically, without stenosis or filling defect. However, inhibition of peristalsis along this segment leads to transient hold-up of urine above the segment, eventually resulting in ureteral dilatation. Typically, primary megaureter leads to massive dilatation of the lower third of the ureter (Fig. 5-34). In patients with severe cases, the entire length of the ureter may be dilated. However, in the majority of patients with primary megaureter, the calyces retain their sharp,

nondilated appearance. This appearance is distinctly different from that of ureteral obstruction, in which blunting of calyces is an early finding that often occurs before ureteral dilatation. The occasional association of megacalicosis (Fig. 5-35), another congenital abnormality, with primary megaureter can complicate diagnosis. Radiographic findings include an increase in number (polycalicosis) and abnormality in shape of the calyces (megacalyces); megacalyces often are squared or laminated in shape, mimicking obstruction. Although primary megaureter and megacalicosis are two distinct entities, the incidence of megacalicosis is increased in patients with primary megaureter. Their coexistence easily is misinterpreted as chronic ureteral obstruction. The increased number of calyces and their characteristic shape in the

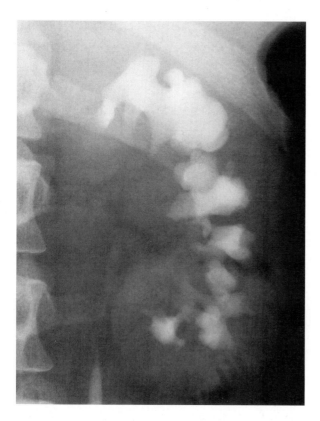

Fig. 5-35 Congenital megacalicosis. This urogram demonstrates an increased number of abnormally shaped calyces. The calyces are squared off rather than concave. There is normal parenchymal thickness. This pattern of abnormalities is typical of congenital megacalicosis.

absence of other findings of obstruction should suggest this association.

Primary megaureter is unilateral in 75% of patients. When unilateral, the left more commonly is affected than the right. Primary megaureter also is more common in men than in women, and it usually is discovered incidentally. Primary megaureter can lead to recurrent urinary infections or, less commonly, urolithiasis. Although the typical appearance of primary megaureter, marked dilatation of the lower third of the ureter without evidence of obstruction, is characteristic, vesicoureteral reflux should be excluded before making a final diagnosis. A radiographic or radionuclide voiding cystourethrogram can be used to exclude vesicoureteral reflux because its management differs from the usual management of primary megaureter.

Ureteral narrowing

The causes of ureteral narrowing are numerous (Box 5-9). It particularly is important initially to try to distinguish intrinsic from extrinsic causes to expedite diagnosis. Intrinsic abnormalities are best evaluated with intra-

luminal procedures, such as endoscopy, brush biopsy, and urine cytology studies. Extrinsic lesions are best evaluated with cross-sectional imaging for characterization and guidance of percutaneous biopsy, if necessary. Figure 5-36 is a diagram of the differing appearances of intrinsic and extrinsic causes of ureteral narrowing. Obviously, these appearances overlap to some extent, but these models serve as guidelines for directing additional evaluation. An intrinsic lesion, such as infiltrating TCC, generally causes an abrupt caliber change with irregularity of the mucosa (Fig. 5-37) in the narrowed area, which is analogous to the apple core lesion seen on barium studies with circumferential colon carcinomas. These infiltrating ureteral tumors lead to irregular circumferential thickening of the ureteral wall and resulting luminal narrowing. Causes of the apple core appearance of ureteral narrowing include urothelial tumors (TCC and SCC) and, less commonly, benign strictures. Benign strictures may be caused by recurrent stone disease, particularly with infection-based stones, and iatrogenic causes, including mechanical and surgical stone extractions or radiation therapy. All of these processes can lead to intrinsic thickening of the ureteral wall with an abrupt transition from normal lumen to narrowed ureteral lumen. This appearance differs from encasement and narrowing of the ureter by extrinsic processes such as those described in Box 5-9. These lesions tend to cause a smooth, gradual tapering of the ureteral lumen, leading to a waist-like appearance of the lumen, with smooth mucosa throughout the narrowed segment (Fig. 5-38). This appearance also is depicted diagrammatically in Figure 5-36.

The features of some of these areas of narrowing may help to determine the underlying diagnosis or to direct additional evaluation of the patient. For example, tapered

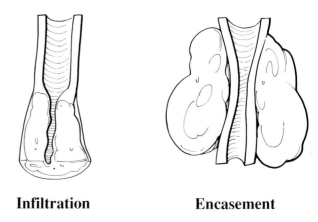

Infiltration   **Encasement**

Fig. 5-36 Diagram of two patterns of ureteral narrowing. Intrinsic, infiltrating lesions, such as transitional cell carcinoma, typically cause abrupt narrowing of the ureter and irregularity of the mucosa. Alternatively, encasement of the ureter by an extrinsic process causes gentle tapering with a waist-like narrowing of the ureteral lumen and normal mucosa.

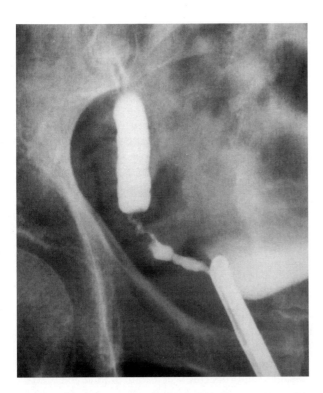

Fig. 5-37   Ureteral narrowing caused by an invasive transitional cell carcinoma (TCC). A retrograde pyelogram in this patient demonstrates mucosal irregularity and abrupt narrowing of the ureter. These features are typical of an infiltrating process such as TCC.

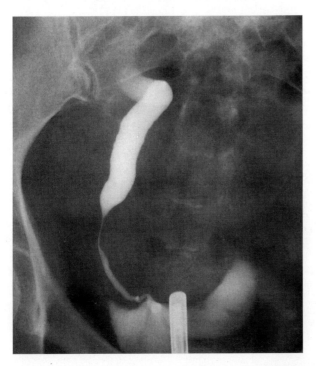

Fig. 5-38   Ureteral narrowing resulting from an extrinsic process. A retrograde pyelogram in this patient with carcinoma of the cervix demonstrates severe ureteral narrowing. The narrowed segment has normal smooth mucosa, and the narrowing is a gentle tapering rather than an abrupt transition. These features are typical of encasement of the ureter by an extrinsic process.

Box 5-12   **Associations with Retroperitoneal Fibrosis**
Common
Idiopathic
Uncommon
Aortic aneurysm
Aortic graft
Retroperitoneal hemorrhage
Urinoma
Abscess
Metastases
Drugs
Bowel disease
Rare
Sclerosing cholangitis
Fibrosing mediastinitis

narrowing of the lower ureters with associated medial deviation and increased lucency in the pelvis is typical of pelvic lipomatosis, which was described previously in this chapter. Similarly, medial deviation of the ureters with ureteral narrowing involving the midureter suggests retroperitoneal fibrosis.

Retroperitoneal fibrosis   Retroperitoneal fibrosis is an interesting disease process. The idiopathic form, also known as Ormond's disease, is found in approximately 50% of these patients. Although the cause of idiopathic retroperitoneal fibrosis is unknown, it often does coexist with inflammatory bowel disease, sclerosing cholangitis, and fibrosing mediastinitis. Known causes of retroperitoneal fibrosis include inflammation originating in the wall of an abdominal aortic aneurysm (the so-called inflammatory aneurysm); vascular grafts; retroperitoneal metastases such as lymphoma, breast carcinoma, or carcinoid tumor; and retroperitoneal hematoma, abscess, urinoma, diverticulitis, or appendicitis (Box 5-12). Other known associations with retroperitoneal fibrosis include certain medications such as ergot alkaloids and hydralazine. Undoubtedly, numerous other etiologies of retroperitoneal fibrosis exist, but regardless of the cause, patients with retroperitoneal fibrosis share many characteristics. The fibrosis tends to begin just lateral to the aorta, therefore, it typically involves the left ureter before the right. As it spreads, the fibrotic process extends to the pericaval region and the interaortocaval area of the retroperitoneum. Although retroperitoneal fibrosis can involve the ureter anywhere between the bladder and the UPJ, it most commonly is centered in the L3–L5 area (Fig. 5-39). On cross-sectional imaging, retroperitoneal fibrosis is a smooth plate-like area of soft tissue (Fig. 5-40) layered around, between, and over the aorta and inferior vena cava. It is unusual for retroperitoneal fibrosis to extend

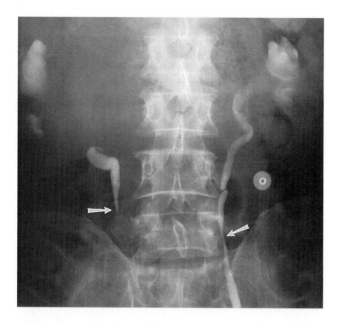

Fig. 5-39 Bilateral ureteral narrowing caused by retroperitoneal fibrosis. Bilateral retrograde pyelograms demonstrate massive hydroureteronephrosis with extrinsic-type ureteral narrowing (arrows) at L5. This is a typical location and appearance of retroperitoneal fibrosis.

toms is insidious. Most often, the degree of hydronephrosis seen with retroperitoneal fibrosis greatly underestimates the degree of renal insufficiency, probably because of the lack of severe pressure increase in the obstructive collecting systems. In addition, it also is typical for passage of ureteral stents to be unusually easy through these smoothly narrowed segments of encased ureter because the ureteral lumen is fixed open by the encasing fibrotic process. Although this fixation inhibits peristalsis, it facilitates stent passage through the ureteral lumen, and although these features are not diagnostic of retroperitoneal fibrosis, they certainly are commonly seen.

Radiation stricture Ureteral narrowing caused by radiation damage to the ureter is another interesting entity. This narrowing develops when pelvic or retroperitoneal neoplasms occur in the same radiation field as a segment of ureter. When a ureteral stricture develops in this area, radiation-induced stricture and recurrent neoplasm are the two major diagnostic considerations. On contrast studies, radiation strictures tend to have an abrupt transition from normal to narrowed ureter (Fig. 5-42), whereas recurrent tumor usually will lead to gradual, tapered narrowing of the ureteral lumen. In addition, the development of radiation strictures usually is delayed at least 12 months after radiation therapy. Hence, earlier development of ureteral narrowing strongly suggests recurrent neoplasm.

Miscellaneous causes of strictures When ureteral strictures result from infections, careful examination of adjacent structures usually will aid in the diagnosis. Involvement of the ureter with tuberculosis always is secondary to renal involvement. Therefore, a careful evaluation of the kidney for signs of tuberculosis (Fig. 5-43), i.e., papillary necrosis, amputated or phantom calyces,

between the aorta and the vertebral bodies. When the aorta is uplifted from the spine by a retroperitoneal mass (Fig. 5-41), lymphoma is a more likely diagnosis than retroperitoneal fibrosis. Retroperitoneal fibrosis is a slow-growing process that encases the ureteral wall and leads to loss of peristalsis in the affected segment. There rarely is ureteral wall invasion, and the mucosa always is spared. Because the ureteral lumen remains patent and obstruction is purely functional, the onset of obstructive symp-

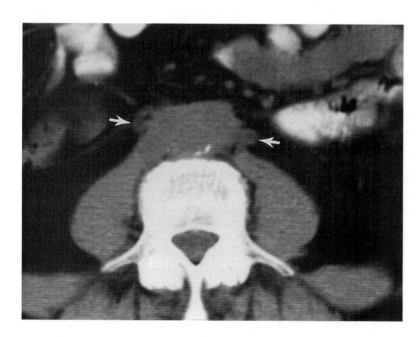

Fig. 5-40 CT of retroperitoneal fibrosis. This uninfused CT scan demonstrates an ill-defined soft-tissue mass surrounding the aorta and vena cava. The ureters (arrows) are drawn into this fibrotic mass.

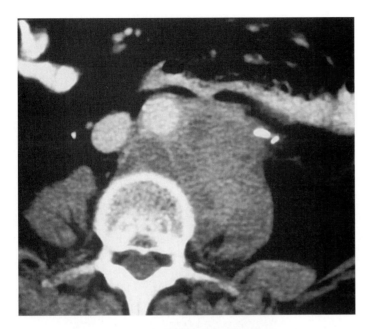

Fig. 5-41   CT of retroperitoneal lymphoma mimicking retroperitoneal fibrosis. This contrast-infused CT demonstrates an ill-defined soft-tissue mass centered around the aorta. A portion of this mass extends behind the aorta and uplifts it away from the spine. In this patient, this mass results from lymphoma. This pattern, although similar to retroperitoneal fibrosis, would be unusual for that benign entity and is more suggestive of malignancy such as lymphoma.

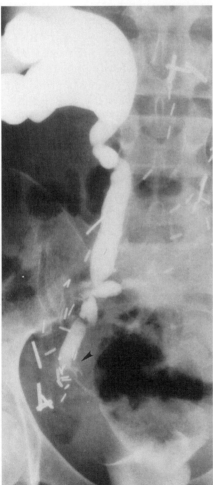

Fig. 5-42   Radiation stricture of the ureter. This intravenous urogram demonstrates an abrupt caliber change in the lower right ureter (arrowhead). This patient had been treated with surgery and radiation for carcinoma of the testes. This stricture developed more than 1 year after radiation therapy to this region.

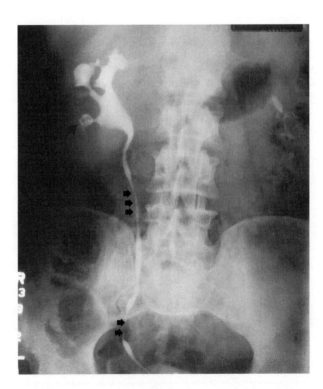

Fig. 5-43   Ureteral strictures from tuberculosis. This intravenous urogram demonstrates multiple ureteral strictures (arrowheads) and a focal area of papillary necrosis (arrow). This is a typical pattern of spread for tuberculosis, which was cultured from this patient's urine.

mucosal ulcerations, or strictures, is important. Alternatively, the spread of schistosomiasis to the ureter always is preceded by bladder involvement. Evidence of cystitis, bladder contraction, and bladder wall calcifications suggests possible schistosomiasis, which can spread via vesicoureteral reflux to the ureters.

Multifocal areas of ureteral narrowing suggest multifocal TCC, tuberculosis, or metastatic disease to adjacent lymph nodes. Infiltrating TCC is less commonly multifocal than is the papillary form. However, TCC would be the most likely diagnosis when multiple intrinsic strictures of a ureter are detected. Alternatively, multiple extrinsic-type strictures suggest metastatic disease encasing the ureter at multiple sites or lymphoma. Lymphoma often involves many retroperitoneal lymph nodes, leading to bilateral ureteral narrowing and associated ureteral deviation from massive adenopathy. However, lymphoma can be indistinguishable from other types of metastatic disease.

Finally, location and clinical history may be helpful in diagnosing other causes of ureteral narrowing. Specifically, patients with diverticulitis often have typical symptoms of abdominal pain and fever. Because the sigmoid colon most commonly is involved with diverticulitis, the lower left ureter is the segment that is narrowed in association with diverticulitis. Alternatively, ureteral strictures associated with regional enteritis (Crohn's disease) usually are in the mid-to-lower right ureter in the area adjacent to the terminal ileum. Strictures from appendicitis occur in the lower right ureter adjacent to the appendix. Endometriosis also can lead to stricturing of the adjacent ureter, which can occur bilaterally and usually is at the level of the uterosacral ligaments in the pelvis, a common site for endometriosis implants. Endometriosis usually is associated with symptoms such as cyclical pelvic pain and dyspareunia.

URETERAL FILLING DEFECTS

Box 5-13 lists numerous causes of ureteral filling defects. This list is long, although many of these entities are rare.

Urolithiasis

When a ureteral filling defect is detected, the list of possible causes must be narrowed for proper patient treatment. The most important step is evaluation of a plain abdominal radiograph with attention to the area of ureteral pathology. Urolithiasis is the most common cause of ureteral obstruction, and 90% of urinary tract stones are radiopaque or visible on a high quality abdominal film. A discussion of the radiographic appearance of urinary tract stone types warrants a slight digression. Pure calcium phosphate stones and calcium monohy-

Table 5-1 Composition of Renal Stones

Composition	Frequency (%)	Radiopacity (0–4)
Calcium phosphate	10	4
Calcium phosphate and oxalate	40	3–4
Calcium oxalate	30	3
Struvite	10	2–3
Cystine	1	1
Uric acid	10	0

drate stones are the most dense per volume of stone (Table 5-1). This fact may be important because pure calcium phosphate stones are less responsive to extracorporeal shockwave lithotripsy (ESWL) than are most other stones. Calcium oxalate dihydrate stones often have a spiculated (Figs. 5-44, 5-45) or dotted configuration that is sometimes compared with the appearance of a mulberry or a child's toy jack. These stones are considered fragile and are fragmented easily with ESWL. Most calcium stones are admixtures of oxalate and phosphate salts with intermediate density and intermediate fragility for ESWL management. Magnesium ammonium phosphate (struvite) stones have low radiopacity or may be completely radiolucent. However, these stones typically complex with calcium phosphate, thereby increasing their radiopacity. These typically are infection-based stones and often grow to become large branched calculi (Fig. 5-46). These stones form in part as a result of urinary

Box 5-13 Ureteral Filling Defects

Intraluminal
  Calculi
  Blood clots
  Sloughed papilla
  Fungus ball
  Mucopus
  Air bubbles
Mucosal
  Neoplasm (benign or malignant)
  Edema
  Leukoplakia
Mural
  Ureteritis cystica
  Hemorrhage
  Malacoplakia
  Endometriosis
  Schistosomiasis
Extrinsic
  Vascular processes

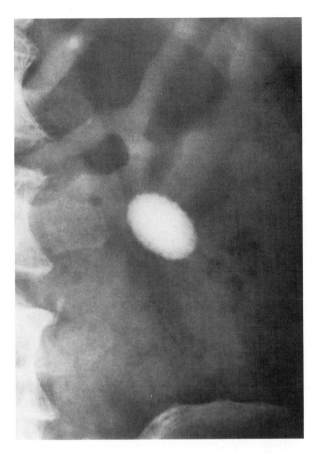

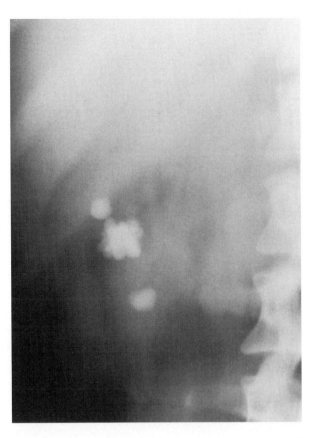

Fig. 5-44   Mulberry stone. This plain abdominal radiograph demonstrates a densely calcified left renal stone. At the edges of the stone, a dotted texture can be appreciated. This appearance is typical of calcium oxalate dihydrate stones.

Fig. 5-45   ''Jack'' stone. Three densely calcified stones are noted in this right kidney. The central stone has spiculated margins and mimics the shape of a toy jack. This is another typical shape for calcium oxalate dihydrate stones.

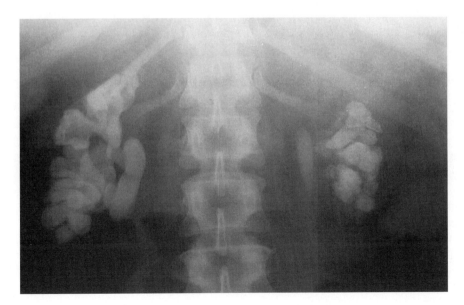

Fig. 5-46   Bilateral branched struvite calculi. This plain abdominal radiograph demonstrates large bilateral infection-based struvite calculi. For their size, these stones are not particularly dense and are composed largely of radiolucent struvite.

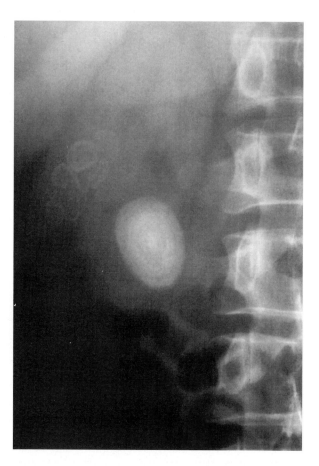

Fig. 5-47 Laminated struvite stone. This radiograph demonstrates prominent laminations in the oval stone in the right renal pelvis. These laminations are typical of an infection-based stone composed largely of struvite. Incidental note is made of multiple gallstones overlying the lateral portion of the right kidney.

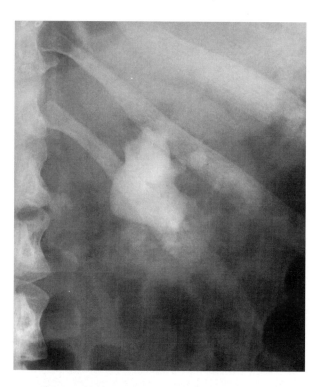

Fig. 5-48 Cystine stone. This abdominal radiograph demonstrates a branched stone in the left kidney. The stone has homogeneous density and has a ground glass or opalescent appearance. These stones tend to be of comparable density as excreted contrast and can be difficult to identify after intravenous injection of contrast material.

infection with bacteria that harbor a urea-splitting enzyme. The enzyme causes alkalinization of the urine, which favors stone formation. The calcium phosphate component of these stones often layers on the struvite and leads to a laminated appearance (Fig. 5-47). Although these stones are fragmented easily with ESWL, their large size and infectious etiology often preclude successful ESWL management. Fragmentation and extraction of these stones via a percutaneous nephrostomy tract is the preferred treatment in most of these patients. Cystine stones contain no calcium and are rendered radiopaque by their sulfur content. They are less opaque than calcium stones of a comparable size and generally have a homogeneous density (Fig. 5-48) similar to that of excreted contrast material. Their appearance typically is described as being opalescent or similar to that of ground glass. Cystine stones are not fragmented easily with ESWL and are considered to be among the least fragile of the urinary tract calculi. Although no cystine stones are very fragile, those with rough surfaces have a fragility similar to that of pure calcium stones, whereas smooth cystine stones are less responsive to ESWL fragmentation.

Radiolucent Filling Defects

When a filling defect is radiolucent, analysis of its appearance (Fig. 5-49) often is helpful to determine its cause (Box 5-13). Lesions that are completely surrounded by contrast material typically are intraluminal processes. Lesions that are inseparable from the ureteral mucosa but have acute angles where the mucosa and mass join typically are mucosa-based abnormalities. Lesions inseparable from the mucosa but with obtuse angles usually are submucosal, intramural ureteral lesions. Finally, lesions with obtuse angles and associated ureteral deviation usually are caused by extrinsic processes indenting the ureter eccentrically. Once categorized, etiologies in each category should be considered, and additional evaluation of the patient can be guided by the likely site of abnormality. For example, lesions that are apparently extrinsic should be evaluated with cross-sectional imaging, whereas intramural and mucosal lesions are best evaluated with some form of intraluminal endoscopy, such as ureteroscopy.

Up to 10% of urinary tract stones are radiolucent on

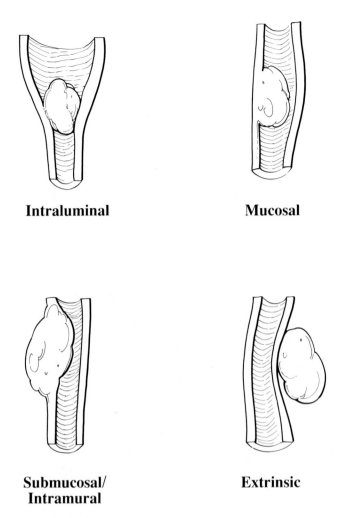

Intraluminal

Mucosal

**Submucosal/
Intramural**

Extrinsic

Fig. 5-49 Diagram outlining classification of ureteral filling defects based on their shape.

abdominal radiographs. These stones are composed of uric acid or xanthine or unmineralized matrix. A radiolucent calculus is the most common cause of a radiolucent ureteral filling defect. If careful comparison with the preliminary film fails to demonstrate a radiopaque stone causing the ureteral filling defect, a radiolucent stone is the most likely diagnosis. This diagnosis can be confirmed by imaging the ureter with CT after complete clearance of intravascular and intraureteral contrast material. All urinary tract calculi are radiopaque (Fig. 5-50) on CT scans. Virtually no ureteral tumors or other causes of ureteral filling defects are homogeneously opaque with uninfused CT scanning. Therefore, CT often is helpful as the next step in evaluation of radiolucent ureteral or calyceal filling defects to distinguish stones from other lesions.

Other causes of filling defects in the ureter bear additional comment. Ureteral blood clots generally originate from renal hemorrhage. The filling defects caused by

ureteral blood clots generally have an elongated shape, as the blood forms a cast of the ureteral lumen (Fig. 5-51). Blood clots may lead to transient ureteral obstruction and symptoms typical of ureteral colic. However, the presence of urokinase in normal urine leads to clot lysis, usually within a matter of hours. Therefore, the appearance of blood clots changes with repeated examinations, and complete resolution often occurs within days of presentation.

Patients who are susceptible to papillary necrosis, particularly patients with diabetes, patients with sickle cell anemia, and abusers of analgesics, may slough a segment or an entire papilla into the urinary tract (Fig. 5-52). Typically, a sloughed papilla has a triangular shape, and its perimeter may calcify. The presence of a ureteral filling defect with calyceal changes of papillary necrosis (Fig. 5-53) strongly suggests a sloughed papilla resulting from papillary necrosis.

Fungal debris or fungus balls can lead to filling defects in the calyces or ureter. Fungal debris has an appearance similar to that of blood clot, i.e., a cast of the calyces (Fig. 5-54) or ureter. The filling defects caused by blood clots or fungal debris within calyces often have been described as the "hand-in-glove" appearance. Blood and fungal debris tend to conform to the shape of their surroundings, and this radiolucent material will be outlined by a thin rim of contrast material in the calyces. Most urinary fungal infections are caused by *Candida* or *Aspergillus* fungi. These typically occur in immunocompromised patients or patients with diabetes. Once the diagnosis has been suggested, it can be confirmed with urine cultures. Infectious debris or frank pus has a similar appearance, mimicking blood or fungal debris. Clinical symptoms and urine cultures are essential for establishing the correct diagnosis.

An air bubble is a well-known cause of a ureteral filling defect. These most commonly are seen as a normal variant in patients with urinary conduit diversions. Typically, ileal conduits allow ureteral reflux, and air bubbles can be refluxed into the ureter or renal collecting systems. In other patients, air bubbles can be introduced by instrumentation (Fig. 5-55 on p. 188), fistula formation with bowel, or a cutaneous fistula. Finally, air bubbles can be introduced into the ureter or collecting system from a gas-producing infection. These infections typically are seen in patients whose diabetes is poorly controlled. Responsible organisms include strains of *Escherichia coli*, *Proteus*, *Klebsiella*, and some strains of fungus. Unlike emphysematous pyelonephritis, gas limited to the lumen of the ureter and renal collecting system is managed primarily nonsurgically. This type of infection, termed *emphysematous pyelitis*, generally can be managed successfully with systemic antibiotics in conjunction with urinary decompression via either retrograde ureteral stinting or percutaneous nephrostomy drainage.

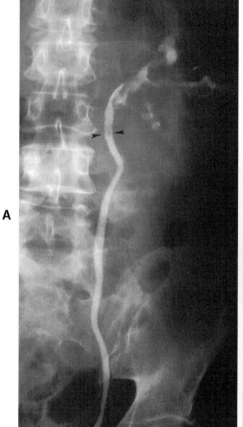

A

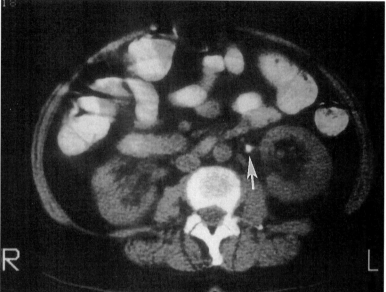

B

Fig. 5-50 Radiolucent stone. **A,** A left retrograde pyelogram demonstrates a focal radiolucent filling defect (arrowheads) in the upper left ureter. **B,** A noncontrast CT scan through this region confirms that this filling defect was caused by a ureteral stone (arrow). This CT appearance is diagnostic of ureteral stones.

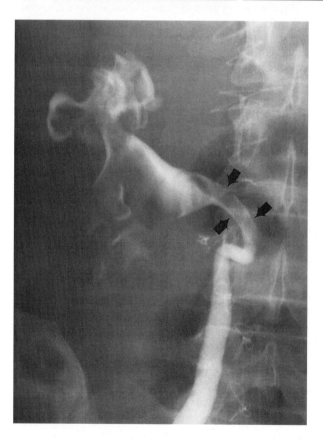

Fig. 5-51 Filling defects caused by blood clots. This film demonstrates an elongated filling defect (arrows) in the upper right ureter and radiolucent material forming a cast of the renal calyces. This is the typical appearance of intraluminal blood, as was the case in this patient who was anticoagulated overzealously.

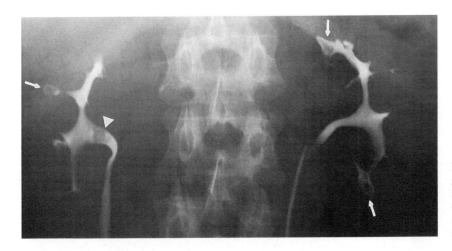

Fig. 5-52 Sloughed papilla. Bilateral retrograde pyelograms demonstrate multifocal papillary necrosis (arrows). A triangular radiolucent filling defect (arrowhead) is noted in the right renal pelvis. This appearance is typical of a sloughed papilla in the renal pelvis.

Mucosal lesions most commonly are caused by urothelial neoplasms. TCC, by far the most common urothelial tumor, exhibits two different growth patterns. Two thirds of TCCs are papillary. They grow into polypoid lesions, extend into the lumen of the urinary tract, and cause radiolucent filling defects. The remaining TCCs infiltrate the urinary tract wall and lead to stricturing, as described previously in this chapter. Another cause of mucosa-based filling defects is ureteral edema. Edema of the mucosa usually is caused by direct irritation, either by passage of a stone or by iatrogenic insult to the ureter. Edema may lead to focal mucosal blisters with a bullous appearance or may be somewhat striated, causing linear filling defects. Removal of the inciting factor, such as a stone or stent, usually results in resolution of the edema within several days or weeks.

Leukoplakia is an uncommon urothelial lesion. This premalignant squamous metaplasia of the urothelium results from chronic irritation of the urinary lining. Leukoplakia most commonly involves the bladder but may involve the ureter or renal collecting system. Typically, leukoplakia is associated with a history of urolithiasis or

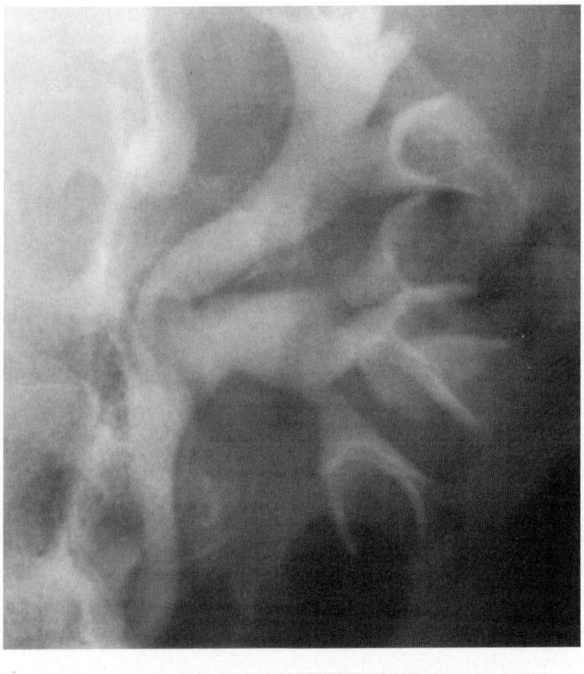

Fig. 5-53 Lobster-claw appearance of papillary necrosis. This intravenous urogram demonstrates another radiographic appearance of papillary necrosis. The peripheral margins of the papilla have necrosed and sloughed, leading to cavities at the papillary tips of the calyces. This causes elongation of the edges of the calyces, leading to a lobster-claw appearance.

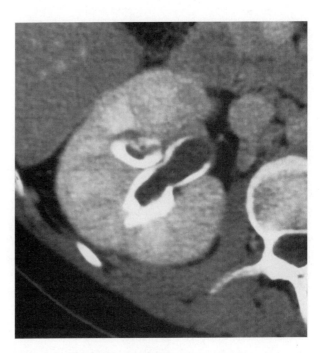

Fig. 5-54 Calyceal fungus debris. This contrast-infused CT scan demonstrates radiolucent material forming a cast of the calyces. This material was fungal debris in this immunosuppressed patient.

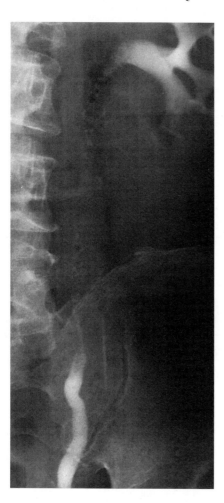

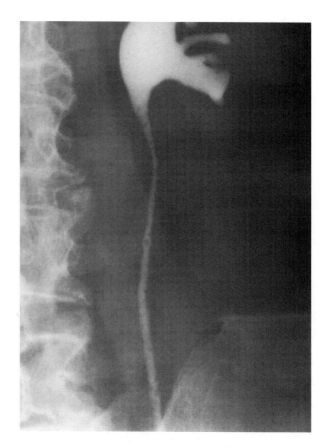

Fig. 5-55 Air bubbles in the ureter causing filling defects. This intravenous urogram was performed after retrograde pyelography. Multiple air bubbles are noted within the upper two thirds of the left ureter, which can be confirmed by changing the patient's position or by close examination of the scout radiograph, which will confirm the presence of air in the ureteral lumen.

Fig. 5-56 Ureteritis cystica. This intravenous urogram of a patient with chronic urinary tract infections demonstrates multiple, smooth, round filling defects in the ureter. Lesions seen in profile have obtuse margins, typical of submucosal location.

chronic urinary tract infection, such as schistosomiasis. When leukoplakia is discovered, SCC of the urothelium usually coexists in an adjacent area of the urinary tract.

Submucosal or mural lesions also can lead to filling defects within the ureter. Ureteritis cystica and pyeloureteritis cystica are rather common postinflammatory causes of filling defects in the urinary tract. They always are associated with chronic urinary tract infections. These sterile submucosal fluid collections are caused by intramural inflammation and lead to encystment and submucosal extension of transitional epithelium. The lesions typically are multicentric, smooth, and round (Fig. 5-56).

Intramural hemorrhage can have a similar appearance, but the patient's history often suggests the correct diagnosis. These patients typically are receiving anticoagulant therapy or have a coagulopathy. Hematuria usually accompanies intramural hemorrhage.

Malacoplakia is a rare, but often discussed, intramural ureteral lesion that occurs secondary to chronic urinary tract infection. These plaque-like, intramural lesions are caused by build-up of defective macrophages. These benign lesions are not premalignant, and the radiographic appearance of these submucosal lesions is nonspecific. Microscopic evaluation of the defective macrophages will reveal incompletely phagocytized *E. coli* bacteria. The intracellular inclusion bodies containing these bacteria are known as Michaelis-Gutmann bodies and are diagnostic of malacoplakia. Malacoplakia can involve the bladder, ureter, collecting system, and renal parenchyma. These lesions tend to regress spontaneously after resolution of the inciting urinary tract infection. Some authors have compared malacoplakia with a localized form, or form *fruste,* of chronic granulomatous disease, another entity with defective macrophage phagocytosis. Endometriosis and schistosomiasis typically lead to strictures of the ureter rather than filling defects. However, either can invade the ureteral wall and lead to focal filling defects impinging on the ureteral lumen. Both entities tend to involve the pelvic ureter; schistosomiasis involves the

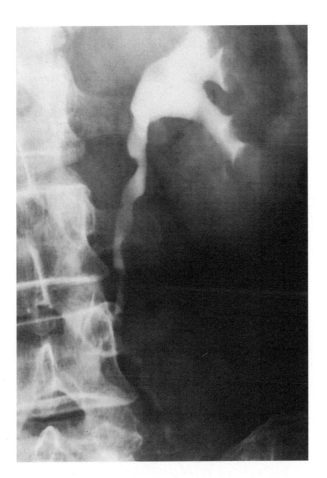

Fig. 5-57 Ureteral notching secondary to enlargement of ureteral arteries. This intravenous urogram demonstrates multiple eccentric indentations on the upper ureter in this patient with severe left renal artery stenosis. These indentations result from enlargement of ureteric vessels, which serve as collaterals to increase blood flow to the kidney.

ureter adjacent to the bladder, and endometriosis involves the ureter adjacent to the uterotubal ligaments, which are several centimeters away from the bladder. Detection of an associated bladder abnormality should suggest schistosomiasis, and typical clinical findings of cyclical pelvic pain generally are present in patients with endometriosis involving the ureter.

Finally, adjacent extrinsic processes may appear as a ureteral filling defect. Crossing vessels often cause ureteral notching (Fig. 5-57) with multiple eccentric indentations on the ureteral lumen. These most commonly are secondary to enlargement of ureteric arteries and veins. These veins and arteries enlarge in patients with renal artery stenosis, hypervascular renal tumors such as RCCs or arteriovenous malformations, or occlusive aortoiliac or venous diseases. Enlargement of gonadal veins also can lead to ureteral indentation. Testicular or ovarian vein varices, ovarian vein syndrome, or thrombophlebitis of the gonadal veins can lead to vascular impressions on the ureteral lumen.

URETERAL TRAUMA

The ureter is the part of the urinary tract least commonly injured when individuals are involved with external trauma. Ureteral and renal pelvic injuries account for less than 1% of all urologic trauma. Unlike other areas of the urinary tract, penetrating injury is the most common mechanism causing ureteral injury. Penetrating injury can lacerate or transect the ureter at any site along its course. Findings indicative of ureteral laceration include urinoma formation, contrast extravasation, and discontinuity of the ureter. More interesting than penetrating injury is ureteral injury as a result of acceleration or deceleration trauma. When ureteral injury results from this type of trauma, ureteral avulsion usually occurs. The most common site of disruption is the UPJ, followed by avulsion of the upper 4 cm of the ureter adjacent to, but below, the UPJ, then the proximal ureter, and the midureter. Interestingly, ureteral avulsion occurs approximately three times more often in children than in adults. In addition, avulsion occurs three times more often on the right than on the left. Ureteral avulsion appears to be caused by sudden hyperextension of the body resulting from sudden acceleration or deceleration. Hyperextension leads to sudden tension on the ureter causing a ''bowstring'' effect. This effect forces the collecting system to snap against the spine, and this may cause ureteral avulsion. This mechanism of injury helps to explain the increased incidence of this type of injury in children. Because of the increased flexibility of the child's body, more severe degrees of hyperextension are possible in children than in adults. More severe hyperextension results in greater tension and avulsive forces on the ureter.

Diagnosing ureteral avulsion is relatively straightforward when it is an isolated injury. However, other serious injuries often obscure the findings caused by avulsion. For instance, severe renal damage may lead to underexcretion of contrast material and urinoma formation. These abnormalities can delay the diagnosis of ureteral avulsion. The classic radiographic tetrad associated with ureteral avulsion includes normal renal excretion of contrast material, normal-appearing calyces, contrast material extravasation at the UPJ or in another area of avulsion, and nonvisualization of the affected ureter below the level of extravasation (Fig. 5-58). Ureteral avulsion can be diagnosed definitively with selective retrograde pyelography when contrast material extravasation occurs and discontinuity of the ureter is evident. Ureteral avulsion may be incomplete, and in these patients, the ureter may heal if it is stented in a timely fashion. In conjunction with stenting, percutaneous urinoma drainage will en-

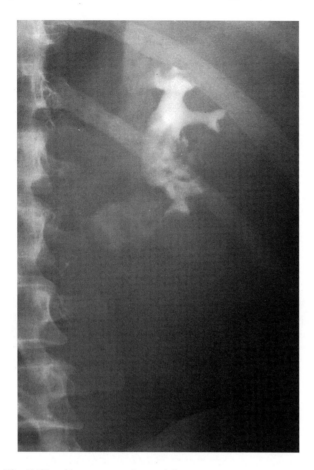

Fig. 5-58 Traumatic avulsion of the ureter. An intravenous urogram in this victim of a motor vehicle accident demonstrates findings typical of ureteropelvic junction (UPJ) avulsion. There is normal contrast excretion from the kidney; the calyces are opacified normally; there is contrast material extravasation at the UPJ; and there is nonvisualization of the ureter below the UPJ. Avulsion was confirmed and repaired surgically in this patient.

courage rapid healing and lessen the risk of ureteral cicatrization. Surgical repair generally is required for complete ureteral avulsion. One additional clinical point about ureteral avulsion is the fact that hematuria may be absent in up to 30% of patients with this type of injury.

SUGGESTED READINGS

Amis ES Jr, Cronan JJ: The renal sinus: an imaging review and proposed nomenclature for sinus cysts, *J Urol* 139:1151-1159, 1988.

Banner MP: Genitourinary complications of inflammatory bowel disease, *Radiol Clin North Am* 25:199-209, 1987.

Bard JL, Klein FA: Ureteropelvic junction avulsion following blunt abdominal trauma, *J Tenn Med Assoc* 83:242-243, 1990.

Bergman H, Friedenberg RM, Sayegh V: New roentgenologic signs of carcinoma of the ureter, *AJR Am J Roentgenol* 86:707-717, 1961.

Birnbaum BA, Friedman JP, Lubat E, et al: Extrarenal genitourinary tuberculosis: CT appearance of calcified pipe-stem ureter and seminal vesicle abscess, *J Comput Assist Tomogr* 14:653-655, 1990.

Bush WH Jr: Radiologic aspects of urolithiasis, *Radiologist* 1:31-43, 1994.

Clark WR, Malek RS: Ureteropelvic junction obstruction. I. Observations on the classic type in adults, *J Urol* 138:276-279, 1987.

Cohen SJ: Ureterocoeles, *Postgrad Med J* 66(suppl 1):S47-S53, 1990.

Cory DA, Tarver RD, Baker MK, et al: Subepithelial pyeloureteric lesions in patients with nephrostomy tubes, *Br J Radiol* 60:449-453, 1987.

Cronan JJ, Amis ES, Zeman RK, et al: Obstruction of the upper-pole moiety in renal duplication in adults: CT evaluation, *Radiology* 161:17-21, 1986.

Cunat JS, Goldman SM: Extrinsic displacement of the ureter, *Semin Roentgenol* 3:188-200, 1986.

Das Narla L, Neal MP Jr, Bulas RV: Prune-belly syndrome, *Applied Radiology* 23:42, 45-46, 1994.

Davidson AJ, Hartman DS: *Radiology of the kidney and urinary tract*, ed 2, Philadelphia, 1994, WB Saunders.

Dean TE, Harrison NW, Bishop NL: CT scanning in the diagnosis and management of radiolucent urinary calculi, *Br J Urol* 62:405-408, 1988.

Dyer RB, Zagoria RJ: Radiological patterns of mineralization as predictor of urinary stone etiology, associated pathology, and therapeutic outcome, *Journal of Stone Disease* 4:272-282, 1992.

Federle MP, McAninch JW, Kaiser JA, et al: Computed tomography of urinary calculi, *AJR Am J Roentgenol* 136:255-258, 1981.

Fein AB, McClennan BL: Solitary filling defects of the ureter, *Semin Roentgenol* 21:201-213, 1986.

Gehr TWB, Sica DA: Case report and review of the literature: ureteral endometriosis, *Am J Med Sci* 294;346-352, 1987.

Hellström M, Jodal U, Mårild S, et al: Ureteral dilatation in children with febrile urinary tract infection or bacteriuria, *AJR Am J Roentgenol* 148:483-486, 1987.

Heyns CF: Pelvic lipomatosis: a review of its diagnosis and management, *J Urol* 146:267-273, 1991.

Honda H, McGuire CW, Barloon TJ, et al: Replacement lipomatosis of the kidney: CT features, *J Comput Assist Tomogr* 14:229-231, 1990.

In der Maur GAP, Puylaert JBCM: Peripelvic renal cysts, hydronephrosis and sinus lipomatosis, *Journal of Medical Imaging* 3:22-26, 1989.

Jorulf H, Lindstedt E: Urogenital schistosomiasis: CT evaluation, *Radiology* 157:745-749, 1985.

Lautin EM, Haramati N, Frager D, et al: CT diagnosis of circumcaval ureter, *AJR Am J Roentgenol* 150:591-594, 1988.

Lucero SP, Wise HA, Kirsh G, et al: Ureteric obstruction secondary to endometriosis: report of three cases with a review of the literature, *Br J Urol* 61:201–204, 1988.

Mindell HJ, Pollack HM: Fungal disease of the ureter, *Radiology* 146:46, 1983.

Narumi Y, Sato T, Hori S, et al: Squamous cell carcinoma of the uroepithelium: CT evaluation, *Radiology* 173:853–856, 1989.

Pedersen-Bjergaard J, Ersbøll J, Hansen VL, et al: Carcinoma of the urinary bladder after treatment with cyclophosphamide for non-Hodgkin's lymphoma, *N Engl J Med* 318:1028–1032, 1988.

Perez LM, Thrasher JB, Weinerth JL, et al: Intermittent ureteropelvic junction obstruction in the adult, *N C Med J* 55:592–595, 1994.

Pfister RC, Papanicolaou N, Yoder IC: The dilated ureter, *Semin Roentgenol* 21:224–235, 1986.

Sarajlif M, Durst-Zivkovif B, Svoren E, et al: Congenital ureteric diverticula in children and adults: classification, radiological and clinical features, *Br J Radiol* 62:551–553, 1989.

Schwartz G, Lipschitz S, Becker JA: Detection of renal calculi: the value of tomography, *AJR Am J Roentgenol* 143:143–145, 1984.

Williamson B Jr, Hartman GW, Hattery RR: Multiple and diffuse ureteral filling defects, *Semin Roentgenol* 21:214–223, 1986.

Winalski CS, Lipman JC, Tumeh SS: Ureteral neoplasms, *Radiographics* 10:271–283, 1990.

Yoder IC, Pfister RC: Periureteral diseases. In Taveras JM, Ferrucci JT, editors: *Radiology: diagnosis, imaging, intervention*, vol 4, Philadelphia, 1986, JB Lippincott.

Yoder IC, Pfister RC, Lindfors KK, et al: Pyonephrosis: imaging and intervention, *AJR Am J Roentgenol* 141:735–740, 1983.

Yousem DM, Gatewood OMB, Goldman SM, et al: Synchronous and metachronous transitional cell carcinoma of the urinary tract: prevalence, incidence, and radiographic detection, *Radiology* 167:613–618, 1988.

Zagoria RJ, Dyer RB, McCullough DL: Angiomyolipoma arising in the renal sinus: a difficult radiologic diagnosis, *Urologic Radiology* 11:139–141, 1989.

The Lower Urinary Tract

The lower urinary tract consists of the bladder and the urethra. Diseases of the lower urinary tract are prevalent and can be potentially debilitating from a medical and a social point of view. The bladder is the most common site of urinary tract infection in women of childbearing age. Symptoms referable to bladder outlet obstruction are among the most common reasons why elderly men are examined by internists and urologists. Traumatic injury to the lower urinary tract or management of such an injury may lead to incontinence or impotence or both. Urinary incontinence may lead not only to skin breakdown and soft-tissue infection but also to social isolation. This chapter presents a practical review of the imaging of common vesical and urethral disease. The chapter is divided into three sections. The first section reviews normal embryology, anatomy, and physiology of the lower urinary tract and briefly reviews urodynamic tests and radiologic protocols used in imaging the bladder and urethra. The second and third sections discuss the pathologic conditions that can affect the bladder and urethra, respectively. To the extent possible, we present this discussion in a radiographic pattern-oriented approach (Boxes 6-1, 6-2). The diseases of the lower urinary tract are presented in a manner that reflects the way practicing radiologists confront disease: as one or more radiographic signs.

LOWER URINARY TRACT: EMBRYOLOGY, ANATOMY, AND PHYSIOLOGY

Embryology of the Bladder and Urethra

During weeks 4 to 7 of gestation, the cloaca is divided into an anterior urogenital sinus and a posterior anorectal canal by the urorectal septum, which grows toward and fuses with the cloacal membrane. At this stage, the urogenital sinus can be divided into the bladder proper, a urethral part, and a phallic part. The bladder is continuous with the allantois through the urachus, which is the tapered, cephalad portion of the urogenital sinus. When the lumen of the urachus is obliterated, a fibrous cord,

or the medial umbilical ligament, connects bladder to umbilicus. The urethral part of the urogenital sinus gives rise to most of the female urethra and to the prostatic and membranous portion of the male urethra. The prostate gland and the female urethral and paraurethral glands develop as evaginations from the urethral part of the urogenital sinus. The phallic part of the urogenital sinus eventually forms the penile urethra in the male subject and a small portion of the urethra and vestibule in the female subject.

The mesonephric ducts and ureteric buds develop separate connections with the urogenital sinus through progressive resorption of the caudal segment of the mesonephric duct. During this process, the openings of these two ductal systems switch craniocaudally so that the ureters enter more cranially than the mesonephric ducts do. The mucosa of the bladder formed by incorporation of these ducts becomes the trigone.

Anatomy of the Bladder

The surface anatomy of the urinary bladder consists of an apex, a superior surface, two inferolateral surfaces, a base or posterior surface, and a neck. The apex of the bladder ends as the medial umbilical ligament. The superior surface of the bladder is the only surface that is covered by peritoneum. The base of the bladder contains the trigone, and the bladder neck is pierced by the internal urethral orifice.

The constituents of the bladder wall from lumen outward are the transitional epithelium or urothelium, the submucosa, the muscular layer, and the serosa. The normal urothelium rarely is more than seven to eight cell layers thick and has the capacity to change shape and alignment to accommodate extremes of bladder volume. The bladder wall often is described as having three muscular coats, but this description is true only around the bladder neck. As a functional unit, the muscular layers of the bladder wall are referred to as the detrusor muscle. The serosal layer is limited to the superior surface of the bladder and is separated from the peritoneal reflection by perivesical fat. The trigone of the bladder, located immediately above and behind the internal urethral orifice, is the functional and anatomic bridge between the ureters and the urethra. It consists of deep and superficial smooth muscle layers. The superficial smooth muscle layer is continuous with the intravesical portion of the distal ureters and with the smooth muscle in the proximal urethra. The deep trigonal smooth muscle melds with the detrusor. The trigone consists of three angles: two posterolateral angles formed by the ureteric orifices and an anteroinferior angle formed by the internal urethral orifice.

The arterial supply of the bladder derives from the superior, middle, and inferior vesical arteries. These arter-

Box 6-3 Normal Male Urethra

Posterior
  Prostatic
    Verumontanum
  Membranous
    External urethral sphincter
    Cowper's gland
Anterior
  Bulbar
    Cowper's duct
  Penile
    Glands of Littré

ies are branches of the anterior division of the internal iliac (hypogastric) artery. The richly vascularized bladder also receives small arteries from the obturator, inferior gluteal, uterine, and vaginal arteries. In the space between the bladder and the adventitia lies a plexus of veins that ultimately join and terminate as the internal iliac vein. This perivesical venous plexus anastomoses with the plexus of Santorini, which drains the penis, prostate, and other perineal organs. Interstitial vesical lymphatics drain into the external iliac, internal iliac, and common iliac lymph node chains.

Anatomy of the Male Urethra

The male urethra is about 20 cm in length and can be discussed in terms of its posterior and anterior parts (Box 6-3; Figs. 6-1, 6-2). The posterior urethra extends from the bladder neck to the urogenital diaphragm and is sub-

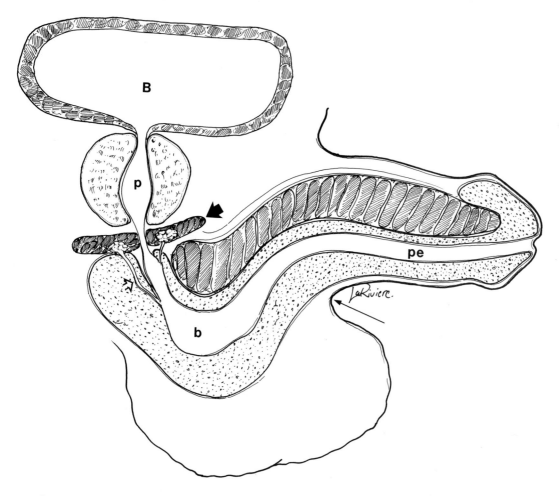

Fig. 6-1 Normal male urethra. The posterior male urethra extends from the bladder (B) to the urogenital diaphragm (black arrow) and consists of the prostatic urethra (p) and the membranous urethra. The anterior urethra extends from the urogenital diaphragm to the external meatus. Cowper's glands are embedded in the urogenital diaphragm, and Cowper's ducts (open arrow) empty into the proximal bulbous urethra (b), the widest part of the anterior urethra. At and distal to the level of the penoscrotal junction (long arrow) is the penile or pendulous urethra (pe).

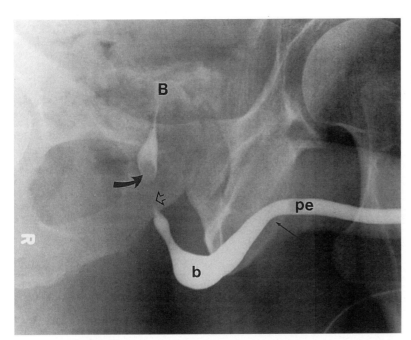

Fig. 6-2 Dynamic retrograde urethrogram of the normal male urethra. The verumontanum appears as a normal filling defect (curved arrow) in the prostatic urethra. The membranous urethra (open arrow) is narrow and marks the site of the external urethral sphincter. The anterior urethra consists of the bulbous (b) and penile (pe) urethra. B = urinary bladder; long arrow = penoscrotal angle.

divided into the prostatic and membranous parts. The prostatic urethra is approximately 3 cm long and traverses the transitional zone of the prostate gland. The verumontanum, or colliculus seminalis, is a mound of tissue that interrupts the otherwise flat posterior wall of the prostatic urethra. The glands of the prostate empty into the prostatic urethra through small lacunae on either side of the verumontanum. At the distal end of the verumontanum is the remnant of the müllerian duct system, the prostatic utricle. Aside the utricle are the paired openings of the ejaculatory ducts. The membranous urethra is the shortest, least distensible, and narrowest part of the male urethra. The muscular wall of the membranous urethra consists of a thin layer of nonstriated muscle and a more prominent outer layer of circularly oriented striated muscle, the external urethral sphincter.

The male anterior urethra extends through the corpus spongiosum from the urogenital diaphragm to the external meatus. The proximal part of the anterior urethra is widest and is referred to as the bulb of the urethra. This bulbar portion of the penile urethra is surrounded by the bulb of the penis and bulbous spongiosus muscle. The accessory sex glands of Cowper are a pair of structures located one on each side of the membranous urethra between the two fascial layers of the urogenital diaphragm. The paired ducts of these glands are about 2 to 3 cm in length and extend forward and slightly medially to enter the proximal bulbous urethra. Cowper's glands are ontogenically homologous to Bartholin's glands in female subjects. During ejaculation, they discharge a clear fluid that acts as a lubricant and that contributes to semen coagulation. At the level of the penoscrotal

junction and distal to it, the anterior urethra is referred to as the penile or pendulous urethra. A focal widening of the penile urethra, the fossa navicularis, normally is found just proximal to the meatus. The mucosa of the penile urethra is pierced by numerous recesses that branch into tubular mucous glands of Littré.

The epithelial lining of most of the prostatic urethra is composed of transitional cells, but it changes from urothelium to stratified columnar epithelium just distal to the opening of the ejaculatory ducts. Stratified columnar epithelium lines the membranous urethra, the bulbar urethra, and the majority of the penile urethra. The epithelium of the fossa navicularis is stratified squamous epithelium and is keratinized at the external meatus.

Anatomy of the Female Urethra

The female urethra is approximately 4 cm in length and extends from the bladder outlet to the perineum adjacent to the anterior wall of the vagina. The female urethra is widest at the bladder neck, and the most distal urethra near the meatus is its narrowest and least distensible part. This natural narrowing creates the "spinning top" configuration of the urethra, a normal finding on micturition urethrography (Fig. 6-3). Small mucous urethral glands (Skene's glands) open along the entire length of the urethra. Groups of these glands drain into one duct, the paraurethral duct, which empties at the lateral margin of the external urethral meatus.

The epithelial lining of the proximal third of the female urethra is urothelium, but that of the distal two thirds is

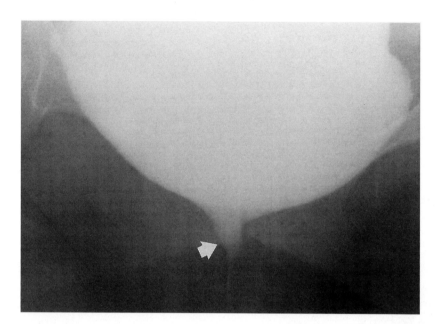

Fig. 6-3   Normal female urethra on voiding cystourethrogram. The normal female urethra (arrow) gradually narrows from the bladder neck to the external orifice.

stratified squamous epithelium. Stratified columnar epithelium lines the periurethral glands of Skene.

Anatomy of the Urethral Sphincters

The urethral sphincters are specialized configurations of muscle that act in synergy with the detrusor muscle to ensure smooth, voluntary expulsion of urine. The inner longitudinal and outer semicircular smooth muscles of the bladder neck surround the entire length of the female urethra and the male posterior urethra. This long muscular sleeve serves as the sphincteric mechanism known as the internal urethral sphincter (smooth sphincter or bladder neck sphincter). The external urethral sphincter is composed of striated muscle and is located at the midurethra in female subjects and at the membranous urethra in male subjects.

Physiology of the Lower Urinary Tract

The lower urinary tract has two main functions: the storage of urine (bladder filling or accommodation) and the volitional expulsion of urine (micturition). The neural modulation of accommodation and micturition is complex, integrating the central and the peripheral nervous systems and the autonomic and somatic nerves.

Accommodation

Somatic and alpha adrenergic efferent neural activity effect contraction of the external and internal urethral sphincters, respectively, thereby increasing intraurethral pressure. Continent intraurethral pressure also is maintained by intraabdominal pressure and adequate thickness and coaptation of the urethral mucosa. Active closure of the bladder outlet occurs with simultaneous inhibition of parasympathetic neural discharge to the bladder body and base, relaxing the detrusor to facilitate bladder accommodation.

Micturition

The first step in micturition involves the inhibition of pudendal nerve efferent activity to the external urethral sphincter and inhibition of sympathetic input to the smooth sphincter. Bladder outlet resistance decreases, which initiates the coordinated contraction of the detrusor by efferent parasympathetic pelvic nerve activity. Expulsion of urine then is driven by the pressure gradient between detrusor and bladder outlet.

DIAGNOSTIC EXAMINATIONS

There are two types of diagnostic examinations that are used to investigate disease of the lower urinary tract: those that primarily evaluate structure and those that evaluate function. Although this division is arbitrary for some examinations, such as the ureteral perfusion test of Whitaker, the majority of diagnostic tests can be categorized accordingly. Imaging studies such as urography, cystography, retrograde pyelography, dynamic retrograde urethrography, sonography, computed tomography (CT), and magnetic resonance (MR) imaging directly evaluate the anatomy of the lower urinary tract. The indications for and methodology of these examinations are discussed in Chapter 1. Many of the medical imaging tests assess only pathophysiology of the lower urinary tract and do so in a nonspecific manner. For instance, the cystographic phase of the intravenous urogram (IVU) frequently is used to assess detrusor function, but its shortcomings in this regard are notable. Evaluation of bladder function through estimates of the postvoiding residual volume is crude and may be misleading. Methodologically, an estimation of the volume of a spherical structure based on a single view clearly is flawed, particularly given the marked variations in bladder configuration. Estimates of prevoiding and postvoiding urinary bladder volume with ultrasonography are more appropriate. The absence of a "significant" postvoiding residual on urography does not necessarily exclude significant bladder outlet obstruction because hypertrophy of the detrusor may be sufficient to compensate for the increased outflow resistance. Furthermore, the presence of a postvoid residual does not always indicate an inability to empty the bladder. The longer the delay between voiding and the postvoiding film, the greater the likelihood that the bladder will be filled by opacified urine from the upper tract.

One method of directly evaluating bladder and lower urinary tract sphincter function is urodynamic testing. Urodynamic tests are a group of clinical examinations designed to measure and record physiologic parameters during bladder accommodation and emptying. The purpose of urodynamic testing is to determine and assess these parameters when the patient is experiencing symptoms of lower urinary tract dysfunction (e.g., urgency, incontinence, slow stream). Cystometry is the measurement of intravesical pressure as it relates to bladder volume during the filling or storage phase. It can be used to assess bladder capacity, compliance, and sensation and the presence of involuntary bladder contractions. Uroflowmetry measures the rate of urine flow during micturition as a function of time. A poor flow rate may result from either a weak bladder contraction or bladder outlet obstruction. Pressure-flow studies combine uroflowmetry and cystometry. A diminished rate of urinary flow in a patient with adequate detrusor pressure suggests that elevated bladder outflow resistance is the cause for poor urine flow. If diminished flow rates result from detrusor inadequacy, contractions of the detrusor may be weak or poorly sustained. A urethral pressure profile is obtained by slowly withdrawing a transducer through the urethra during micturition urethrography. In healthy subjects, the recorded pressure within the bladder and proximal urethra are the same during micturition, but there is a drop in pressure at the level of the membranous urethra. The myoneural integrity of the striated urethral sphincter can be tested by positioning a concentric electrode in the periurethral striated sphincter to record the sphincter electromyogram. During normal micturition, electrical activity in the striated sphincter completely disappears approximately 1 second before the onset of voluntary detrusor contraction. Dyssynergia can be as-

sessed by simultaneously measuring bladder pressure and striated sphincter electromyographic activity.

Box 6-4 Focal Filling Defect of the Bladder Wall

Common
  Neoplasm (malignant)
  Stone ± mural edema
  Blood clot
  Enlarged prostate gland
Uncommon
  Focal cystitis*
  Ureterocele
  Neoplasm (benign)
  Endometriosis
  Fungus ball

*"Herald" lesion, bullous cystitis, cystitis cystica and glandularis, and malacoplakia

FOCAL MURAL FILLING DEFECT

Malignant Neoplasms of the Bladder

When radiographic evidence of a focal filling defect of the bladder wall is discovered (Box 6-4), the work-up is directed to exclude neoplasms (Table 6-1; Box 6-5). Malignant neoplasms of the bladder account for 4% of all malignancies. The incidence of bladder cancer peaks in those aged 50 to 69 years, and the disease occurs more often in men than in women (3:1 ratio). Malignant neoplasms of the bladder can be grouped broadly into two categories: the carcinomas or epithelial neoplasms and the mesenchymal or nonepithelial neoplasms. Approximately 95% of all malignant bladder cancers are carcinomas. Epithelial cancers of the bladder can be characterized by pattern of growth, by malignant cell type, and by the degree of cellular differentiation (i.e., tumor grade). Bladder tumors can be either papillary, sessile, or invasive in growth pattern. As a general rule, papillary tumors are less likely than invasive or sessile neoplasms to metastasize, although papillary tumors have the trou-

Table 6-1 Bladder Tumors

Type	Common	Uncommon
Malignant	Transitional cell carcinoma Squamous cell carcinoma	Adenocarcinoma
Benign	Leiomyoma Fibroepithelial polyp	Hemangioma Pheochromocytoma Adenoma

Box 6-5 Carcinoma of the Bladder

Most common cancer in the urinary tract
90% transitional cell carcinoma
75% superficial papillary lesions; 25% invasive
Upper tract metachronous tumors in 2%–3%
Superficial cancers recur, and 15% progress to invasive
Etiologies: chemical carcinogens (acrolein, aromatic
    amines, nitrosamines) and cigarette smoking

blesome tendencies to be multifocal and to recur after initial management. Epithelial bladder malignancies also are classified by cell type: urothelial (transitional cell), squamous, or glandular (adenocarcinoma). About 90% of all malignant tumors of the bladder originate from the transitional cell urothelium; 5% are squamous cell tumors, and 2% are adenocarcinomas. Nonepithelial neoplasms make up less than 5% of malignant bladder neoplasms. The most common of these tumors is leiomyosarcoma, followed by lymphoma. Rhabdomyosarcoma of the bladder is more common in children aged 2 to 6 years. Malignant tumors originating from neighboring or distant organs also can involve the bladder wall secondarily. Carcinoma of the prostate may infiltrate along the posterior urethra or bladder neck or through the trigone. Cancer of the cervix or uterus involves the posterior wall of the bladder in the midline, whereas invasion from a malignancy of the sigmoid colon or rectum usually involves the left lateral bladder wall. Cancers of the stomach or breast are the most common distant malignancies to metastasize to the bladder.

Several risk factors have been implicated in the development of bladder cancer. Exposure to industrial carcinogens, cigarette smoking, and abuse of analgesics are associated with an increased risk of transitional cell tumors of the urinary tract. Pelvic irradiation for gynecologic malignancies also may be associated with a higher risk of bladder cancer. An association also exists between schistosomiasis of the urinary tract and squamous cell cancer of the bladder; approximately 50% of the malignant tumors associated with schistosomiasis are of this cell type. Chronic irritation and infection of the bladder caused by neurogenic bladder, long-term catheter drainage, or recurrent cystitis also result in an increased incidence of squamous metaplasia and cancer. Urothelial atypia or dysplasia is considered to be a premalignant condition, and some types of metaplastic and proliferative cystitis (cystitis glandularis) are considered precursors of cancer. Adenocarcinoma of the bladder occurs with greater frequency in urachal remnants and bladder exstrophy.

Tumor stage, as ascertained before management, is the most important prognostic factor. The depth of invasion through the bladder wall is an excellent predictor of recurrence, metastatic disease, and survival. Of the several staging algorithms proposed, the Jewett-Strong-Marshall and TNM classifications are most widely used (Table 6-2). Carcinoma in situ (CIS) is neoplastic transformation of the epithelium without extension into the bladder lumen or through the basal membrane into the lamina propria. Superficial transitional cell carcinoma (TCC) is a papillary neoplasm confined to the mucosa or extending into the lamina propria but without invasion of the muscular layer. Approximately 50% of patients with superficial papillary and 90% with CIS have recurrences within 2 years after initial treatment. However, recurrences usually can be controlled with transurethral bladder resection, and muscle-invasive tumors develop in only 10% to 15% of patients. Patients with muscle-invasive tumors have a poor prognosis. Most of the tumors already have infiltrated the bladder muscularis at initial presentation. Once the muscularis has been invaded, lymphatic and distant spread often follows. Five-year survival rates reflect the importance of depth of invasion: for superficial muscle-invasive tumors, 30% to 80% of patients survive 5 years, whereas for deep muscle-invasive tumors, the 5-year survival rate is 10% to 20%. Distant metastases to the lungs and mediastinum, liver, and bone are as common as local recurrence in treatment failures among patients with muscle-invasive tumors.

Like prognosis, management of urinary bladder carcinoma is determined by depth of neoplastic invasion of the

Table 6-2 Carcinoma of the Urinary Bladder: The Jewett-Strong-Marshall and TNM Staging Systems

Jewett-Strong-Marshall stage	TNM stage	Description
0	TIS	Carcinoma in situ
0	TA	Papillary tumor, noninvasive
A	T1	Papillary tumor, lamina propria invasion
B1	T2	Superficial muscle invasion
B2	T3A	Deep muscle invasion
C	T3B	Perivesical fat invasion
D1	T4A	Invasion of contiguous viscera
D1	T4B	Invasion of pelvic or abdominal wall
D2	N4	Regional lymphadenopathy
D2	M1	Distant metastases

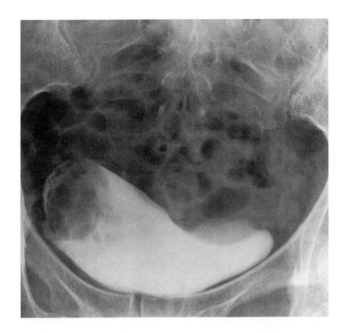

Fig. 6-4 Urogram during the cystographic phase demonstrates a large, polypoid intraluminal mass along the lateral wall of the bladder. At surgery, a papillary transitional cell carcinoma was removed; there was no evidence of deep muscle invasion.

bladder wall and by extent of local and distant metastases. Superficial bladder cancers (TA or T1) are managed with local fulguration. Muscle-invasive tumors (T2 or T3) are managed with total cystectomy, and if local or distant metastases are extensive, palliative radiation or chemotherapy is offered.

Plain abdominal radiography is of little value in the detection of bladder cancer but it may reveal focal calcification associated with a papillary bladder tumor in 0.7% to 6.7% of patients.

Intravenous urography often is performed when bladder carcinoma is suspected. Its ability to demonstrate small tumors is limited. Standard and micturition cystography and the cystographic phase of IVU are notoriously insensitive. In one study, only 60% of known bladder tumors were detected with standard urography. When bladder cancers are visible on urography, an irregular, polypoid or sessile filling defect is seen most often (Fig. 6-4). Early and postvoid films of the bladder are helpful. The bladder trigone and posterolateral bladder walls are the most frequent sites of origin of TCCs; carcinoma originates in 2% of bladder diverticula. Mural infiltration leads to bladder wall thickening and poor distensibility. The presence of ureterovesical junction obstruction and hydroureter usually implies muscle invasion by the neoplasm (Fig. 6-5). Detection of multifocal disease of the upper urinary tract and hydronephrosis secondary to obstruction of a ureteral orifice is an additional reason for obtaining a urogram (Fig. 6-6). Synchronous and metachronous upper tract tumors are discovered with approximately 2% and 7% of primary bladder carcinomas, respectively. Patients with synchronous or metachronous upper tract disease have a higher prevalence of multifocal and recurrent vesical cancer.

Transabdominal, transrectal, and intravesical sonography have been used to evaluate lesions of the bladder wall and lumen. Meticulous technique and adequate bladder distention are essential for optimal transabdominal sonography. The location and size of the tumor have the greatest impact on detection with sonography. Tumors larger than 1 cm and distant from the bladder neck area are easier to image and have a relatively higher rate of detection, approaching 85% (Fig. 6-9A on p. 203). Infiltrating tumors also are more likely than superficial ones to be detected. Tumors larger than 3 cm in diameter or those with associated calcification more often are overstaged. Sonography is limited in its ability to depict extension of disease beyond the bladder wall and usually cannot detect nodal metastases. Wall edema, prominent mural folds, inflammation, muscular hypertrophy, blood clots, and postoperative changes can further reduce the specificity of ultrasound examination for the detection and staging of bladder malignancies (Fig. 6-7 on p. 202).

Computed tomography and MR imaging currently are the imaging modalities of choice for the staging of bladder neoplasms. CT is an excellent method for assessing neoplastic invasion of the pelvic viscera and side wall. Lymphadenopathy and distant metastases also can be demonstrated well. Identification of the primary lesion is more difficult in the areas of the bladder neck and dome. Limitations exist in that with CT, inflammatory, postoperative, or postradiation edema or fibrosis cannot be distinguished from tumor. In addition, accurate assessment of the depth of invasion of the bladder by tumor is not possible with CT (Fig. 6-8 on p. 202). Most published reports suggest that accurate staging of tumors confined to the vesical wall is not feasible (stages A to B2 or TIS to T3A). Although microscopic invasion of the perivesical fat is impossible to detect, in many institutions, microscopic perivesical fat disease with no other involvement is managed with radical cystectomy and lymph node dissection, as if it were stage B2 disease. An overlap between stages B and C, therefore, seems to be unavoidable. Stage B sometimes is overstaged, and stage C sometimes is understaged. In general, the accuracy of CT for bladder cancer staging ranges between 40% and 90%, with a mean accuracy of 75%.

The accuracy of CT for detecting nodal metastases varies from 50% to 90%. The only morphometric criterion that is used to define tumor infiltration of lymph nodes is size. Size thresholds above which tumor involvement is suggested are a maximal length of 13 mm and a maximal

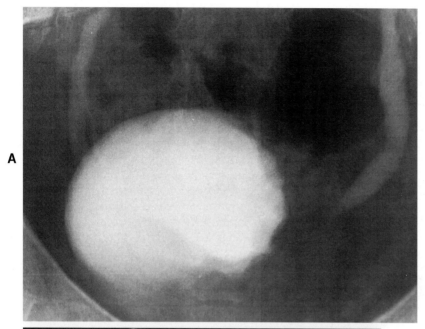

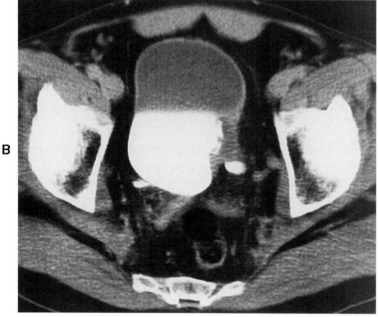

Fig. 6-5   Infiltrative bladder cancer on urogram and computed tomography (CT). **A,** A broad, sessile filling defect with a lobulated margin is seen along the lateral wall of the bladder on this urogram. There is asymmetric dilatation of the left ureter. **B,** CT demonstrates that the bladder cancer originates at the left ureterovesical junction and is of slightly lower density than the normal bladder wall. Obstruction of the ureter at the ureterovesical junction implies muscle invasion by the tumor. (Case courtesy of Mark S. Ridlen, MD)

short axis diameter of 10 mm. Enlargement of a node, however, is not tantamount to metastasis, and, conversely, normal-sized nodes may harbor disease. Radiographic detection of disease in nodes of normal size requires lymphangiography. Because of its invasive nature and the false-positive and false-negative rates of 10% to 30%, lymphangiography may be performed if CT results are normal or equivocal for nodal disease. Percutaneous fine-needle biopsy of enlarged or borderline nodes may be necessary for more accurate nodal staging.

Magnetic resonance imaging is expected to circumvent several of the limitations associated with CT. The use of an endorectal surface coil has improved MR imaging of the prostate and seminal vesicles and provides excellent images of the bladder base and neck. Although the intravenous administration of gadolinium-pentetic acid (DTPA) is emerging as a useful complement to MR imaging of the bladder, unenhanced T_2-weighted images often display the bladder wall with clarity, resulting from contrast between the urine-filled lumen and the soft tissues of the bladder wall. In addition, the striking contrast between the bright perivesical fat and the intermediate signal intensity bladder wall permits evaluation of the bladder contour on T_1-weighted images. On T_1-weighted

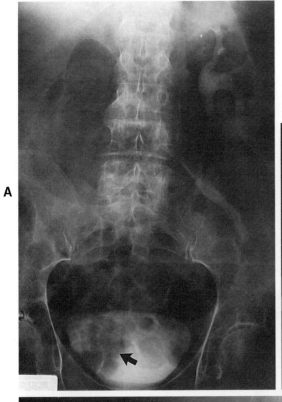

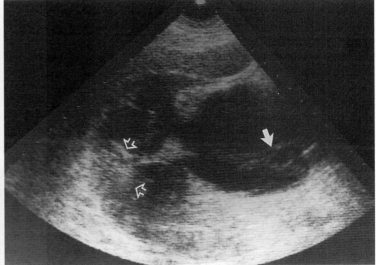

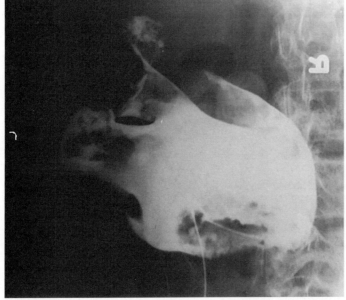

Fig. 6-6   Synchronous transitional cell carcinoma (TCC) of the upper and lower urinary tract. **A,** The anteroposterior film from a urogram shows a large, lobulated filling defect in the bladder (arrow). There was no opacification of either the right kidney or ureter during this examination. **B,** Transverse sonogram of the right kidney demonstrates echogenic masses in the markedly dilated renal pelvis (solid arrow) and in multiple dilated calyces (open arrows). **C,** Antegrade pyelography shows multiple irrregular filling defects in the dilated renal collecting system. There was completed obstruction of the kidney at the ureteropelvic junction. Multifocal TCC was diagnosed at nephroureterectomy.

images, most bladder neoplasms are of equal or slightly higher signal intensity than the bladder wall and of lower intensity than the perivesical fat (Fig. 6-9B). Lesions smaller than about 8 mm may not be demonstrated with MR imaging. On T_2-weighted images, the same neoplasms are of higher signal intensity than the normal bladder wall, and therefore they are easier to distinguish from it (Fig. 6-9C). Deep muscle invasion is seen as focal or more extensive disruption of the low signal intensity of the bladder wall by tumor on T_2-weighted images. Deeper invasion into the perivesical fat appears as focal or extensive infiltration of the high-signal intensity fat (Fig. 6-10 on p. 204). Likewise, invasion of adjacent organs by tumor can be assessed by demonstrating extension of the process from the bladder wall to the pelvic structures (stage T4A). Like CT, MR imaging currently relies on

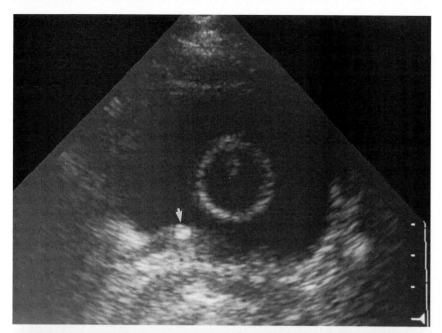

Fig. 6-7 Ureterovesical junction secondary to calculus. In an adult with painless hematuria, an ill-defined filling defect and mild dilatation of the right ureter were noted on intravenous urography (not shown). Transverse sonogram of the bladder demonstrates mural edema that mimics a focal bladder mass around a small calculus (arrow) at the ureterovesical junction. A Foley catheter is in the bladder.

Fig. 6-8 Staging of bladder wall invasion with CT. **A,** A pedunculated mass originates from the focally thickened inferolateral wall of the bladder. There is increased attenuation of the perivesical fat (arrow) adjacent to this mass. At total cystectomy, tumor invasion of the perivesical fat was seen (stage C disease). **B,** There is a broad-based, sessile mass originating from the inferolateral wall of the bladder. Increased density is seen in the perivesical fat (open arrow) lateral and posterior to the bladder mass. At surgery, deep muscle invasion was found, but there was no infiltration of tumor into the perivesical fat (stage B2 disease).

A

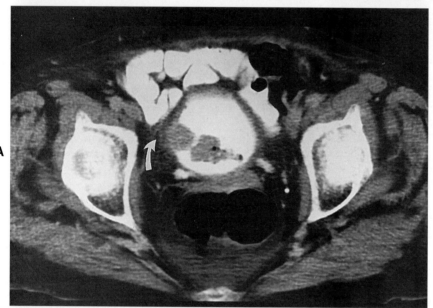

B

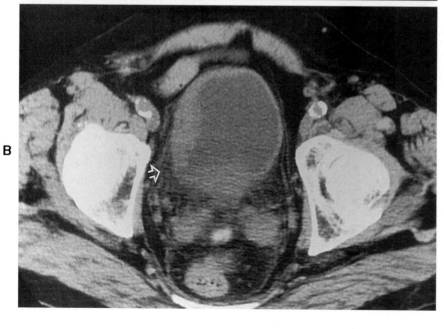

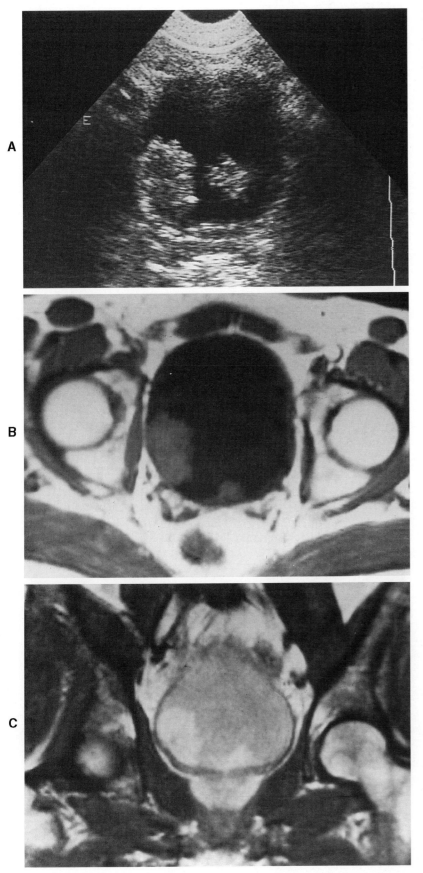

Fig. 6-9   Sonography and magnetic resonance (MR) imaging of multifocal, papillary bladder cancer. **A,** Transverse sonogram of the bladder demonstrates two papillary, endophytic masses. The right inferolateral wall of the bladder appears intact. **B,** On a transaxial spin–echo T_1-weighted image (repetition time = 400 msec; echo time = 15 msec), both masses are hyperintense compared with the bladder wall and hypointense relative to perivesical fat. **C,** On a coronal proton density-weighted image (repetition time = 2000 msec; echo time = 40 msec), the tumors are hyperintense compared with the bladder wall. This case illustrates the typical appearance of bladder cancer on MR imaging. (Case courtesy of Jeffrey M. Brody, MD)

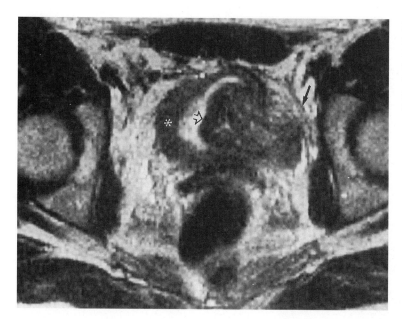

Fig. 6-10 MR imaging of perivesical fat infiltration by transitional cell carcinoma. There is diffuse thickening of the bladder wall (*) on this transverse T$_2$-weighted image. A large mass (open arrow), which is slightly hyperintense compared with the bladder wall, invades the perivesical fat extensively (arrow) and has grown to the sidewall of the left hemipelvis.

nodal size for diagnosis of metastatic disease. Several published series comparing CT with MR imaging for the staging of bladder neoplasms indicate more accurate staging with MR imaging, which is superior for the detection of invasion of adjacent organs, but MR imaging and CT are equally accurate for evaluating perivesical fat infiltration. Particularly for tumors of the bladder dome or base, MR imaging is superior. MR imaging and CT are comparable in staging metastases to regional lymph nodes.

Bladder neoplasms have been imaged before and after relaxivity enhancement. After the intravenous administration of gadopentetate dimeglumine, early and relatively greater enhancement of mucosa, submucosa, and neoplasm is demonstrated when compared with the muscle layer of the bladder wall (Fig. 6-11). Hence, one of the advantages of contrast-enhanced MR imaging is the improved detection of small tumors (7 mm). Areas of necrosis also are differentiated easily from viable tumor tissue after the paramagnetic contrast medium is given.

Benign Neoplasms of the Bladder

Transitional cell papilloma is a rare urothelial neoplasm that can be difficult to distinguish from low-grade papillary carcinomas. These tumors most often originate singly and are 0.5 to 2 cm in diameter. Papillomas are attached superficially to the mucosa of the bladder by a fine stalk (Fig. 6-12). Resection is the management of

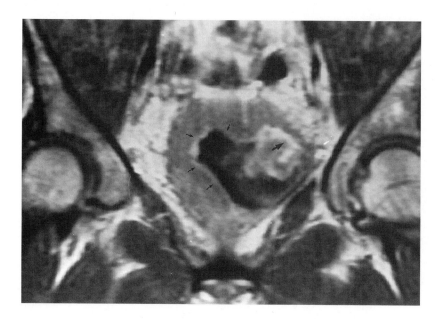

Fig. 6-11 Contrast-enhanced MR imaging of bladder carcinoma. Coronal T$_1$-weighted image of the bladder shows serpentine enhancement of a bladder cancer (arrow) where it invades the deep layer of the bladder wall. Note the linear enhancement of the bladder mucosa and submucosa (small arrows).

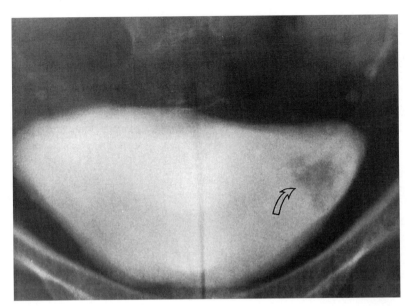

Fig. 6-12   Transitional cell papilloma. Coned-down view of the bladder demonstrates a focal filling defect with a lobulated margin (open arrow) near the left ureterovesical junction. There is nothing specific about the radiographic appearance of this rare benign neoplasm, which cannot be distinguished from papillary transitional cell carcinoma.

choice because as many as 10% of papillomas may develop ultimately into invasive carcinoma if left unmanaged. Leiomyoma is the most common benign bladder neoplasm of mesenchymal origin. This tumor presents as an isolated, well-defined intramural mass that may be up to several centimeters in size. Leiomyomas are encapsulated and are oval to spheroid. Other benign tumors of the bladder include pheochromocytoma (Fig. 6-13), hemangioma, lipoma, neurofibroma, hamartoma, and nephrogenic adenoma, all of which are rare.

DIFFUSE THICKENING OF THE BLADDER WALL

The most common causes of diffuse bladder wall thickening are bladder nondistention, pancystitis, and trabeculation (Box 6-6).

Trabeculation

Trabeculation of the bladder wall is observed most commonly in patients with bladder outlet obstruction or neurogenic bladder. Radiographically, trabeculation is generalized irregularity of the inner or luminal contour of the bladder when the bladder is filled with urine. Bladder wall thickening resulting from detrusor contraction or incomplete relaxation is normal in an underfilled bladder. Cystometry has shown a strong association between radiologic trabeculation of the bladder and detrusor instability, defined as a pressure rise of more than 15 cm water during bladder filling. In the absence of detrusor instability, outflow obstruction with high intravesical pressure produces the same effect on the detrusor and,

therefore, trabeculation. Trabeculation was once thought to result from work hypertrophy of the detrusor muscle in response to an increase in bladder outflow resistance. This opinion was based on the frequent correlation of trabeculation with bladder outlet obstruction, particularly when it resulted from benign prostatic hyperplasia. However, histologic studies of trabeculated bladders have found infiltration of detrusor smooth muscle by connective tissue elements and not muscle hypertrophy.

As previously noted, trabeculation often accompanies other radiologic evidence of bladder outlet obstruction. Benign prostatic hyperplasia is the most common cause of this obstruction, although prostate adenocarcinoma and prostatitis also may cause narrowing of the prostatic urethra. Stricture of the urethra is another cause of bladder outlet obstruction. In addition to trabeculation, several other radiologic findings may be present to suggest the diagnosis of bladder outlet obstruction at the level of the prostate gland (Fig. 6-14). These signs include 1) prostatic impression on the base of the bladder, 2) hook-

---

Box 6-6   Causes of Generalized Bladder Wall Thickening

Common
  Nondistention
  Trabeculation
  Pancystitis
Uncommon
  Hemorrhage or edema
  Infiltration by carcinoma

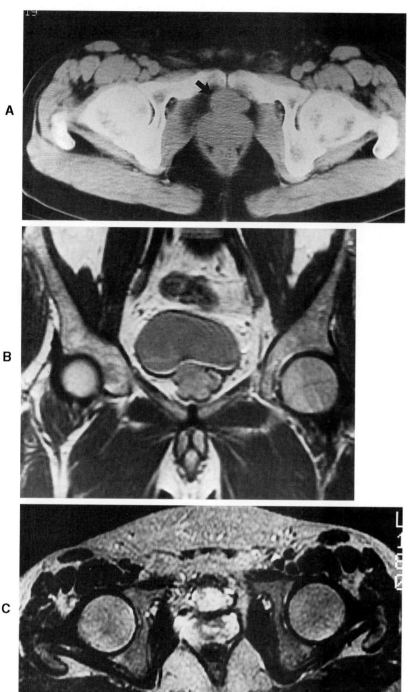

Fig. 6-13   Pheochromocytoma of the bladder. The patient complained of palpitations and dizziness during micturition. **A,** CT demonstrates a soft-tissue mass (arrow) anterior to the apex of the prostate gland. **B,** Coronal, T$_1$-weighted, spin–echo MR imaging (repetition time = 1000 msec; echo time = 20 msec) shows an exophytic, lobulated mass that originates from the base of the bladder. **C,** The mass is hyperintense compared with fat and isointense to the peripheral zone of the apex of the prostate on a transverse, T$_2$-weighted MR imaging (repetition time = 2200 msec; echo time = 80 msec).

ing or "J" configuration of the juxtavesical ureters caused by elevation of the trigone, and 3) large postvoid residual.

Cystitis

Cystitis is inflammation of part or all of the urinary bladder wall. For simplicity of discussion, we have classified cystitis according to etiology (Box 6-7). The term *cystitis* often is combined with a clinical descriptor, especially if the etiology is multifactorial or unknown (Box 6-8). For instance, viral, radiation, or cyclophosphamide cystitis may manifest as a hemorrhagic cystitis (i.e., cystitis accompanied by significant, and frequently gross, hematuria). Bullous cystitis refers to fluid-filled collections of edema fluid in the submucosa (Fig. 6-15). Polypoid cystitis is a reactive urothelial hyperplasia that protrudes

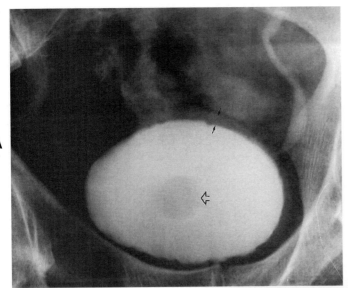

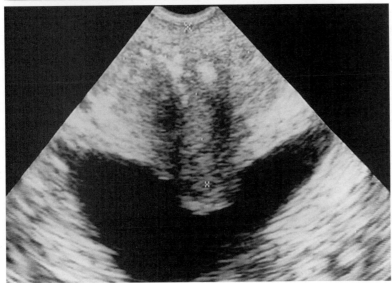

Fig. 6-14   Bladder wall trabeculation caused by benign prostatic hyperplasia. **A,** Coned-down view of the bladder from a urogram demonstrates diffuse thickening of the bladder wall (small arrows), which has a finely lobulated contour. A focal, rounded filling defect (open arrow) is seen next to a large prostatic impression along the base of the bladder. **B,** Sonography of the bladder in the transverse plane demonstrates focal enlargement of the subcervical (Albarran) lobe of the prostate as the cause of the rounded filling defect.

Box 6-7   Classification of Cystitis by Etiology

Infectious
    Bacterial (including malacoplakia)
    Viral
    Protozoal (Schistosomiasis)
    Fungal (Candida)
Noninfectious
    Irritative or mechanical (foreign body such as
        indwelling Foley catheter or bladder stone;
        perivesical inflammatory process)
    Toxic (cyclophosphamide)
    Radiation
    Allergic (interstitial; eosinophilic)

Box 6-8   Clinicopathologic Descriptors of Cystitis

Acute
Chronic
Hemorrhagic
Bullous
Emphysematous
Polypoid
Cystitis cystica
Cystitis glandularis
Squamous metaplasia
Alkaline encrustation

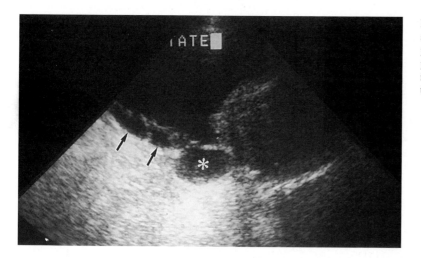

Fig. 6-15   Sagittal sonogram of the bladder demonstrates bullous cystitis. An elderly patient with benign prostatic hyperplasia presented with severe pelvic pain. Sonography showed multiple echo-poor areas in the wall of the trabeculated bladder. At cystoscopy, these were focal areas of bullous edema. * = saccule.

into the lumen of the bladder as a polyp-like growth (polypoid pseudotumor). The terms *cystitis cystica, cystitis glandularis,* and *cystitis follicularis* refer to particular histopathologic variants of chronic cystitis, which may be better characterized as forms of urothelial metaplasia. One of the more common ways of describing cystitis refers to its duration. Acute cystitis refers to bladder inflammation of recent symptomatic onset and rather short duration. Radiographically, a completely normal-appearing bladder is not uncommon, despite the presence of cystoscopic abnormalities such as ulcerations, petechiae, or erythema. Chronic cystitis implies that an inflammatory process of longer duration (many months to years) has resulted in a bladder with thickened walls and of small capacity. Bladder compliance often is decreased in patients with chronic cystitis, and elevated intravesical pressures may cause ureteral dilatation and vesicoureteral reflux. Although the inflammatory process often affects the entire bladder wall (pancystitis), occasionally cystitis is more marked or at least more radiographically apparent focally. The result may be a focal lesion that is indistinguishable radiographically from bladder carcinoma (Box 6-9). A common example is bullous edema, which frequently accompanies pancystitis of various causes. Mechanical cystitis, often resulting from irrita-tion by a foreign body such as a catheter, is a focal process in many patients.

Infectious cystitis

Bacterial cystitis is the most frequent type of infectious cystitis encountered in developed countries. The usual pathogens include *Escherichia coli, Klebsiella,* and *Pseudomonas*. Bacterial cystitis most often occurs in women who are sexually active and is thought to result from retrograde deposition of bacterial flora that normally inhabit the vagina. In women, routine radiographic evaluation is not indicated unless cystitis is recurrent or difficult to eradicate. In men, cystitis usually occurs as a consequence of bladder outlet obstruction, typically benign prostatic hyperplasia or neurogenic bladder. Evaluation of the bladder and urethra is indicated with the first episode of bacterial cystitis in men to exclude lower urinary tract anomalies or obstruction. In most patients with acute bacterial cystitis, the bladder appears normal when evaluated with cystography, ultrasonography, or CT. However, severe forms of bacterial cystitis may be accompanied by mural thickening, which may be irregular or nodular (Fig. 6-16). Mural edema may appear hypoechoic on sonograms or hypodense on CT. Emphysematous cystitis, an unusual manifestation of bacterial cystitis, is discussed later in the chapter.

An unusual manifestation of recurrent bacterial infection is malacoplakia, a granulomatous inflammatory process that affects the urinary bladder and lower ureter. This disease tends to occur in immunoincompetent patients and is associated with *E. coli* urinary tract infections. The proffered pathogenesis of malacoplakia is deficient function of lysosomes in macrophages, causing a chronic and ineffective response to urinary tract infection. Soft, yellowish plaques are seen on the surface of the bladder with cystoscopy. With IVU or cystography, malacoplakia usually appears as multiple raised but sessile

Box 6-9   Focal Mural Abnormalities Attributed to Cystitis

Bullous edema
"Herald" lesion
Polypoid pseudotumor
Cystitis cystica or cystitis glandularis
Malacoplakia

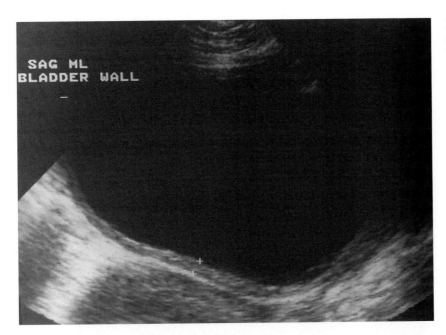

Fig. 6-16   Bladder sonogram in the sagittal plane shows diffuse thickening of the bladder wall in a patient with dysuria and pyuria.

filling defects, 5 to 10 mm in diameter. Central umbilication of these flat lesions may be seen, and there is a predilection for involvement of the bladder base. When malacoplakia is found in the lower ureter, there may be contiguous areas of stricture.

Viral cystitis more often is an affliction of childhood in which dysuria and gross hematuria follow viremia. The causative agent is adenovirus 11 in children and influenza virus type A in adults. Cystographic findings often indicate an aggressive cystitis. The capacity of the urinary bladder is decreased markedly, and mural nodularity may take the form of multiple polypoid filling defects. Differentiating viral cystitis from sarcoma botryoides can be difficult. An important distinguishing feature is reduced bladder capacity; in patients with rhabdomyosarcoma, the bladder capacity is normal or increased.

Schistosomiasis of the urinary bladder is a frequent cause of lower urinary tract disease in patients in underdeveloped countries. Its clinical and radiologic manifestations are discussed in the section on bladder lumen and wall calcification (Fig. 6-17).

Tuberculous infection of the genitourinary tract follows hematogenous dissemination from the lung or, less often, from the skin or gastrointestinal tract. Cystitis usually follows infection of the kidney and ureter and can be seen in 10% to 20% of patients with chronic urinary tract tuberculosis. Focal, irregular mural filling defects caused by mucosal tuberculomas may be seen early in the course of tuberculous cystitis and can simulate neoplasia. If the infectious process proceeds unchecked, transmural involvement occurs and may result in fibrosis and associated reduction in bladder capacity. Bizarre vesi-

cal configurations may be observed in chronic tuberculous cystitis when the fibrotic process is nonuniform. Vesicoureteral reflux and ureteral obstruction frequently accompany reduced vesical compliance. Radiographically visible calcification is present in approximately 10% of patients; if present, extensive tuberculous changes in the kidney and ureter usually are apparent.

Noninfectious cystitis

The main causes of noninfectious cystitis can be divided into four main pathogeneses: mechanical, toxic or drug-related, radiation-related, and allergic. Mechanical cystitis implies that there is contact irritant either within or external to the bladder. Because the cause of inflammation rarely involves the entire bladder, mechanical cystitis is frequently a focal process. Common irritants within the bladder lumen include an indwelling Foley catheter, a bladder stone, or surgery-related foreign bodies such as suture material. Paravesical disease, such as diverticulitis, pelvic abscess, regional enteritis, prostate cancer, or gynecologic malignancy, also can incite bullous edema and focal bladder wall-thickening or nodularity caused by inflammation (see Fig. 6-25A on p. 217). Such a focal inflammatory response of the adventitial and muscular layers of the bladder has been referred to as the herald lesion.

Cyclophosphamide management can cause a cystitis that may be associated with fulminant, gross hematuria in 4% to 12% of patients. Clinically, symptoms of bladder irritation may develop within days after drug administration. Blood clots may appear as intraluminal filling defects (Fig. 6-18A). With cystography, the bladder wall appears

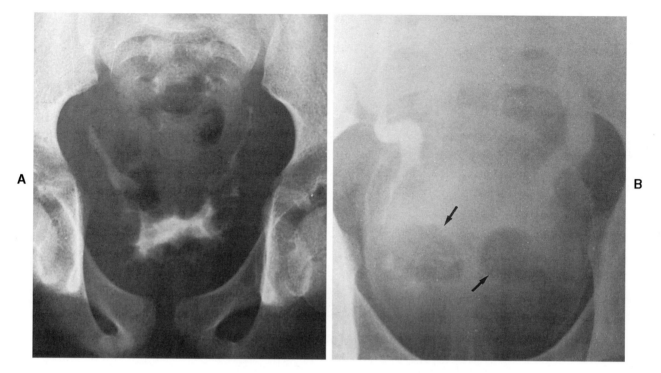

Fig. 6-17 Bladder schistosomiasis. **A,** Coned-down view of the bladder from an intravenous urogram demonstrates diffuse, multinodular thickening of the bladder wall, markedly reduced bladder capacity, and fixed dilatation of the distal right ureter. **B,** In another case of schistosomiasis, there is nodular thickening of the bladder wall, particularly near the ureterovesical junction, and several large polypoid filling defects (arrows).

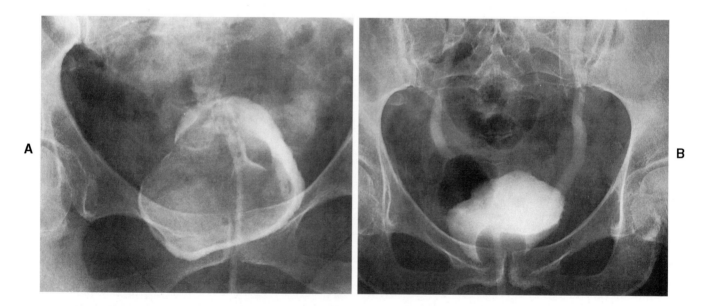

Fig. 6-18 Fulminant hemorrhagic cystitis in a 62-year-old patient with gross hematuria and dysuria. **A,** Cystogram demonstrates a large filling defect consistent with a blood clot. **B,** A urogram performed 4 weeks later shows nodular thickening of the bladder that has a reduced capacity.

thickened, and nodular filling defects are seen. In later stages, a contracted bladder can be seen, and the development of bladder wall fibrosis is irreversible (Fig. 6-18B).

Interstitial cystitis is an idiopathic pancystitis that often occurs in patients with allergies. Interstitial cystitis has been associated with polyarteritis nodosa, rheumatoid arthritis, and systemic lupus erythematosus; many patients have a strong atopic history. The diagnostic triad consists of chronic irritative voiding symptoms, sterile urine, and cystoscopic demonstration of urothelial ulcers or petechiae. In the early phase, the bladder usually appears normal on cystography. In later phases, the bladder becomes contracted, and capacity is reduced. Nodular thickening of the bladder wall may be demonstrated as bladder fibrosis ensues.

Several complications of chronic cystitis can produce a radiographic picture that is indistinguishable from bladder carcinoma. As a result of long-standing inflammation, clusters of hyperplastic urothelial cells called Brunn's nests may form in the submucosa of the bladder wall. When necrosis occurs in the center of these cell clusters, fluid-filled pseudocystic structures are formed; this condition is referred to as *cystitis cystica*. When Brunn's nests form into glandular structures, the condition is termed *cystitis glandularis*. Cystic or glandular metaplasia is indicative of mucosal instability, which often is reversible. In contrast to submucosal urothelial hyperplasia, squamous metaplasia is a change in the urothelium of the bladder wall to keratin-producing squamous cells. White patches, or leukoplakia, may cap mucosal foci of squamous metaplasia and are evident cystoscopically. The hyperplastic and metaplastic changes tend to occur earliest and to predominate in the trigone and base of the bladder.

OUTPOUCHING OF THE BLADDER WALL

Common and uncommon outpouchings of the bladder wall are listed in Box 6-10.

Box 6-10   Outpouching of the Bladder Wall

Common
  Diverticulum and saccule
  Cystocele
  Herniation of the bladder
Uncommon
  Urachal diverticulum

Box 6-11   Bladder Diverticula

Result from bladder neck or urethral obstruction
Congenital: Hutch diverticulum
Can cause ureteral obstruction or reflux
Urinary stasis may lead to stones or cystitis
Carcinoma in approximately 2%

Diverticula

Diverticula are focal herniations of the urothelium and submucosa through naturally weak sites in the bladder wall (Box 6-11). When acquired, diverticula frequently develop in the setting of chronic elevation of intravesical pressure. These herniations tend to occur next to the ureteral orifices. Diverticula are important clinically as a potential cause of urinary stasis, ureteral obstruction, and vesicoureteral reflux. Large diverticula may exert extrinsic mass effect on the bladder or may displace or obstruct the pelvic ureters. Lateral deviation of the lower ureters may be caused by bladder diverticula, but medial displacement is more common (Fig. 6-19). Radiographically, diverticula are outpouchings that have smooth inner walls, unlike the trabeculated bladder from which they originate. They may be as small as several centimeters and rarely enlarge to a size greater than that of the native bladder (Fig. 6-20). Outpouchings of the bladder

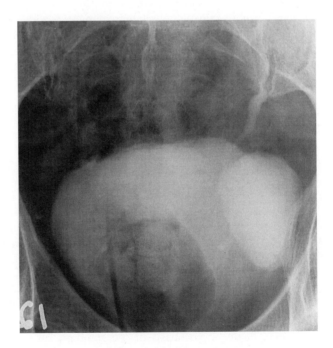

Fig. 6-19   A smooth-walled diverticulum originates from the lateral wall of the bladder and displaces the left ureter medially.

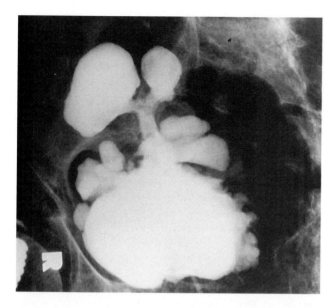

Fig. 6-20 Oblique, coned-down cystogram shows multiple large and small diverticula. Outpouchings of the bladder that are smaller than 2 cm are called saccules.

wall that are smaller than 2 cm often are referred to as saccules rather than diverticula, although the pathogenesis is the same (Fig. 6-15). Filling defects in diverticula may be caused by stones or, rarely, carcinoma (Fig. 6-21). Diverticula communicate with the bladder lumen by a channel that may be narrow and imperceptible. Diverticula may be demonstrated by cystography when they are not seen on the cystographic phase of the IVU. They also may be more conspicuous after voluntary bladder emptying as a result of the combination of increased filling and decreased emptying that occurs with the high intravesical pressures associated with voiding. The relative evacuation of contrast-laden urine from a diverticulum after bladder emptying is important, because it may influence the decision to treat patients surgically, especially those with recurrent urinary tract infections.

Cystocele

Cystocele is abnormal descent of the bladder with prolapse into the vagina. The trigone and bladder neck usually prolapse together, but occasionally only the trigone is involved (Fig. 6-22). Concomitant prolapse of the bladder and urethra (cystourethrocele) frequently is present with stress urinary incontinence. In addition, cystocele can be associated with bladder outlet obstruction or hydronephrosis, especially when the degree of prolapse is severe. The cystographic diagnosis of cystocele is best made on the basis of the standing lateral view rather than the supine anteroposterior view. On a standing lateral film, cystocele is defined as any part of the bladder that reaches the level of the inferior pubic

rami during straining. Cystoceles are graded from minimal to severe according to the degree of descent of the bladder. Prolapse of up to 2 cm below the superior pubic margin defines a mild cystocele, whereas a cystocele that descends below the level of the rami is severe.

Bladder Herniation

Herniation of the bladder through a pelvic or abdominal opening is an unusual cause of a small or asymmetrically shaped bladder associated with a focal area of outpouching (Fig. 6-23). Herniation through the inguinal or femoral canal occurs in more than 95% of all patients, and those with inguinal hernias outnumber femoral hernias two to one. In adults, the majority of bladder herniations result from age-related weakening of the supportive structures of the abdominal wall. Such herniations are more likely to occur in the presence of bladder outlet obstruction and secondary vesical distention. In infants aged less than 1 year, transitory, small inguinal herniations can be seen in as many as 9% of patients undergoing voiding cystourethrography (VCUG) or IVU. These "bladder ears" are a normal variant in infants and are of little clinical significance. In most patients, bladder herniation is asymptomatic and is discovered incidentally during herniorrhaphy. Inadvertent bladder perforation may occur in this setting. Other patients present with a classic history of two-stage voiding: the patient empties the bladder proper first but then must compress manually the herniated bladder.

Bladder hernias usually are less than 2 to 2.5 cm in size but occasionally can be massive. The wall of the hernia is smooth, unless the hernia is complicated by lithiasis or inflammation. The lateral and inferior aspect of the bladder herniates anteriorly and inferiorly in patients with inguinal canal herniation. Radiographic position may impact on the ability to demonstrate bladder hernias; one study showed that films acquired with the patient in the erect and prone position were more likely than conventional supine views to demonstrate herniations. Continuity with the bladder may be demonstrated more readily with cystography than with IVU, especially when the neck of the hernia is narrow or is unopacified because of a nondependent position.

INTRAVESICAL OR INTERSTITIAL AIR

The most common reason for the radiographic finding of air within the lumen of the bladder is recent catheterization or instrumentation (Box 6-12). The two important pathologic conditions that must be considered are fistula to bowel or vagina and infectious pancystitis caused by a gas-forming infection.

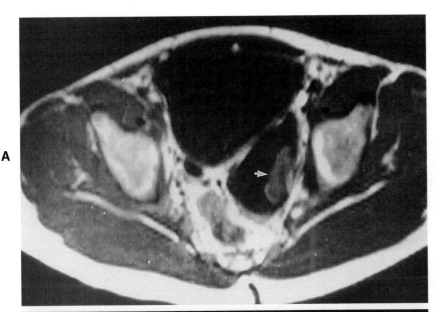

A

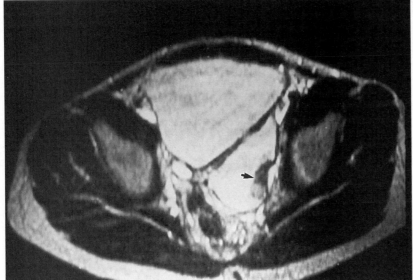

B

Fig. 6-21   Magnetic resonance (MR) imaging of a sarcoma originating in a diverticulum. T_1-weighted (**A**) and T_2-weighted (**B**), transverse MR images demonstrate a large diverticulum originating from the left inferolateral wall of the bladder. There is an endophytic mass (arrow) growing from the thickened lateral wall of this diverticulum. Leiomyosarcoma was resected at surgery.

Box 6-12   Causes of Air in the Lumen or Wall of the Urinary Bladder

Common
   Iatrogenic (recent catheterization or
     instrumentation)
   Fistula from bowel or vagina
Uncommon
   Emphysematous cystitis

Vesicoenteric Fistula

In addition to pneumaturia, a fistula from either small bowel or colon may cause chronic infectious cystitis or fecaluria (Box 6-13). These symptoms often dominate the clinical presentation of vesicoenteric fistula. Colovesical fistula may develop in as many as 2% of patients with diverticulitis. Other common causes of colovesical fistula include carcinoma of the colon and regional enteritis or Crohn's colitis. Carcinoma of the rectosigmoid is complicated by colovesical fistula more often than is cecal carcinoma. Enterovesical fistula has been reported in as many as 5% of adults and 10% of children with regional enteritis. Rectosigmoid diseases that lead to fistula formation involve the left and posterior bladder wall (Fig. 6-24 on p. 216). Conversely, infectious or inflammatory processes originating from the cecum, appendix, or distal small bowel tend to affect the right side of the bladder, either anteriorly or laterally.

Fistulas from bladder to bowel can be difficult to demonstrate by cystoscopic or radiologic methods. Fistulous

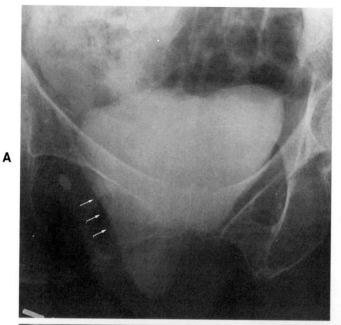

A

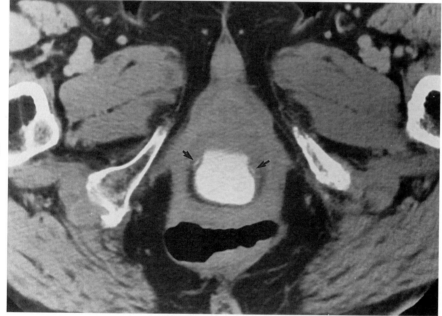

B

Fig. 6-22 Cystocele (trigonocele). **A,** Oblique urogram during the cystographic phase shows marked focal prolapse of the bladder base (arrows = distal right ureter). **B,** CT demonstrates the ureters (arrows) entering the trigone, which has prolapsed to the level of the ischial tuberosities.

connections are diagnosed with cystography and barium enema in only 30% to 60% of patients; the accuracy of cystoscopy is similar. VCUG should be performed with steep oblique or full lateral views when vesicointestinal fistula is suspected clinically. The most common cystographic findings include focal mural irregularity or extrinsic mass effect (Fig. 6-25A). Radiography of centrifuged urine to detect traces of radiopaque barium (Bourne test) has been advocated as an adjunct to an otherwise nondiagnostic barium enema examination. CT has been reported to be sensitive for identifying enterovesical fistu-

las. Optimal CT technique requires the administration of oral and rectal contrast; intravenous contrast material should not be administered (Fig. 6-25B). Bladder catheterization or cystoscopy before CT should be avoided to eliminate iatrogenic introduction of air. The diagnostic signs of enterovesical fistula on CT include the identification of intravesical air or contrast, focal bladder wall-thickening of more than 2 mm, contiguous bowel wall-thickening of more than 3 mm, and the presence of an air-containing, paravesical soft-tissue mass (Fig. 6-26 on p. 218).

Box 6-13 Causes of Fistula Between Bladder and Bowel

Common
  Iatrogenic
  Diverticulitis
  Carcinoma of the rectum or sigmoid colon
  Regional enteritis or Crohn's colitis
Uncommon
  Complication of radiotherapy
  Pelvic inflammatory disease
  Pelvic abscess (appendicitis)
  Neoplasms of the bladder
  Schistosomiasis or tuberculosis
  Cervical cancer

Vesicovaginal Fistula

Vesicovaginal fistulas most often are a complication of pelvic surgery but can result from locally advanced cancer of the cervix or bladder. Gynecologic surgery, particularly abdominal hysterectomy and vaginal surgery, and urologic surgery are the leading causes of postoperative vesicovaginal fistula. Rarer causes include obstetric injury, radiation therapy, foreign body (Foley catheter), and tuberculous or bilharzial cystitis. The clinical hallmark of vesicovaginal fistulas is continuous urinary incontinence. Voiding cystourethrography often is used successfully to demonstrate these fistulas, which are delineated on steep oblique or lateral views (Fig. 6-27 on p. 219). Vaginoscopy or speculum examination after

cystoscopic instillation of indigo carmine or milk in the urinary bladder can be used for direct visualization of a fistula.

Emphysematous Cystitis

Emphysematous cystitis is a rare form of bacterial cystitis that tends to occur in patients with poorly controlled diabetes. Emphysematous cystitis usually occurs in the setting of urinary stasis and with *E. coli* or, less frequently, *Aerobacter aerogenes* or *Candida* infections. Management with appropriate antibiotics and control of diabetes usually is effective. Radiographically, gas (carbon dioxide) is seen within the wall of the bladder and may be present within the bladder lumen. The pattern of air within the bladder wall may be linear, streaky, or multicystic. Proximal spread of mural gas to the ureters and renal pelves has been reported.

CALCIFICATION IN THE BLADDER WALL OR LUMEN

Common and uncommon causes of mural or luminal bladder calcification are shown in Box 6-14 on p. 218.

Bladder Stones

Like nephrolithiasis, bladder stones have a propensity to form when urinary stasis and infection are present. A discrete nidus on which stones can form and grow, such as a Foley catheter balloon, suture material, or pubic hairs, may coexist but is not necessary. Uric acid stones predominate in the setting of bladder outlet obstruction;

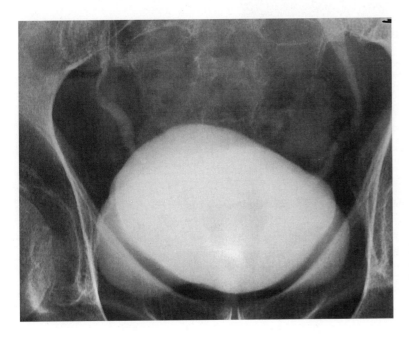

Fig. 6-23 Small femoral herniations of the bladder. Anteroposterior view during the cystographic phase of an intravenous urogram demonstrates bilateral focal outpouchings of the inferolateral bladder wall consistent with small bladder herniations. The patient was asymptomatic.

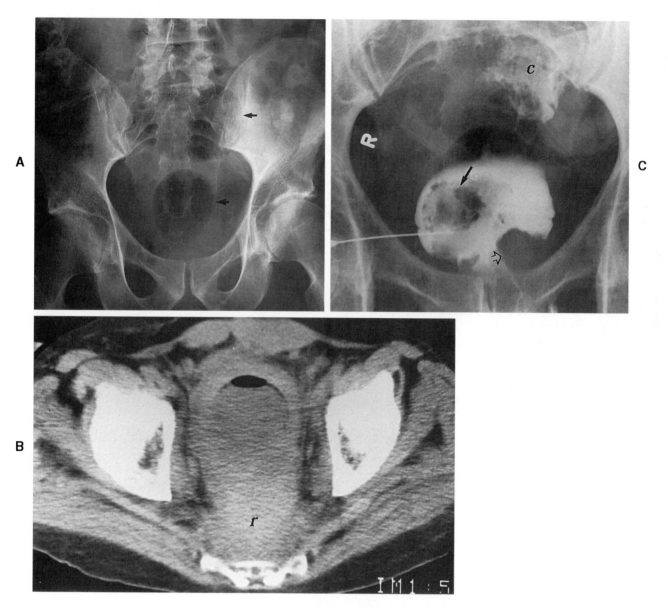

Fig. 6-24   Rectovesical fistula and bladder obstruction caused by recurrent rectal carcinoma. **A,** Abdominal plain film demonstrates two large pockets of air (arrows) in the pelvis. **B,** Uninfused CT shows a presacral mass (r). Obliteration of retrovesical fat suggests invasion of the posterior bladder wall. There is intravesical air and diffuse thickening of the bladder wall. **C,** Percutaneous cystogram demonstrates two filling defects: one resulting from purulent debris (arrow) and another resulting from invasive recurrent rectal cancer (open arrow). There is contrast opacification of sigmoid colon (c).

magnesium ammonium phosphate and apatite stones tend to occur when there is urinary tract infection, particularly with *Proteus* species. Given the propensity for urinary stasis and infection, stone formation in bladder diverticula is not unexpected. Patients with bladder stones may present with microscopic hematuria, suprapubic pain, or interruption of the stream resulting from intermittent bladder neck obstruction; however, many patients are asymptomatic. Of particular concern in patients with asymptomatic bladder stone disease is the development of squamous cell carcinoma (SCC) in areas of the bladder that are chronically inflamed because of mechanical irritation. If sufficiently calcified, stones in the bladder may be visible in whole or in part on a plain film (Fig. 6-28). Therefore, small uric acid stones often are undetectable, especially when compared with

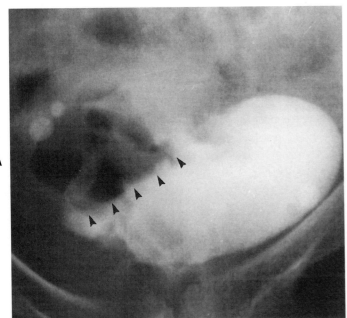

A

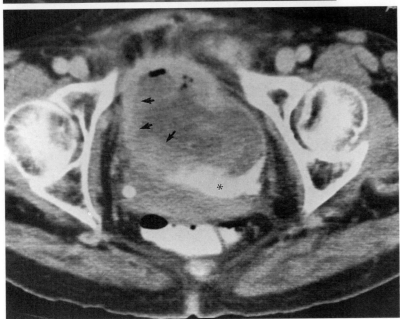

B

Fig. 6-25   Enterovesical fistula caused by regional enteritis. **A,** Coned-down view of the bladder from an intravenous urogram shows extrinsic mass effect and a lobular margin of the superolateral margin of the bladder (arrowheads). **B,** Uninfused CT demonstrates thickening of the bladder wall (arrows) and intravesical contrast (*) and air.

larger uric acid and struvite stones. In the patient positioned supine, bladder stones tend to rest in the midline; laterally positioned stones, especially if there are several faceted stones in close proximity, suggest location within a diverticulum. A large, nonopaque calculus with rim calcification can simulate bladder wall calcification on plain abdominal radiographs. Stones usually are less dense than contrast-opacified urine and therefore appear as filling defects on cystographic examinations or the cystographic phase of IVU (Fig. 6-29 on p. 220). Differentiation of stone from mural-based mass can be accom-

plished if mobility is shown on plain film or sonograms. In rare cases, CT may be needed to distinguish bladder stones from calcifications of the uterus, rectal wall, or prostate gland.

Schistosomiasis

Worldwide, schistosomiasis is the most frequent cause of bladder wall calcification. Of the three major species, *Schistosoma haematobium* is the primary schistosome that infects the lower urinary tract. These blood flukes

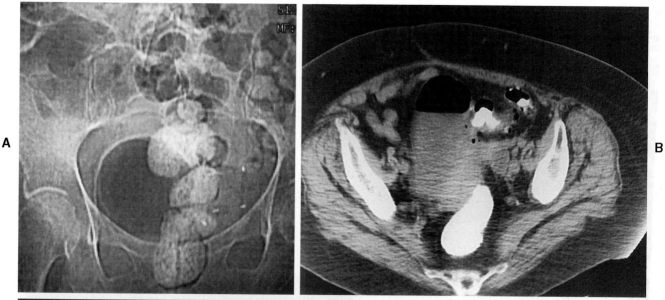

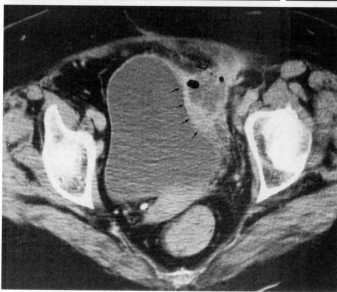

Fig. 6-26   Colovesical fistula secondary to diverticulitis. **A,** Digital image of the pelvis shows a large air collection in the pelvis next to the contrast-opacified rectum. **B,** Uninfused CT shows intravesical air. **C,** At a more caudal level, CT demonstrates focal bladder wall-thickening (small arrows) adjacent to an inflamed segment of sigmoid colon (open arrow).

Box 6-14   Mural or Luminal Bladder Calcification

Common
  Bladder stone
  Transitional cell carcinoma (0.5%)
  Cystitis (infectious and noninfectious:
    schistosomiasis, tuberculous, radiation,
    cyclophosphamide)
Uncommon
  Foreign body–associated encrustation
  Amyloidosis

---

live in the portal and mesenteric veins and migrate through the systemic veins to reach the lower urinary tract, prostate gland, and lower gastrointestinal tract. The female schistosome deposits her eggs in small venules of the bladder wall. Granuloma formation, obliterative endarteritis, and fibrosis are the histopathologic responses to these deposited ova. The earliest finding of bladder schistosomiasis on cystography is an indistinct, blurred bladder wall contour, resulting from submucosal edema. Small, flat filling defects may be seen and are attributed to bilharzial polyps. The characteristic manifestation of schistosomiasis is sheet-like or eggshell calcification in the submucosa of the bladder and ureteral walls

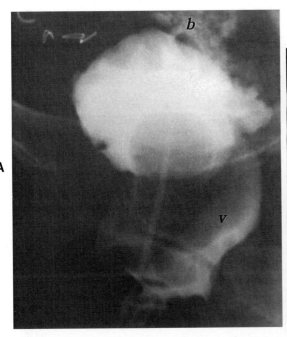

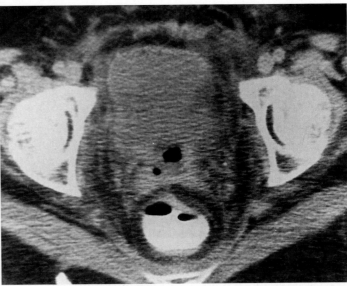

A

B

b

v

Fig. 6-27   Vesicovaginal and vesicoenteric fistulas after radiation therapy for local recurrence of cervical cancer. **A,** Oblique view from a cystogram demonstrates abnormal opacification of the vagina (v) and small bowel (b). **B,** Uninfused CT shows pockets of air in a fluid-distended vagina. The fat plane between the posterior bladder wall and vagina is indistinct.

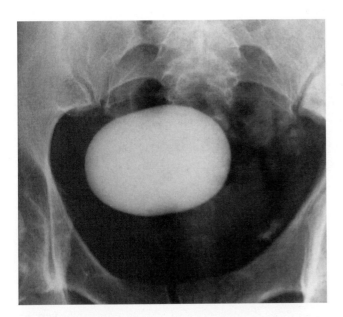

Fig. 6-28   Coned-down view of the pelvis shows a large and densely calcified bladder stone. The calculus enlarged from 5 mm to 5 cm in approximately 7 years.

(Fig. 6-30). However, the pattern of calcification is variable and may be dense and wavy or serpiginous. Typically, the entire bladder wall is involved, although the base of the bladder may be involved earliest. Approximately 50% of patients with bladder schistosomiasis have calcification that is visible on plain film. Despite the extensive nature of the calcification, bladder capacity is normal, and with voiding, the calcified bladder contracts. Any of the bladder carcinomas may complicate chronic schistosomiasis, but SCC is cited most frequently. Single or multiple asymmetric or irregular filling defects or focal disruption of mural linear calcification should raise suspicion concerning this malignant complication. Radiographic changes also may be seen in the ureters. Persistent opacification of the lower third of the ureters on IVU is an early finding and may progress to fixed dilatation (Fig. 6-17). Multiple focal strictures may develop and always are present in the lower ureters first. The combination of dilatation and tortuosity caused by stricture or reflux has been described as the "snakehead" appearance of the distal ureter. Progressive proximal ureteral involvement with strictures and intervening dilatation creates a beaded appearance of the ureters, which is outlined by linear calcification in about 15% of patients.

Bladder Carcinoma

The incidence of radiographically detected calcification in bladder tumors has been estimated at 0.5%. When calcification is associated with a mass in the bladder, neoplasm must be excluded. TCCs and SCCs most often are associated with dystrophic calcification, which is focal and can be linear, punctate, or coarse in pattern

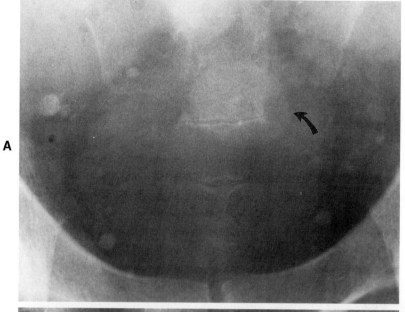

Fig. 6-29 Uric acid bladder calculus. **A,** In addition to multiple phleboliths, a coned-down view shows a 2.5-cm calcification (curved arrow) in the midline of the pelvis. **B,** A focal filling defect (curved arrow), corresponding to the calcification, is seen on this urogram. In addition, there is a second filling defect caused by an enlarged prostate gland . This was a uric acid stone, which occurs more often in the setting of bladder outlet obstruction. (Case courtesy of Mark S. Ridlen, MD)

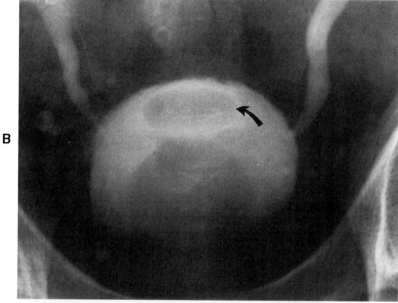

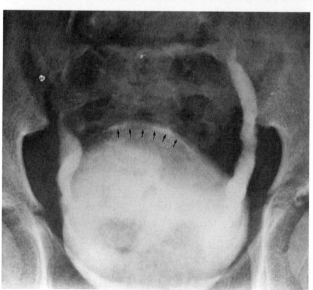

Fig. 6-30 Eggshell calcification of vesical schistosomiasis. Coned view of the bladder shows fine, eggshell or sheet-like calcification of the bladder wall (arrows). Persistent opacification of the distal ureter is an early finding of this disease.

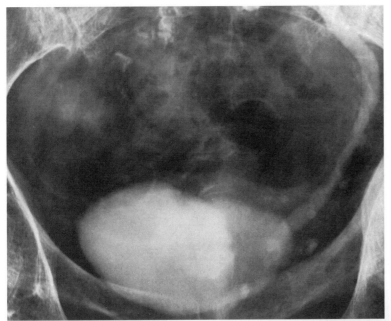

A

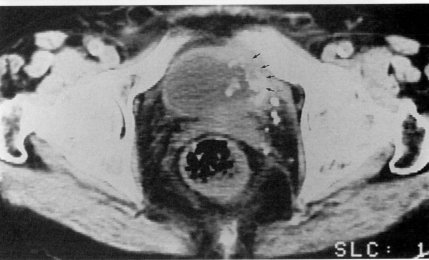

B

Fig. 6-31 Calcification of a bladder carcinoma. **A,** A coned-down view from a urogram shows a large filling defect along the superior and inferolateral walls of the bladder. In addition, there is obstruction of the left ureter. **B,** Uninfused CT shows linear, plaque-like calcifications (arrows) in a part of the extensive bladder wall mass. An invasive transitional cell carcinoma was found at surgery.

(Fig. 6-31). Benign mesenchymal tumors, such as hemangioma (Fig. 6-32), and 70% of urachal carcinomas may have radiographically detectable calcification.

Alkaline Encrustation Cystitis

Inflammatory bladder wall lesions that contain focal areas of necrosis may undergo dystrophic calcification. This type of calcification is more likely to occur in the environment of alkaluria, which fosters the precipitation of calcium phosphate or struvite salts. Thus, urinary tract infection with *Proteus* species or other coliforms that elaborate urease, together with focal or diffuse areas of bladder necrosis, may result in bladder wall calcification attributable to alkaline encrustation cystitis. Bladder necrosis leading to alkaline encrustation may occur with

antecedent radiotherapy, cyclophosphamide management, mitomycin C instillation, or, more rarely, bacterial cystitis alone. Calcifications, which are not always seen radiographically, manifest in a variety of patterns, including linear or coarse and nodular (Fig. 6-33). The calcifications seen with alkaline encrustation cystitis regress and disappear with resolution of the underlying infection.

Miscellaneous

Tuberculous cystitis may be associated with bladder wall calcification late in its course. By the time it is apparent radiographically, there is evidence of extensive upper tract tuberculosis and prostatic calcification. Tuberculous vesical calcification could be confused with bilharziasis, but the latter begins in the bladder and progresses

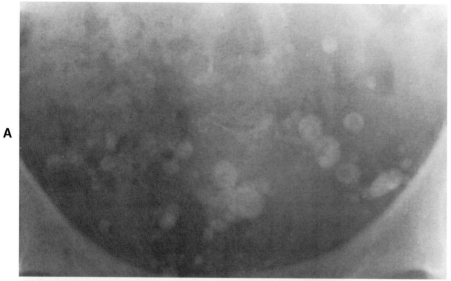

A

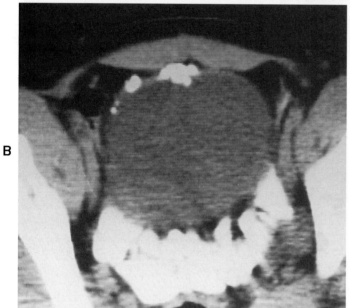

B

Fig. 6-32 Calcification of a mesenchymal bladder tumor. **A,** Plain film coned-down to the pelvis demonstrates multiple round calcifications, many of which have central radiolucent areas. **B,** Uninfused CT of the bladder shows round calcifications, isolated and clustered, in focally thickened bladder wall. Hemangioma of the bladder wall was removed at surgery.

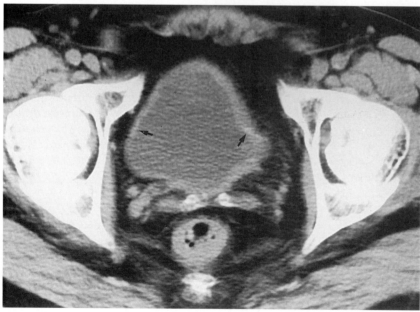

Fig. 6-33 Alkaline encrustation cystitis in patient with *Proteus* cystitis after radiation therapy. In addition to diffuse bladder wall thickening, uninfused CT demonstrates faint linear areas of mural calcification (arrows).

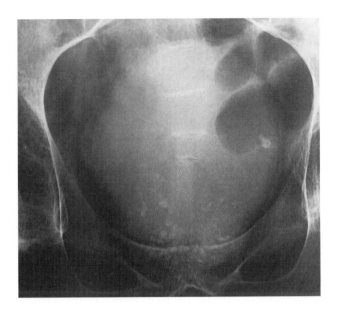

Fig. 6-34 Coned-down view of the bladder from an intravenous urogram shows multiple calcifications overlying the base of the bladder. On transrectal sonography, extensive calcification of the seminal vesicles and prostate gland was found.

proximally, whereas the converse pattern typifies urinary tract tuberculosis. As mentioned previously, a rim-calcified bladder stone or Foley balloon encrustation may mimic mural calcification. Calcifications in the prostate gland or seminal vesicles also can mimic bladder base calcification, particularly when the prostate gland is enlarged (Fig. 6-34).

EXTRINSIC COMPRESSION OR DISPLACEMENT OF THE BLADDER

Common and uncommon causes of extrinsic compression or displacement of the bladder are listed in Box 6-15.

Pelvic Hematoma and Urinoma

A pelvic hematoma large enough to compress or displace the bladder most often occurs after blunt or penetrating trauma to the pelvis and rarely as a complication of pelvic surgery (Fig. 6-35). Blood from laceration of the internal iliac artery or perivesical venous plexus can accumulate in the pelvis, causing compression and superior displacement of the urinary bladder. If trauma results in extraperitoneal bladder rupture, extravasated urine also may contribute to the mass effect of blood. Standard cystography or pelvic CT will demonstrate the compression of the lateral walls of the bladder, which typically is symmetric, and the elevation of the bladder base (Fig. 6-36). Osseous pelvic ring fracture or diastasis of the

---

Box 6-15	Extrinsic Compression or Displacement of the Bladder

Common
    Pelvic hematoma and urinoma*
    Pelvic mass (abscess or tumor)
    Bladder diverticulum
Uncommon
    Lymphadenopathy†
    Postoperative or radiation change
    Inferior vena cava thrombosis†
    Pelvic lipomatosis*
    Iliopsoas muscle hypertrophy*

*Pear-shaped bladder.
†Tear-drop bladder.

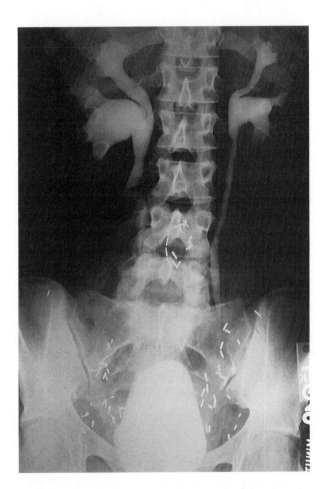

Fig. 6-35 Pear-shaped bladder. The pear-shaped and teardrop bladder looks like the top of a rocket! Think of the mnemonic LAUNCH: lymphoma/lipomatosis, abscess, urinoma, nodes, collateral veins (inferior vena cava obstruction), and hematoma. (Case and mnemonic courtesy of Jeffrey M. Brody, MD)

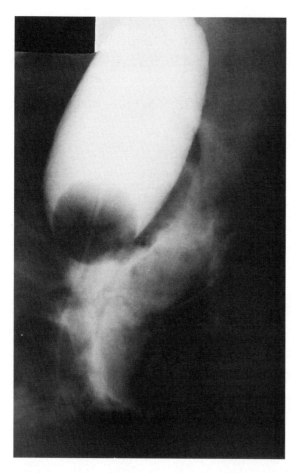

Fig. 6-36   Compression and displacement of the bladder because of pelvic hematoma and urinoma. Left posterior oblique view from a cystogram shows extrinsic compression of the bladder and extravasation of contrast from a type 2 complete tear of the posterior urethra.

pubic symphysis or sacroiliac joints also may be evident (Fig. 6-37).

Bladder Diverticulum

During the cystographic phase of IVU, an unopacified bladder diverticulum may cause focal bladder displacement. Typically, one also may see focal medial deviation of the ureter ipsilateral to the diverticulum. The diverticulum often is demonstrated on urographic postvoid or delayed views, but it may require cystography, ultrasonography, or CT evaluation for confirmation (Fig. 6-38).

Pelvic Lipomatosis

Pelvic lipomatosis is a rare disease characterized by infiltration of the true pelvis by benign adipose tissue. Pelvic lipomatosis occurs most frequently in a specific group of patients: middle-aged, usually overweight, black men with a history of hypertension. Clinical symptoms

are nonspecific and include abdominal or low back pain, urinary frequency, urinary tract infection, or constipation. Increased radiolucency in the pelvis may be recognized on the plain film of the pelvis. Characteristic radiologic signs have been reported on urograms, barium enema examinations, and CT scans. The bladder has a strikingly abnormal configuration, similar to that of a gourd or inverted pear (pear-shaped bladder) with narrowing most prominent inferiorly or in the midportion. The bladder base is elevated, and bladder capacity is reduced. In addition, the pelvic ureters may be displaced, and the proximal ureter may be dilated. Obstruction of the urinary tract is a complication of this disease that occurs in approximately 40% of patients. The rectum and sigmoid colon are elongated and narrowed, but the colonic mucosal pattern is intact. The retrorectal space also is enlarged. CT confirms the profusion of adipose tissue in the pelvis and its mass effect on the bladder and bowel.

Inferior Vena Cava Obstruction

Pelvic collateral channels enlarge subsequent to obstruction of the middle and lower inferior vena cava (IVC) and can deform the urinary bladder by compression. These collateral channels include the ascending lumbar, gonadal, superior hemorrhoidal, and ureteric veins. In adults, the most common cause of IVC obstruction is tumor thrombosis. Renal, pancreatic, or adrenal carcinomas may secondarily invade the IVC. Abdominal sepsis, trauma, or cephalad extension of thrombus from the femoroiliac veins also may result in bland thrombosis of the IVC. The urogram demonstrates compression and superior and anterior displacement of the bladder, resulting from the mass effect of pelvic venous collaterals and soft-tissue edema. The ureters below L3 may be notched or displaced medially or anteriorly by periureteral collateral veins.

Miscellaneous

Iliopsoas hypertrophy, a rare cause of symmetric narrowing of the upper third of the bladder, tends to occur most often in young black men with narrow bony pelves. Unless massive, pelvic lymphadenopathy is not typically associated with bladder compression. Thus, extensive pelvic lymphoma or, rarely, lymphogenous spread of prostate carcinoma may cause extrinsic mass effect on the bladder.

BLADDER RUPTURE

Rupture of the urinary bladder most often occurs in the setting of pelvic trauma, but occasionally it is sponta-

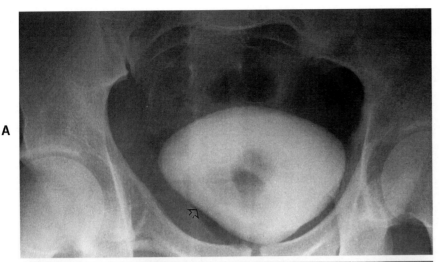

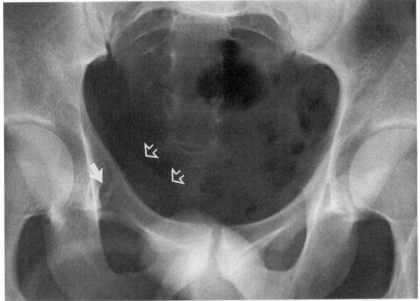

Fig. 6-37 Small pelvic hematoma that causes extrinsic compression of the bladder. **A,** Cystogram after pelvic trauma demonstrates extrinsic mass effect (arrow) on the right inferolateral wall of the bladder. **B,** Review of the plain film shows medial displacement of the obturator internus shadow (open arrows) and a nondisplaced fracture of the acetabulum (arrow). (Case courtesy of Jeffrey M. Brody, MD)

neous. Bladder rupture is classified according to the site of extravasation and is described as being either intraperitoneal, extraperitoneal, or both (Table 6-3). The management of intraperitoneal bladder rupture requires immediate surgery for exploration and bladder closure because extravasated urine is absorbed quickly by the peritoneum and may cause uremia. Extraperitoneal rupture, in contrast, can be managed by urethral or suprapubic catheter drainage of the bladder. Accurate diagnosis is imperative and is facilitated by imaging in the majority of patients.

The occurrence of posttraumatic bladder rupture depends on the degree of bladder distention, the nature of the inciting injury, and the presence of underlying bladder abnormality. The distended bladder is more likely than the collapsed bladder to rupture with blunt trauma. Fracture of the pelvis, particularly when it involves the anterior osseous ring, should raise the suspicion of lower

Table 6-3   Characterization of Bladder Rupture on Computed Tomography Scan

Intraperitoneal	Extraperitoneal
Lateral pelvic recesses (lateral paravesical recesses superior to bladder)	Perivesical space (extends anterior and superior to bladder to level of umbilicus)
Midline pouch of Douglas (posterior to bladder and anterior to rectosigmoid)	Retrorectal or presacral space

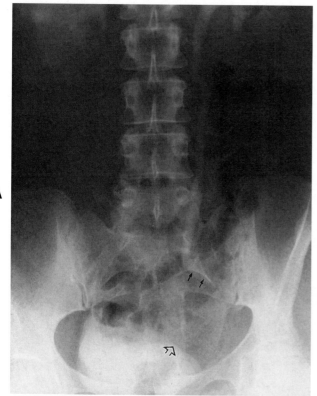

A

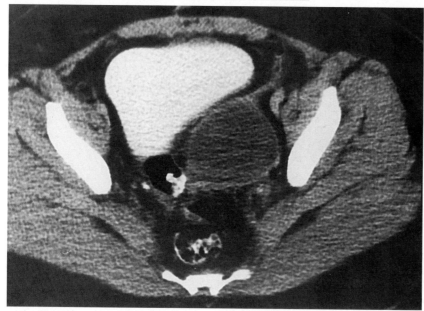

B

Fig. 6-38 Displacement of the bladder and ureter by a pelvic mass. **A,** Anteroposterior view from an intravenous urogram demonstrates extrinsic mass effect on the superior surface of the bladder (open arrow). There is lateral displacement (small arrows) and partial obstruction of the left ureter. Although medial displacement of the ureter is more common, bladder diverticulum was diagnosed. **B,** Infused CT shows a hypodense pelvic mass that did not opacify with contrast material. An endometrial cyst was removed at surgery. (Case courtesy of Mark S. Ridlen, MD)

urinary tract injury. Bladder injuries occur in 7% of patients with traumatic separation of the symphysis pubis and fractures of the pubic rami. Cesarean section and transurethral resection of the bladder may be complicated by iatrogenic bladder rupture. Spontaneous rupture occurs when there is a lesion that attenuates the bladder wall, such as tumor, cystitis, perivesical inflammation, bladder outlet obstruction, neurogenic bladder, or injury related to therapeutic radiation.

Standard cystography with views of the bladder after drainage of contrast material is the time-honored test for evaluation of bladder trauma. Cystography is optimized with complete filling of the bladder; 300 to 400 cc of a dilute contrast material should be used to distend the bladder. Exclusion of injury to the urethra always is important before transurethral catheterization of the bladder for cystography. Extravasation of contrast material isolated to the perivesical space is the hallmark of extra-

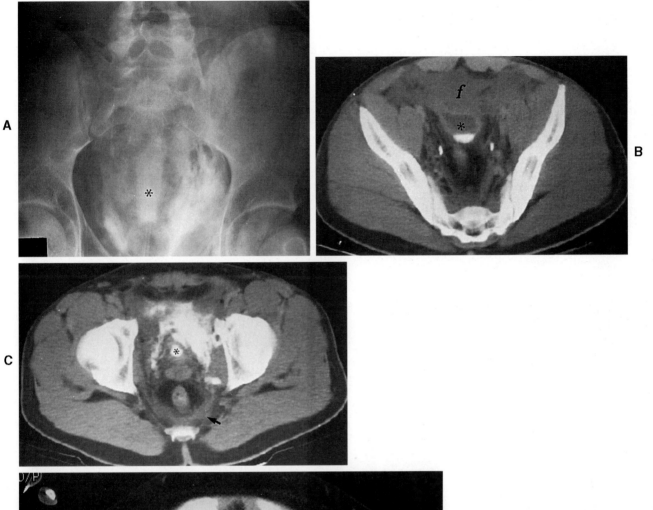

Fig. 6-39 Extraperitoneal rupture of the bladder. **A,** Anteroposterior view of the pelvis from cystogram shows extravasated contrast material that has jagged, irregular margins. There is marked extrinsic compression and elevation of the bladder (*). Bowel loops are not outlined by contrast. **B,** CT scan demonstrates free fluid in the prevesical space (f). **C,** CT scan at a more caudal level demonstrates fluid in the retrorectal space (arrow) and extravasated contrast material in the anterior and lateral perivesical spaces (* = collapsed and compressed bladder). **D,** In another patient with extraperitoneal bladder rupture, extravasated contrast is seen in the prevesical and lateral perivesical spaces. Extravasated urine or contrast material can extend to the level of the umbilicus in the prevesical space (* = collapsed bladder containing air).

peritoneal rupture (Figs. 6-36, 6-39A). Fracture of the anterior ring of the pelvis accompanies this form of bladder rupture in 90% of patients with related trauma. The site of the bladder defect frequently is the anterolateral

bladder wall, and opinions differ as to whether fracture fragments are the cause of this laceration. The extravasated contrast material often collects close to the bladder and may have sharp but irregular margins, described as

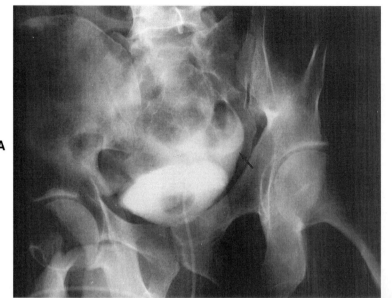

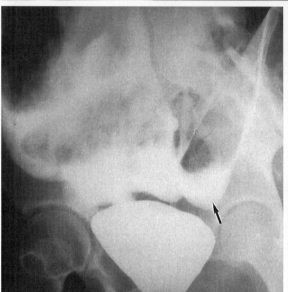

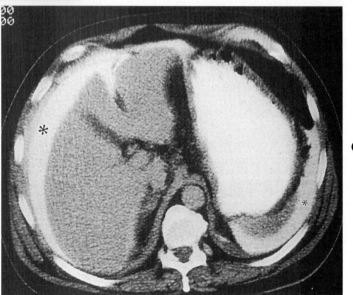

Fig. 6-40   Intraperitoneal bladder rupture. **A and B,** Cystograms from two different patients with intraperitoneal bladder rupture. Described as "cloud-like," extravasated contrast material outlines bowel loops and can be seen in the lateral paravesical recesses (arrow) and paracolic gutter. **C,** CT demonstrates extravasated contrast material (*) in the peritoneal space around the liver and spleen. (Case courtesy of John J. Cronan, MD)

flame-shaped. If the urogenital diaphragm is violated, contrast material may spread into the perineum, thigh, or scrotum. Intraperitoneal rupture is typified by delineation of intraperitoneal organs, such as small bowel loops or the liver edge, by extravasated contrast material. Contrast material extravasated in the peritoneal space has a homogeneous and cloud-like appearance (Fig. 6-40A, B). A horizontal rent along the peritonealized dome of the bladder, the mechanically weakest site, is the usual location of the bladder defect. Blunt trauma is the cause, and pelvic fracture accompanies this form of bladder perforation in 75% of patients. The use of cystography in the diagnosis of bladder rupture is not without problems. Pelvic fracture fragments, mast suit, spine board, and oral contrast material from CT may create diagnostic ambiguities.

Contrast-enhanced pelvic CT has been used increasingly and successfully in the diagnosis and characterization of posttraumatic bladder rupture. Recent studies conclude that the technically optimal contrast CT examination equals standard cystography in diagnostic accuracy and often is more valuable in the detection of pelvic fractures and soft-tissue injuries. Several technical points for the use of CT in the diagnosis of bladder rupture are worthy of mention. First, the bladder must be distended with contrast material to optimize the sensitivity. This distention can be accomplished either by direct instillation of a dilute contrast solution into the bladder or by clamping the intravesical Foley catheter before the start of scanning. Second, delayed CT imaging (obtained 15 to 30 minutes after the study is completed) ensures that sufficient intravenous contrast material has been excreted by the kidneys and collected in the catheter-clamped bladder to distend it adequately. In addition, delayed images help to differentiate unopacified bowel loops from perivesical fluid collections associated with bladder rupture.

The distribution of extravasated fluid and contrast material in the pelvis and abdomen is crucial for classifying the bladder rupture as intraperitoneal or extraperitoneal. Intraperitoneal fluid may collect in the midline pelvis within the pouch of Douglas, posterior to the bladder and anterior to the rectosigmoid colon. It also may be found in the lateral pelvic recesses superior to the bladder and in the pericolic space or around loops of small bowel. Extraperitoneal pelvic fluid can be found in the prevesical, perivesical, or retrorectal spaces. Fluid superior to the bladder in the prevesical space extends superiorly and anteriorly to the level of the umbilicus (Fig. 6-39D). Pelvic fluid or extravasated contrast material that is lateral to the bladder or behind the rectum is in the extraperitoneal space (Fig. 6-39B–D).

NEUROMUSCULAR DISORDERS

Neuromuscular disorders of the lower urinary tract stem from lesions of the cerebrum, spinal cord, or peripheral nerves, which compromise normal bladder accommodation or micturition. A neurogenic or neuropathic bladder has lost the capacity to fill, store, or empty urine under voluntary control because of a neuromuscular disorder. Several pathophysiologies of neurogenic bladder have been described, and one or a combination of these mechanisms may explain the dysfunction in patients (Box 6-16). Detrusor hyperactivity manifests by involuntary bladder contractions that cause phasic increases in detrusor pressure. These intermittent contractions interfere

---

Box 6-16   Neuromuscular Disorders of the Lower Urinary Tract

Spastic bladder
    Detrusor hyperreflexia and sphincter synergy
    Central nervous system disease or local bladder or
        pelvic irritation
Sphincter dyssynergia
    Detrusor hyperactivity and bladder–sphincter
        dyssynergia
Flaccid bladder
    Detrusor areflexia with or without infravesical
        obstruction caused by bladder prolapse
    Injury or disease of the conus, cauda equina, sacral
        nerve roots, or peripheral nerves

---

with bladder relaxation during urine collection and compromise the storage function of the bladder. When caused by neurologic disease, bladder hyperactivity is termed detrusor hyperreflexia; when idiopathic, it is referred to as detrusor instability. Hyperactivity also may be secondary to reduced bladder compliance. Injury to the lower motor neurons that innervate the bladder (i.e., the preganglionic and postganglionic parasympathetic neurons) results in detrusor areflexia. This adynamic bladder also is referred to as a flaccid or motor paralytic bladder. Synergy refers to the coordinated relaxation of the urethral sphincters that occurs during bladder contraction. Striated sphincter dyssynergia and smooth sphincter or bladder neck dyssynergia is the inappropriate contraction of the external and internal sphincters, respectively.

The clinical expression of neuromuscular disorders includes incontinence, pressure, urgency, frequency, and urinary retention. Urinary incontinence is the involuntary loss of urine. Different types of urinary incontinence described on the basis of the pattern, cause, or pathophysiology of the involuntary urine loss include stress, precipitous, continuous, and overflow urinary incontinence. Urgency is the strong desire to void, either because of discomfort (pressure) or because of the fear of involuntary urine loss.

Lesions of the anteromedial frontal lobes, those of the medial aspect of the sensorimotor cortex, and some lesions of the cerebellum and basal ganglia may cause neuromuscular disorders of the lower urinary tract through their effect on the pontomesencephalic micturition center. The functional effect of the cerebrum on the brain stem micturition center is one of detrusor inhibition. Loss of inhibition may result in detrusor hyperreflexia, but the micturition reflex remains intact, and there is sphincter synergy. Cerebral infarction, neoplasm, penetrating brain trauma, Parkinson's disease, dementia of the Alzheimer's type, multiple sclerosis, and normal pressure hydrocephalus are the more common etiologies of the so-called uninhibited neurogenic bladder. Involuntary detrusor contraction is the most common cause of precipitous incontinence in the elderly, but it does not always result from cerebral or cerebellar disease. Spastic bladder also may result from local bladder or pelvic irritation by infection, inflammation, fecal impaction, neoplasms, uterine prolapse, or prostatic hypertrophy. Bladder hyperreflexia may manifest radiographically as serrations of the bladder mucosa, which is seen earliest along the posterior bladder wall, or as a prominent interureteric indentation (Fig. 6-41). Bladder serration during voiding correlates well with cystometric evidence of bladder contraction. Bladder capacity is small because of uncontrolled contractions, and the contour of the bladder is persistently rounded. The bladder wall usually is smooth; bladder trabeculation is unusual with this form

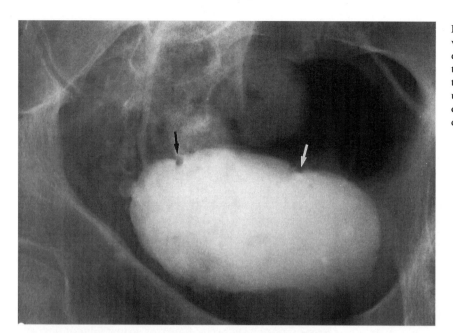

Fig. 6-41   Bladder hyperreflexia in a patient with multiple sclerosis who presented with frequency, urgency, and urge incontinence. Cystometry showed uninhibited detrusor contractions. Cystographic phase of an intravenous urogram shows a rounded and slightly trabeculated bladder with prominent interureteric indentations (arrows).

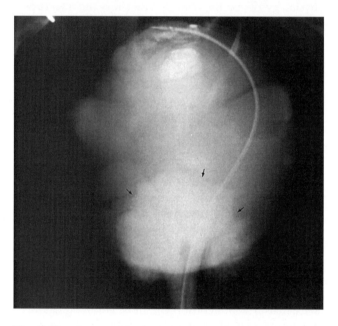

Fig. 6-42   Patient with chronic urinary retention and overflow incontinence. The bladder neck appeared normal at cystoscopy, but cystometry revealed smooth sphincter dyssynergia. Cystogram demonstrates a markedly distended bladder, which contained 5 L of urine (arrows = extensive calcification of the seminal vesicles).

of neurogenic bladder but may be seen occasionally in patients with long-standing disease.

Injuries of the spinal cord at or above T12 result in a pattern of neuromuscular dysfunction typified by detrusor hyperreflexia and bladder–sphincter dyssynergia. Patients with these disorders have no bladder sensation and cannot voluntarily initiate micturition. Incontinence results either because of low-volume bladder hyper-

reflexia or because of urinary retention and overflow incontinence (Fig. 6-42). In addition to posttraumatic spinal cord injury, patients with multiple sclerosis and 10% of patients with lumbar disc disease may have this type of neuromuscular injury. Radiographic findings include those associated with bladder hyperreflexia and marked bladder neck dilatation during detrusor contractions resulting from striated sphincter dyssynergia. Secondary bladder and upper tract changes are more likely to occur when bladder outlet obstruction and high-pressure detrusor dysfunction are long standing. With chronic bladder outlet obstruction, detrusor hypertrophy and bladder trabeculation may occur. Stones may form within the bladder or on foreign bodies, such as an indwelling Foley catheter. SCC is more likely to occur in the neurogenic bladder, particularly in the setting of bladder stones and chronic cystitis. Upper tract sequelae of neurogenic bladder include ureterectasis, reflux, and loss of parenchymal tissue as a result of stone disease, reflux, or obstruction.

Disease of the conus medullaris, cauda equina, sacral nerve roots, or peripheral nerves may result in loss of bladder sensation and contraction, the so-called autonomous neurogenic bladder. Extensive injury to the pelvic nerves may complicate abdominoperineal resection or radical hysterectomy, diabetic neuropathy, alcoholic neuropathy, or tumor infiltration (Fig. 6-43). Detrusor inadequacy implies insufficient detrusor tone to overcome normal intraurethral resistance. Vesical pressures may exceed intraurethral pressures only at high bladder volume, resulting in overflow incontinence. The volume of the flaccid bladder can be increased moderately to markedly. Although a smooth bladder with a large capac-

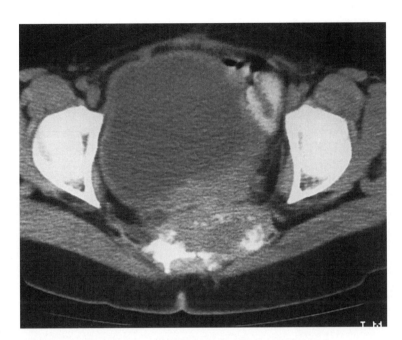

Fig. 6-43   Autonomous neurogenic bladder as a result of sacral and peripheral nerve invasion caused by metastatic endometrial carcinoma. CT scan demonstrates destruction of the lower sacrum and infiltration of the pelvic soft tissues by tumor. There is dilatation of the bladder caused by areflexia and infravesical obstruction.

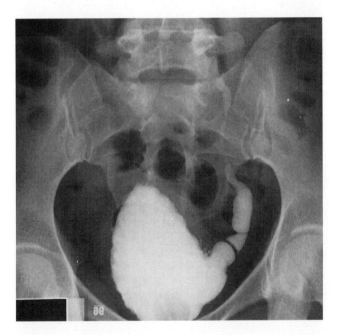

Fig. 6-44   Pine tree bladder. Anteroposterior view from a cystogram demonstrates an elongated and trabeculated bladder. There is left ureteral reflux. Upper tract sequelae of chronic neurogenic bladder include ureterectasis, reflux, and loss of renal parenchymal tissue.

ity is the typical appearance of a flaccid bladder, other patterns can occur. Once described as typical for the lower motor neuron type of bladder lesion, the "pine tree" configuration can be found in patients with either detrusor hyperreflexia or detrusor areflexia. The pathogenesis of the "pine tree" configuration is infravesical obstruction and impaired bladder sensation. During se-

vere overdistention, focal weak areas of the bladder yield, leading to trabeculation, sacculation, and eventually the pine tree configuration (Fig. 6-44).

Stress incontinence more often is the manifestation of inadequacy of one or both of the urethral sphincters than of a neuromuscular disorder. It most often occurs when a sudden increase in intraabdominal pressure results in an unequal transmission of pressure to the bladder and urethra. When support to the vesical neck is lost so that it descends to a position outside of the abdominal cavity, intravesical pressure may transiently exceed urethral pressure with stress, and urine leakage will occur. In women, diminution of striated muscle tone associated with aging, multiparity, or surgery (particularly vaginal hysterectomy) can cause incompetence of the pelvic floor, sometimes referred to as hypermobility of the bladder neck and urethra. Radiographically, the normal bladder base is at or cephalad to the level of the superior margin of the pubic symphysis, and it may descend as much as 1.5 cm with stress. Women with stress incontinence may have a vesical neck that is closed at rest but is low-lying. With stress, the vesical neck and proximal urethra will descend more than 2 cm and may open (Table 6-4; Fig. 6-45). Surgery for patients with stress incontinence caused by abnormal bladder descent includes urethropexy with or without retropubic suspension. The other mechanism by which stress incontinence occurs is incompetence of the urethral sphincter resulting from weakness or deformity. Sphincter weakness may be caused by periurethral inflammation, lumbosacral spondylolisthesis, lesions of the cauda equina, or peripheral neuropathy. Sphincter deformity most often is a complication of surgery and is the most common cause of

A

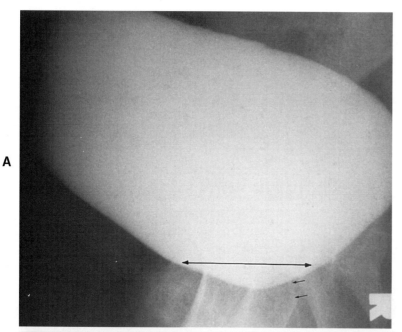

B

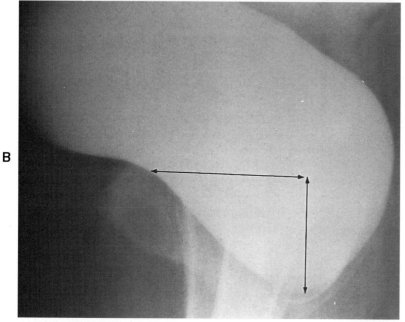

Fig. 6-45 Type IIA stress incontinence. **A,** At rest, a lateral view of the bladder shows the bladder base 0.8 cm below the superior margin of the pubic symphysis (horizontal line). A urethral catheter (small arrows) denotes the bladder neck. **B,** With straining, the bladder base descends 5.5 cm (vertical line) below the superior margin of the symphysis (horizontal line), and there was leakage of urine.

Table 6-4   Grading of Stress Incontinence*

	AT REST			WITH STRESS (COUGH/VALSALVA)		
Type	BB shape	BN-PU	BN-PU location	BN-PU opens?	BN-PU descends?	Urine leak
0	Flat	Closed	At or above SM-SP	Yes	Yes	No
I	Flat	Closed	AT or above IM-SP	Yes	< 2 cm	Yes
IIA	Flat	Closed	Above IM-SP	Yes	≥ 2 cm	Yes
IIB	Flat	Closed	Below IM-SP	Yes	May not	Yes
III	Cone shape	Open				

*Adapted from Blaivas JG, Olsson CA: Stress incontinence: classification and surgical approach, *J Urol* 139:727–731, 1988.

BB = bladder base; BN-PU = bladder neck–posterior urethra; SM-SP = superior margin of the symphysis pubis; IM-SP = inferior margin of the symphysis pubis.

Extraperitoneal remnant of allantois and umbilical
  arteries
Anomalies of closure: patent urachus, umbilical sinus,
  diverticulum, and urachal cyst
Often discovered because of secondary infection
Urachal adenocarcinoma: low attenuation components
  resulting from mucin; dystrophic calcification in
  70%; poor prognosis and transmural invasion occurs
  early

urinary incontinence in men. After radical prostatectomy, 5% to 10% of men become incontinent. Radiographically, the weakened female urethral sphincter is diagnosed when an upright cystogram demonstrates an open proximal urethra at rest in the absence of a detrusor contraction. In these patients, the treatment of choice is a pubovaginal sling, particularly in those who have recurrent stress incontinence despite urethropexy, or a sphincter prosthesis.

URACHAL ANOMALIES

The urachus is the tapered, ventrocephalic terminus of the fetal bladder, which communicates with the allantois at the level of the umbilicus (Box 6-17). It undergoes spontaneous closure by the middle of the second trimester, and the median umbilical ligament is its obliterated, fibrous remnant. The urachus is an extraperitoneal structure that is bordered anteriorly by the transversalis fascia and posteriorly by the peritoneum. Histologic study of

urachal remnants reveals an epithelial lining of transitional cells, although columnar metaplasia is seen in one third of specimens.

There are four anomalies of the urachal closure: patent urachus, umbilical urachal sinus, vesicourachal diverticulum, and urachal cyst. Congenital anomalies of the lower urinary tract often occur with the urachal anomalies. For example, patent urachus may occur with posterior urethral valves or complete urethral atresia. Urachal diverticulum is more common in patients with bladder outlet obstruction and may be complicated by stone formation or carcinoma (Fig. 6-46). Infection, the most common complication of the urachal anomaly, often precipitates its clinical presentation.

Urachal carcinoma is an extremely rare malignancy. Nearly 90% of urachal malignancies are adenocarcinomas, and one third of all primary bladder adenocarcinomas originate from urachal tissue. Discharge of blood or mucus from the umbilicus may occur, and the discovery of gross or microscopic mucus in the urine suggests the diagnosis. The location of the urachal tumor is supravesical and often midline, immediately posterior to the linea alba. In 60% of patients, the urachal adenocarcinoma contains low-attenuation components attributed to collections of mucin, and in 70% of patients, dystrophic calcification can be seen. The prognosis for patients with urachal adenocarcinoma is worse than for those with other bladder carcinomas because local invasion frequently has occurred before the diagnosis is suspected.

URINARY DIVERSIONS

Urinary diversions are surgical procedures designed to redirect the flow and collection of urine from the

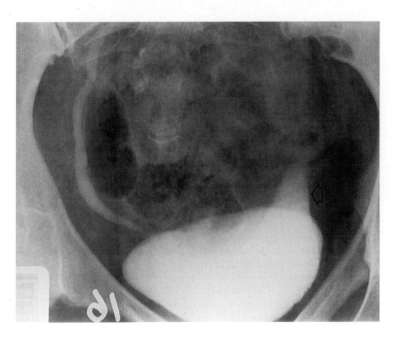

Fig. 6-46   Urachal diverticulum demonstrated by urography. Coned-down, oblique view shows contrast material in a cone-shaped diverticulum (open arrow) from the apex of the bladder.

bladder. The four most common clinical indications for urinary diversion are 1) management of muscle-invasive bladder cancer, 2) loss of the storage function of the bladder because of neurogenic bladder or congenital anomalies of the lower urinary tract, 3) medically or psychosocially incapacitating urinary incontinence, and 4) intractable symptoms referable to bladder abnormalities.

Box 6-18   Ileal Loop Complications

Early
    Obstruction (often at the ureteroileal anastomosis)
    Extravasation (anastomosis or at base of the loop)
Late
    Chronic pyelonephritis (resulting from chronic
        obstruction or reflux)
    Nephrolithiasis
    Obstruction (stenosis of ureter, loop, or stoma)

As the paradigm for a refluxing, noncontinent diversion, the ileal conduit uses a short segment of distal ileum for collection of urine. Typically, this segment is supplied by the ileocolic artery or a suitable large branch of the terminal superior mesenteric artery. One end of the isolated ileal segment is closed and is secured to either the sacral promontory or the retroperitoneum near the aortic bifurcation. The other end drains externally through a stoma typically placed in the right lower quadrant. This configuration permits continuous drainage of urine into a collecting device attached to the skin. End-to-side ureteroileal anastomoses are made approximately 2 to 3 cm above the closed end of the loop. Unless an antireflux mechanism is created, free vesicoureteral reflux is expected. To complete the anastomosis between the loop and the left ureter, the latter must pass under the base of the sigmoid mesentery, and, therefore, it is more likely than the right ureter to be angulated or under tension.

The radiologist must be aware of several complications of ileal diversion surgery, which can be classified by the expected time of occurrence (Box 6-18). Early postopera-

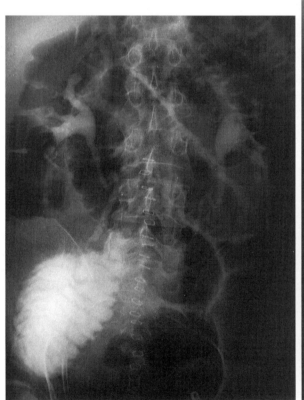
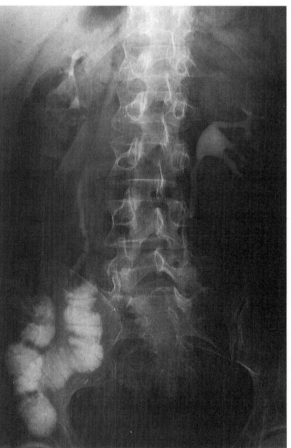

Fig. 6-47   Ileal conduit in the postoperative period. **A,** Routine intravenous urogram performed 6 days after construction of an ileal loop shows mild ureteropyelocaliectasis. The ileal loop also is dilated and is edematous. There is an adynamic ileus. **B,** Three months later, repeat urogram demonstrates a normal collecting system and ileal loop.

tive complications include obstruction and extravasation of urine. Both of these complications occur most often at the ureteroileal anastomosis, although extravasation also may be seen from the base of the loop. Late complications include chronic pyelonephritis, stone disease, neoplasm, and urinary obstruction caused by stenosis of the ureter, loop, or stoma. Chronic pyelonephritis occurs in 10% to 33% of patients and results from either chronic obstruction or reflux. Urinary tract infection plays a central role in the development of nephrolithiasis, which occurs in about 5% of diverted patients. Stone impaction causing obstruction at a narrowed ureteroileal anastomosis is a common presentation. Ureteral stricture resulting from fibrosis is a relatively late complication with an incidence of 5% to 7%. Predisposing factors include ischemia, radiation therapy, and urine extravasation. In nearly 20% of patients undergoing cystectomy for bladder cancer, severe ureteral epithelial atypia occurs. In up to 33% of patients, metachronous urothelial cancer in the ureter or renal pelvis may develop after cystectomy and urinary diversion. This complication should be suspected in any patient with ureteral stenosis, and it may be either an early or a late complication.

The ileal conduit usually is first studied radiologically about 10 days after surgery. IVU is performed to assess ureteral dilatation and the presence of extravasation (Fig. 6-47). Abdominal and pelvic CT is performed as a confirmatory examination when extravasation or abscess is suspected clinically or on the basis of IVU results, and it can be used to direct percutaneous drainage. Direct contrast instillation into the ileal loop is not performed routinely during the immediate postoperative period, although it is an invaluable examination any time thereafter when stenosis at the ileoureteral anastomosis is suspected. Renal ultrasonography or urography is used to follow renal parenchymal changes.

The continent urinary diversion is becoming increasingly popular because it removes the stigma of an external collection appliance and provides an effective alternative for the patient who is unable to maintain dryness with a conduit diversion. Some continent diversions open to the abdominal wall, but others can be constructed to permit emptying per urethra. The goals of the continent diversion are to create 1) a continence mechanism permitting facile intermittent emptying by self-catheterization, 2) a large capacity (500 to 1000 cc) and low pressure reservoir for urine collection, and 3) an antireflux mechanism at the anastomosis of the pouch and ureter. Continent reservoirs can be constructed from the terminal ileum and cecum together (Indiana, King, Mainz, and Penn techniques) or from the small bowel alone (Kock and Camey techniques). Incontinence, excessive leakage of urine at the stoma, and difficulty with catheterization are the most common late complications and may occur

---

Box 6-19   Urethral Stricture

Infectious or inflammatory
  Nongonococcal urethritis, gonococcus, or rarely
    tuberculosis
  Bulbar urethra
  Multiple and serial strictures
Iatrogenic (surgery, instrumentation, catheterization)
  Membranous urethra or penoscrotal junction
Traumatic
  Occurs after complete rupture
  Solitary, short stricture

---

in up to 18% of patients. Early and other late complications are similar to those described for the ileal loop.

STRICTURE OF THE URETHRA

The etiology of the urethral stricture is best determined from the clinical history and the patient's age (Box 6-19). The purpose of the radiographic evaluation is to assess the length, location, multiplicity, and severity of the urethral stricture, and to identify concomitant lesions that may complicate urethral obstruction.

Gonococcal and Nongonococcal Urethritis

Venereal infection of the male urethra with *Neisseria gonorrhoeae* begins in the mucosa and periurethral glands of Littré. Mucosal infection causes symptoms of dysuria and urethral discharge, but the presence and severity of these symptoms vary. Local extension of the infection to the posterior urethra, seminal vesicles, or epididymis occurs frequently in the untreated patient and rarely may occur in the patient who seeks prompt treatment. Nongonococcal urethritis (NGU) is diagnosed when urethral inflammation is present but *N. gonorrhoeae* cannot be detected by means of stain or culture. *Chlamydia trachomatis* and *Ureaplasma urealyticum* most commonly are cited as the cause of NGU, although other, less common pathogens may be responsible. The course of nongonococcal urethritis is more chronic and indolent than that of gonococcal urethritis, and postinflammatory strictures complicate 0.5% to 5% of patients with NGU.

When a patient has persistent or recurrent urethritis that appears to be unresponsive to antimicrobial treatment, urethral stricture or one of its complications, and prostate infection should be investigated. Stricture formation after an adequate course of appropriate antibiotics is thought to be uncommon, although it is estimated that

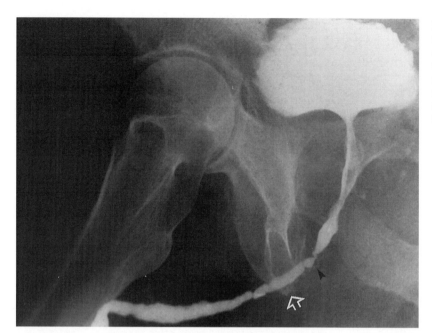

Fig. 6-48   Urethral strictures after gonococcal urethritis. Retrograde urethrogram demonstrates serial, short strictures of the anterior urethra. Urethral stricture resulting from infection or inflammation tends to be multiple and tends to involve the bulbar urethra. Cowper's duct (arrowhead) and glands of Littré (open arrow) are opacified. (Case courtesy of Mark S. Ridlen, MD)

in North America, 40% of urethral strictures are infectious in etiology. The proximal bulbar urethra is the site of stricture in 70% of patients with gonococcal urethritis because of the rather high concentration of periurethral glands in this area and the dependent position of this portion of the male urethra. Infectious strictures can be multiple and short or several centimeters long. Serial strictures are common. The glands of Littré may be opacified on urethrography in the presence of such strictures because of inflammatory dilatation of duct ostia. Backfilling of ducts or glands that empty into the urethra proximal to a stricture may be an important clue to the urodynamic significance of a stricture (Fig. 6-48). Gonococcal urethritis may incite mucosal hyperplasia, resulting in polypoid urethritis or urethritis cystica, which appears as flat, nodular filling defects that may be difficult to distinguish from carcinoma.

Tuberculous Urethritis

Urethral inflammation caused by *Mycobacteria tuberculosis* is reported to occur in only 2% of men with upper urinary tract tuberculosis. Antecedent traumatic or infectious urethral stricture is thought to be necessary for its development. However, direct extension of tuberculosis from the prostate gland to the prostatic urethra or from the perineal tissues to the bulbar urethra has been reported. Advanced tuberculosis of the urethra and periurethral tissues can produce the "watering can" perineum, which describes the radiographic appearance of multiple fistulous tracts from the urethra to the perineal soft tissues.

Iatrogenic Stricture

Stricture formation may complicate urethral surgery, instrumentation, or catheterization. Iatrogenic strictures most often occur in parts of the urethra that are anatomically fixed and narrow (i.e., the membranous urethra and the penoscrotal junction of the anterior urethra). No characteristic radiographic appearance of these strictures has been established; an iatrogenic stricture can be focal and short, multifocal, or long (Fig. 6-49).

Trauma

Traumatic stricture usually occurs after complete transection of the urethra, whereas partial laceration more likely heals without significant narrowing. As many as 97% of patients with injuries to the posterior urethra develop strictures requiring repeated dilatations or urethroplasty, regardless of initial treatment. The stricture that develops usually is solitary, less than 2 cm in length, and flanked by segments of urethra that are normal in caliber (Fig. 6-50). Typically, these strictures form more rapidly than inflammatory strictures.

Neoplasm

Stricture formation rarely is the sole manifestation of a urethral carcinoma, however, carcinoma should be suspected when stricture formation occurs in an elderly patient with no previous medical history of urethral surgery, instrumentation, or infection.

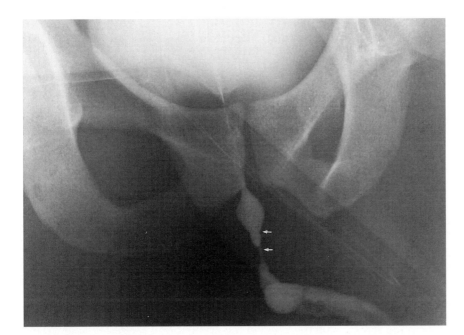

Fig. 6-49 Strictures of the urethra after instrumentation. Two strictures (arrows) of the membranous urethra developed several months after multiple failed attempts to catheterize the bladder. Iatrogenic strictures tend to occur where the urethra narrows.

Complications of Urethral Stricture

When severe, stricture formation can result in symptoms of urethral obstruction that prompt the patient to seek medical attention. Urethral obstruction may cause several other complications that can overshadow the inciting stricture (Box 6-20). Periurethral abscess and pseudodiverticula may form on the high-pressure side of the stricture (Fig. 6-51). Fistula formation, urinary extravasation, or venous intravasation also may occur, and any of these can be demonstrated readily with dynamic retrograde or micturition urethrography. False passages

are tracts that exit one part of the urethra, extend through the periurethral tissue, and reenter an adjacent segment of the urethra. These tracts develop after surgery or attempted dilatation of a stricture.

TRAUMATIC INJURY TO THE URETHRA

Injury to the male urethra should be suspected in a patient who is unable to void after pelvic trauma, when the bladder is distended on physical examination, and particularly when there is blood at, or bleeding from,

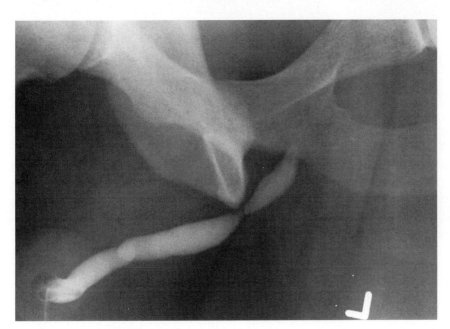

Fig. 6-50 Traumatic stricture of the urethra. Retrograde urethrogram demonstrates a focal, tight stricture of the bulbar urethra that developed 4 weeks after a straddle injury.

Box 6-20   Complications of Urethral Obstruction Secondary to Stricture

Periurethral abscess
Pseudodiverticula
Fistula
Extravasation of urine
Venous intravasation
False passages
Back-filling of ducts and glands

the urethral meatus. Transurethral catheterization of the bladder without confirming urethral integrity is strongly discouraged, because blind catheterization may complete a partial urethral tear or may enlarge a hematoma. Retrograde urethrography can be performed safely in the setting of pelvic trauma and is a reliable method for establishing and characterizing urethral injury in male patients. In contrast, rupture or avulsion of the female urethra is observed only after very severe pelvic injury, likely because it is short and relatively mobile. Traditionally, traumatic injury to the male urethra has been described by location, because the pathophysiology of posterior urethral rupture differs from that of anterior urethral rupture.

Posterior Urethra

Trauma to the posterior urethra occurs in approximately 10% of patients with fractures of the anterior bony pelvis. The shear force associated with pelvic fracture may disrupt the urethra and may cause severe injury to other parts of the lower genitourinary tract. Initially, the posterior urethral laceration is managed with suprapubic cystostomy for 3 to 6 months. Retrograde urethrography with steep oblique views is the initial diagnostic study of choice, although posterior urethral injuries can be imaged with CT or MR imaging. The goal of the radiologic evaluation is to assess the integrity of the urethra and, if there is urethral rupture, to identify its site and determine its severity. Colapinto and McCallum have proposed one classification system of posterior urethral injuries based on the presence and pattern of contrast extravasation (Table 6-5). Injury that produces urethral contusion or laceration but does not involve the full thickness of the urethral wall is referred to as a type 1 injury. On urethrograms, the posterior urethra appears intact but may be elongated. Type 2 injury, the most common variety, is the classic urethral rupture at the apex of the prostate, which spares the urogenital diaphragm. With urethrography, extravasated contrast material is localized to the retropubic extraperitoneal space, and the bulbar urethra is intact (Fig. 6-36). In type 3 injury, the urogenital diaphragm is disrupted, and extravasated contrast material is permitted to collect in the

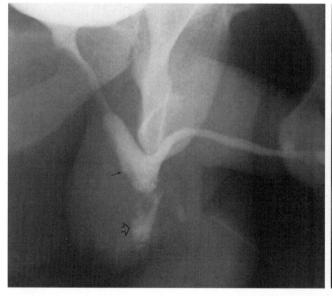
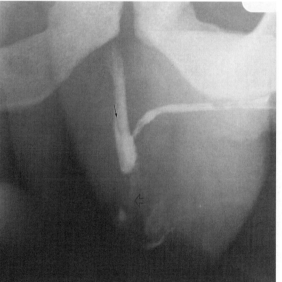

Fig. 6-51   Pseudodiverticulum and scrotal fistulas after urethroplasty. Oblique **(A)** and anteroposterior **(B)** retrograde urethrograms show a wide-mouthed diverticulum that originates from the bulbar urethra (small arrow). Unlike the normal bulbar urethra, the diverticulum has an indistinct margin on the oblique view. At surgery, linear and globular contrast collections (open arrows) were scrotal fistulas.

Table 6-5   Classification of Injury to the Male Posterior Urethra*

Type of injury	Injury to membranous urethra	FINDINGS WITH DYNAMIC RETROGRADE URETHROGRAPHY		
		Bulbar urethra	Contrast extravasation in perineum	Contrast extravasation in retropubic space
I	Contusion or partial tear	Stretched or normal	No	No
II	Complete rupture above UGD	Stretched or normal	No	Yes
III	Complete rupture above and below UGD	Ruptured	Yes	No

*Adapted from McCallum RW, Colapinto V: *Urological radiology of the adult male lower urinary tract*, Springfield, IL, 1976, Charles C Thomas.
UGD = urogenital diaphragm.

perineum. Not only is the posterior urethra ruptured at the apex of the prostate, but concomitant injury to the bulbar urethra is frequent (Fig. 6-52).

In addition to identifying the site of injury, the severity of partial or complete laceration also should be assessed during retrograde urethrography. Partial or incomplete posterior urethral rupture is implied when some retrograde filling of the bladder is achieved during urethrography. When extravasation from the posterior urethra occurs and when the bladder cannot be filled, the laceration is assumed to be complete. Type 2 injuries of the posterior urethra can be either partial or complete, but type 3 ruptures usually are complete. The distinction between partial and complete laceration is important because complete rupture, which is about twice as common as

partial laceration, is more likely to heal with formation of a short (<2 cm) stricture. Urethroplasty frequently is required for repair. In contrast, partial lacerations often heal uneventfully. If stricture does form after partial rupture, it can be repaired by dilatation or urethrotomy in most patients. The most serious consequences of traumatic disruption of the posterior urethra or its management are impotence and incontinence, which occur in 12% and 2% of patients, respectively, even with optimal treatment of the urethral injury.

Anterior Urethra

Injury to the anterior urethra may follow blunt perineal trauma in which the bulbar urethra and corpora spongiosum are crushed against the inferior aspect of the osseous anterior pelvic ring. Pelvic fracture typically is not associated with these straddle injuries. The most common cause of anterior urethral injury is iatrogenic, e.g., after instrumentation or attempted catheterization. As with posterior urethral injuries, the severity of anterior urethral lacerations can be classified as partial or complete. In partial injury, contrast material extravasation is seen during urethrography, but some continuity of the urethra is maintained, and the urethra proximal to the injury site can be opacified (Fig. 6-53). An abrupt discontinuity of the urethra at the site of extravasation is seen in complete urethral rupture, and no contrast material flows into the proximal urethra. In either situation, prominent opacification of the penile corpora and draining veins can be confusing if not anticipated. Stricture can complicate the healing of partial or complete anterior urethral lacerations.

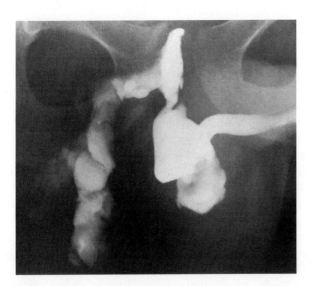

Fig. 6-52 Type 3 complete tear of the posterior urethra. Retrograde urethrogram demonstrates extravasation of contrast material into the perineum from the prostatic urethra. There also is a tear of the bulbar urethra. Type 3 tear is likely the most common injury in patients with urethral transection resulting from pelvic fracture. Note diastasis of the symphysis pubis.

FILLING DEFECTS IN THE URETHRA

Common and uncommon causes of filling defects in the urethra are listed in Box 6-21.

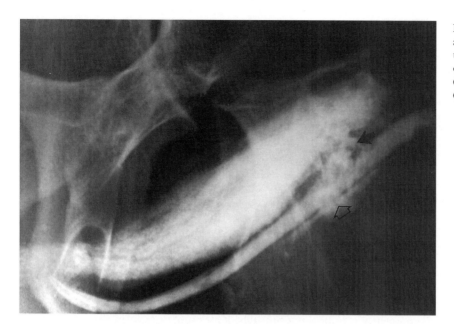

Fig. 6-53 Partial tear of the anterior urethra after blunt trauma to the perineum. Retrograde urethrogram demonstrates extravasation of contrast material into the corpus spongiosum (open arrow) and the corpus cavernosum (solid arrow) from a tear of the penile urethra.

Urethral Stone Disease

Urethral calculi occur when renal or bladder stones migrate into the urethra. These migrant stones are 10 times more common than stones that form de novo in the urethra. Migrant stones are more likely to cause symptoms associated with sudden urethral obstruction; the patient may experience dysuria, a poor urinary stream, or recurrent episodes of urethritis. Anatomy that predisposes patients to primary urethral stone formation includes diverticula or pseudodiverticula and urethral stricture (Fig. 6-54). It is unusual for primary urethral stones to cause acute symptoms because they are formed slowly or are sequestered in diverticula.

Technical and interpretive errors account for the observation that only 40% of urethral stones are diagnosed with plain film and IVU. The area inferior to the symphysis often is neglected during radiographic interpretation or is excluded on the routine overhead film. Hence, voiding cystourethrography, retrograde urethrography, and cystourethroscopy are the best methods for diagnosing urethral stones. The majority of urethral stones are radiopaque and may appear as fixed or mobile filling defects at dynamic retrograde urethrography. The calculus most often is found in a midurethral diverticulum in the female patient, and in the male patient it is discovered frequently in the bulbar or prostatomembranous urethra (Fig. 6-55).

Carcinoma of the Female Urethra

Carcinoma of the urethra is the only epithelial malignancy of the urinary tract that occurs more frequently in women (Box 6-22). The peak age range in which these neoplasms present is 40 to 60 years. Chronic irritation and inflammation likely incite malignant epithelial change because benign inflammatory lesions, such as fibrous polyps and caruncle, may be discovered synchronously. Patients present with urethral bleeding, dysuria, frequency, perineal pain, or urethral obstruction. SCC, which occurs in 75% of patients, is the most common

---

Box 6-21 Filling Defects in the Urethra

Common
  Calculus
  Polyp
Uncommon
  Carcinoma
  Condylomata acuminata
  Polypoid urethritis
  Malacoplakia
  Urethritis cystica
  Metastases
  Amyloidosis

Box 6-22 Urethral Carcinoma

2 to 5 times more common in women
Two thirds originate from bulbomembranous urethra
Associated with stricture of anterior urethra
Squamous cell carcinoma found in 75%; transitional
  cell carcinoma in 15%

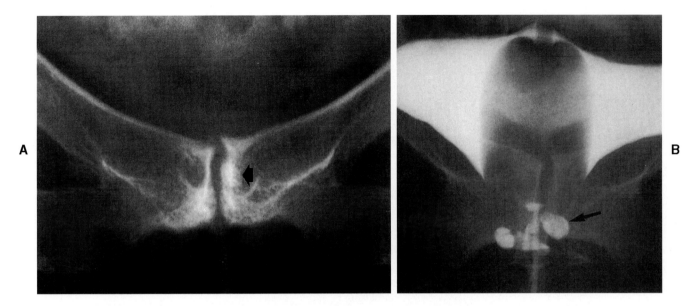

Fig. 6-54   Urethral calculus in a diverticulum. **A,** Coned-down plain film shows an oval calcification (arrow) overlying the pubic symphysis. **B,** Double balloon urethrogram demonstrates two diverticula in the midurethra. The stone is a faint filling defect (arrow) in the left-sided diverticulum.

histopathologic type, followed by TCC. Adenocarcinoma is the most common malignancy to occur in a urethral diverticulum, which reflects the origin of diverticula from infection and abscess formation in paraurethral Bartholin's glands. Urethral carcinomas appear as single or serial irregular filling defects within the urethra on positive-pressure urethrography. Stricture is infrequent. The extent of local tumor invasion and lymph node involvement can be evaluated by CT or MR imaging (Fig. 6-56). Lymphogenous spread occurs before hematogenous dissemination in most patients. Carcinomas that originate in the distal third of the female urethra preferentially spread to the superficial and deep inguinal nodes, whereas those originating from the proximal two thirds spread to the external and internal iliac node groups preferentially (Fig. 6-57).

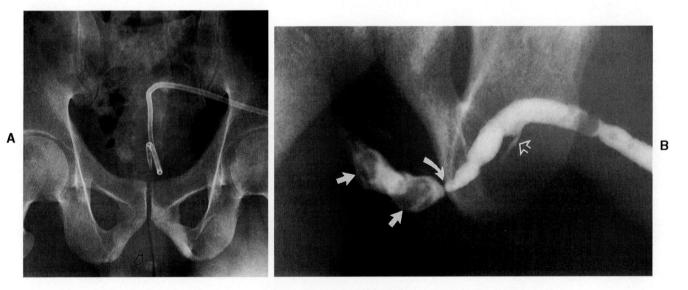

Fig. 6-55   Urethal calculi on the high-pressure side of a stricture. **A,** Plain film demonstrates calculi in the pelvis (arrow) and perineum (open arrow) of a 44-year-old man with bladder-outlet obstruction that required suprapubic cystostomy. **B,** Coned-down, magnified oblique view from a retrograde urethrogram demonstrates two filling defects (arrows) in the bulbar urethra proximal to a tight stricture (curved arrow). There is opacification of Cowper's duct (open arrow).

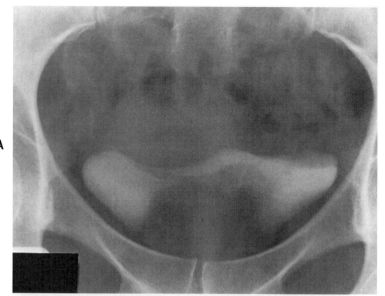

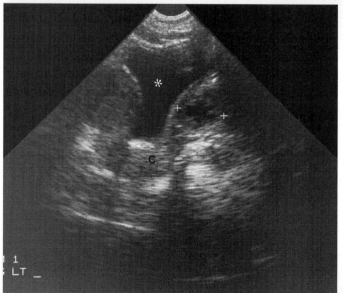

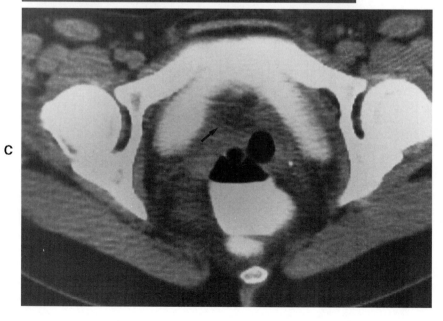

Fig. 6-56 Squamous cell carcinoma of the urethra in a 43-year-old woman with hematuria and perineal pain. **A,** Coned-down urogram during the cystographic phase demonstrates a large filling defect along the floor of the bladder (female prostate sign). **B,** Sagittal sonogram shows a mass (between electronic markers) that does not originate from the bladder wall (c = cervix; * = bladder lumen). **C,** Infused CT demonstrates extrinsic displacement of the bladder neck by a low-density mass (arrow); no lymphadenopathy was seen. (Case courtesy of Isabel C. Yoder, MD)

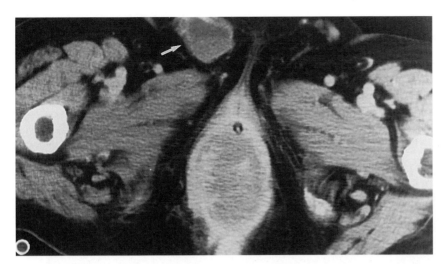

Fig. 6-57   Spread of perineal carcinoma to the inguinal lymph nodes. Infused CT of the pelvis shows a large hypodense mass in the perineum, which had invaded and obstructed the distal urethra. In the right inguinal region, there is a large necrotic lymph node (arrow). Tumors that originate from or that invade the distal third of the female urethra preferentially spread to the inguinal nodes.

Carcinoma of the Male Urethra

Carcinoma of the male urethra is almost exclusively a disease of the older population, occurring predominantly in men aged more than 50 years. Two risk factors predispose to the development of urethral carcinoma: a medical history of chronic urethral inflammation or sexually transmitted disease and urethral stricture, which is seen in up to 75% of patients. The onset of symptoms is insidious; initial clinical complaints include poor urinary stream, serosanguinous discharge, or hematuria. Almost 80% of all urethral carcinomas are SCCs. Two thirds originate in the bulbar or membranous urethra, and the majority of the remaining carcinomas are found in the anterior urethra, especially the fossa navicularis. TCC accounts for 15% of urethral carcinomas; in most patients, it originates in the posterior urethra. An association also exists between TCC of the prostatic urethra and previous transurethral resection of bladder carcinoma. The diagnosis of urethral carcinoma is made on urethroscopy or urethrography. Carcinoma appears as an irregular filling defect, which may be eccentric or circumferential. This diagnosis also should be suspected when the margin of a stricture is irregular or poorly defined. Spread of carcinoma almost always is initially lymphogenous. Carcinomas of the penile urethra spread to the deep inguinal and external iliac lymph nodes. Bulbar and posterior urethral carcinomas involve the internal iliac or obturator nodes before spread occurs to more proximal nodal stations.

Benign Neoplasm

A fibrous polyp (also known as a congenital urethral polyp or fibroepithelial polyp) consists of a fibrovascular connective tissue core that is lined by urothelium. This lesion usually is discovered in children but can occur in young adults. Fibrous polyps usually are pedunculated,

and the base of the stalk originates near the verumontanum. The polyp itself appears as a well-defined, smooth, finger-like filling defect, approximately 1 to 1.5 cm in length. Mobility of the polyp with urination is demonstrable as the force of the urinary stream carries the polyp distally (Fig. 6-58). Hence, patients may present with bladder outlet obstruction or intermittent interruption of the urinary stream. Transitional cell and squamous cell papillomas are benign mesenchymal growths that are lined by urothelium and metaplastic squamous cells, respectively. These lesions usually are discovered in patients aged 20 to 40 years. Symptoms include hematuria, local pruritus, and urethral discharge. Papillomas mostly are found at the fossa navicularis and parameatal area in male patients and at the distal third of the urethra in female patients, in whom they are referred to as urethral caruncles. Transitional cell papillomas also may be found in the prostatic urethra and can be associated with papillomas in the urinary bladder. At urethrography, papillomas can appear as single or multiple smooth, sessile filling defects.

Condylomata Acuminata

Condylomata acuminata, or venereal warts, are caused by a DNA-virus of the papilloma family and are transmitted by sexual contact. Dermal papillomas of the genitalia and around the anus can spread to the urethra, vagina, and rectum. As many as 5% of patients with penile condylomata also may have urethral lesions, which usually are limited to the anterior urethra. In addition, condylomata acuminata precede or are present in up to 16% of patients with SCC of the vulva. The appearance of condylomata acuminata images is that of multiple, sessile filling defects of the anterior urethra. An associated stricture, although typical of carcinoma, is atypical with condylomata acuminata.

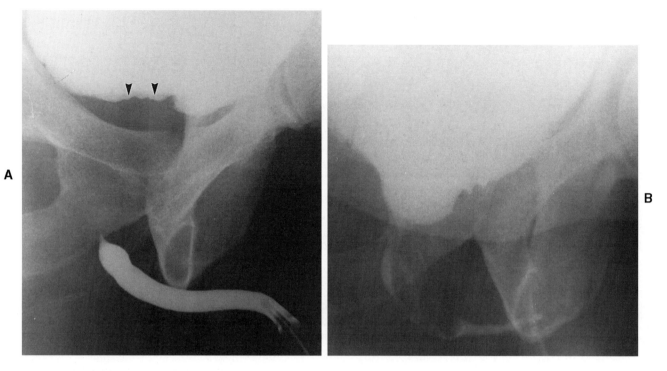

Fig. 6-58   Prolapsing fibrous polyp of the posterior urethra. **A,** Percutaneous cystogram shows a slightly lobulated filling defect (arrowheads) near the bladder neck. A normal anterior urethra is demonstrated with retrograde urethrography, but the posterior urethra could not be opacified. **B,** Voiding cystourethrogram shows an oblong, polypoid filling defect in the posterior urethra. Fibrous polyps can be long and pedunculated; the force of the urinary stream may cause antegrade prolapse and urethral obstruction.

Metastases to the Urethra

In male and female patients, bladder and colorectal carcinomas can involve the urethra through extensive local spread. Prostate, cervical, and vaginal cancers also may invade the urethra secondarily.

URETHRAL OUTPOUCHING OR TRACT

Common and uncommon causes of paraurethral outpouching or tract are listed in Box 6-23.

Acquired Diverticulum (Pseudodiverticulum)

Urethral diverticulum may be either a congenital or an acquired lesion. Congenital saccular diverticulum is a rare lesion of the midpenile urethra that may cause high-grade obstruction in children. After posterior urethral valves, it is the most common cause of urethral obstruction in male infants. It frequently is difficult to distinguish congenital diverticulum from an anterior urethral valve. In contrast with the congenital urethral diverticulum, the

acquired diverticulum presents in adults. An acquired diverticulum also is termed a pseudodiverticulum because it is lined by fibrous tissue or inflammatory cells rather than urothelium. There are several possible reasons why acquired diverticula form. The most common explanation is infection and abscess formation in female paraurethral glands, which decompress into the urethra. Similarly, a prostatic abscess also may form a pseudodiverticulum if it spontaneously drains into the urethra. Patients who are catheterized for an extended time may

---

Box 6-23   Paraurethral Outpouching or Tract

Common
    (Pseudo)diverticulum
    Fistula
Uncommon
    Cowper's duct or gland
    Glands of Littré
    Müllerian remnants (utricle or müllerian cyst)

develop a diverticulum as a result of pressure necrosis, which is an erosion of the inferior wall of the bulbar urethra at the penoscrotal junction as a result of an improperly worn Foley catheter. Pseudodiverticula also may form on the high-pressure side of a urethral stricture. Stasis of urine within a diverticulum creates a suitable environment for stone formation and urinary tract infection.

Diverticula may be suspected on films of the bladder taken during IVU because a diverticulum of sufficient size may elevate the base of the bladder (the "female prostate" sign). In the female patient, double balloon urethrography is the best examination for detecting a urethral diverticulum and is more accurate than cystourethroscopy (Figs. 6-54, 6-59). The acquired diverticulum most often is located posteriorly to the midurethra in female patients and at the penoscrotal junction in male patients. It will appear as either a unilocular or multilocular, round, and sharply marginated collection of contrast material separate from, but adjacent to, the urethra. It is important to search for an associated urethral stricture distal to the diverticulum. Perineal fistula also

may be demonstrated, especially when acquired diverticula occur after trauma or urethritis (Fig. 6-51).

Fistula

Urethral fistula may form if there is an impediment to closure and healing after urethral rupture or laceration. This impediment may be elevated intraurethral pressure that occurs proximal to an obstruction. Rectal or gynecologic surgery, obstetric injury, and radiation therapy also have been implicated in urethral fistula formation. Fistulas from the urethra may end blindly in the soft tissues of the perineum, or they may communicate with another structure such as colorectum or vagina, with pelvic organs such as the uterus, or with the skin of the perineum or penis.

Voiding urethrography, dynamic retrograde urethrography, or fistulography can demonstrate these abnormal passages from the urethra. The fistula itself usually is an irregular tract or cavity that can have a variety of shapes and sizes (Fig. 6-51). As with a urethral diverticulum, it is important to seek a coexistent abnormal process, such as a stricture or carcinoma, that may have incited fistula formation.

Cowper's Duct and Gland

Paired Cowper's ducts enter the ventral surface of the perineal portion of the bulbous urethra. The length of the duct varies from a few millimeters to 6 cm, and duct width varies from 1 mm to 6 to 8 mm. The ducts extend backward adjacent to the undersurface of the bulbar urethra as far back as the urogenital diaphragm, in which Cowper's glands are embedded. The ducts have a gentle curvature and a smooth contour. Opacification of Cowper's duct or gland during retrograde urethrography may accompany a stricture distal to, or urethral inflammation around, the opening of the duct at the bulbar urethra (Figs. 6-48, 6-55B). Opacification of the duct or the duct and gland should not be misinterpreted as evidence of a urethral diverticulum or fistula, particularly in the setting of a urethral stricture.

Müllerian Remnants

The paramesonephric or müllerian duct system regresses in the male subject as a result of an inhibiting substance produced by the developing testis. A cranial remnant of the duct may persist as the appendix testis and Müller's tubercle; the caudal tip of the duct remains as the verumontanum. Incomplete obliteration of the caudal part of the ductal system may give rise to tubular, vagina-like structures or cysts lying between the bladder and rectum. The prostatic utricle has come to be viewed as the homologue of the uterus (utriculus masculinus)

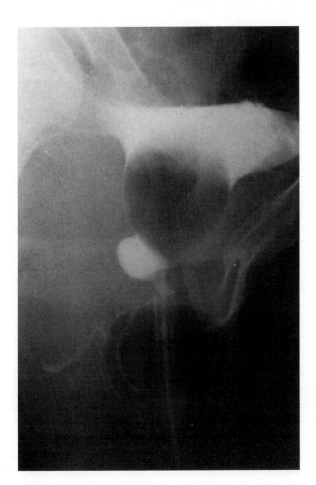

Fig. 6-59 Typical appearance of a urethral diverticulum on double-balloon urethrogram. Oblique view shows a unilocular, well-defined collection of contrast posterior to the midurethra.

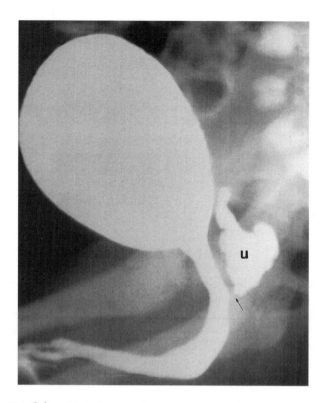

Fig. 6-60 Utriculus masculinus in a patient with congenital adrenal hyperplasia and pseudohermaphroditism. Oblique view from a voiding cystourethrogram demonstrates an outpouching (u) dorsal to the prostatic urethra. Its shape is similar to that of a uterine cavity. A narrow tract (arrow) connects it to the prostatic urethra.

and, therefore, a derivative of the caudal remnant of the paramesonephric ducts. The utricle may become visibly enlarged with maldevelopment of genitalia, as in hypospadias, cryptorchidism, or intersex states. Müllerian duct cysts are thought to occur when there is incomplete closure of a part of the paramesonephric duct or when cystic dilatation of the utricle occurs as a result of obstruction and accumulation of prostatic secretions. In contrast to the utricle, müllerian duct cysts occur most often in patients with no congenital anomalies and with normal genitalia. The majority of müllerian cysts and enlarged prostatic utricles are asymptomatic, but, occasionally, stagnant urine in the utricle leads to infection and stone formation. Mass effect from a müllerian cyst may cause frequency, urinary obstructive symptoms, infertility, or deep perineal pain during micturition or defecation.

The prostatic utricle can be seen on retrograde or voiding urethrography, transrectal sonography, CT, or MR imaging. It appears as an outpouching that extends proximally from the verumontanum, maintaining a narrow tract with the prostatic urethra (Fig. 6-60). It can be millimeters to several centimeters in length. The müllerian cyst may be imaged on a urethrogram when extrinsic mass effect on the posterior urethra is noted; in general, however, there is no direct communication with the

prostatic urethra. These cysts are located posteriorly to the prostate and most often are midline in position. Müllerian duct cysts must be differentiated from cysts of the seminal vesicle, ejaculatory duct, and prostate. Transrectal sonography or MR imaging with an endorectal surface coil is best suited to this task.

SUGGESTED READINGS

Aldrete J, ReMine W: Vesicoenteric fistula: a complication of colonic cancer. Long-term results of its surgical treatment, *Arch Surg* 94:627, 1967.

Amis E, Newhouse J, Olsson C: Continent urinary diversions: review of current surgical procedures and radiologic imaging, *Radiology* 168:395–401, 1988.

Barentsz J, Rujis S, Strijk S: The role of MR imaging in carcinoma of the urinary bladder, *AJR Am J Roentgenol* 160:937–947, 1993.

Bowie W: Nongonococcal urethritis, *Urol Clin North Am* 11:55–63, 1984.

Buy J, Moss A, Guinet C, et al: MR staging of bladder carcinoma: correlation with pathologic findings, *Radiology* 169:695–700, 1988.

Colapinto V, McCallum R: Injury to the male posterior urethra in fractured pelvis: a new classification, *J Urol* 118:575–580, 1977.

Currarino G, Fuqua F: Cowper's glands on urethrogram, *AJR Am J Roentgenol* 116:838–842, 1972.

Dalal S, Siegel J, Burgess A: Pelvic fractures in multiple trauma: classification by mechanism is key to pattern of organ injury, resuscitative requirements and outcome, *J Trauma* 29:981–1002, 1984.

Dooms G, Hricak H, Crooks L, et al: Magnetic resonance imaging of lymph nodes: comparison with CT, *Radiology* 153:719–728, 1984.

Doringer E, Joos H, Forstner R, et al: MR imaging of bladder carcinoma: tumor staging and gadolinium contrast behaviour, *Fortschr Röntgenstr* 154:357–363, 1991.

Gibod L, Katz M, Cochand B, et al: Lymphography and percutaneous fine needle node aspiration biopsy in the staging of bladder cancer, *J Urol* 132:24–26, 1984.

Goldman S, Fishman E, Gatewood O, et al: CT in the diagnosis of enterovesical fistula, *AJR Am J Roentgenol* 144:1229–1233, 1985.

Harrison W: Gonococcal urethritis, *Urol Clin North Am* 11:45–53, 1984.

Hillman B, Silver M, Cook G, et al: Recognition of bladder tumors by excretory urography, *AJR Am J Roentgenol* 138:319–323, 1981.

Husband J, Olliff J, Williams M, et al: Bladder cancer: staging with CT and MR imaging, *Radiology* 173:435–440, 1989.

Kane N, Francis I, Ellis J: Value of CT in the detection of bladder and posterior urethra injury, *AJR Am J Roentgenol* 153:1243–1246, 1989.

Karamchandani M, West Jr C: Vesicoenteric fistulas, *Am J Surg* 147:681–683, 1984.

Liebskind A, Elkin M, Goldman S: Herniation of the bladder, *Radiology* 106:257, 1973.

Lis L, Cohen A: CT cystography in the evaluation of bladder trauma, *JCAT* 14:386–389, 1990.

Neuerburg J, Bohndorf K, Sogn M, et al: Urinary bladder neoplasms: evaluation with contrast-enhanced MR imaging, *Radiology* 172:739–743, 1989.

Nordling J, Meyerhoff H, Oleson K: Cysto-urethrographic appearance of the bladder and posterior urethra in neuromuscular disorders of the lower urinary tract, *Scan J Urol Nephrol* 16:115–124, 1982.

Rholl K, Lee J, Heiken J, et al: Primary bladder carcinoma: evaluation with MR imaging, *Radiology* 163:117–121, 1987.

Shah P, Whiteside C, Milroy E, et al: Radiological trabeculation of the male bladder—a clinical and urodynamic assessment, *Br J Urol* 53:567–570, 1981.

Tachibana M, Baba S, Deguchi N, et al: Efficacy of gadolinium-diethylenetriaminepentaacetic acid-enhanced magnetic resonance imaging for differentiation between superficial and muscle-invasive tumor of the bladder: a comparative study with computerized tomography and transurethral sonography, *J Urol* 145:1169–1173, 1991.

Umerah B: The less familiar manifestations of schistosomiasis of the urinary tract, *Br J Radiol* 50:105–109, 1977.

Ward J: Diagnosis and treatment of colovesical fistulas, *Surg Gynecol Obstet* 130:1082–1090, 1970.

Webster G, Mathes G, Selli C: Prostatomembranous urethral injuries: a review of the literature and a rational approach to their management, *J Urol* 130:898–902, 1983.

Yousem D, Gatewood O, Goldman S, et al: Synchronous and metachronous transitional cell carcinoma of the urinary tract: prevalence, incidence, and radiologic detection, *Radiology* 167:613–618, 1988.

The Female Genital Tract

Medical imaging has assumed an increasingly important role in the diagnostic evaluation of gynecologic disease, which in part, is because sonography and MR imaging can provide high-resolution and multiplanar imaging of the female reproductive tract without exposing the ovaries to ionizing radiation. In this chapter, gynecologic radiology is reviewed in two parts. The first part is an overview of the embryology, anatomy, and physiology of the female reproductive tract. In addition, the sonographic method for measuring the ovary and uterus and normal values for these measurements are discussed. The second part of the chapter reviews the imaging of selected gynecologic diseases, including congenital anomalies, pelvic pain, ovarian cyst, infertility, and gynecologic oncology.

THE NORMAL FEMALE REPRODUCTIVE TRACT

Embryology of the Ovary

Large primordial germ cells appear with other cells in the wall of the yolk sac at about 3 weeks gestation. After migrating along the dorsal mesentery of the hindgut, these germ cells collect along the urogenital ridge in cortical sex cords. Among the non-germ cell population of the sex cords are granulosa and theca cells. It appears that two X chromosomes must exist for normal ovarian development to occur. For example, in Turner's syn-

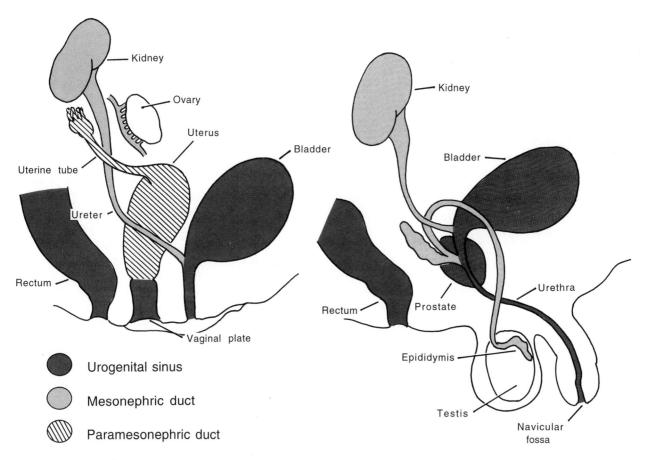

Fig. 7-1   Derivatives of embryonic urogenital structures. The vestigial remnant of the paramesonephric (müllerian) duct in the male subject is the appendix of the testis. The vestigial remnants of the mesonephric (wolffian) duct and tubule in the female subject include the duct of Gartner (in the anterolateral vagina) and the paroophoron and epoophoron (adjacent to the uterus in the broad ligament or mesosalpinx). (Modified from Moore KL: *Before we are born: Basic embryology and birth defects,* ed 2, Philadelphia, 1983, W. B. Saunders.)

drome (45XO), rudimentary ovarian remnants or streak ovaries are found; however, when there are multiple XX chromosomes, the presence of a Y chromosome favors testicular differentiation of the gonad, as in Klinefelter's syndrome (47XXY).

Embryology of the Genital Ducts

The upper vagina, cervix, uterus, and uterine (fallopian) tubes are formed from the paramesonephric or müllerian ducts (Fig. 7-1). The cranial end of each duct opens into the coelomic cavity and will become the ostia of the uterine tubes. The caudal end of the two paramesonephric ducts crosses dorsally to the mesonephric ducts and approximates in the midline. The distal point of fusion is called the müllerian tubercle. The tubercle meets the urogenital septum to form the uterovaginal primordium.

Degeneration of the mesonephric, or wolffian, ducts begins during the second trimester of pregnancy in the

female fetus. Vestigial remnants of these ducts may persist in the anterolateral vagina (Gartner's duct cyst or Gartner's duct) or adjacent to the uterus within the broad ligament or mesosalpinx (paroophoron or epoophoron).

Anatomy of the Female Genital Tract

The uterus

The uterus is a thick-walled muscular organ that lies in the true pelvis between the bladder anteriorly and the rectosigmoid posteriorly. It consists of an inner mucosa (endometrium), a middle muscular layer (myometrium), and an outer serosa (perimetrium). The uterus is divided at the internal os into the corpus and cervix; the fundus and cornua are parts of the corpus uteri. The fallopian tubes insert at the cornua, and the fundus is the dome of the corpus, located superior to the cornua. The uterine cervix projects into the vagina and separates the vagina into anterior, posterior, and two lateral fornices. The arterial supply of the uterus comes primarily from the

Box 7-1   Endometrial Stripe Thickness

Outer-to-outer margin on sagittal image
Proliferative phase—up to 11 mm
Secretory phase—up to 16 mm
Mean normal in postmenopause 4-8 mm
May increase to 12 mm with hormone replacement
   therapy
Postmenopausal bleeding and endometrial stripe
   thickness is
   < 5 mm, then biopsy yield is low (endometrial
      atrophy)
   > 8 mm, then biopsy (polyps, hyperplasia, or
      carcinoma)

uterine artery, a branch of the anterior trunk of the internal iliac artery. The uterine arteries anastomose extensively with each other across the midline through arcuate arteries and reach the hilum of the ovary to join the ipsilateral ovarian artery.

The uterus is connected to the bladder, rectum, and pelvic walls by ligaments. The broad ligaments are peritoneal folds that extend from the lateral sides of the uterus to the pelvic walls. The fallopian tubes and uterine arteries lie in the leaves of the broad ligament, and the ovary is attached posteriorly by the mesovarium.

The size of the uterus varies with patient age, parity, and the menstrual cycle. The relative contribution of the fundus, corpus, and cervix to the length of the uterus varies with menstrual status. In the neonate, the size of the uterine fundus may be equal to or slightly larger than that of the cervix. However, in the infant or prepubertal girl, the corpus is much smaller than the cervix, which may contribute two thirds to five sixths of the uterine length. In the premenstrual girl, the anteroposterior dimension of the cervix may be twice that of the uterine body. At menarche, growth of the uterine corpus accelerates relative to that of the cervix, so that in the mature woman, the fundus and body constitute two thirds of the uterine length.

Various measurements of the uterus can be obtained from hysterosalpingography, sonography, computed tomography (CT), and MR imaging. Sonography often is used to ascertain the linear dimensions of the uterus, and from these, the volume and weight of the uterus can be estimated. The length and height (maximal anteroposterior diameter) of the uterus are measured on the midline sagittal image. The appropriate sagittal plane on which to measure uterine length and height is the one in which the maximal length of the central endometrial echo complex is seen. The length measurement is the distance between the top of the uterine fundus and the external cervical os; uterine height is the maximal perpendicular to the length measurement. The width of the uterus is measured in a transverse plane orthogonal to the sagittal plane in which the height was measured. For the nulliparous woman, the normal upper limits of uterine dimensions are length, 9 cm; width, 5 cm; and height, 4 cm. The ranges of linear dimensions for the postmenopausal uterus are length, 6.0 ± 1.2 cm; height, 2 ± 1 cm; and width, 3 ± 1 cm.

The appearance of the normal central endometrial echo complex varies with the menstrual cycle and can be measured in the sagittal plane by transabdominal sonography (Box 7-1). In the early proliferative phase, the endometrium appears as a single, echogenic line. In the midfollicular phase, three longitudinal lines can be seen in the center of the uterus. The outer lines represent the echo-interface between the myometrium and endometrium, and the central line is the uterine canal. Within 48 hours of ovulation, the trilaminar appearance of the endometrium disappears, indicating the onset of the secretory endometrium. The distance between the outer lines of the endometrial echo complex can be measured (outer-to-outer border), and cycle-specific normal limits have been established for each phase: menstrual, 2 to 3 mm; early proliferative, 5 ± 1 mm; periovulatory, 10 ± 1 mm; and late secretory, up to 16 mm (Fig. 7-2). In the

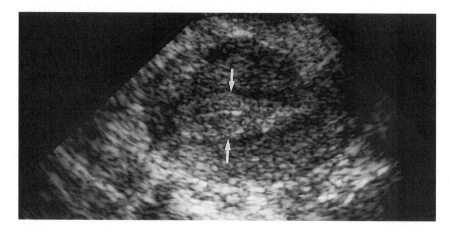

Fig. 7-2   Endometrial echo complex. The distance between the outer lines of the echogenic endometrial echo (arrows) is measured on a sagittal endovaginal sonogram. In postmenopausal women, this distance should not exceed 8 mm.

postmenopausal woman, the width of the hyperechoic interface should be no thicker than 8 mm, although in women who are receiving estrogen, the normal endometrium may measure up to 12 mm.

The ovary

The internal structure of the ovary consists of an outer, thick cortex surrounding a vascular medulla. The cortex contains ovarian follicles, corpora lutea, and stroma. The medulla is composed of fibrous stroma and multiple vessels. The ovaries are attached to the posterosuperior surface of the broad ligament, and the fimbriae of the uterine tube lie near the superior pole of the ovary. In nulliparous women, the ovary usually is situated in the ovarian fossa (Waldeyer's fossa); the ovarian fossa is bounded by the external iliac vein superiorly, the obliterated umbilical artery anteriorly, and the internal iliac artery and ureter posteriorly. The ovarian artery originates from the aorta just inferior to the renal arteries. The arteries reach the ovarian hilum through the suspensory ligament of the ovary. The ovarian veins course parallel to the arteries; the left ovarian vein empties into the left renal vein, and the right ovarian vein empties into the inferior vena cava just inferior to the right renal vein.

The size of the ovary is determined from orthogonal linear dimensions, and because ovaries vary in shape, ovarian volume is considered the most accurate method for comparing ovarian size. The length and height (anteroposterior dimension) of the ovary traditionally are measured from a parasagittal plane. The length is designated as the maximal dimension of the ovary in a parasagittal plane, and the height is measured in the same plane. Finally, the width is measured in a transverse plane, which is orthogonal to that in which the length and height were determined. The volume of the ovary then is estimated by using the formula for a prolate ellipsoid: volume (cc) = 0.52 × length × height × width. Cohen et al report a mean ovarian volume of 9.8 cm^3 (95% confidence value, 21.9 cm^3) during the fertile years. The mean for the postmenopausal woman was 5.8 cm^3 (95% confidence value, 14.1 cm^3). There does not appear to be a significant change in the volume of the adult ovary during the menstrual cycle unless a dominant follicular cyst develops. There also is no statistically significant difference between the size of the left ovary and that of the right ovary.

In two thirds of healthy postmenopausal women, the ovaries can be identified on sonograms; therefore, simple sonographic visualization of the postmenopausal ovary does not imply abnormality. Full atresia of the ovaries does not occur until an average of 4 years after cessation of menses. The postmenopausal ovary should not be considered abnormal unless the volume of the ovary is either twice the contralateral ovary or that of an age-matched control subject. Postmenopausal ovaries identified at surgery are not demonstrated by transvaginal sonography (TVS) in about 20% of patients; TVS can identify most ovaries larger than 1.5 cm in diameter. Numerous studies have shown that the incidence of carcinoma in small, completely cystic ovarian lesions is extremely low. As a general rule, a unilateral cystic adnexal mass in postmenopausal women that is smaller than 5 cm, contains no septations or mural nodules, and is not associated with ascites has a negligible incidence of malignancy. It should be noted that most of these studies were done with transabdominal ultrasound techniques. Many cysts that appear unilocular on transabdominal ultrasound evaluation may have fine internal echoes or thin septations on TVS studies.

Either transabdominal or TVS provides a noninvasive means for directly monitoring follicular development, ovulation, and corpus luteum formation in spontaneous and induced cycles. The range of the mean follicular diameter before ovulation is 20 to 25 mm. The corpus luteum may appear as a spherical, predominantly cystic mass containing a highly echogenic portion or as a septated, cystic mass containing elements of varying echogenicity. The diameter of the corpus luteum should not exceed 40 mm unless complicated by cyst formation or hemorrhage.

Fallopian (uterine) tubes

The fallopian (uterine) tube is a muscular conduit that lies in the upper margin of the broad ligament. The fallopian tube measures 7 to 12 cm and is divided into four parts: interstitial, isthmus, ampulla, and infundibulum. The interstitial (intramural) part is contained in the uterine wall, is the narrowest part of the tube, and ends as the uterine ostium. The medial third of the tube is the cord-like isthmus, which inserts at the cornua of the corpus uteri. The isthmus is continuous laterally with the wider and more tortuous ampulla. The infundibulum is the expanded end of the ampulla and terminates as the peritoneal opening at the fimbriated end of the tube. One of these fimbria is attached to the superior pole of the ovary.

Physiology of the Ovary, Menstrual Cycle, and Menopause

Physiology of the ovary

Primordial germ cells originate from endodermal cells lining the yolk sac and migrate to the genital ridge adjacent to the mesonephric kidney (Fig. 7-3). By the end of the first trimester, the ovary begins to produce estrogen, and some oogonia in the ovarian cortex begin to develop into primary oocytes. Oocyte proliferation and division are suspended after the first meiotic division until puberty. Under the influence of the pituitary gonadotropins, follicle-stimulating hormone (FSH), and luteinizing hor-

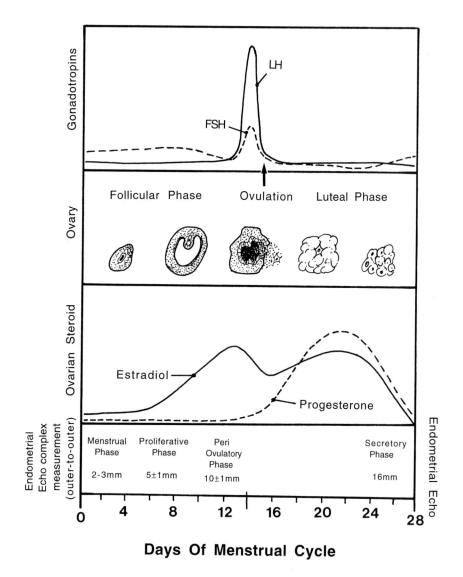

Days Of Menstrual Cycle

Fig. 7-3 The normal menstrual cycle. A normal ovulatory cycle is divided into a follicular and a luteal phase; the corresponding cyclic changes in the endometrium are the proliferative and the secretory phases, respectively. The follicular phase begins with the menses and ends in the preovulatory surge of luteinizing hormone (LH). During this phase, the maturing follicle secretes increasing amounts of estrogen that result in the proliferation of endometrial glands. Increasing blood estradiol levels result in the midcyle surges of LH and follicle stimulating hormone (FSH). The luteal phase begins with the LH surge and ends on the first day of menses. The preovulatory LH surge initiates structural changes in the maturing graafian follicle that culminate in ovulation. After ovulation and under the influence of LH, the granulosa cells of the ruptured follicle undergo luteinization. Luteinized granulosa cells form the corpus luteum, which produces large amounts of progesterone and some estradiol. Progesterone stimulates endometrial glandular cells to secrete glycogen and mucus.

mone (LH), the final maturation of ovarian follicles begins at puberty. The endocrinologic hallmark of puberty is an increased secretion of FSH and LH, possibly because of the increased production of luteinizing hormone-releasing hormone (LHRH) by the hypothalamus, and a pulsatile pattern of LH secretion. An enhancement of gonadotropin secretion by the pituitary gland leads to an increase in ovarian estrogen secretion, and this, in turn, results

in the anatomic changes of puberty. The culmination of puberty is the onset of cyclic menses. A critical body mass of approximately 48 kg and a specific combination of body water and fat are required for menses to occur.

Under the influence of pituitary gonadotropins, a few primary follicles begin to mature, and at about day 7 of the menstrual cycle, one follicle becomes dominant. The follicle consists of the oocyte, surrounding granulosa cells, and a basement membrane that separates the follicle from interstitial cells. Maturation of the dominant follicle involves accelerated growth of the granulosa cells and enlargement of the fluid space, called the antrum, within the follicle. Ovulation is the rupture of the thinned follicular wall and expulsion of the ovum. After ovulation, remnant granulosa and theca cells of the follicle accumulate lipid and a yellow pigment, forming the corpus luteum. After a period of 14 ± 2 days, the corpus luteum atrophies, forming a fibrous scar called the corpus albicans. However, if pregnancy occurs, chorionic gonadotropins from the developing placenta avert atresia of the corpus luteum, which produces progesterone to support the gestation.

Physiology of the menstrual cycle

The menstrual cycle is defined as the time between the onset of menstrual bleeding from one period to the next. The average cycle length is 28 ± 3 days, and the mean duration of menstrual hemorrhage is 4 ± 2 days. The menstrual cycle can be divided into a follicular, or proliferative, phase (days 5 to 14) and the luteal, or secretory, phase (days 15 to 28). The secretion of pituitary gonadotropins is under negative feedback control by the action of ovarian estradiol on hypothalamic production of LHRH; however, the positive feedback of estradiol at the pituitary gland produces the midcyle LH surge.

At the end of one menstrual cycle, circulating levels of estrogen and progesterone wane because of attrition of the oocyte and corpus luteum, respectively. Consequently, circulating levels of FSH begin to increase, and this process initiates maturation of a dominant follicle and the follicular phase of the menstrual cycle. Approximately 9 days before the midcycle surge of LH, estradiol levels begin to rise in response to increased production of this hormone by granulosa cells in the dominant follicle. Subsequent to the rising levels of estradiol, glandular growth of the endometrium begins. Just before ovulation, a peak in the secretion of estradiol elicits the LH surge. Ovulation occurs approximately 24 hours after the LH surge.

At the onset of the luteal phase, gonadotropin levels are low, and plasma progesterone levels begin to increase steadily. A second peak in the serum level of estradiol occurs during the luteal phase, and rising levels of progesterone and estradiol perpetuate endometrial growth (the secretory phase). Concurrent with increasing progesterone levels, the basal body temperature increases 0.4°C during the luteal phase. Near the end of the luteal phase, plasma estradiol and progesterone levels decrease. This decrease causes intense vasospasm of endometrial spiral arterioles; hemorrhage and desquamation of the endometrium ensue as a result of ischemic necrosis. The first day of the cycle begins with the onset of bleeding. Concomitant with the fall in estradiol and progesterone levels, FSH secretion by the pituitary gland increases, and another follicle is recruited for maturation.

Physiology of the menopause

The menopause indicates the final menstrual period and occurs during the climacteric, a phase in normal female aging between the reproductive and nonreproductive stage. Currently, the average age of onset of menopause in the United States is 51.4 years. After the menopause, plasma gonadotropin levels begin to rise because of a decrease in estrogen production by the ovaries. Reduced production of estradiol is related directly to a steady decline in the number of ova. The ovaries of postmenopausal women are small, and stromal cells predominate. Plasma gonadotropin levels peak approximately 5 to 10 years after the onset of menopause and remain constant until the eighth to ninth decade, when levels begin to fall.

The most common symptoms that accompany menopause are vasomotor instability, atrophy of the epithelium, osteoporosis, and a decrease in breast size. Atrophy of the endometrium, urethral mucosa, vaginal mucosa, and skin occurs secondary to estrogen deficiency.

FUNDAMENTALS OF GYNECOLOGIC RADIOLOGY

Congenital Anomalies

Anomalies of müllerian duct formation and fusion

The most common congenital uterine anomalies occur as a result of malfusion of the müllerian, or paramesonephric, ducts and have a prevalence of about 2% to 3%. The spectrum of anomalies includes varying degrees of uterine or vaginal fusion and uterine septal resorption, which may be associated with cornual atresia or hypoplasia. The American Fertility Society has endorsed the classification proposed by Buttram, which divides these anomalies into classes with similar clinical features, management, and prognosis (Fig. 7-4). Class I anomalies include agenesis or hypoplasia of the vagina, uterus, or uterine tubes, either alone or in combination. The unicornuate uterus represents the Class II müllerian anomaly and results from either agenesis or incomplete development of one müllerian duct. If there is a coexistent rudimentary horn, it may or may not have a central cavity, and if a cavity does exist, that cavity may or may not communicate with the unicornuate uterus. The Class III anomaly results from the complete lack of fusion of the müllerian ducts (uterus didelphys). There are two separate uteri and cervices of normal size, and there also may be a longitudinal septum in the upper vagina. The bicornuate uterus, which represents the Class IV anomaly, results from partial failure of müllerian duct fusion.

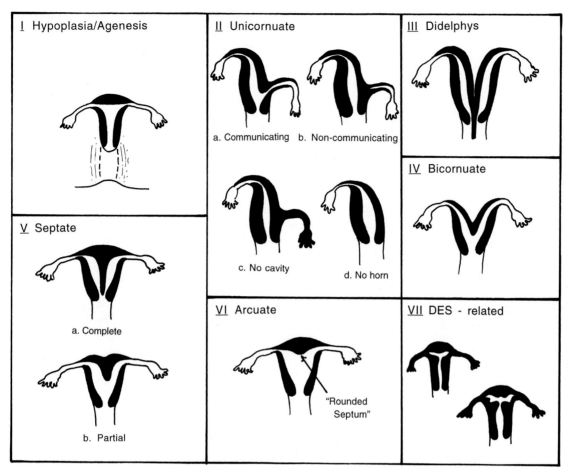

Fig. 7-4   American Fertility Society Classification of müllerian anomalies. (Modified from the American Fertility Society classifications of adnexal adhesions, distal tubal occlusion, tubal occlusion secondary to tubal ligation, tubal pregnancies, müllerian anomalies and intrauterine adhesions, *Fertil Steril* 49:944–955, 1988; and from Buttam VC Jr, Gibbons WE: Müllerian anomalies: a proposed classification (an analysis of 144 cases), *Fertil Steril* 32:40–47, 1979. Reproduced with permission of the American Society for Reproductive Medicine.)

The tissue dividing the two cornua is composed of myometrium and may extend to the internal os (uterus bicornus unicollis) or to the external os (uterus bicornus bicollis). The arcuate uterus (Class IV) may represent a mild form of the bicornuate uterus in which the uterine cavity is divided only partially. The septate uterus is designated Class V and is the most common müllerian anomaly. A fibrous septum may divide the endometrial cavity (partial septate uterus) alone or may extend into the endocervical canal (complete septate uterus).

Approximately 25% of women with uterine anomalies have fertility problems, such as difficulty maintaining a normal pregnancy or spontaneous abortion. Some have obstetric complications, such as premature birth, abnormal uterine activity during delivery, abnormal fetal presentation, and dystocia. Others present with abdominal pain or mass resulting from hematocolpos, hematometra, or hematosalpinx. The turgid uterus or vagina may ob-

struct the ureter. Concomitant anomalies of the urinary tract can accompany these disorders. When there is partial unilateral development, a high incidence of unilateral renal anomalies coexists. In virtually all reported cases of uterus didelphys with atresia of one vagina, ipsilateral renal agenesis coexists. Conversely, 50% of all women with unilateral renal agenesis have associated genital tract anomalies. Other abnormalities of the urinary tract, such as horseshoe kidney, pelvic kidney, and collecting system duplication, occur with increased incidence with complete müllerian agenesis.

From a diagnostic perspective, it is critical to distinguish anomalies in which reconstructive management requires transabdominal surgery from those in which this approach may not be necessary. In general, unicornuate and bicornuate uteri require the transabdominal approach, whereas uterine anomalies that either do not require management or can be managed with hystero-

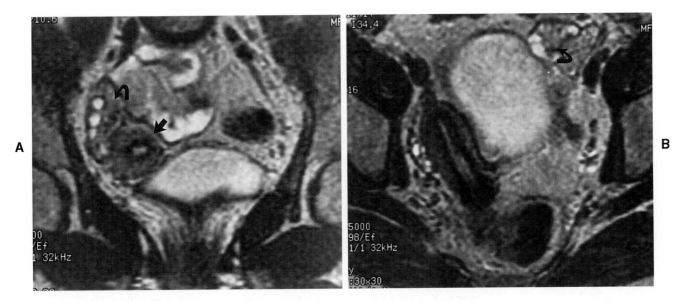

Fig. 7-5   Magnetic resonance imaging of unicornuate uterus (Class II müllerian anomaly). Coronal **(A)** and transverse **(B)** fast spin–echo T$_2$-weighted images (repetition time = 5000 msec; effective echo time = 98 msec) demonstrate a cigar-shaped uterus (arrow) located to the right of midline. The signal intensity of the endometrium, junctional zone, and outer myometrium are normal. There is no evidence of a rudimentary left horn (curved arrows = normal ovaries).

scopic metroplasty include the arcuate, septate, and didelphus uteri. In particular, the septate uterus can be managed with hysteroscopic excision of the septum.

Hysterosalpingography, ultrasonography, MR imaging, laparoscopy, and surgery have been used to evaluate suspected müllerian duct anomalies. Of the minimally invasive or noninvasive techniques, hysterosalpingography is the traditional technique for investigating the anatomy of the uterine cavity. However, this evaluation only can be accomplished if the endometrial cavity is patent and if it communicates with the cervical canal. Furthermore, hysterosalpingography does not demonstrate the external morphology of the uterine fundus. Transabdominal sonography is used to detect müllerian duct anomalies in early pregnancy, but it may not be as accurate as endovaginal sonography for characterizing these anomalies in the nongravid uterus. The major advantage of endovaginal sonography and MR imaging is that they are reliable methods to evaluate the external contour of the fundus and the tissue between uterine hemicavities.

The diagnosis of müllerian anomaly Classes I, II, III, and VI is not as difficult a problem as the diagnosis of Classes IV and V. Uterine atresia or hypoplasia (Class I) is diagnosed when there is no identifiable uterine tissue, and hypoplasia is suggested when an infantile uterus is seen with an intercornual distance less than 2 cm. With MR imaging, these small uteri have no discernible zonal anatomy on T$_2$-weighted images. The volume of the unicornuate uterus (Class II) is decreased because it consists of a single horn with normal endometrial and myometrial

width (Fig. 7-5). If a second horn is present, it is rudimentary. In uterus didelphys (Class III), widely bifurcated uterine horns are separated by a deep fundal cleft. Cervical duplication, which is detected on pelvic examination, also is a feature of this anomaly. The arcuate uterus (Class VI) may be a normal variant. A smooth and often subtle indentation of the fundal endometrial contour is the only abnormality. There is no division of the uterine cornua, and the external fundal contour is convex.

The septate uterus (Class V) may be difficult to distinguish from the bicornuate uterus (Class IV), particularly if the division of the bicornuate uterus does not involve the cervix (Table 7-1). This distinction is important for the selection of the appropriate surgical approach. In many patients, the distinction between bicornuate and septate uterus cannot be made with hysterosalpingography because neither the external fundal contour nor the

Table 7-1   Differentiating Bicornuate from Septate Uteri

	Bicornuate	Septate
Depth of fundal cleft	> 1 cm	≤ 1 cm
Intercornual angle	≥ 105°	≤ 75°
Intercornual distance	> 4 cm	≤ 4 cm
Intercornual tissue	Myometrial tissue	Fibrous or myometrial tissue

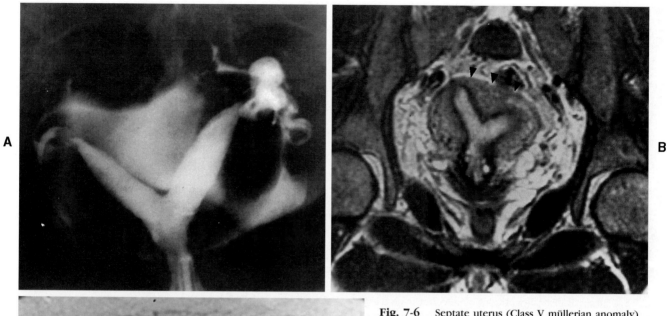

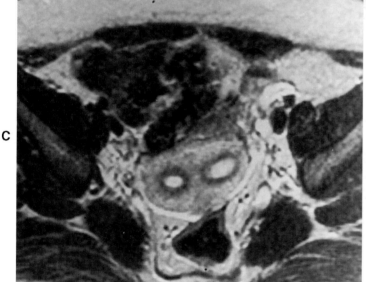

Fig. 7-6 Septate uterus (Class V müllerian anomaly). **A,** Hysterosalpingogram shows distinct uterine cornua, separated by an indeterminate intercornual angle of 85°. The oblique coronal T₂-weighted fast spin–echo image **(B)** demonstrates a flat fundal contour (arrowheads), which is consistent with septate uterus. The oblique coronal and the oblique transverse image **(C)** clearly show myometrial tissue between the cornua.

nature of the dividing tissue can be defined by this technique. In contrast, endovaginal sonography and MR imaging can be used to define the external contour of the fundus. In the septate uterus, the fundal contour may be normal, or flat, or it may have a slight concave indentation 1 cm or less in depth (Fig. 7-6). In contrast, bicornuate and didelphys uteri may have a deep fundal concavity (Fig. 7-7). The fundal cleft of a bicornuate uterus is deeper than 1 cm. Another distinguishing feature is the intercornual angle, or the angle defined by the medial margin of the endometrial hemicavities. In bicornuate and didelphic uteri, the intercornual angle is at least 105° on hysterosalpingogram, whereas in septate uteri, this angle is 75° or less. On T₂-weighted coronal oblique images

prescribed orthogonally to the long axis of the uterus, the intercornual distance is 4 cm or less in the septate uterus. In bicornuate or didelphys uteri, this intercornual distance is more than 4 cm. Finally, the nature of the tissue separating the two endometrial hemicavities has been used to distinguish septate and bicornuate uteri, although there is no consensus on this point. For some authorities, a fibrous septum defines the septate uterus, whereas a myometrial septum occurs only in a bicornuate uterus. Others have found myometrium and fibrous tissue in the dividing tissue of septate uteri. If the mass dividing the endometrial canals is isoechoic or isointense to myometrium, it is assumed to be myometrial in composition. If the bifurcating tissue is fibrous, it will appear hypo-

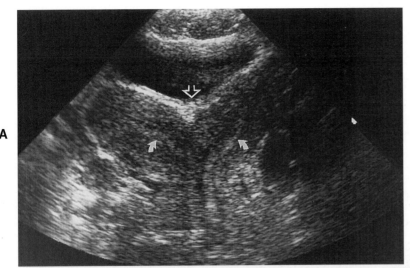

A

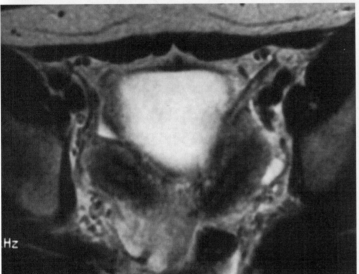

B

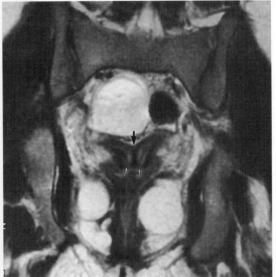

C

Fig. 7-7 Uterus didelphys (Class III müllerian anomaly). **A,** Coronal sonogram of the uterus shows widely separated endometrial echoes (arrows). There is no uterine tissue between each cornua, which creates a deep fundal concavity (open arrow). Transaxial **(B)** and coronal **(C)** T$_2$-weighted images demonstrate the prominent fundal concavity (black arrow) and separate cervices (white arrows). (From Mayo-Smith WW, Lee MJ: MR imaging of the female pelvis, *Clin Radiol* 50: 667–676, 1995.)

echoic compared with myometrium on endovaginal sonography, and it will appear hypointense on all MR imaging sequences.

Diethylstilbestrol exposure in utero

Diethylstilbestrol is a synthetic estrogen that was used during the 1950s and 1960s to prevent miscarriage. This drug has been associated with congenital anomalies of the female genital tract in the offspring of exposed women; these anomalies have been designated as Class VI müllerian anomalies. These uterine anomalies have been associated with reduced fecundity, premature delivery, and ectopic pregnancy. Reported uterine dysmorphisms include hypoplasia, irregular short strictures of the uterine corpus, and a T-shaped uterine cavity (Box 7-2; Fig. 7-8). These anomalies of uterine shape are demonstrable on hysterosalpingography and MR imaging.

Box 7-2   Uterine Anomalies Resulting from Diethylstilbestrol

Generalized hypoplasia
Irregular short strictures of uterine corpus
T shape
Vaginal and cervical carcinomas
Increased spontaneous abortion and premature birth
Not associated with urinary tract abnormalities

For example, on T$_2$-weighted MR images, generalized uterine hypoplasia may be seen, or there may be localized areas of junctional zone thickening, leading to focal indentations or a "T" shape. In addition to uterine hypoplasia and dysplasia, in utero exposure to diethylstilbestrol

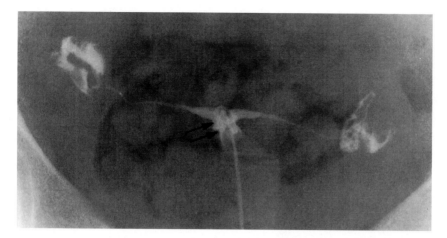

Fig. 7-8   Small, T-shaped uterus in a patient with infertility with a history of diethylstilbestrol exposure. Catheter hysterosalpingogram demonstrates a small uterine cavity with focal strictures (small arrows) of the uterine corpus. Note the normal appearance of the fallopian tubes.

is associated with vaginal and cervical adenosis (i.e., glandular epithelial metaplasia), dysmorphic fallopian tubes, and an increased risk of clear-cell adenocarcinoma (Fig. 7-9).

Pelvic Pain

Painful menstruation, or dysmenorrhea, which affects 50% of women, may be primary or may be secondary to organic pelvic disease. Primary dysmenorrhea typically occurs with menstruation and lasts 2 to 3 days. Crampy lower abdominal pain is common and usually responds to nonsteroidal anti-inflammatory drugs or oral birth control pills. In contrast, dysmenorrhea caused by organic abnormalities is less often temporally related to menses, develops in older women, and may be associated with other signs and symptoms, such as abnormal bleeding or infertility. Uterine causes of secondary dysmenorrhea include leiomyoma, adenomyosis, uterine polyps, uterine malformations, or cervical stenosis. Extrauterine causes include pelvic inflammatory disease and endometriosis.

Endometriosis and Adenomyosis

Endometriosis   Endometriosis is a benign, but potentially debilitating, disease in which endometrial tissue is

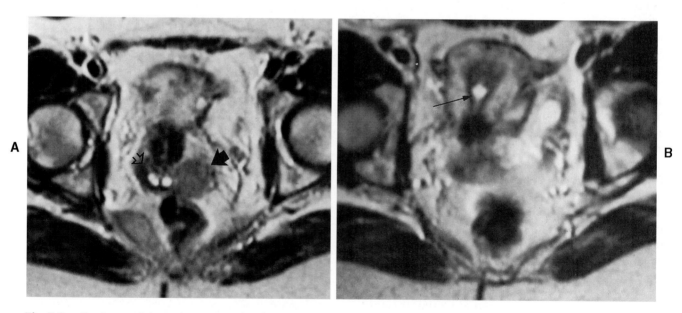

Fig. 7-9   Carcinoma of the vagina associated with diethylstilbestrol exposure. **A,** On a transverse T$_2$-weighted fast spin–echo MR image (repetition time = 3883 msec; effective echo time = 102 msec), there is a 3-cm exophytic mass (arrow) originating from the superolateral recess of the vagina, next to the cervix (open arrow). This mass was surgically proven to be a poorly differentiated endometrioid carcinoma of the vagina. **B,** On a more cephalic image, a small endometrial cavity (arrow) is seen.

Box 7-3   Endometriosis

Associated with infertility
Predilection for ovary, cul-de-sac, retrovaginal septum,
    broad ligament
Poorly imaged implants
Endometrioma (endometrial cyst, chocolate cyst)
Paratubal adhesions

found outside the uterus (Box 7-3). Up to 40% of patients with endometriosis have endometrial implants within the myometrium, a condition called *adenomyosis*. The pathogenesis of endometriosis is not defined, but it likely results from implantation of desquamated menstrual endometrium. Like normal endometrium, endometrial implants undergo cyclic changes from menstrual hormonal influence. Repetitive episodes of desquamation and hemorrhage incite inflammation and fibrosis, leading to adhesions. An estimated 15% of women are afflicted by endometriosis or adenomyosis, which can cause chronic pelvic pain, dysmenorrhea, infertility, vaginal spotting, dyspareunia, and irregular bleeding. Endometriosis has been found in up to 50% of women who undergo surgery for infertility; endometrial implants may cause tubal scarring or adnexal adhesions, and there is an increased incidence of luteal phase defects and luteinized unruptured follicle syndrome in patients with endometriosis.

Pelvic sites for which endometriosis has a predilection include the ovaries, the peritoneum of the cul-de-sac, the rectovaginal septum, and the broad ligament. About 60% of women have ovarian involvement, and in most patients, both ovaries are involved. Endometrial implants typically are very small, frequently less than 5 mm in diameter. When these implants become walled off and undergo cyclical hemorrhage, a cystic mass can result and is termed an *endometrioma*. The endometrioma begins as a small cyst, which is filled with thick, dark fluid with the consistency of motor oil. This fluid is composed of chronic by-products of hemorrhage and desquamated endothelium. The cyst wall may thicken as a result of reactive fibrosis. A tender, fixed mass may form and may be difficult to distinguish from a hemorrhagic ovarian cyst, tubovarian complex or abscess, benign or malignant ovarian neoplasm, hemorrhagic corpus luteum, or ectopic pregnancy. When endometriosis involves peritoneal surfaces, it can incite cicatrization and can cause obstruction of the gastrointestinal or urinary tracts and fixed retroversion of the uterus.

Of all patients with untreated endometriosis, approximately 50% will either have their symptoms improve or remain the same over 6 months, and the others' conditions will deteriorate. When necessary, medical therapy of endometriosis includes the use of progesterone acetate, a combined oral contraceptive, or danazol, which is an androgen derivative. Conservative surgical techniques based on ablation and excision are tried when medical therapy is unsuccessful. Symptomatic endometriomas (6 cm or larger in diameter) and adhesions are managed surgically.

Endometriosis is occult to many imaging tests because implants are sessile and typically smaller than 3 to 5 mm. In some patients, the only sequela of endometriosis and cyclical hemorrhage is fibrosis, and in the absence of a distinct mass, results of the ultrasound examination will be essentially normal. The sonographic appearance of an endometrioma is variable and nonspecific (Box 7-4). Sonographically detected endometriomas are 3 to 20 cm in diameter, and the majority are located in the adnexa or cephalad to the uterine fundus. Posterior acoustic enhancement can almost always be demonstrated in endometriomas, which are either predominantly or completely cystic. Internal, low-level echoes are thought to result from blood and desquamated tissue (Fig. 7-10). Endometrial cysts usually have thin walls and may be multilocular or septated. The presence of paratubal adhesions suggests the diagnosis of endometriosis and can be diagnosed with hysterosalpingography. When these adhesions are present, the fallopian tube will be convoluted or tethered into a fixed position. With hysterosalpingography, loculated contrast material may pool within pseudocavities created by adhesions, creating a peritubal halo effect (Fig. 7-11).

Although laparoscopy is widely considered the procedure of choice for diagnosis, staging, and follow-up evaluation, MR imaging has been used to monitor the progress of managed endometriosis once the diagnosis has been made. MR imaging also is of value when pelvic laparoscopy is limited by dense adhesions from either previous surgery or extensive endometriosis. MR imaging also has been used to detect endometriosis and, in particular, endometrial cysts, with a sensitivity between 70% and 80%. Endometrial cysts are characterized by the presence of a variegated signal-intensity pattern, which reflects variable stages of hemorrhage. Endometriomas appear as

Box 7-4   Imaging of Endometrial Cysts

Multiple or multilocular
Uniform medium-level internal echoes, intense
    posterior shadowing
T_1-weighted image—hyperintense, no change with fat
    saturation
T_2-weighted image—shading, hypointense rim
Differential diagnosis: hemorrhagic ovarian cyst or
    corpus luteum cyst

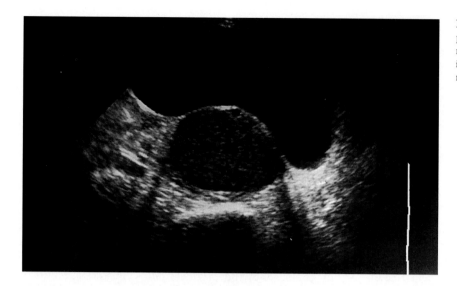

Fig. 7-10 Endometrial cyst on ultrasonography. Sagittal image shows a well-circumscribed mass with thin walls. The mass has uniform internal, low-level echoes, and there is posterior acoustic enhancement.

loculated collections containing areas of short T_1 and long T_2. In adnexal cysts, predominantly high signal intensity on T_1-weighted images may result from protein or blood content. Fat saturated–T_1-weighted MR imaging may increase the conspicuity of hemorrhagic adnexal cysts and may permit distinction from the rarer dermoid cyst. Prominent shading is seen within endometrial cysts on T_2-weighted images. Shading refers to the presence of hypointense signal, usually mixed with hyperintense signal, in areas that are hyperintense on T_1-weighted images (Fig. 7-12). This shading has been attributed to the high viscosity of fluid within the endometrial cyst rather than to the presence of blood products. Multiple or multilocular cysts on T_1-weighted images also are typical of endometriomas; this situation has been explained by the propensity of endometrial cysts to perforate cyclically. Repetitive hemorrhage creates daughter cysts and results

in the characteristic finding of multiple or multilocular cysts, which adhere to each other and to neighboring organs. The presence of a hypointense rim caused by chronic hemorrhage also is observed more commonly with endometriomas than with other hemorrhagic adnexal masses, such as hemorrhagic ovarian cysts or corpus luteum cysts. Less often, solid pelvic masses may result from endometriosis. These masses tend to be of intermediate signal intensity with punctate areas of high-signal intensity on T_1-weighted images and of low-signal intensity on T_2-weighted images. Enhancement is characteristic. Like endometrial cysts, these masses are found in or near the cul-de-sac and can involve the rectum or bladder wall.

Adenomyosis Adenomyosis is the presence of ectopic endometrial tissue and stroma in the myometrium, which induces an overgrowth of surrounding uterine

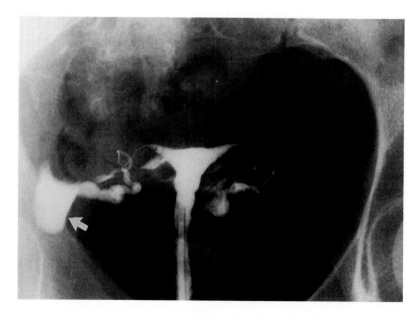

Fig. 7-11 Paratubal adhesions. Hysterosalpingogram demonstrates pooling of contrast material (arrow) near the fibria of the right tube.

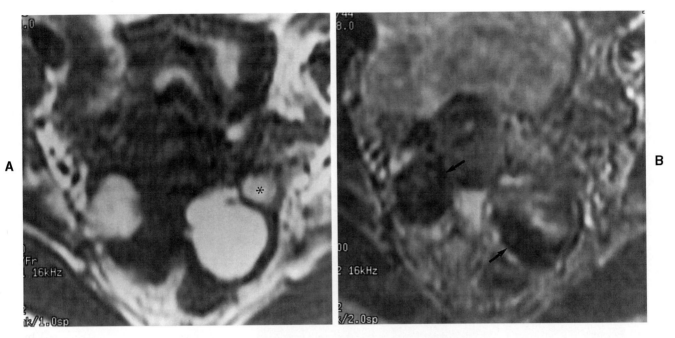

Fig. 7-12   MR imaging of endometrial cysts. **A,** Transverse T$_1$-weighted image (repetition time = 400 msec; echo time = 12 msec) of the lower pelvis shows multiple hyperintense masses that remained hyperintense on a fat-saturated T$_1$-weighted image. A smaller daughter cyst (*) is associated with the larger mass. **B,** The T$_2$-weighted transverse image (repetition time = 2500 msec; echo time = 80 msec) shows areas of marked decrease in signal intensity (arrows) in both masses, referred to as "shading."

smooth muscle. There are focal and diffuse forms. On TVS, adenomyosis may be demonstrated with one or more of the following signs: (1) ill-defined myometrial mass, (2) asymmetrically thickened myometrial wall, or (3) focal increased myometrial echogenicity (Fig. 7-13). Adenomyosis can be difficult to distinguish from leiomyoma on ultrasound evaluation, but distinguishing features are present on MR images (Table 7-2). Although myomas typically are round, focal adenomyosis is oval or elongated. Adenomyosis also is less well defined than leiomyomas and always is contiguous with the junctional zone, which is frequently thicker than 12 mm (Fig. 7-14). Margins are shaggy, and an irregular interface between endometrium and adenomyosis is typical. T$_2$-weighted images will show a relatively homogeneous, low-intensity mass, but the signal intensity is not as uniform or as low in intensity as with leiomyomas. There may be sparse, small, high-intensity foci within an adenomyoma on T$_1$- and T$_2$-weighted images, which represent hemorrhage in endometrial islands (Fig. 7-15 on p. 264). Other areas that are bright on T$_2$-weighted images but are not seen on T$_1$-weighted images represent small foci of nonhemorrhagic endometrial tissue.

Pelvic inflammatory disease

Pelvic inflammatory disease (PID) comprises a wide spectrum of multibacterial infectious diseases of the lower genital tract, uterus, uterine tubes, ovary, or pelvic peritoneum (Box 7-5). Clinical criteria include lower abdominal pain, vaginal discharge, cervical motion tenderness, adnexal tenderness, and supportive laboratory signs of infection, such as fever, leukocytosis, and elevation of the sedimentation rate. Venereal infection of the fallopian tubes or ovaries is common and frequently there is evidence of infection with *Neisseria gonorrhoeae, Chlamydia trachomatis,* or both. Intrauterine contraceptive devices predispose to nonvenereal infection with *Actinomyces israelii*. The infection usually begins as cervicitis, which ascends to involve secondarily the endometrial

Table 7-2   Differentiating Leiomyoma and Adenomyosis

	Leiomyoma	Adenomyosis
Margin	Well-defined	Ill-defined
Focality	Focal	Focal or diffuse
T$_2$-signal intensity	Hypointense*	Small hyperintense foci†
Thickened junctional zone	No	Yes

*Unless degeneration is present.
†May be present, but not necessarily.

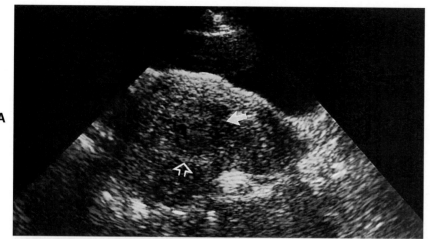

A

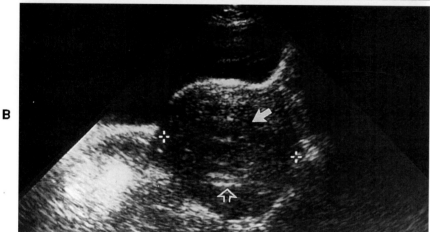

B

Fig. 7-13   Sonography of focal adenomyosis. Sagittal (**A**) and transverse (**B**) images of the uterus demonstrate a focal hypoechoic area (arrow) anterior to the central endometrial echo (open arrow). The presence of small (2 to 6 mm) myometrial cysts associated with abnormal echogenicity of the myometrium would increase the specificity of this appearance for adenomyosis.

cavity and fallopian tubes (canalicular spread). An infectious salpingitis may be the full extent of disease or, via tubal spillage, peritoneal spread of infection may result in a local peritonitis and oophoritis. Adnexal adhesions may cause fusion of the inflamed tube and ovary, termed a *tuboovarian complex*. Necrosis of the phlegmonous mass may result in a tuboovarian abscess. Initial management of PID includes aggressive therapy with broad-spectrum antibiotics. When fever, leukocytosis, and pain persist despite intravenous antibiotic administration, surgery has been the traditional alternative, although tuboovarian complex and abscess have been managed effectively with percutaneous catheter drainage. Potential sequelae of tubal inflammation, particularly if recurrent or severe, are infertility and ectopic pregnancy caused by tubal stricture or dysmotility. Other problems that may result from chronic PID include recurrent pelvic pain, menometrorrhagia, and dyspareunia.

Because PID has a relatively high prevalence among women of child-bearing age, transabdominal sonography and TVS have been used most often for diagnosis and follow-up evaluation. Up to one third of patients with clinical signs or symptoms of PID have normal ultrasound examination results, possibly because disease is early or mild. A variety of sonographic findings have been ascribed to PID. The inflamed uterus may be enlarged and ill defined. In patients with infectious endometritis, excessive fluid may be present in the endometrial cavity, or the central endometrial echo complex may be indistinct (Fig. 7-16). Because normal fallopian tubes are 1 to 4 mm in diameter, they are not identified consistently

---

Box 7-5   Pelvic Inflammatory Disease

Canalicular spread
Cervicitis
Endometritis
Salpingitis
Hydrosalpinx or pyosalpinx
Tuboovarian complex
Tuboovarian abscess

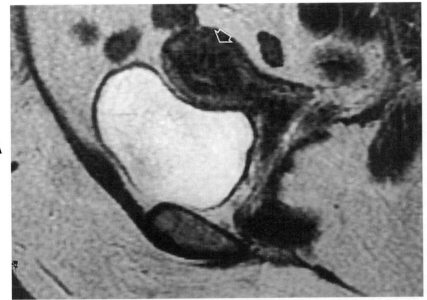

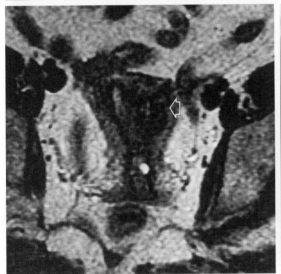

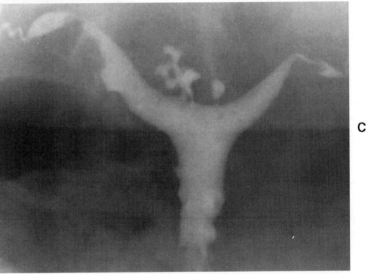

Fig. 7-14 Typical appearance of focal ad-enomyosis on MR imaging and hysterosal-pingography. Sagittal (**A**) and oblique trans-verse (**B**) fast spin–echo T_2-weighted images (repetition time = 5000 msec; effec-tive echo time = 104 msec) of the uterus show an ill-defined area of inhomogeneous decreased signal intensity (open arrow), which contains small high-signal intensity foci. **C**, Single and grouped globular collec-tions of contrast material extend from the endometrial cavity into fundal myometrium on the hysterosalpingogram.

on TVS, and in many patients, mild tubal erythema and salpingitis are undetectable. Hydrosalpinx is the dilata-tion of the ampullary segment of the tube that accompa-nies distal obstruction; pyosalpinx refers to purulent in-fection of a dilated tube. Abnormal tubes are distended with fluid, may be folded or septated, and can have thick, echogenic walls (Fig. 7-17). In some patients, it may be difficult to differentiate hydrosalpinx or pyosalpinx from bowel loops or distended pelvic veins. The absence of peristalsis or flow in hydrosalpinx can be documented on Doppler sonography. Cystic adnexal masses also may mimic hydrosalpinx on ultrasound evaluation. The ova-ries may be enlarged or may appear poorly defined. Heterogeneous adnexal masses on transabdominal sonograms may represent hydrosalpinx, tuboovarian complex, or abscess. The improved visualization of tubal

and ovarian inflammation with TVS may allow differentia-tion of these different stages of PID.

Adhesions and loculated fluid collections in the ad-nexa or cul-de-sac can complicate chronic or recurrent PID. Pelvic peritoneal adhesions may result from PID, previous pelvic surgery, or endometriosis. The "sliding sign" describes en bloc motion of adherent organs on sonograms when simultaneous pressure is applied to the pelvic organs with the examiner's free hand. This motion occurs because adhesions tether the ovary and tubes to surrounding viscera. On hysterosalpingography evalua-tion, adhesions may manifest as loculated collections of spilled contrast material that fail to disperse around loops of pelvic bowel (Fig. 7-18 on p. 266).

Computed tomography also has been used to examine patients with complicated PID, particularly when ade-

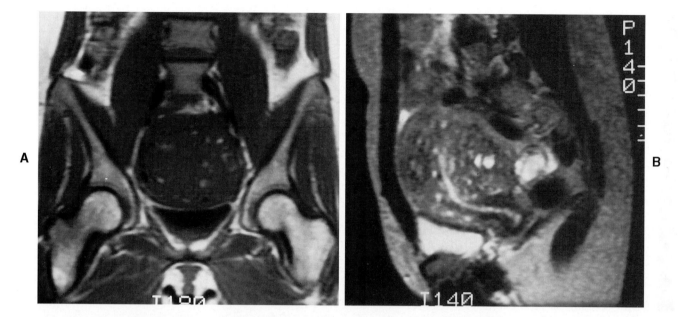

Fig. 7-15 MR imaging of diffuse adenomyosis. **A,** Multiple, punctate foci of increased signal intensity are seen in an enlarged uterus on a coronal T_1-weighted image. **B,** A sagittal T_2-weighted image shows diffuse thickening of the junctional zone that contains small hyperintense foci. These areas of increased signal intensity on T_1- and T_2-weighted images are thought to represent hemorrhage in ectopic endometrial tissue. (From Mayo-Smith WW, Lee MJ: MR imaging of the female pelvis, *Clin Radiol* 50:667-676, 1995.)

quate information is unobtainable with sonography. Findings include bilateral, low-attenuation adnexal masses with irregularly thickened walls, which represent the tuboovarian complex, and an enlarged, ill-defined uterus. Hydrosalpinx may appear as a complex, fluid-filled, multicystic mass. Secondary findings include pelvic ascites, thickening of the uterosacral ligaments, and increased density within the pelvic fat caused by inflammation. Ureterectasis may result from the inflammatory process. Although the appearance of PID on CT images is not specific, other focal inflammatory processes in the pelvis are less frequently bilateral.

Tuboovarian abscess

In approximately 1% of women who are treated for acute salpingitis, the condition progresses to tuboovarian abscess. Patients with tuboovarian abscess usually are ill and may present with pelvic pain, marked adnexal tenderness, high fever, nausea, and emesis. Clinically and radiographically, tuboovarian abscess can be difficult to distinguish from ovarian torsion, incomplete septic abortion, diverticular or other pelvic abscess, and appendicitis. Patients usually are treated with intravenous hydration, analgesics, and broad-spectrum antibiotics. Treatment by surgery or interventional radiology is neces-

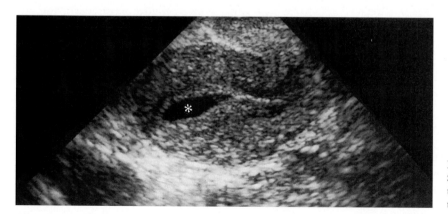

Fig. 7-16 Ultrasonography of endometritis. Sagittal image of the uterus demonstrates a thickened endometrial echo and focal distention of the endometrial cavity by fluid (*).

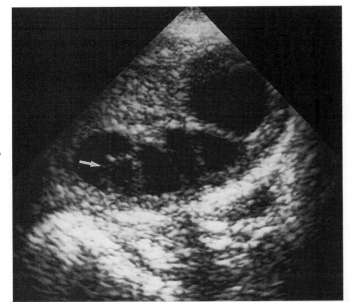

A

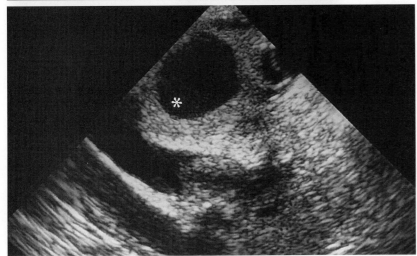

B

Fig. 7-17 Pyosalpinx in an 18-year-old woman with an adnexal mass and purulent cervical discharge. Transverse (**A**) and parasagittal (**B**) pelvic sonograms demonstrate a septated, tubular adnexal mass. The walls of the septations are thick and echogenic (arrow), and purulent debris is seen in the dilated tubal ampulla (*).

sary only if the patient's symptoms fail to respond clinically within 72 hours after the administration of antibiotics or if abscess rupture is suspected.

Ultrasonography is the primary imaging test used to detect suspected PID or tuboovarian abscess. Sonography identifies either a cystic, solid, or heterogeneous adnexal mass in more than 90% of patients with clinically diagnosed tuboovarian abscess. The ovary frequently is enlarged (volume, >14 cm³), and normal ovarian morphology is unrecognizable in most patients (Fig. 7-19). In patients with severe cases, there may be irregular septations and fluid–debris levels that distort the adnexa completely.

Computed tomography may demonstrate a tubular or spherical mass, containing single or many focal areas of hypoattenuation. Thick walls and septations are com-

mon, and internal bubbles of gas also may be present. The inflammatory nature of these masses is suggested by the loss of distinct fat planes between the mass and pelvic viscera and by thickening of the uterosacral ligaments (Fig. 7-20). Dilatation of one or both ureters also is a common finding on CT, and regional lymphadenopathy also may be present. The differential diagnosis of these CT findings includes infected ovarian cyst or dermoid tumor, ovarian cystadenoma, endometriosis, pelvic hematoma, and, rarely, ectopic gestation. A pelvic abscess engulfing the fallopian tubes or ovaries may have a similar appearance.

Ovarian torsion

Torsion of the adnexa affects all age groups and has been reported in utero. An adnexal mass predisposes to

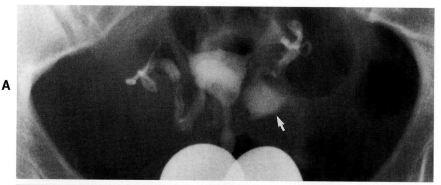

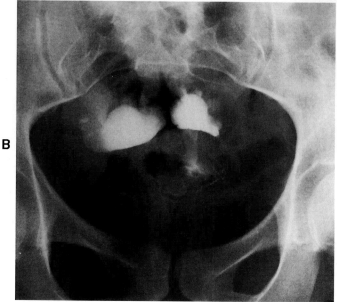

Fig. 7-18 Adnexal adhesions. **A,** Early film from a hysterosalpingogram shows normal fallopian tubes. Contrast material from the left tube is beginning to pool next to the left fallopian tube (arrow). **B,** A late film after evacuation of contrast material from the uterine cavity shows two persistent, focal collections of contrast material caused by pelvic adhesions.

torsion. Other putative preconditions include an excessively long or tortuous mesosalpinx or mesosalpingeal vessels, tubal spasm, and previous surgery. Mechanical torsion compromises lymphatic and venous drainage of the adnexa initially, producing passive congestion. Venous thrombosis and hemorrhage ensue, eventually compromising arterial perfusion and leading to complete infarction. The diagnosis of ovarian torsion is in the differential diagnosis of a painful solid pelvic mass, with or without free pelvic fluid (Box 7-6). In some patients with adnexal torsion, sonography, CT, or MR imaging will show multiple 8- to 10-mm cysts, which represent dilated germinal follicles in the cortex of a markedly enlarged ovary (Fig. 7-21). Enlargement of these follicles is thought to result from fluid transudation from the congested ovarian stroma. The ovary may be so enlarged that it assumes a midline position behind the urinary bladder. On CT or MR images, the torsed ovary may have a beaked or serpentine protrusion at the apex of the twist. In addition, a torsed and edematous pedicle and engorged, straight vessels may be draped around the ovary. After administration of contrast material, CT of the torsed ovary may show an adnexal mass with prominent peripheral hyperattenuation resulting from vascular congestion. The attenuation of the torsed ovary may be heterogeneous, as a result of variable perfusion. Doppler interrogation of suspected ovarian torsion may be valuable, although results are mixed because of variable degrees of vascular compromise.

Box 7-6   Ovarian Torsion

May be extrapelvic mass in prepubertal girls
Multiple 8- to 10-mm cortical cysts in an enlarged
  ovary
Beaked or serpentine protrusion at site of twist
Surrounded by engorged, straight vessels
Color Doppler flow and enhancement variable

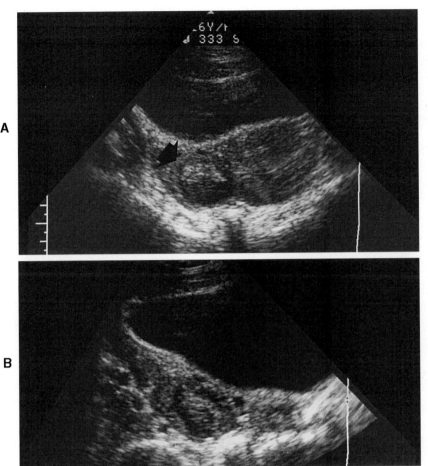

Fig. 7-19   Tuboovarian abscess in a 22-year-old woman with fever and right lower quadrant pain. A solid adnexal mass (arrow) is demonstrated on oblique transverse (**A**) and sagittal (**B**) pelvic ultrasonograms. At surgery, hyperechoic areas within the mass were foci of acute hemorrhage.

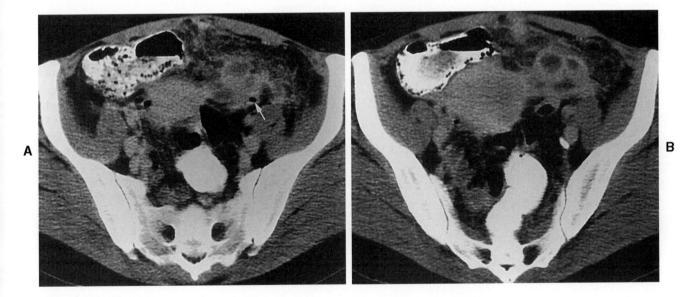

Fig. 7-20   Computed tomography (CT) of tuboovarian abscess. **A** and **B,** CT scans demonstrate a heterogeneous left adnexal mass containing multiple areas of low attenuation and a gas bubble (arrow). The fat planes around the mass are indistinct and suggest an inflammatory etiology. On other images, there was hydrometra and pelvic ascites. (Courtesy of Mark S. Ridlen, MD.)

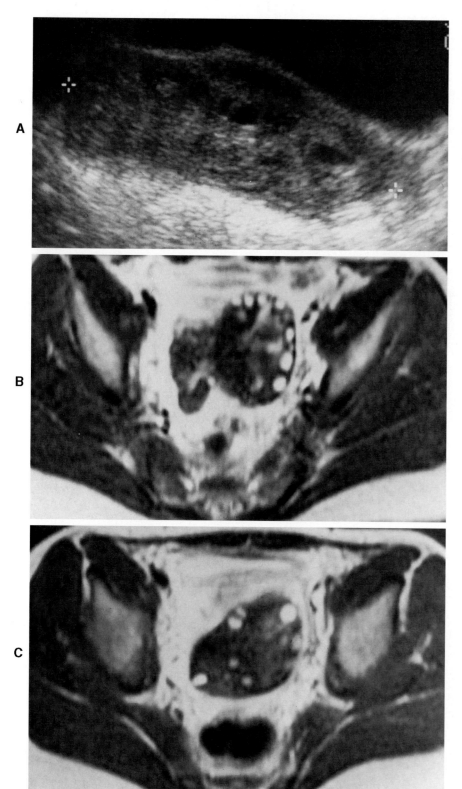

Fig. 7-21 Torsion of the ovary. A 10-year-old girl presented with intermittent, severe abdominal pain and constipation. **A,** Sagittal pelvic sonogram shows a 9.5-cm solid midline mass containing a few small, peripheral cysts. **B** and **C,** Transverse, T₂-weighted MR images (repetition time = 2000 msec; echo time = 80 msec) demonstrate a markedly enlarged left ovary with multiple small cortical follicles, a typical appearance of a torsed ovary. (Case courtesy of Michael T. Wallach, MD.)

Uterine leiomyoma

Uterine leiomyoma is a benign smooth-muscle tumor that is detected in almost 20% of women (Box 7-7). An increased prevalence and rate of growth have been reported in blacks. These tumors are estrogen-dependent, hence, there is an increased prevalence of leiomyomas in patients with diseases associated with hyperestrogenism, such as endometrial hyperplasia, endometrial cancer, anovulatory states, and granulosa–theca tumors. Gynecologic symptoms that are attributed to fibroids include menorrhagia, metrorrhagia, pelvic pain, dyspareunia, dysmenorrhea, infertility, and symptoms related to pressure on adjacent pelvic organs. About 5% of leiomyomas are associated with irritative urinary tract symptoms, acute or chronic urinary retention, or ureteral compression, however, the majority of fibroids are asymptomatic.

Fibroids generally are classified by location with respect to the uterine wall. Therefore, leiomyomas are described as submucous (submucosal), intramural, or subserosal. An intramural location is most common. The prevalence of infertility and excessive bleeding is highest for patients with submucosal leiomyoma, which can be managed with hysteroscopic myomectomy (Fig. 7-22). Pedunculated subserosal fibroids may present as adnexal masses and may be difficult to distinguish from ovarian metastases or fibromas (Fig 7-23). Rarely, a pedunculated subserosal fibroid may detach from the uterus and develop as a separate mass in the broad ligament (intraligamentous leiomyoma). Myomas can also originate in the cervix (Fig. 7-24).

Rapid enlargement, degeneration, neoplastic transformation, and growth during pregnancy are several other complications of leiomyomas. The natural history of unmanaged leiomyomas is such that regression, or at least stabilization, occurs after menopause; however, hyaline, cystic, hemorrhagic, or fatty degeneration of leiomyomas may occur. Rarely, leiomyomas may become infected or may undergo sarcomatous transformation, a complication in 0.5% of patients. Being estrogen-sensitive, leiomyomas may enlarge or degenerate during pregnancy. Approximately 10% of women who are pregnant and have uterine fibroids must be hospitalized during the pregnancy for related complications. Pain generally is not a feature unless the uterus is markedly enlarged or the fibroid undergoes acute infarction or carneous degeneration during pregnancy (Fig. 7-25). Large myomas can interfere with the growth of the fetus and, when located in the lower uterine segment, may cause dystocia.

Complication related to uterine leiomyoma is one of the most common indications for major surgery in women. Indications for myomectomy include abnormal uterine bleeding and intractable pain, dysmenorrhea, in-

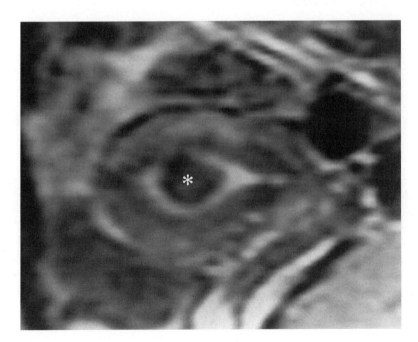

Fig. 7-22   A submucosal fibroid on MR imaging. A sagittal T_2-weighted image of the uterus (repetition time = 2033 msec; echo time = 80 msec) demonstrates a pedunculated, hypointense mass (*) that protrudes into the uterine cavity. Although these leiomyomas are the least common, they more often are the cause of dysmenorrhea or infertility.

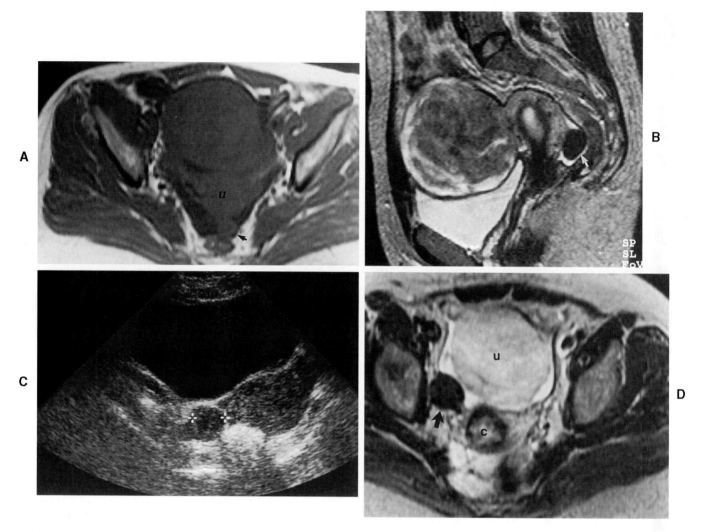

Fig. 7-23   The hypointense adnexal mass. **A,** A large mass in the midline of the pelvis is demonstrated on a transverse, T_1-weighted MR image (repetition time [TR] = 600 msec; echo time [TE] = 12 msec). There also is a small mass (arrow) posterior to the uterus. Both masses are isointense compared with the uterus. A small amount of pelvic ascites also is seen. **B,** On a sagittal, turbo spin–echo, T_2-weighted image (TR = 4861 msec; effective TE = 96 msec), the large mass anterior to the uterus has a broad attachment to the anterior wall of the uterus and is consistent with a degenerating subserosal leiomyoma. The smaller, uniformly hypointense mass posterior to the uterus is another subserosal fibroid. **C,** In another patient, oblique transverse sonogram demonstrates a solid adnexal mass (electronic markers) next to the uterine fundus. **D,** On a transverse T_2-weighted MR image (TR = 2000 msec; TE = 80 msec), this mass is uniformly hypointense (arrow = adnexal mass; u = uterine fundus; c = cervix). A 2.2-cm fibrothecoma of the right ovary was removed.

fertility, enlargement after menopause, rapid increase in size, and irritative urinary tract symptoms. Myomectomy may be performed by either operative hysteroscopy or laparotomy. Hysteroscopic myomectomy is reserved for small submucous leiomyomas, and an open operative approach is elected when the fibroid is intramural, subserous, or pedunculated. In addition to surgery, gonadotropin-releasing hormone (GnRH) agonists combined with hormone-replacement therapy are under investigation for management of symptomatic leiomyomas.

The sonographic appearance of a uterine fibroid depends on its relative composition of muscle and fibrous tissue and on the presence and nature of degeneration (Box 7-8). These masses may be difficult to detect with ultrasonography because of variable patterns of echogenicity; prospective sensitivity of sonography for the detection of uterine fibroids is as low as 60% and is low particularly for isoechoic fibroids in a retroverted uterus. The majority of fibroids are intramural and appear as focal hypoechoic masses that frequently distort the contour

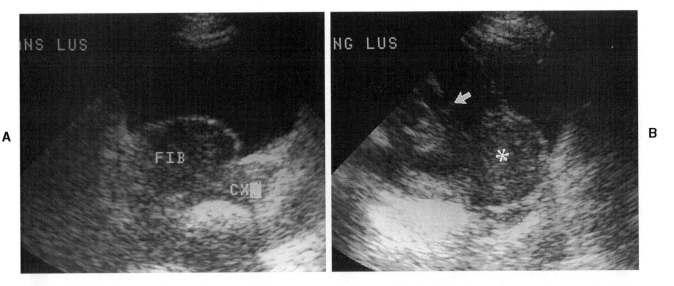

Fig. 7-24   Cervical fibroid in a gravid uterus. **A,** Transverse ultrasound image shows a solid mass originating from the anterior wall of the cervix (FIB = fibroid; CX = cervix). **B,** Sagittal image shows the lower uterine segment (arrow) and the paracervical mass (*). Leiomyoma originating from the lower uterine segment or cervix may enlarge during pregnancy and mechanically impede vaginal delivery.

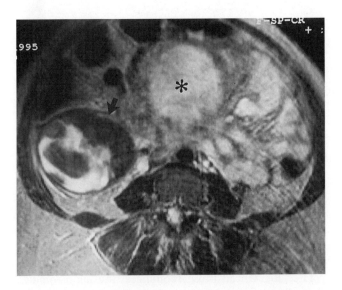

Fig. 7-25   Hyaline degeneration of a subserosal fibroid. A patient, who was 32 weeks pregnant, presented with increasingly severe pain in the right lower quadrant. A transverse turbo spin–echo T$_2$-weighted MR image (repetition time = 4914 msec; effective echo time = 96 msec) demonstrates a heterogeneous mass (arrow) in the right lower quadrant, adjacent to the gravid uterus (*). The mass was removed at cesarian section and was found to be a subserosal fibroid with extensive hyaline degeneration.

Box 7-8   Imaging of Leiomyoma

Submucous, intramural, subserosal, or combination
Plain radiography
    Coarse, popcorn calcification
    Nonspecific soft-tissue mass, sometimes large
Ultrasonography
    Hypoechoic focal mass or globular enlargement of
        uterus
    Acoustic shadowing resulting from calcification
    Irregular anechoic area resulting from degeneration
Hysterosalpingography
    Submucous—focal endometrial filling defect
    Intramural—enlargement or deformation of
        endometrial cavity
    Subserosal—no signs, or displacement of uterine
        cavity
Computed tomography
    Uniform attenuation of a globular, enlarged uterus
    Heterogeneous or hypodense as a result of
        degeneration
    Coarse, dystrophic calcification
Magnetic resonance imaging
    T$_1$-weighted image isointense or hypointense
        compared with myometrium
    T$_2$-weighted image homogeneous hypointense
    T$_2$-weighted image heterogeneous or hyperintense as
        a result of degeneration

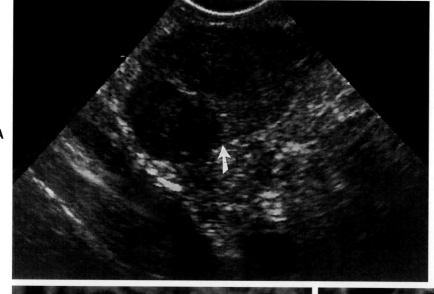

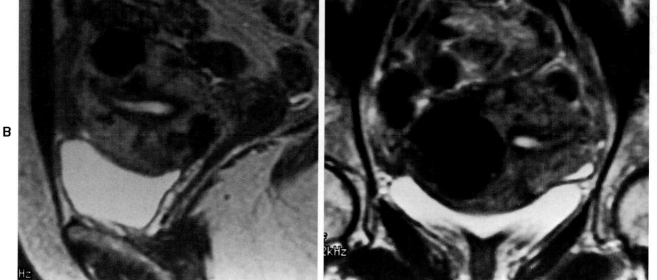

Fig. 7-26 Sonography and MR imaging of uterine leiomyoma. **A,** Sagittal sonogram shows a single, well-defined hypoechoic mass originating from the dorsal myometrium in a patient with an enlarged uterus. Note the beak of the normal myometrium (arrow) at the margin of the intramural leiomyoma. On fast spin–echo T$_2$-weighted MR imaging, multiple hypointense myometrial masses and the endometrium are demonstrated on sagittal (**B**) and coronal (**C**) images. Often, MR imaging demonstrates more leiomyomas than sonography and shows more clearly the location of the tumor relative to the endometrium.

of the uterus (Fig. 7-26). Increased echogenicity of some myomas is attributed to either relatively more fibrous tissue or calcification. Irregular anechoic areas within large myomas are ascribed to hyaline or cystic degeneration. By transabdominal sonography, it may not be possible to distinguish submucosal and intramural fibroids. Distortion of the endometrial echo by a submucosal fibroid is easier to identify on endovaginal sonography. The location of a fibroid before surgery is best determined by MR imaging or hysterosalpingography. A pedunculated or exophytic subserosal leiomyoma may simulate a solid adnexal mass because the echogenicity of leiomyomas and solid ovarian tumors can be indistinguishable (Fig. 7-23).

Magnetic resonance imaging has become an important adjunctive examination in the evaluation of the suspected uterine leiomyoma, particularly when sonographic results are equivocal because of coexistent adnexal disease, when the myoma is large, or when the patient is obese. On T$_2$-weighted images, the location of the myoma relative to the endometrium is well defined (Figs. 7-22, 7-23, 7-26). On all pulse sequences, the leiomyoma is characteristically well circumscribed, being sharply demarcated from surrounding myometrium. This sharp demarcation is caused by either a pseudocapsule composed of areolar tissue or by compressed myometrial tissue. Leiomyomas are entirely or predominantly hypointense compared to myometrium on T$_1$-weighted images, al-

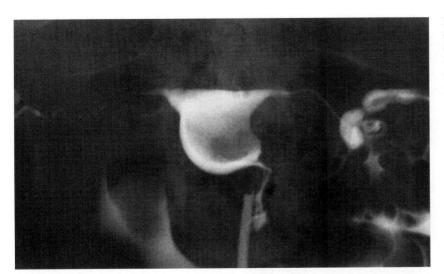

Fig. 7-27 Submucosal mass demonstrated on hysterosalpingogram. A smooth filling defect with an acute angle margin distorts the endometrial cavity. A submucosal leiomyoma or endometrial polyp might have this appearance.

though they may be isointense. On T_2-weighted images, these tumors are entirely or predominantly hypointense compared with myometrium. A heterogeneous or speckled appearance on T_2-weighted images, with small or large focal areas of increased signal intensity, is consistent with hyaline and cystic degeneration (Figs. 7-23, 7-25). Nevertheless, the essential distinguishing feature is that leiomyomas are predominantly or entirely hypointense compared with myometrium on T_2-weighted images. With the exception of ovarian fibroma, no other solid adnexal or pelvic mass has this signal intensity profile. Uterine masses that are predominantly hyperintense on T_2-weighted images may represent degenerated leiomyomas, and they may not be distinguished from malignant tumors.

Hysterosalpingography has been used to determine the location of a leiomyoma before myomectomy. A submucosal fibroid appears as a well-defined smooth filling defect with obtuse margins in the endometrial cavity (Fig. 7-27). Intramural leiomyomas are suggested when the lumen of the uterus is normal but distorted because of displacement.

In the evaluation of leiomyoma, the role of CT is secondary to that of sonography and MR imaging. An enlarged uterus frequently is the only sign of uterine leiomyoma on the noncontrast CT scan because these neoplasms usually are isodense relative to myometrium in the absence of cystic or carneous degeneration. The enlarged uterus containing one or more eccentric leiomyomas may have a lobulated contour or, in about 10% of myomas, focal calcification that can be speckled, streaked, or whorled. After intravenous contrast material administration, leiomyomas usually are isodense compared with enhanced myometrium because they enhance to the same degree as normal smooth muscle. Irregular and nonenhancing central areas of decreased density may occur when leiomyomas undergo cystic or carneous degeneration. It may not be possible to distinguish benign degeneration of a leiomyoma from sarcomatous transformation in the absence of lymphadenopathy or evidence of pelvic viscera or muscle invasion.

The Ovarian Cyst

Functional and physiologic cysts

The follicular cyst, corpus luteum or lutein cyst, and theca lutein cyst are termed collectively *functional cysts* because they originate from an alteration in the development or regression of the ovarian follicle or its derivatives. A follicular or follicle cyst, the most common type of functional ovarian cyst, occurs when a maturing follicle fails to regress after oocyte demise. Because the natural history of these cysts is to regress during a subsequent menstrual cycle, expectant follow-up examination is recommended in the premenopausal woman. Rarely, spontaneous hemorrhage into an ovarian cyst may present with acute pelvic or abdominal pain (Fig. 7-28). The more typical hemorrhagic cyst is the corpus luteum cyst, which develops if the corpus luteum fails to regress within 14 days after ovulation. Follicular and lutein cysts often are incidental findings because they are asymptomatic unless complicated by hemorrhage or torsion. Theca lutein cysts, unlike the other functional cysts, usually are bilateral because they develop when human chorionic gonadotropin (hCG) levels are increased abnormally (Box 7-9). As many as 50% of all cases occur with gestational trophoblastic disease, and theca lutein cysts also may develop during administration of fertility drugs (ovarian hyperstimulation).

Follicular cysts typically are 1 to 2 cm and rarely ex-

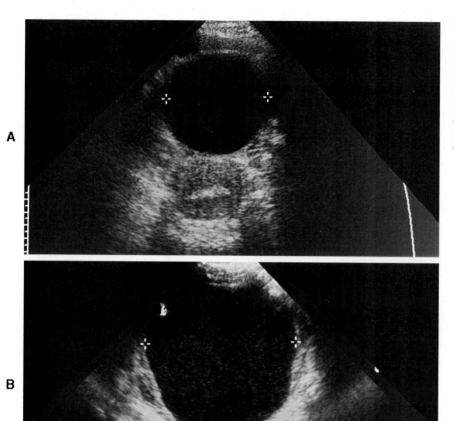

Fig. 7-28 Characterization of a hemorrhagic cyst with endovaginal sonography. A 5-cm simple cystic mass was seen on a follow-up transabdominal sonogram. **A,** The initial ultrasound examination was done 6 weeks before this study and showed a 2-cm simple cyst. **B,** Additional evaluation with endovaginal sonography demonstrates fine internal echoes, suggesting internal hemorrhage. At surgery, a hemorrhagic ovarian cyst was removed.

ceed 6 cm in diameter. Uncomplicated follicular cysts are sonographically simple, unilocular, and well defined. On CT evaluation, these cysts typically are well circumscribed and of uniform low attenuation. However, thin septations, focal thickening of the wall, or increased attenuation may be observed in up to one third of patients. Follicular cysts may change in size on serial examinations. In contrast, lutein cysts frequently are complicated by hemorrhage and may appear predominantly, but not entirely, cystic. There may be solid material along the dependent wall of a cystic mass or radiating from the center of the cyst. A corpus luteum cyst also can be predominantly solid and indistinguishable from neoplasms. Theca lutein cysts usually are larger than other types of functional cysts and frequently are bilateral and multilocular.

Polycystic ovary disease

Polycystic ovary disease (PCOD) epitomizes chronic anovulation in the setting of acyclic production of estrogen (Box 7-10). This syndrome is characterized clinically by amenorrhea or oligomenorrhea, infertility, hirsutism, and obesity. Endocrinologic investigation reveals an LH-to-FSH ratio of more than 2 and increased androgen levels. Acyclic production of estrone results in appropriately elevated levels of LH and decreased levels of FSH. Increased plasma levels of LH lead to stimulation of ovarian theca and stroma, and decreased FSH levels are responsible for chronic anovulation. Although the original pathologic description of the ovaries by Stein and Leventhal was that of enlarged and multicystic ovaries, the diagnosis of PCOD is based primarily on the characteristic endocrinologic profile because a variety of pathologic findings subsequently have been described, none of which is pa-

---

Box 7-9   Theca Lutein Cysts

Result from elevated β human chorionic gonadotropin
  levels
Fertility drugs
Gestational trophoblastic disease
Multiple gestations
Hydrops fetalis

thognomonic. In the classic description, the ovaries are enlarged and sclerotic with a thickened capsule. Multiple subcapsular follicular cysts are identified, and the ovarian stroma is hyperplastic. Conversely, multicystic ovaries may be seen in patients with anorexia nervosa and other forms of hypothalamic amenorrhea, congenital adrenal hyperplasia, virilizing neoplasms of the ovary or adrenal gland, and hypothyroidism, and in premenarchal girls.

Transvaginal sonography and MR imaging have been used to distinguish the polycystic ovary from the healthy one. The classic polycystic ovary is enlarged and echogenic and contains an increased number of smaller-than-normal follicles crowded at its surface. In general, the polycystic ovary contains twice the number of antral follicles, which usually are less than 4 mm in diameter, and has twice the volume of the normal ovary

(Fig. 7-29). When compared with healthy control subjects, Pache and others reported a statistically significant decrease in the mean follicular diameter (3.8 mm vs. 5.1 mm), increase in mean follicular number (9.8 vs. 5.0), increase in average ovarian volume (9.8 mL vs. 5.9 mL), and increase in stromal echogenicity in the polycystic ovary. However, with respect to ovarian volume and follicular number, there is considerable overlap with healthy subjects; in almost one third of patients with clinical and endocrinologic evidence of PCOD, the ovaries are normal in volume.

Ovarian cyst in the postmenopause

The occurrence of any ovarian cyst in postmenopausal women has, until recently, been considered abnormal and an indication for surgery. However, more recent work supports the concept that simple cystic lesions of the ovary, especially those less than 5 cm in diameter, are not likely to be malignant. Asymptomatic, simple adnexal cysts may be seen in up to 20% of postmenopausal women. Although no clear relationship has been established between the presence of cysts and treatment with hormone replacement, some authorities have noted that up to 40% of women who take sequential estrogen and progesterone have ovarian cysts, and that at follow-up examination in many of these women, cysts may appear de novo or may increase in size. Ovarian cystic disease can be dynamic because as many as 60% of the cysts disappear or change in size. In addition to the presenting size and growth of an adnexal cyst, other factors

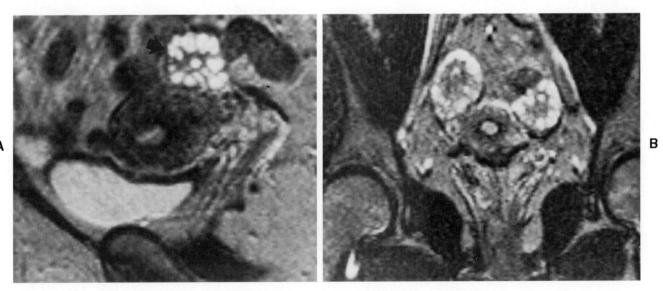

Fig. 7-29   Polycystic ovary disease on MR imaging. **A,** A right parasagittal turbo spin-echo T_2-weighted image (repetition time [TR] = 5000 msec; effective echo time [TE] = 96 msec) shows the multiple follicles crowded at the surface of the ovary (arrow). **B,** A coronal spin-echo T_2-weighted MR image (TR = 2370 msec; TE = 80 msec) demonstrates a similar appearance of the right ovary.

that can be used to assess the malignant potential of a cystic mass include the Doppler resistive index and serum CA-125 levels. In general, patients who have a normal CA-125 level and ovarian cysts that are 4 cm or less in diameter with a normal resistive index can be followed. Surgical exploration is recommended for patients with larger cysts, complex cysts with mural or septal nodules, and cysts with prominent diastolic flow on duplex scanning.

Infertility

Infertility is defined as the inability to conceive after 12 months of unprotected intercourse. Infertility is termed primary when there have been no successful previous pregnancies and secondary when a previous conception has occurred. This distinction is of little clinical importance because, with the exception of tubal occlusion, endometriosis, and oligoazoospermia, similar etiologies are responsible for infertility, whether primary or secondary. The causes of infertility can be divided into those attributed to each partner; in 5% to 10% of couples, no explanation can be found after extensive investigations (Box 7-11). Approximately 55% of infertility is related to female factors, which can be subclassified into abnormalities of ovulation, peritoneum, cervical mucous consistency, tubal patency, and endometrial function. Abnormalities of male endocrine function or spermatogenesis account for 35% of infertility. Infertility may result either from one major deficiency, such as tubal occlusion, or from a combination of minor deficiencies, as is true in 40% of patients.

Cervical factor

Immediately before ovulation, the cervix produces a watery mucus that promotes and maintains the viability of sperm. Simple physical evaluation of this fluid during the immediate preovulatory phase assesses the amount and clarity of this mucus. The cervical mucus also is evaluated 6 to 8 hours after intercourse in the postcoital (Sims-Huhner) test. In addition, the number and motility of spermatozoa that have entered the cervical canal are assessed. Because it is essential to evaluate the cervical mucus in the preovulatory phase, sonography has been used to monitor follicular development and to detect ovulation.

Endometrial factor

Abnormalities of the uterine endometrium are seldom the cause of primary or secondary infertility. More often, congenital müllerian anomalies, submucosal leiomyoma, or endometrial polyps are the cause of habitual first-trimester spontaneous abortion. Anatomic abnormalities, such as congenital anomalies, synechiae, or leiomyoma, may interfere with the normal function of the uterus by impeding zygote implantation and development. The radiologic evaluation of the uterus for these abnormalities includes hysterosalpingography, ultrasonography, and MR imaging.

Congenital anomalies of uterine formation are common causes of habitual abortion, but they rarely cause primary infertility. Septate uteri have the highest prevalence of spontaneous abortion, followed by unicornuate and bicornuate uteri. Arcuate uteri and uterus didelphys do not have a significantly higher risk of fetal wastage, especially compared with the other congenital anomalies.

Leiomyomas likely interfere with normal reproductive function of the uterus because of mechanical factors. Large myomas may obstruct the cervical canal or the intramural segment of the fallopian tubes. Distortion of the endometrial cavity may impair sperm transport. Implantation may be impeded by a submucosal fibroid, but more often, the abnormal vascular supply of an adjacent myoma will not permit development of sufficient vascular support for a pregnancy to proceed normally.

Intrauterine adhesions or synechiae can obstruct the endometrial cavity and sperm transit or zygote implantation. Asherman's syndrome refers to persistent amenorrhea and secondary sterility, which is caused by intrauterine adhesions or synechiae. Synechiae most often are the sequelae of therapeutic curettage, but they also may follow severe endometritis. Although occasionally diagnosed by TVS, the presence and extent of intrauterine adhesions are evaluated most commonly with hysterosalpingography or hysteroscopy. On hysterosalpingography evaluation, thick or thin, linear, irregular filling defects may reduce the effective size of the endometrial cavity (Fig. 7-30). Extensive synechiae may prevent uterine filling with contrast material. Intrauterine synechiae appear as tissue bridges within the endometrial cavity on TVS or as serpentine, echogenic endometrial irregularities, surrounding small cystic areas.

Box 7-11   Infertility

Female factors (~55%)
  Cervical
  Endometrial
  Tubal
  Peritoneal
  Ovulatory
Male factors (~35%)
  Endocrine
  Spermatogenesis

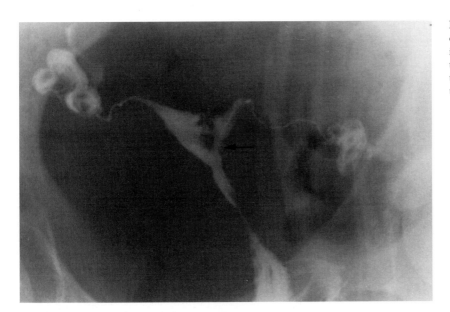

Fig. 7-30 Intrauterine adhesions or synechiae. On a hysterosalpingogram, polypoid filling defects with jagged margins project into the endometrial cavity. The wall of the endometrium is slightly irregular (small arrow). At hysteroscopy, adhesions were resected.

Tubal factors

Tubal stenosis or occlusion most often occurs at the fimbria, but midsegment and isthmic narrowings also are observed. PID, endometriosis, and intrauterine device use are the most common predisposing conditions for occlusive tubal disease; however, in 50% of patients, no clear predisposing factor can be identified. Midsegment occlusion almost always is secondary to tubal sterilization surgery; rarer causes include salpingitis isthmica nodosum (SIN) or tuberculous salpingitis. With SIN, numerous small diverticula extend from the lumen into the wall of the isthmic segment (Fig. 7-31). Frequently, patients have a history of PID, and both fallopian tubes are affected in 80% of patients. Isthmic diverticulosis can be seen in some patients with tuberculosis, and in these patients,

there is ampullary contraction and adnexal calcification. Isthmic–cornual stenosis can occur congenitally or can be related to myomata, previous infection, or endometriosis. Tubal obstruction most commonly is diagnosed when free intraperitoneal spillage of contrast material cannot be demonstrated with hysterosalpingography. Spasm from pelvic pain may be the cause of a false-positive result of hysterosalpingogram.

Between 60% and 80% of patients with tubal obstruction are treated successfully with microsurgical tuboplasty, a more effective alternative to conventional surgical techniques. Fallopian tube catheterization entails selective catheterization of the ostium of the fallopian tube with an angiographic catheter. Passage of the guidewire through the tube separates intraluminal adhesions,

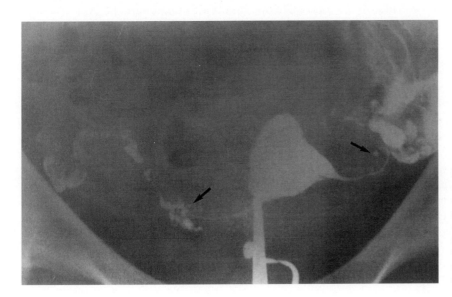

Fig. 7-31 Salpingitis isthmica nodosa (tubal diverticulosis) on hysterosalpingogram. Typical findings for salpingitis isthmica nodosa are seen on this left posterior oblique film. Small, clustered collections of contrast material (arrows) extend from the tubular lumen into the wall of both fallopian tubes. Obstruction of the fallopian tube often accompanies this disease.

and contrast instillation clears the tube of detritus. This procedure restores functional or anatomic tubal patency in up to 90% of patients, and there is a subsequent pregnancy rate of up to 30%.

Peritoneal factors

Pelvic adhesions or endometriosis can impair fertility by interfering with the normal transport function of the fallopian tubes. Peritubular adhesions may obstruct the fallopian tube, cause tubal dysmotility, or impede the entry of the oocyte into the tube. Diagnostic laparoscopy remains the mainstay for the diagnosis of endometriosis because it identifies previously unsuspected pelvic abnormality in 30% to 50% of women with unexplained infertility.

Ovulatory factors

The simplest screening tests for the initial evaluation of ovulation are the basal body temperature and the midluteal serum level of progesterone. The thermogenic effects of progesterone cause a 0.4°F elevation of the body temperature at ovulation. The midluteal concentration of progesterone usually is above 10 ng/mL during cycles in which conception is possible. Ultrasonography also can be used in the initial evaluation of the patient with infertility for the detection of ovulation or luteal phase defect, but more often it is used to monitor women in whom ovulation is being induced or whose oocytes are being collected for in vitro fertilization. For example, one of the serious complications of ovulation induction is related to excessive stimulation of the ovaries. The hyperstimulation syndrome, or exudation of large amounts of fluid into the peritoneal and pleural cavities, may accompany stimulated ovarian enlargement. The premature development of several large follicles or more than 10 follicles of intermediate size, together with an increase in the estradiol concentration, indicates that gonadotropins should be withheld to avert ovarian over-stimulation.

Male factors

The evaluation of factors that relate to the male partner and may contribute to infertility begins with the analysis of semen for a reduction in the quality and quantity of sperm. Patients with an absence of sperm in the ejaculate are subclassified into those with either a low-volume (< 1 mL) or normal volume (≥ 1 mL) ejaculate. The differential diagnosis of azospermia with a low-volume ejaculate includes retrograde ejaculation and obstruction of the distal seminal duct system, such as urethral stricture, stenosis of the ejaculatory duct, or agenesis of either the seminal vesicles or vas deferens. Intrinsic testicular failure and epididymal obstruction are causes of azoospermia or oligospermia and a normal-volume ejaculate.

Transrectal sonography can be used to detect congenital or acquired obstruction of the distal genital duct system and is an accurate and noninvasive alternative to vasography. Lesions that can be detected by transrectal sonography include unilateral or bilateral absence of the vasa deferentia, seminal vesicle cysts, seminal vesicle atrophy with or without dystrophic calcification, and midline prostatic cysts that can obstruct the ejaculatory ducts. Scrotal ultrasonography is used occasionally to confirm testicular atrophy or varicocele, which may be suggested by results of the physical evaluation.

Gynecologic Oncology

Cancer of the ovary

Although it is the sixth most common cancer among female patients in the United States, ovarian cancer is the leading cause of death from gynecologic cancer because it often is locally advanced or disseminated at presentation. Many patients are asymptomatic or complain of nonspecific symptoms like lower abdominal discomfort, fullness, irregular menses, or dyspareunia. Rarely, severe abdominal distress may occur if the tumor is torsed or ruptures. Patients with ovarian cancer in advanced stages may have abdominal pain, increased abdominal girth because of ascites, or, rarely, vaginal bleeding.

Based on tissue type of origin, there are four predominant histopathologic types of ovarian cancer: epithelial, germ cell, sex cord–stroma, and metastatic (Box 7-12). Epithelial cancers are derived from peritoneal mesothelial cells and comprise about 65% of all ovarian neoplasms and the majority of all ovarian malignancies. Three major subtypes of epithelial ovarian neoplasms include serous, mucinous, and endometrioid (Box 7-13). Increased serum concentrations of CA-125, a high-molecular weight glycoprotein, can be detected in 80% of patients with epithelial ovarian neoplasms. Serous tumors are the most common type of epithelial ovarian neoplasm; the majority are either benign (60%) or borderline-malignancy (15%) cystadenomas; the remainder are malignant cystadenocarcinomas (Box 7-14; Fig. 7-32). Borderline tumors are carci-

---

Box 7-12 Ovarian Malignancy— Histologic Types and Frequency

Epithelial—65%
Germ cell—25%
Sex cord–stroma—5%
Secondary or metastatic—5%
Gonadoblastoma—rare

nomas of low malignant potential that present cytologic features of malignancy, such as mitosis or nuclear abnormalities, but do not invade the stroma. Mucinous tumors are slightly less common than serous forms (Box 7-15; Fig. 7-33). Ninety-five percent of mucinous tumors are benign or of borderline malignancy. A rare complication of malignant mucinous cystadenocarcinoma occurs after rupture. Gelatinous material implants on peritoneal surfaces and causes mass effect in a condition known as pseudomyxoma peritonei.

Germ cell tumors make up the majority of ovarian tumors that occur in infants and children and 25% of all ovarian tumors (Box 7-16). The most common neoplasm of this cell type is the benign cystic teratoma or dermoid cyst, which makes up 95% of all germ cell tumors (Box 7-17). Benign teratomas may contain well-differentiated tissue from skin or dermal appendages, such as hair and teeth (Fig. 7-34). Metaplastic sebaceous glands can produce fat or oil (Fig. 7-35 on p. 282). Immature tissue elements are found in the rarer malignant teratoma, and even more unusual is dedifferentiation of a benign teratoma to squamous cell carcinoma (SCC). The most common malignant germ cell tumor is the dysgerminoma, an ovarian counterpart of testicular seminoma. The majority of these tumors occur in patients aged 10 to 30 years. The tumors are confined to the ovaries at the time of diagnosis and are radiosensitive. The endodermal sinus, or yolk sac, tumors are the rarest germ cell tumors and may retain the capacity to produce hormones. Choriocarcinomas produce HCG; endodermal sinus tumors pro-

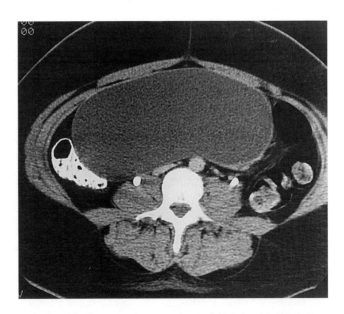

Fig. 7-32   Serous cystadenoma. Abdominal CT demonstrates a large cystic mass in an obese patient. There were no septations or mural nodules, and the nonenhancing wall of the mass is uniformly thin. Most serous epithelial ovarian tumors are benign and may present as a large, unilocular cyst. (Case courtesy of Mark S. Ridlen, MD.)

duce alpha-fetoprotein, and both hormones may be produced by embryonal-cell carcinomas.

Five percent of ovarian neoplasms are derived from the sex cords and specialized stroma of the developing gonad (Box 7-18 on p. 282). In order of descending frequency, benign tumors of this category include the fibroma–thecoma, granulosa cell tumor, and Sertoli-Leydig cell tumor. The ovarian fibroma is a nonfunctioning tumor that can be complicated by ascites; Meig's syndrome is the occurrence of ascites and a right pleural effusion with this benign tumor. Fibromas also have been associated with the basal cell nevus syndrome. Tumors that originate from specialized ovarian stroma retain the potential to secrete estrogen or progesterone. Consequently, functional granulosa cell and thecal cell tumors may be associated with precocious puberty, endometrial carcinoma, endometrial hyperplasia, or cystic diseases of the breast. Sertoli-Leydig cell tumors are less common and

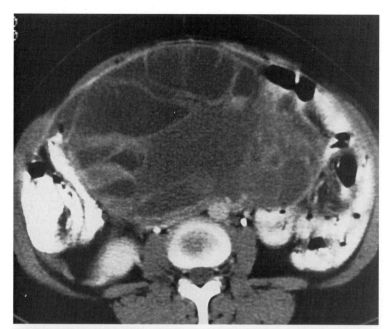

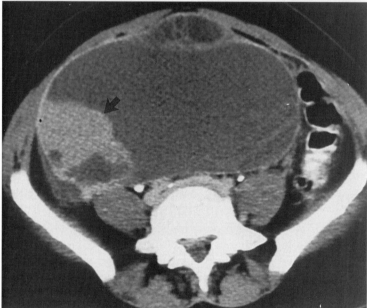

Fig. 7-33 Mucinous cystadenocarcinoma of the ovary. Infused CT scans of the abdomen show a large, heterogeneous mass with solid and complex cystic components. Heterogeneous density of the cystic component reflects the variable content of mucin in this malignant tumor. There was contrast enhancement of the solid mural mass (arrow) and portions of the tumor wall.

Box 7-16 Germ Cell Tumors

Twenty-five percent of all ovarian tumors
Teratoma or dermoid cyst
Two percent of all ovarian malignancies: malignant germ-cell tumor
Rare functional tissue: stroma ovarii causing hyperthyroidism

---

Box 7-17 Dermoid Cyst (Mature Cystic Teratoma)

Originates from primordial germ cell
Two-thirds of ovarian tumors in girls aged 15 years or younger
Fifteen percent bilateral
Complications: torsion, trauma, infection, rupture
Malignant transformation in 1% to 2%; squamous cell carcinoma
Sebaceous plug or dental parts

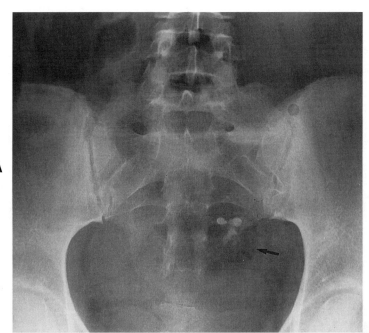

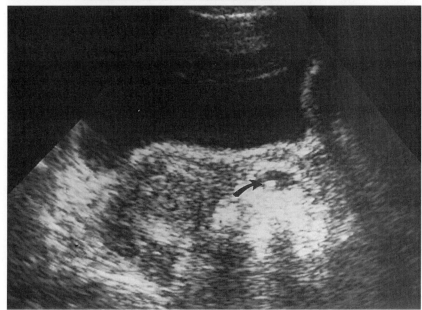

Fig. 7-34   Benign cystic teratoma containing dental elements. **A,** Coned-down view of the pelvis shows a faintly radiolucent mass (arrow) that is associated with tooth-like calcifications. **B,** Sonography in the transverse plane shows an intensely echogenic left adnexal mass. The dental parts appear as a small echogenic focus (curved arrow) with posterior acoustic shadowing.

may cause masculinization as a result of the production of testosterone or testosterone-like hormones.

Five percent of ovarian neoplasms are caused by metastasis from primary cancers of the gastrointesinal tract, breast, lymphatic system, or pelvic viscera (Box 7-19). The Krukenberg tumor is a specific histologic type of bilateral metastatic ovarian adenocarcinoma featuring mucin-filled "signet ring" cells (Fig. 7-36). Transcoelomic spread to the ovary is the primary mode of metastasis for mucinous cancers of the stomach or colon. Krukenberg tumors tend to be large (often > 8 cm in diameter), particularly if predominantly cystic, and bilateral ovarian

masses. Peritoneal carcinomatosis and lymphadenopathy also may be seen.

A typical mode of dissemination is exfoliation of ovarian tumor cells into the peritoneal cavity, followed by the development of ascites, peritoneal nodules, and serosal implants. Lymphatic spread is less common, although ovarian cancer can involve the pelvic and paraaortic lymphatics. In contrast with other gynecologic malignancies, the lymphatic dissemination of ovarian cancer generally involves the renal hilar lymph nodes initially rather than the pelvic lymph nodes. Hematogenous spread occurs relatively late, if at all; only about 2% to 3% of patients

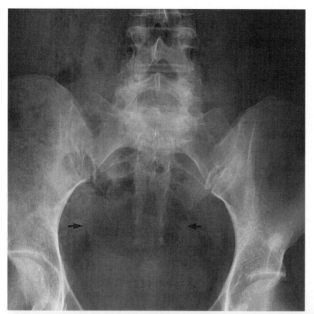

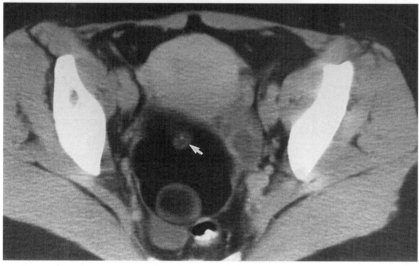

Fig. 7-35   Dermoid cyst. **A,** Plain film of the pelvis shows a radiolucent mass (arrow) in the midpelvis. **B,** A large, predominantly fatty mass is demonstrated on CT. Nodules or plugs originate from the wall of the mass, and there is a small focus of calcification in the dermoid plug on the anterior tumor wall (arrow). These findings are typical of an ovarian dermoid cyst containing sebaceous material.

have liver or pulmonary metastatic disease at presentation. Frank invasion of viscera or bowel is atypical, but encasement and compression are observed more frequently (Fig. 7-37).

Staging of ovarian cancer is important because it determines the treatment options offered to the patient (Box 7-20). Patients with early stage disease or no gross evidence of extraovarian disease are treated with bilateral salpingo-oophorectomy (BSO), abdominal hysterectomy, infracolic omentectomy, and staging biopsies of the pelvic peritoneum, omentum, bowel serosa, and retroperitoneal lymph nodes. In patients with advanced stages of disease, in addition to BSO, total abdominal hysterectomy, and omentectomy, debulking surgery is performed to reduce as much of the tumor burden as possible. After primary cytoreductive surgery, combination chemother-

---

Box 7-18   Sex-Cord or Stromal Tumors

Fibroma–thecoma (Meig's syndrome; estrogen
   production)
Granulosa cell tumor (estrogen production)
Sertoli-Leydig tumor (testosterone production)

Box 7-19   Metastases to the Ovary

Krukenberg tumors (signet ring cells)
   Mucinous adenocarcinoma from stomach or colon
Breast carcinoma
Lymphoma

apy, frequently consisting of cis-platinum and cyclophosphamide, also is administered. After systemic chemotherapy, second-look laparotomy often is performed to evaluate for residual disease, but the efficacy of this procedure is controversial.

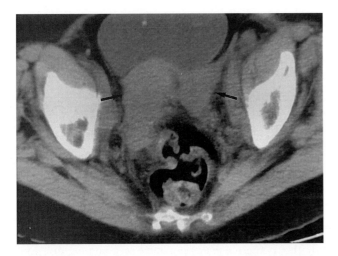

Fig. 7-36 Krukenberg tumor. CT of the pelvis demonstrates bilateral, solid ovarian masses (arrows) in an elderly woman with gastric adenocarcinoma. Pathology revealed mucin-filled signet ring cells typical for this diagnosis.

Evaluation of the adnexal mass

For the patient with a suspected pelvic mass, ultrasonography is the accepted initial examination (Box 7-21; Table 7-3). The objectives of the ultrasound evaluation are (1) to determine if an adnexal mass is present; (2) if a mass is present, to ascertain the organ of origin; (3) to characterize the mass as completely cystic, cystic but with atypical features, or solid; and (4) to determine if there is concurrent disease that would suggest an ovarian malignancy, such as abdominal or pelvic ascites, lymphadenopathy, ureterocaliectasis, or liver metastases. For the objectives of detection and characterization, CT and

Box 7-20	**Staging of Ovarian Carcinoma**
Stage I	Growth limited to ovaries
	IA One ovary
	IB Both ovaries
	IC With ascites
Stage II	Pelvic extension
Stage III	Extrapelvic intraperitoneal or omental metastases, or positive nodes
Stage IV	Distant metastases

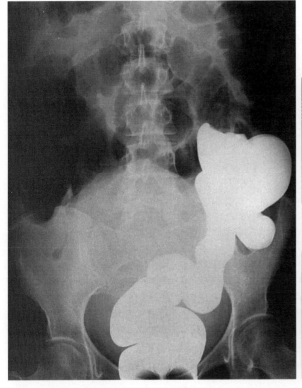

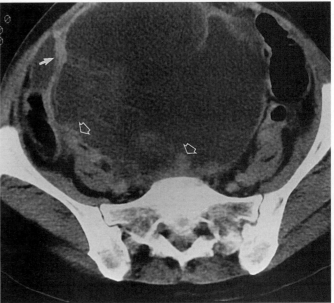

Fig. 7-37 Colonic obstruction caused by serosal implants from metastatic mucinous cystadenocarcinoma. **A,** Complete mechanical obstruction at the level of the mid-descending colon is demonstrated with barium enema. Note the lower abdominal mass. **B,** CT scan demonstrates a large abdominal mass with solid and dense cystic components, mural nodularity (open arrows), and thick septations (arrow). At surgery, multiple serosal implants were removed.

Box 7-21 Goals of Radiologic Evaluation of a Suspected Pelvic Mass

Is there a pelvic mass? What is its size and volume?
What is the organ of origin?
Is the mass a simple cyst, an atypical cyst, or predominantly solid?
Is there associated disease, such as ascites, lymphadenopathy, ureterocaliectasis, or liver masses?

MR imaging are of secondary importance to ultrasonography, although these tests are comparable with ultrasound in diagnostic accuracy. Either CT or MR imaging may be useful when the mass is so large as to defy characterization by sonography results. Patient habitus, particularly obesity, also may make the transabdominal ultrasound study suboptimal.

In general, sonographic evaluation is well suited to characterize an ovarian mass as a typical cyst, an atypical cyst, or a solid mass. The features of a typical cyst are absence of internal echoes and a uniform, nonnodular wall; posterior acoustic enhancement also can be seen. The likely etiologies for a completely cystic mass of the ovary are functional cyst, serous cystadenoma, and benign dermoid cyst (Boxes 7-22, 7-23). Of the functional cysts, follicular cyst most often is unilocular and completely cystic. Corpus luteum cysts frequently are complicated by hemorrhage or dependent debris. Serous cystadenoma is frequently a unilocular, cystic mass, but it may be bilocular with a thin (< 3 mm wide), regular septation or may have a partially calcified rim. Papillary projections alone are rare (Fig. 7-38). Benign dermoid cysts are either unilocular or septated masses, but they can be distinguished from other cystic masses when specific, mature tissues are recognized, such as fat or sebum and dental parts. In most patients, the classification of an ovarian mass as a "simple cyst," particularly if the mass is 5 cm or less in diameter, directs treatment toward

---

Table 7-3 Guidelines for Management of an Adnexal Mass

Type of mass	Size	Management
Typical cyst	< 2.5 cm	No follow-up evaluation
Typical cyst	2.5–5 cm	Follow-up sonography at 4–6 weeks
Atypical cyst	≤ 5 cm	Follow-up sonography at 4–6 weeks
Any cyst	> 5 cm	Laparoscopy or surgery
Solid mass	Any size	Laparoscopy or surgery

Box 7-22 Completely Cystic Adnexal Mass

Functional cyst (follicular or corpus luteum cyst)
Paraovarian or broad-ligament cyst
Serous cystadenoma

---

observation. Repetition of sonography during the next or subsequent menstrual period usually suffices for the follow-up evaluation of lesions in this class.

Atypical cystic masses include hemorrhagic functional cyst, endometrioma, cystic teratoma, serous cystadenoma, and mucinous cystadenoma (Box 7-24). Findings that would characterize an atypical cyst include bilocular or multilocular form, outer wall or septations that are uniformly thick and less than 3 mm, and homogeneous internal echoes. These masses should not have a solid mural component.

Ovarian neoplasms other than those discussed, whether benign or malignant, have prominent mural nodules or are predominantly or completely solid masses (Box 7-25, Fig. 7-39). Unlike its benign counterpart, serous cystadenocarcinoma more often is a multilocular mass with multiple papillary projections and septations. Papillary excrescences and echogenic material also are prominent components of mucinous cystadenocarcinoma. Other criteria that suggest a borderline or malignant tumor include irregular solid component, a nodular wall, thick or nodular septa, and endocystic or exocystic vegetations (Fig. 7-40). Soft-tissue components associated with a predominantly cystic mass should be considered more suspicious if contrast enhancement is demonstrated on either CT or MR images. Other lesions that are partly or entirely solid include tuboovarian abscess, torsion, or, rarely, an ectopic gestation (Fig. 7-41). Ovarian lesions that are not simple cysts often are explored surgically, particularly if other findings on imaging or laboratory tests (i.e., elevated CA-125 levels) suggest an ovarian malignancy (Box 7-26).

Although characterization of pelvic mass traditionally has been based on morphology, duplex sonography also has been explored as a method to improve characterization (Box 7-27). Neovessels associated with tumors can be distinguished from normal vessels by an irregular, meandering course, paucity of smooth muscle in the

---

Box 7-23 Multicystic Adnexal Mass

Hydrosalpinx
Theca lutein cysts
Polycystic ovary

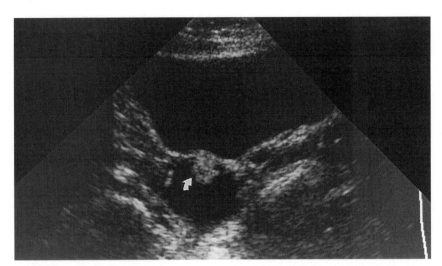

Fig. 7-38   Serous cystadenoma of the ovary in a 32-year-old woman with a palpable adnexal mass. Sagittal image from a pelvic ultrasound examination shows a papillary projection (arrow) from the wall of a predominantly cystic adnexal mass.

A

B

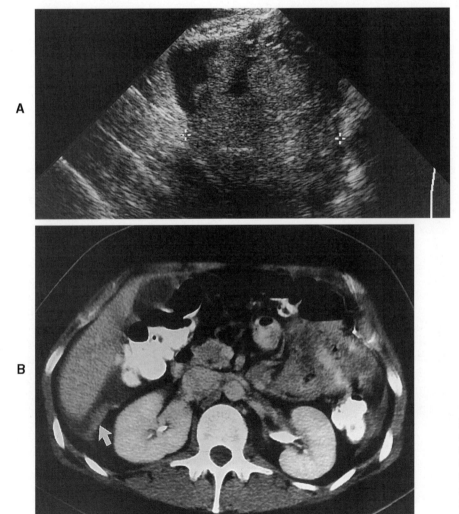

Fig. 7-39   Solid adnexal mass in a 21-year-old woman with pelvic pain and increasing abdominal girth. **A,** Pelvic sonogram demonstrates a 6.7-cm predominantly solid right ovarian mass. **B,** Infused CT of the abdomen shows ascites and a peritoneal implant (arrow) along the anterior renal fascia. The ovarian mass surgically was proven to be a dysgerminoma.

Box 7-24   Atypical Cyst*

Hemorrhagic cyst
Endometrioma
Cystic teratoma
Serous cystadenoma
Mucinous cystadenoma

*Features of an atypical cyst: non-nodular wall, bilocular or multilocular, septations and wall thickness less than 3 mm, and uniform internal echoes.

Box 7-25   Predominantly or Completely Solid Adnexal Mass

All other ovarian carcinomas and metastasis to ovary
Cystic teratoma or dermoid cyst
Tuboovarian abscess
Ovarian torsion
Ovarian ectopic pregnancy
Subserosal leiomyoma

A

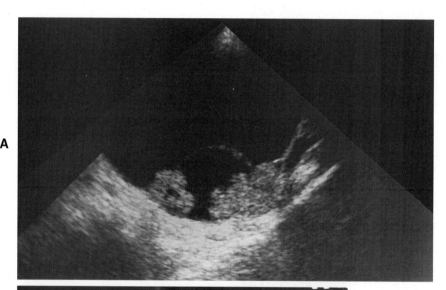

B

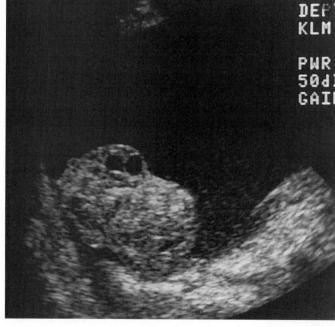

Fig. 7-40   Sonographic findings of predominantly cystic masses that suggest a borderline or malignant tumor. **A,** Papillary projections and septations are seen in a patient with borderline serous cystadenocarcinoma. **B,** In another patient, ultrasonography demonstrates an endocystic vegetation and echogenic fluid in a mucinous cystadenocarcinoma.

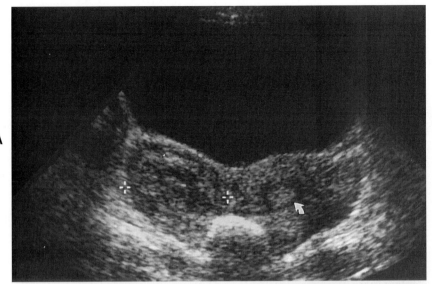

A

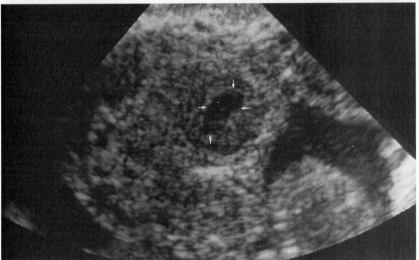

B

Fig. 7-41 Ovarian ectopic gestation presenting as a solid adnexal mass. A 15-year-old girl presented with right lower quadrant pain. **A,** Transverse pelvic sonogram shows a solid right adnexal mass, denoted by electronic markers. Note the decidual reaction of the endometrium (arrow). **B,** Endovaginal sonogram in the sagittal plane shows a gestational sac (small arrows) containing an embryo with cardiac activity. Intense blood flow was identified around the gestational sac by color Doppler sonography (not shown).

Box 7-26 Adnexal Mass: Criteria Suggesting Malignancy
Growth Solid or predominantly solid Diameter more than 5 cm Irregular cystic spaces, suggesting necrosis Mural or septal thickness greater than 3 mm

Box 7-27 Adnexal Mass: Doppler Evaluation
Neovessels lack smooth muscle in media, hence, low resistance Abnormal flow is nonpulsatile and continuously fluctuating Thresholds: pulsatility index less than 1.0 and resistive index less than 0.4 for malignancy False-positive: inflammatory mass, endometrioma, hydrosalpinx, hemorrhagic corpus luteum

vessel media layer, arteriovenous shunting, and pooling of blood in amorphous, sinusoid-like lakes. The theory that supports the use of Doppler sonography is that tumor neovascularity is associated with increased diastolic flow because of decreased resistance to flow from a paucity of smooth muscle within the media of neoplastic vessels. The technique calls for gray-scale and color

Doppler evaluation of the ovarian mass, main ovarian vessels, and adnexal branches of the uterine vessels for areas of abnormal flow. Abnormal flow is identified as continuously fluctuating color rather than the pulsatile color seen with normal arteries. Spectral analysis of iden-

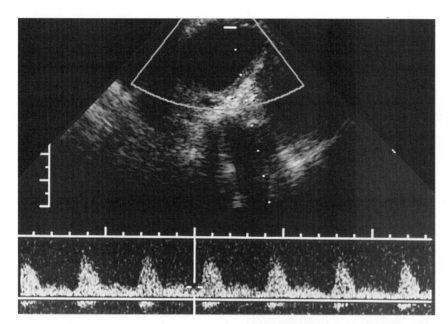

Fig. 7-42 Doppler sonography of a 5-cm predominantly cystic ovarian mass. Flow was demonstrated in the wall of the mass. Spectral analysis revealed a peak systolic velocity of 22 cm/sec, end diastolic velocity of 6 cm/sec, pulsatility index of 1.1, and resistive index of 0.73. At surgery, a serous cysadenoma was removed.

tified vascular flow and calculation of a pulsatility index (PI = peak systolic velocity − end diastolic velocity/ mean velocity) or resistive index (RI = peak systolic velocity − end diastolic velocity/peak systolic velocity) is performed. Some investigators have found that malignant masses tend to have abnormal flow in the center of the mass, a PI less than unity, and higher maximum systolic velocity. In many benign masses, flow tends to be identified best in the periphery of the mass, the maximal systolic velocity is low, the PI is 1.0 or more, and a dicrotic notch is identified (Fig. 7-42). Others have characterized ovarian masses based on an RI in the ovarian branch of the uterine artery and have found that an RI more than 0.7 indicates a benign mass, whereas an RI less than 0.4 indicates a malignant mass. RI values between 0.4 and 0.7 are equivocal. Some benign masses, such as inflammatory masses, pyosalpinx, endometriomas, and hemorrhagic corpus luteum cysts, also may show a low impedance flow pattern, suggestive of malignancy.

For characterization of an ovarian mass, the use of contrast material has been shown to increase the accuracy of MR imaging. In 1991, Stevens et al established primary and secondary criteria for differentiating benign from malignant ovarian masses. The primary criteria used to characterize ovarian lesions include (1) lesion size more than 4 cm in diameter, (2) solid or predominantly solid lesion, (3) cystic space in the tumor consistent with necrosis, (4) cystic lesion with thickness of wall or septa more than 3 mm, and (5) presence of mural nodularity or mass. With the exception of the first criterion, evaluation of all of these criteria is better accomplished on contrast-enhanced images. Secondary criteria that suggest malignancy include (1) pelvic side wall extension, (2) presence of ascites, (3) presence of implants on peri-

toneal, mesenteric, or omental surfaces, and (4) lymphadenopathy. In particular, implants are made more conspicuous with contrast enhancement. According to this system, a mass should be considered malignant if two of the five primary criteria are present or if a single ancillary criterion is found.

An important part of the characterization of a suspicious ovarian mass is the assessment of the pelvis and abdomen for ascites, uretetopelvocaliectasis, and lymphadenopathy. An evaluation of the liver for metastatic foci also may yield important information about the nature of a pelvic mass. Whereas pelvic ascites can be associated with benign or malignant tumors, abdominal ascites suggest a malignant tumor and peritoneal metastases. Two notable exceptions to this rule are the association of abdominal ascites with benign ovarian fibroma (Meig's syndrome) and ovarian torsion.

Computed tomography and MR imaging have shortcomings in the evaluation of staging of ovarian neoplasms, particularly in the detection of peritoneal implants or omental metastases 1 to 1.5 cm or less in size. In contrast, surgery is diagnostic and therapeutic. The relatively poor sensitivity of CT and MR imaging in identifying minimal pelvic and abdominal disease precludes its use as a substitute for second-look surgery. On CT, peritoneal implants appear as focal soft-tissue masses along the lateral peritoneum or in the subdiaphragmatic spaces (Fig. 7-43). Mesenteric disease may manifest on CT scans as poorly defined nodular masses. With neurovascular invasion, a stellate pattern can be seen in the root of the mesentery. There is a spectrum of findings that suggest omental disease. Small nodules of soft tissue may pepper the fat anterior to bowel, or large, cakelike masses can be seen wedged between colon and the

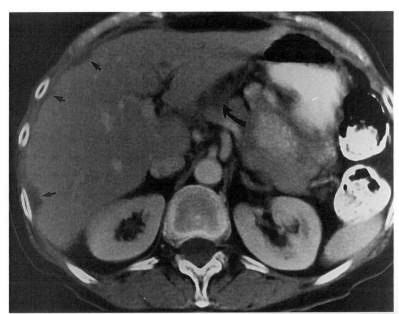

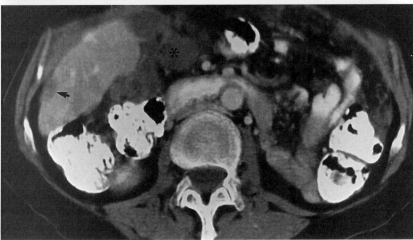

Fig. 7-43   Peritoneal metastases from ovarian carcinoma. Contrast-enhanced CT scans of the abdomen demonstrate small hypodense masses (small arrows), which result in a scalloped liver margin. Larger focal masses were noted along the gastrohepatic ligament (curved arrow) and in the omentum (*). There were relatively little ascites, and a large pelvic mass also was present.

anterior abdominal wall or small bowel. Serosal implants may appear as nodular thickening or spiculation of the bowel wall on barium-contrast radiography, CT, or MR imaging.

Cancer of the uterine corpus

Hyperplasia of the endometrium   Endometrial hyperplasia is overgrowth of the normal uterine endometrium under the hormonal influence of persistently high levels of estrogens unopposed by progesterone. This condition may occur physiologically during periods of infrequent ovulation. It also may occur when exogenous estrogens are administered to postmenopausal women with PCOD and with estrogen-producing ovarian neoplasms. Younger patients with anovulatory cycles often have a mild and reversible form of cystic endometrial hyperplasia. In contrast, older patients tend to have adenomatous hyperplasia. The majority of such hyperplasias, those

without atypia, have a low risk of progression to endometrial carcinoma: 1% for simple and 3% for complex hyperplasia without atypia. Endometrial hyperplasia should be suspected when there is prolonged or irregular menses or postmenopausal bleeding. The diagnosis is made by endometrial biopsy, but in many patients, curettage must be performed to exclude endometrial cancer. Hysterosalpingography of endometrial hyperplasia may show an irregular, micronodular endometrial contour (Fig. 7-44).

Endometrial polyp   A polypoid mass originating in the endometrium may represent a true polyp of endometrial tissue, pedunculated submucous fibroid, or endometrial carcinoma. Endometrial polyps may cause endometrial hemorrhage, although the majority of polyps are discovered incidentally. Ten percent of endometrial polyps in postmenopausal women are malignant. Endometrial polyps are managed with hysteroscopic excision (Fig. 7-45).

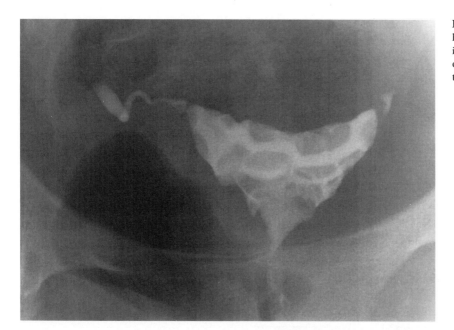

Fig. 7-44   Cystic endometrial hyperplasia on hysterography. An early film in which the uterine cavity is underfilled with contrast material demonstrates multiple polypoid filling defects typical of diffuse endometrial hyperplasia.

Endometrial carcinoma   Endometrial cancer is the most common gynecologic malignancy. It predominantly afflicts postmenopausal women, and only 5% of tumors occur in women aged less than 40 years. Prolonged stimulation of the endometrium by unopposed estrogens is a major risk factor. Nearly 90% of patients with endometrial cancer present with abnormal vaginal bleeding. Although there are several histopathologic types of endometrial cancer, about 85% of patients have adenocarcinoma. Sarcomas of the uterus are considerably more rare than carcinomas and have a poorer prognosis, because they disseminate earlier and tend to be discovered at a more advanced stage. Sarcomatous transformation occurs in 0.5% of leiomyoma, yet, because of the high prevalence of leiomyoma, leiomyosarcoma is the most common uterine sarcoma (Fig. 7-46). Like carcinomas, sarcomas frequently cause vaginal bleeding in postmenopausal women.

Several factors bias the prognosis of endometrial carcinoma, including the histologic grade of the neoplasm, the depth of myometrial invasion, and the presence of metastatic lymphadenopathy. Of these various factors, the depth of myometrial invasion is important. For example, the prevalence of malignant lymphadenopathy increases from 3% among patients with tumor tissue confined to the endometrium or superficial myometrium to 46% when endometrial cancer invades the outer myometrium. The American Cancer Society staging system of carcinoma of the uterine corpus reflects the common routes of spread by direct extension into the cervix and through the myometrium into the pelvis (Box 7-28). Rarely, direct extension may involve the parametrium, vagina, bladder, and rectum. Lymphatic spread to aorto-

caval and pelvic lymph nodes occurs after deep myometrial invasion or when the tumor is poorly differentiated. Hematogenous metastases to the liver, lungs, or brain usually are a late finding of incurable disease.

Accurate staging is important for deciding among various management options. Primary management of Stage I disease is total abdominal hysterectomy and BSO. Adjuvant radiation therapy is offered to patients with poorly differentiated tumors or to those whose tumor has invaded beyond the inner third of the myometrium. Patients with gross enlargement of the cervix and Stage II disease receive radiation therapy before abdominal hysterectomy. More advanced stages of endometrial cancer may be managed palliatively with surgery and radiation therapy; hormonal therapy or chemotherapy also may be added on an individual basis.

Transabdominal sonography and TVS have been used

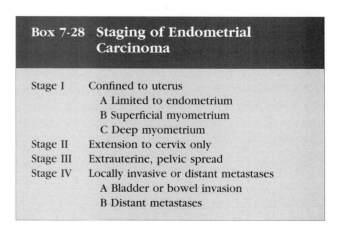

Box 7-28	Staging of Endometrial Carcinoma
Stage I	Confined to uterus
	A Limited to endometrium
	B Superficial myometrium
	C Deep myometrium
Stage II	Extension to cervix only
Stage III	Extrauterine, pelvic spread
Stage IV	Locally invasive or distant metastases
	A Bladder or bowel invasion
	B Distant metastases

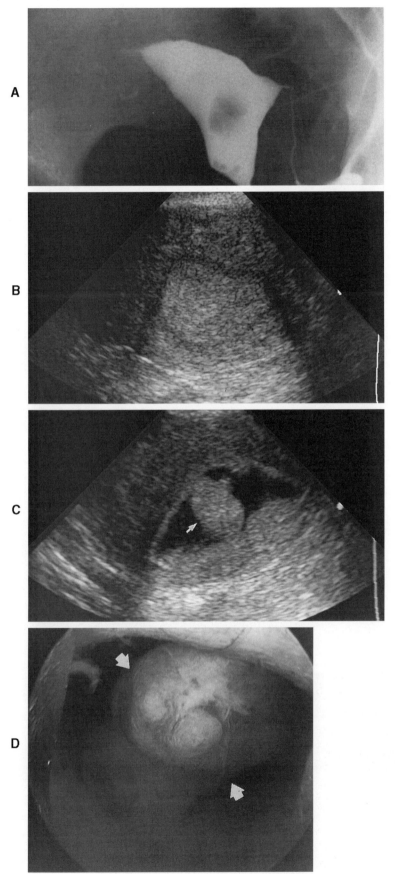

Fig. 7-45   Hysterosonogram of an endometrial mass in a 34-year-old woman with primary infertility. **A,** Hysterosalpingogram shows a filling defect projecting into the endometrial cavity. **B,** Endovaginal sonogram demonstrates a marked increase in the size and echogenicity of the endometrium. **C,** Repeat sonogram after instillation of sterile saline through a balloon catheter inserted into the endometrial cavity (hysterosonography) shows a 2.5-cm echogenic polypoid mass (arrow) originating from thickened endometrium. **D,** At hysteroscopy an endometrial polyp (between arrows) was removed.

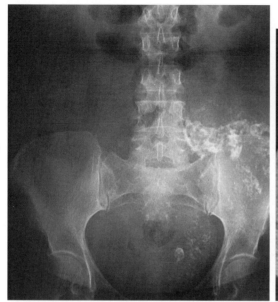

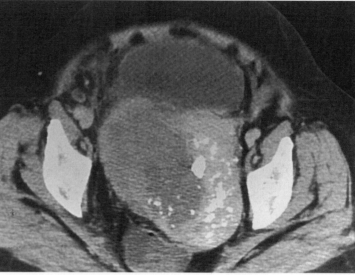

Fig. 7-46 Sarcomatous transformation in a degenerating uterine leiomyoma. **A,** Plain film of the abdomen demonstrates sheet-like coarse and flocculent calcifications in the left lower abdomen and pelvis in an elderly patient with abdominal pain, weight loss, and increasing abdominal girth. **B,** On CT, the calcifications were contained in the wall of a 15-cm necrotic mass. At surgery, this mass was a leiomyosarcoma, and multiple degenerating fibroids also were found in the hysterectomy specimen.

to evaluate the uterus when cancer of the endometrium is suspected clinically. As a general rule, the central endometrial echo should be no thicker than 8 mm in postmenopausal women. However, the normal endometrium may measure up to 12 mm in postmenopausal women who are being treated with exogenous estrogens. The appearance of the central endometrial echo stripe on ultrasound images has been correlated with the likelihood of yielding diagnostically significant endometrial tissue in a patient with suspected endometrial carcinoma. The presence of a linear, thin endometrial echo less than 5 mm in anteroposterior diameter is associated with the

diagnosis of "tissue insufficient for diagnosis." Presumably, vaginal hemorrhage in these patients results from atrophic epithelium, which is prone to superficial ulceration and bleeding. When the echogenic endometrium is thicker than 5 mm, in 35% of patients, significant histologic tissue including hyperplastic endometrium, polyp, and malignancy, may be recovered during curettage (Fig. 7-47). Ultrasonography also has been used to stage the depth of myometrial invasion. The inner myometrium appears as a hypoechoic layer around the echogenic endometrium. If this layer is intact but focally thinned, superficial myometrial invasion should be suspected.

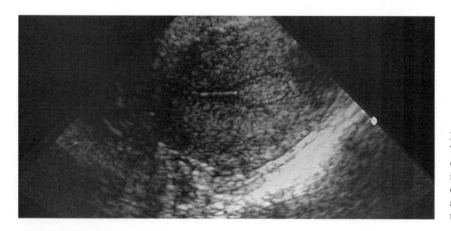

Fig. 7-47 Stage IA endometrial carcinoma. Transverse ultrasonogram of the uterine fundus demonstrates a focal, echogenic mass originating from the endometrium. The outer hypoechoic zone of the endometrium is thinned but appears intact. At surgery, carcinoma limited to the endometrium was found.

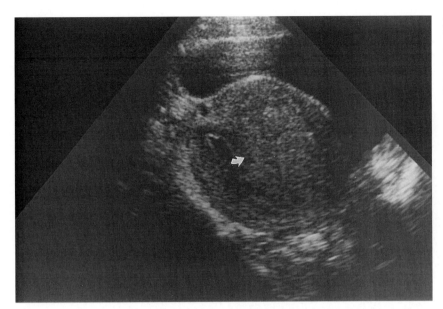

Fig. 7-48   Staging of endometrial carcinoma by ultrasonography. Sagittal image shows obliteration of the hypoechoic inner myometrium consistent with deep myometrial invasion. Note the normal inner myometrium (arrow) and a small amount of fluid in the endometrial cavity.

Obliteration of the hypoechoic layer implies deep myometrial invasion (i.e., more than 50% of the myometrium has been invaded by endometrial cancer) (Fig. 7-48). The depth of myometrial invasion has been quantified by measuring the distance from the endometrial lumen to the most distal interface between tumor and myometrium. When this value is divided by the total thickness of the uterine myometrium, the percentage of myometrial invasion can be estimated. Myometrial invasion is suspected when this value exceeds 30%. Pitfalls to these sonographic staging criteria include normal thinning of the junctional zone in postmenopausal women, uterine fibroids, endometrial cavity distention by blood or secretions, and myometrial distortion by large, exophytic polypoid tumors.

Computed tomography is used commonly for documenting the extent of local extrauterine disease and for evaluating for retroperitoneal, visceral, and pulmonary spread of endometrial carcinoma. Compared with the increased density of the myometrium after contrast administration, endometrial carcinoma is typically a hypodense mass. There may be signs of secondary obstruction of the cervical os, such as hydrometra. As with cervical cancer, parametrial extension is suggested when "stranding" or "dirty fat" is observed in adnexal fat (Fig. 7-49). Although CT has been effective in evaluating parametrial

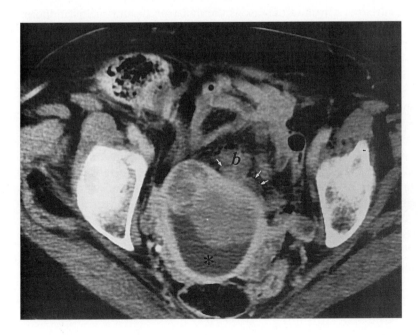

Fig. 7-49   Stage IVA endometrial adenocarcinoma. A hypodense, endophytic mass originates from the anterior wall of the uterine corpus. The fat plane along the anterior uterine wall is indistinct (small arrows). Marked enlargement of the uterus results from tumor and hydrometra (*). At surgery, the tumor had spread into the parametrium and serosa of the small bowel (b). (Case courtesy of Mark S. Ridlen, MD)

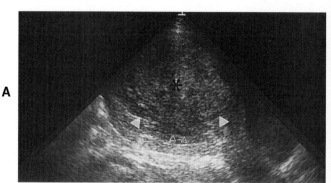

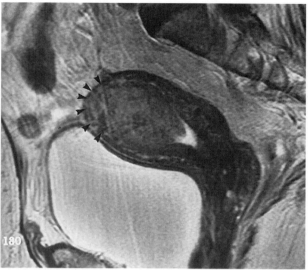

Fig. 7-50   Ultrasonography and MR imaging of deep myometrial invasion of endometrial carcinoma. **A,** Sagittal ultrasound image shows a large endometrial mass (*). Deep myometrial invasion is suggested by focal interruption (open triangles) of the inner myometrium (closed triangles). **B,** On a sagittal fast spin–echo T_2-weighted image (repetition time = 5000 msec; effective echo time = 90 msec), the tumor is relatively hyperintense compared with myometrium. There is marked thinning of the fundal myometrium (arrowheads) at the site of deep myometrial invasion.

and lymphogenous spread of endometrial carcinoma, it has not been as accurate in assessing the depth of myometrial invasion.

On noncontrast MR imaging, the signal intensity of endometrial cancer may be similar to that of normal endometrium. Therefore, detection may rely on the presence of subtle secondary signs, such as widening or lobularity of the endometrial contour. Myometrial invasion (Stage IB) is suggested by disruption or discontinuity of the junctional zone. Unfortunately, focal areas in which the junctional zone is indistinct may be seen normally in postmenopausal women. When the junctional zone is not visible, but the interface between endometrium and myometrium is sharp and smooth, invasion is unlikely. In contrast, an irregular endometrial–myometrial interface is consistent with myometrial invasion. Deep myometrial invasion (Stage IC) is suggested when a mass of high-signal intensity on T_2-weighted images extends through the junctional zone into the outer myometrium (Fig. 7-50). However, when the objective is to stage endometrial carcinoma, contrast-enhanced MR imaging is more accurate than the noncontrast examination. Contrast-enhanced MR imaging permits more accurate assessment not only of tumor volume but also of depth of tumor invasion. After administration of gadopentetate dimeglumine, there is variable enhancement of endometrial carcinomas. In some patients, enhancement is greater than that of normal endometrium and myometrium, thereby increasing conspicuity. In other patients, endometrial carcinoma has lower signal intensity than

normal myometrial tissue on gadolinium-enhanced T_1-weighted MR images.

Gestational trophoblastic disease

Gestational trophoblastic disease (GTD) refers to a diverse group of diseases that share the capacity to produce chorionic gonadotropins (βhCG). GTD refers not to one but to a spectrum of diseases consisting of hydatidiform mole, chorioadenoma destruens or invasive mole, and choriocarcinoma. Toward the benign spectrum of disease is the molar pregnancy or hydatidiform mole. Molar pregnancies exhibit neither myometrial invasion nor metastasis. Complete or classic hydatidiform mole is characterized by hydropic enlargement of chorionic villi, which create multiple vesicles of variable size. The majority of hydatidiform moles are complete moles. Complete moles rarely are associated with fetal tissue and have a karyotype of 46 XX. In contrast, the partial or incomplete mole presents with a dysmorphic and frequently triploid fetus. In 80% of patients, the karyotype of the molar tissue is 69 XXY. A completely healthy fetus with a coexisting molar pregnancy can occur, but it is less common than a partial molar pregnancy.

The malignant forms of GTD are chorioadenoma destruens, a locally invasive, but nonmetastatic, molar pregnancy, and choriocarcinoma. Chorioadenoma destruens represents less than 10% and choriocarcinoma represents about 5% of GTD. The pathology of chorioadenoma destruens is marked by the presence of vesicular chorionic villi that show gross or microscopic evidence of myometrial invasion. Choriocarcinoma is the malignant form of GTD in which hematogenous dissemination to the lungs, brain, liver, kidneys, and gastrointestinal tract can occur. Unlike the other forms of GTD, choriocarcinoma does not necessarily follow a gestational event; nongestational forms of choriocarcinoma originate de novo in either the ovary or the testicle. Choriocarcinoma is characterized pathologically by the lack of any recognizable villous structure. Syncytial and cytotrophoblastic cells are interspersed between areas of hemorrhage and necrosis.

Hydatidiform mole usually presents with heavy, painless vaginal bleeding during the first trimester of pregnancy. Vaginal passage of hydropic placental tissue also may occur. Occasionally, toxemia before 24 weeks of gestation or severe hyperemesis gravidarum are presenting features. The physical examination may reveal a uterine size that is too large for gestational age in 50% of patients or an ovarian mass caused by theca lutein cysts. βhCG titers are elevated disproportionately for the gestational age. Management of choice of hydatidiform mole is suction evacuation, followed by curettage of the uterus. The βhCG level should return to normal within 3 months. Malignant forms of GTD should be suspected if the βhCG level fails to return to normal or increases after uterine evacuation, if the theca lutein cysts fail to regress, or if vaginal bleeding persists.

Sonography has been used to detect GTD and to evaluate local and distant metastatic disease. Ultrasonography also can be used to examine the patient with persistently elevated or rising βhCG levels after treatment of molar pregnancy. Particularly during the second trimester, the sonographic appearance of molar pregnancy is characteristic. The uterus is enlarged, and hydropic changes in molar villi produce multiple small, echolucent areas 3 to 10 mm in diameter (Fig. 7-51). These small cystic spaces may not be evident during the first trimester when molar tissue may appear as a homogeneously echogenic endometrial mass (Fig. 7-52). Foci of hemorrhage or ischemic necrosis may appear as focal, irregular hypoechoic, or anechoic areas. The differential diagnosis includes hydropic placental degeneration after incomplete abortion, myxoid or carneous degeneration of a leiomyoma, retained products of conception, and endometrial proliferative disease. It is important to evaluate the uterus for fetal membranes or parts, which would suggest partial mole.

Myometrial invasion or the presence of abdominal metastatic disease is seen with the malignant forms of GTD and can be evaluated with sonography. Myometrial invasion is suggested by focal myometrial thinning adjacent to vesicle-containing tissue (Fig. 7-53 on p. 298). Multiple anechoic channels can be seen deep within myometrial tissue, and Doppler endovaginal sonography shows that many of these spaces represent dilated spiral arteries with abnormally increased systolic and diastolic flow on spectral analysis. Malignant GTD also is suggested

by the presence of irregular hypoechoic areas representing hemorrhage, necrosis, or both. It is important to remember that echolucent hydropic villi will be seen with chorioadenoma destruens but not in patients with choriocarcinoma. Patients with choriocarcinoma also may have local pelvic or distant metastases to the liver and kidney at the time of diagnosis (Figs. 7-53C and D).

Under the trophic influence of βhCG, theca lutein cysts develop in approximately 25% of patients with GTD. These cysts present a sonographic picture of bilateral, multiple, multiloculated anechoic spaces that enlarge the ovaries. It is important to document the resolution of theca lutein cysts after evacuation of the uterus because failure to resolve after 3 to 4 months suggests the presence of residual or metastatic disease.

Cancer of the uterine cervix

Although the incidence of cancer of the cervix has declined over the past several decades, it remains the most common malignancy in women aged less than 50 years and is the third most common gynecologic cancer. The overwhelming majority (90%) of cervical cancers are SCCs, whereas 10% are adenosquamous or adenocarcinomas. Although cervical cytology correlates with the histopathologic diagnosis, colposcopic biopsy is necessary for the definitive diagnosis. The colposcope is a stereoscopic binocular microscope used to detect areas of cervical dysplasia for biopsy. Dysplastic epithelium appears white under the colposcope after surface application of acetic acid. Punch biopsies are taken from suspicious areas, and endocervical curettage also is performed.

Preinvasive cervical cancer usually does not produce symptoms. Invasive cervical cancer is accompanied by abnormal vaginal bleeding in 80% of patients. Several risk factors for cervical cancer have been identified. There is a strong link to infection with the human papilloma virus. Cervical cancer is more prevalent in patients of lower socioeconomic status, in patients with multiple sexual partners, and in those who were aged less than 20 years at first coitus. Young age at first pregnancy and high parity also are risk factors.

Staging of cervical cancer plays an important role in management selection (Box 7-29). Carcinoma in situ and microinvasive cervical cancer can be managed with superficial ablative techniques. Stage IA cervical cancer is managed definitively with radical hysterectomy, and Stages IB and IIA are managed with radical hysterectomy and preoperative radiation therapy. Radical hysterectomy entails removal of the uterus, along with adjacent parts of the vagina and bladder and the uterosacral and cardinal ligaments. Primary radiation therapy also can be used to manage early and locally advanced cervical cancer. Pelvic exenteration with reconstruction is reserved for patients with local recurrence after radiation therapy or those with primary disease unresponsive to initial surgery or

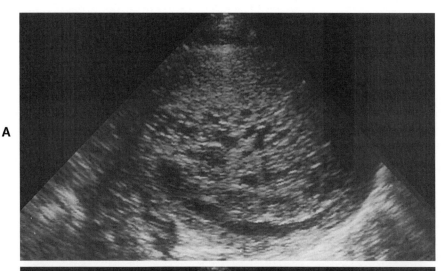

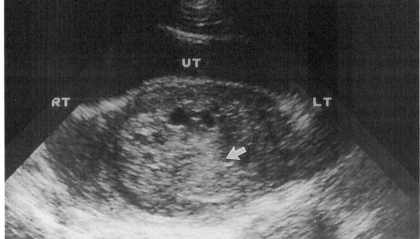

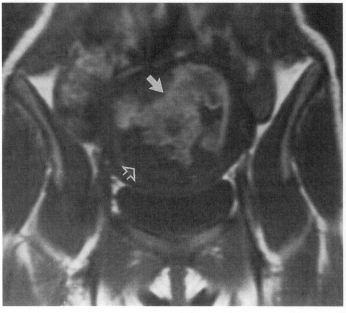

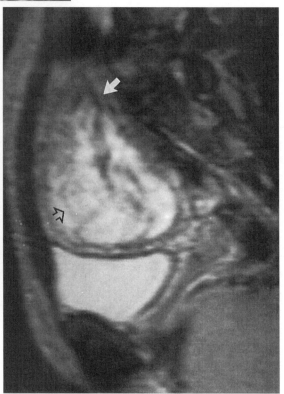

Fig. 7-51 Hydatidiform mole complicated by hemorrhage. **A** and **B**, Transverse endovaginal sonograms show enlargement of the uterus because of a solid mass containing multiple small cystic spaces. This appearance is typical of a molar pregnancy. However, there also was a focal hyperechoic area (arrow) intermixed with molar tissue. **C**, Coronal T_1-weighted MR image (repetition time [TR] = 400 msec; echo time [TE] = 20 msec) shows molar tissue that is isointense to muscle (open arrow), although small hypointense cystic areas can be seen. The hyperintense signal (arrow) represents subacute hemorrhage into molar tissue. **D**, Molar tissue (arrow) is hyperintense on a sagittal T_2-weighted image (TR = 3000 msec; TE = 80 msec), and hemorrhage is relatively hypointense (open arrow).

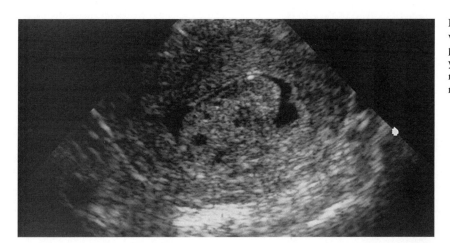

Fig. 7-52 Early molar pregnancy. Transverse endovaginal sonogram demonstrates a predominantly solid endometrial mass in a 24-year-old woman with a positive pregnancy test result. In the first trimester, molar gestations may not have hydatidiform features.

combined surgical treatment, chemotherapy, and radiation therapy.

Because local spread of the tumor is most characteristic of cervical cancer, detection of invasion to the vagina, parametria, and pelvic side wall is important. Prognostic variables in cervical cancer include the histopathology and grade of the tumor, location within the cervix, transverse diameter, depth of stromal invasion, and extracervical pelvic invasion. Because lymphogenous metastasis to pelvic and paraaortic lymph nodes is more common than hematogenous dissemination, lymph node involvement is another prognostic factor.

As the sonographic appearance of cervical cancer frequently is isoechoic with that of normal cervical tissue, enlargement of the cervix may be the only sign of cancer on transabdominal and transrectal sonograms. If cancer obstructs the cervical canal, hydrometra may be detected with transabdominal, endovaginal, or transrectal sonography. Because cervical cancer is identified frequently on the basis of the physical examination and after histologic screening, ultrasonography plays a minor role in cancer detection. Staging of cervical cancer is a more important objective of imaging. Transrectal ultrasonography can be used to stage disease of the parametrium with 87% accuracy, which is superior to that of the clinical examination, but accurate staging of pelvic and retroperitoneal lymph nodes remains elusive. The tumor-infiltrated parametrium, which is normally hypoechoic on transrectal sonograms, is replaced by tissue with sonoreflective properties similar to that of tumor in the cervix. False-positive diagnosis occurs when concurrent disease, such as endometriosis or chronic PID, causes parametrial fibrous or inflammatory changes that can mimic invasive tumor on ultrasound examinations.

Computed tomography traditionally has been used to evaluate the primary tumor and to stage the spread of cervical carcinoma. The cervical cancer primary tumor typically causes enlargement and heterogeneous contrast enhancement of the cervix (Fig. 7-54). Secondary obstruction of the endocervical canal may result in endometrial distention and hydrometra. Parametrial spread of tumor is suggested when the lateral margins of the cervix are poorly defined and irregular or when there is an eccentric soft-tissue mass. Increased density and strands of soft tissue in the paracervical fat also suggest Stage IIB disease (Fig. 7-55). Spread to the side wall of the pelvis is suggested when soft tissue extends to within 3 mm of the obturator internus and pyriformis muscles. Extension of the cervical primary tumor to either the bladder or the rectum, designated Stage IVA, is diagnosed when the fat planes around these viscera are obliterated. Thickening or nodularity of the bladder or rectal wall or a focal intraluminal mass also suggests locally advanced disease (Fig. 7-56 on p. 300). Ureteral dilatation also may accompany locally invasive cervical cancer and rarely is the presenting manifestation of this disease. Cervical carcinoma usually first affects the external and internal iliac lymph nodes, followed by the paraaortic nodes. Pelvic lymph nodes larger than 1.5 cm are suspicious for metastatic disease, but lymph nodes may be enlarged for

Box 7-29	**Staging of Cervical Carcinoma**
Stage 0	Preinvasive carcinoma
Stage I	Carcinoma confined to the cervix
Stage II	Carcinoma extends beyond the cervix, but not to pelvic wall
	A No parametrial involvement
	B Parametrial involvement
Stage III	Carcinoma extends beyond cervix
	A To, but not into, pelvic wall
	B Onto pelvic wall; ureter involved
Stage IV	Carcinoma extends beyond true pelvis or invades bladder or rectum

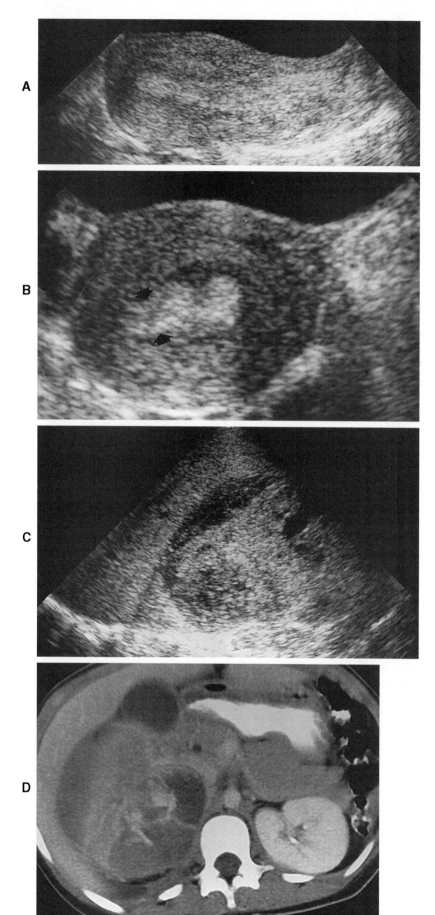

Fig. 7-53 Choriocarcinoma metastases to the kidney. Sagittal (**A**) and transverse (**B**) sonograms of the uterus demonstrate an echogenic mass that completely fills the endometrial cavity. On the transverse image, there is invasion into the inner myometrium (between arrows). **C,** Sagittal sonogram of the right renal fossa demonstrates a hyperechoic mass and no reniform tissue. **D,** Infused abdominal CT shows a large mass of mixed attenuation that has destroyed the right kidney and filled the pararenal spaces. Biopsy of this mass revealed choriocarcinoma.

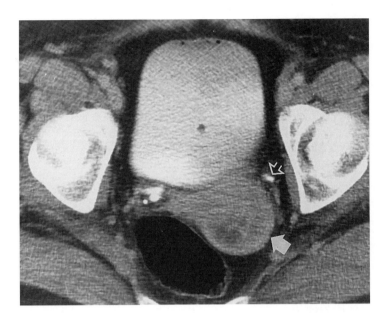

Fig. 7-54   Stage IIA cervical carcinoma on infused CT. There is enlargement and heterogeneous enhancement of the cervix (arrow). The margins of the cervix are well defined, and the distal left ureter (open arrow) is normal. At surgery, there was no parametrial spread of cervical carcinoma.

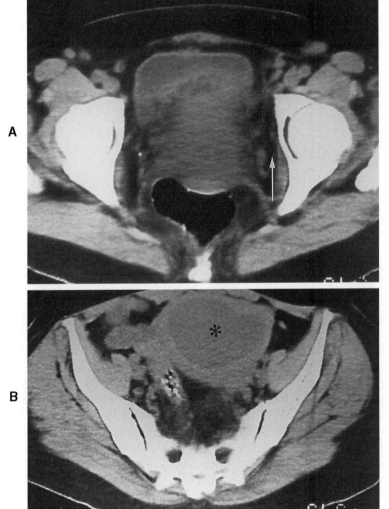

Fig. 7-55   CT findings on parametrial cervical cancer. **A,** Noncontrast pelvic CT demonstrates marked enlargement of the cervix, which has poorly defined margins; however, the fat planes (arrow) next to the obturator internus muscles are intact. This finding suggests spread to the parametrium but not to the pelvic wall. **B,** Secondary obstruction of the cervical canal results in hydrometra (*).

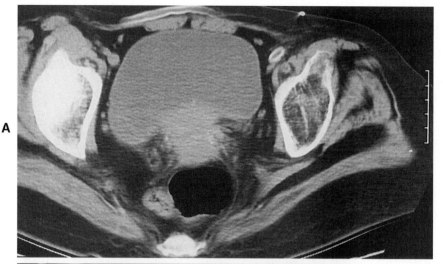

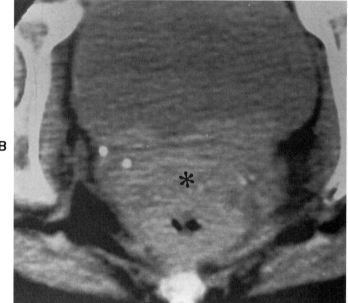

Fig. 7-56   Stage IVA cervical carcinoma. **A,** Noncontrast CT of the pelvis demonstrates loss of the retrovesical fat plane adjacent to a cervical soft tissue mass. The bladder wall is focally thickened at the site of tumor invasion. **B,** In another patient, there is more diffuse thickening of the bladder wall contiguous with a cervical carcinoma (*). In this patient, locally invasive tumor also has spread to the rectal serosa.

reasons other than metastasis, such as reactive hyperplasia or lipid infiltration. Conversely, microscopic neoplastic infiltration may be found in nodes of normal size. The reported accuracy of CT for the staging of cervical cancer ranges between 60% and 90%.

Cervical cancer also can be detected and staged with T_2-weighted MR imaging, because this cancer is imaged as a mass of relatively high-signal intensity compared with that of the cervical stroma, which usually is of uniformly low-signal intensity. The cervical stroma is composed of compact collagen tissue and, therefore, is of uniformly low-signal intensity on T_2-weighted images and on postcontrast T_1-weighted images. The glandular elements lining the endocervical canal are of increased signal intensity on T_2-weighted images and on the postcontrast T_1-

weighted images because these elements show marked enhancement. On T_2-weighted images, an intact low-signal intensity peripheral ring of tissue around the endocervical canal is a reliable indication that cervical stromal transgression and parametrial invasion are not present (Fig. 7-57). The staging accuracy of body-coil MR imaging for parametrial invasion ranges between 75% and 85%.

Cervical cancer can be restaged accurately after radiation therapy with MR imaging. Response to radiation is typified by reduction in size and significant decrease in signal intensity on T_2-weighted images. Conversely, tumors that do not respond to radiotherapy generally are large at the outset (i.e., larger than 50 cm³ in volume) and retain a high-signal intensity relative to that of the adjacent cervical stroma. Similarly, recurrent tumor can

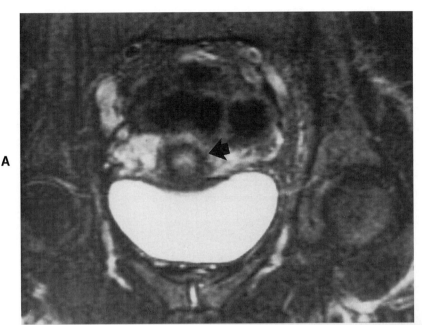

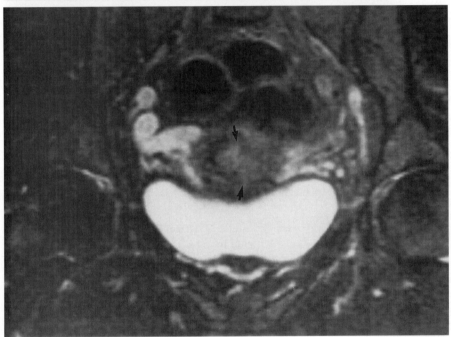

Fig. 7-57 Small cervical carcinoma on MR imaging. **A,** Oblique transverse, fast spin–echo, T₂-weighted fat-saturated image of the cervix (repetition time = 6000 msec; effective echo time = 98 msec) shows an intact, uniformly hypointense ring of stromal tissue (arrow). **B,** At a more caudal level, the stromal ring is disrupted focally (small arrows) by a mass that is isointense with endocervical tissue. At surgery, a 1.5-cm adenosquamous carcinoma was removed. The tumor had invaded 1.2 cm of the cervical wall, which was 2 cm thick.

be differentiated from radiation fibrosis because tumor tends to present as a focal mass that is hyperintense to pelvic side-wall muscle and fat on T₂-weighted images. Therefore, MR imaging, unlike CT or ultrasonography, can enable assessment of response to radiotherapy and distinction between residual and recurrent tumor in most patients. However, the distinction based on relative signal intensity may be less reliable within 6 months of radiotherapy, when vascularized or edematous granulation tissue may mimic residual tumor in signal intensity.

SUGGESTED READINGS

Ascher S, Arnold L, Patt R, et al: Adenomyosis: prospective comparison of MR imaging and transvaginal sonography, *Radiology* 190:803–806, 1994.

Athey P, Diment D: The spectrum of sonographic findings in endometriomas, *J Ultrasound Med* 8:487–491, 1989.

Bourne T, Campbell D, Steer C, et al: Transvaginal colour flow imaging: a possible new screening technique for ovarian cancer, *BMJ* 299:1367–1370, 1989.

Buttram VJ: Müllerian anomalies: a proposed classification (an analysis of 144 cases), *Fertil Steril* 32:40–46, 1979.

Buy J-N, Ghossain M, Sciot C, et al: Epithelial tumors of the ovary: CT findings and correlation with ultrasound, *Radiology* 178:811, 1991.

Carrington B, Hricak H, Nuruddin R, et al: Müllerian duct anomalies: MR imaging evelution, *Radiology* 176:715–720, 1990.

Cohen H, Tice H, Mandel F: Ovarian volumes measured by ultrasound: bigger than we think, *Radiology* 177:189–192, 1990.

Fleischer A, Dudley B, Entman S, et al: Myometrial invasion by endometrial carcinoma: sonographic assessment, *Radiology* 162:307–310, 1987.

Fleischer A, Rodgers W, Rao B: Assessment of ovarian tumor vascularity with transvaginal color Doppler sonography, *J Ultrasound Med* 10:563–568, 1991.

Flueckiger F, Ebner F, Psochauko H, et al: Cervical cancer: serial MR imaging before and after primary radiation therapy—a 2-year followup study, *Radiology* 184:89–93, 1992.

Ghossain M, Buy J-N, Ligneres C, et al: Epithelial tumors of the ovary: comparison of MR and CT findings, *Radiology* 181:863, 1991.

Goldstein S, Nachtigall M, Snyder J: Endometrial assessment by vaginal ultrasonography before endometrial sampling in patients with postmenopausal bleeding, *Am J Obstet Gynecol* 163:114–123, 1990.

Graif M, Itzchak Y: Sonographic evaluation of ovarian torsion in childhood and adolescence, *AJR Am J Roentgenol* 150:647–649, 1988.

Hamper U, Sheth S, Abbas F, et al: Transvaginal color doppler sonography of adnexal masses: differences in blood flow impedance in benign and malignant lesions, *AJR Am J Roentgenol* 160:1225–1228, 1993.

Hricak H, Hamm B, Semelka R, et al: Carcinoma of the uterus: use of gadopentetate dimeglumine in MR imaging, *Radiology* 181:95, 1991.

Hricak H, Lacey C, Sandles L, et al: Invasive cervical carcinoma: comparison of MR imaging and surgical findings, *Radiology* 166:623–631, 1988.

Innocenti P, Pulli F, Savino L, et al: Staging of cervical cancer: reliability of transrectal US, *Radiology* 185:201–205, 1992.

Jain K: Prospective evaluation of adnexal masses with endovaginal gray-scale and duplex and color Dopper ultrasound: correlation with pathologic findings, *Radiology* 191:63–67, 1994.

Kimura I, Togashi K, Kawakami S, et al: Ovarian torsion: CT and MR imaging appearances, *Radiology* 190:337–341, 1994.

Kuligowska E, Baker C, Oates R: Male infertility: role of transrectal ultrasound in diagnosis and management, *Radiology* 185:353–360, 1992.

Levine D, Gosink B, Wolf S, et al: Simple adnexal cysts: the natural history in postmenopausal women, *Radiology* 184:653–659, 1992.

Pache T, Wladimiroff J, Hop W, et al: How to discriminate between normal and polycystic ovaries: transvaginal ultrasound study, *Radiology* 183:421–423, 1993.

Pellerito J, McCarthy S, Doyle M, et al: Diagnosis of uterine anomalies: relative accuracy of MR imaging, endovaginal sonography, and hysterosalpingography, *Radiology* 183:795–800, 1992.

Reuter K, Daly D, Cohen S: Septate versus bicornuate uteri: errors in imaging diagnosis, *Radiology* 172:749–752, 1989.

Siegelman E, Outwater E, Wang T, et al: Solid pelvic masses caused by endometriosis: MR imaging features, *AJR Am J Roentgenol* 163:357–361, 1994.

Sironi S, Colombo E, Villa G, et al: Myometrial invasion by endometrial carcinoma: assessment with plain and gadolinium-enhanced MR imaging, *Radiology* 185:207–212, 1992.

Sironi S, De Cobelli F, Scarfone G, et al: Carcinoma of the cervix: value of plain and gadolinium-enhanced MR imaging in assessing degree of invasiveness, *Radiology* 188:797–801, 1993.

Stark J, Siegel M: Ovarian torsion in prepubertal and pubertal girls: sonographic findings, *AJR Am J Roentgenol* 163:1479–1482, 1994.

Stevens S, Hricak H, Stern J: Ovarian lesions: detection and characterization with gadolinium-enhanced MR imaging at 1.5 T, *Radiology* 181:481, 1991.

Taylor K, Schwartz P: Screening for early ovarian cancer, *Radiology* 192:1–10, 1994.

Togashi K, Nishimura K, Sagoh T, et al: Carcinoma of the cervix: staging with MR imaging, *Radiology* 171:245, 1989.

Togashi K, Ozasa H, Konishi I, et al: Enlarged uterus: differentiation between adenomyosis and leiomyoma, *Radiology* 171:531, 1989.

Weber T, Sostman H, Spritzer C: Cervical carcinoma: determination of recurrent tumor extent versus radiation changes with MR imaging, *Radiology* 194:135–139, 1995.

Weinreb J, Barkoff N, Megibow A, et al: Value of MR imaging in distinguishing leiomyomas from other solid pelvic masses when sonography is indeterminate, *AJR Am J Roentgenol* 154:295, 1990.

The diagnosis and management of diseases of the male
genital tract have changed significantly in recent years
as a direct result of technologic advances in medical
imaging and interventional radiology. The purpose of this
chapter is to present medical imaging of the male genital
tract in the context of selected clinical problems. The
first part of the chapter reviews the embryology, anat-

omy, and physiology of the male genital tract. Medical
imaging of the male genital tract then is presented as a
series of eight clinical topics. The first four topics relate to
medical imaging of the testis and scrotum: (1) atraumatic
scrotal pain, enlargement, or mass; (2) staging of testicular carcinoma; (3) trauma to the scrotum; and (4) undescended testicle. The next three topics cover disease of
the prostate: (1) the prostate nodule and enlargement,
(2) staging of prostatic carcinoma, and (3) prostatodynia
and fever. The final clinical topic is erectile dysfunction.

EMBRYOLOGY, ANATOMY, AND PHYSIOLOGY OF THE MALE GENITAL TRACT

Embryology

Upper urinary tract

Three pairs of excretory organs develop from the intermediate mesoderm: pronephros, mesonephros, and
metanephros. The pronephros is a rudimentary and transient organ from which the primary nephric duct is derived. The mesonephric tubules fuse with the mesonephric or wolffian duct, an extension of the primary nephric
duct. The metanephros forms the definitive renal unit
and is composed of the metanephric duct, or primitive
ureter, and metanephrogenic tissue. By the process of
mutual induction, the developing permanent kidney
(metanephros) induces the development of the ureteral
bud, an outpouching from the wolffian duct. As the urogenital sinus and rectum are being formed from the division of the cloaca by the urorectal fold, the caudal ends
of the metanephric ducts (ureters) undergo resorption.
As a result, the paired caudal ends of the wolffian and
metanephric ducts develop separate openings into the
urogenital sinus. Additional division of the urogenital sinus into the bladder and urethra is accompanied by a
rotation in the relative positions of these ducts so that

the metanephric duct orifice empties into the bladder and assumes a more cranial and lateral position than the wolffian ducts, which empty into the prostatic urethra.

Internal genitalia

The internal genitalia are derived from the wolffian (mesonephric) and müllerian (paramesonephric) ducts that are side-by-side in early embryos of both sexes. In men, the müllerian ducts largely degenerate, and the wolffian ducts differentiate into epididymides, ductus deferens, seminal vesicles, and ejaculatory ducts. In women, the müllerian ducts develop into the upper part of the vagina, the uterus, and the paired fallopian or uterine tubes; the wolffian ducts regress. In both sexes, the external genitalia and urethra develop from the urogenital sinus and the genital tubercle, folds, and swellings. In the absence of the hormonally functional testis, the phenotypic sex develops along female lines. Masculinization results from the action of hormones from the fetal gonad, whereas female development does not require the presence of a gonad. As the fetal gonad descends from the abdomen to the pelvis, it is enveloped by a peritoneal diverticulum called the *processus vaginalis*. The processus vaginalis is attached to the gubernaculum, which also attaches the fetal gonad to the scrotal swelling. The testes remain near the deep inguinal ring until the third trimester and usually enter the scrotum before birth. A part of the processus vaginalis persists as the tunica vaginalis.

The prostate gland is derived from urethral epithelium, which is induced to form ductular structures by mesenchymal cells from the urogenital sinus. The prostatic utricle develops from the epithelium of the urogenital sinus, wolffian ducts, and müllerian ducts. In the male fetus, the cranial portions of the müllerian ducts involute as a result of the secretion of an antimüllerian factor by the Sertoli cells of the testes. The most caudal remnant persists as a well-defined tube that unites with the posterior wall of the urogenital sinus to form the utricular plate.

Anatomy

The normal testis is an ovoid gland that measures 3.5 to 4 cm in length and 2 to 3 cm in width and is invested by a fibrous capsule called the *tunica albuginea*. The mediastinum testis is a thick, vertical invagination of this fibrous capsule along the posterosuperior margin of the testis and is the site where the spermatic cord enters the testicle. Each testis is divided into cone-shaped lobules, organized so that the apices converge on the mediastinum (Fig. 8-1). Each lobule is composed of branching seminiferous tubules that coalesce to enter the mediastinum testis and, through a series of anastomoses, form 12 to 20 efferent ductules.

The ductal system of the testis continues as the epidid-

ymis, a conduit 6 to 7 cm in length that lies posteriorly and laterally to the testicle. The head of the epididymis (globus major), which is lateral to the upper pole of the testis, normally is 7 to 8 mm in diameter and is connected to the upper testicular pole by the efferent ductules (Fig. 8-1). The body and tail of the epididymis extend inferiorly along the margin of the testicle and normally decrease in diameter to 1 to 2 mm. The appendices of the testis (hydatid of Morgagni) and the appendix of the epididymis are functionless embryonic remnants of the paramesonephric and mesonephric ducts, respectively. The vas deferens, or deferent duct, is the distal continuation of the tail of the epididymis (Fig. 8-2). It ascends in the posterior part of the spermatic cord but leaves the cord at the deep inguinal ring. It extends anteriorly to the external iliac artery and then curves obliquely downward to enter the true pelvis. After crossing the ureter, it continues a descending course between the posterior surface of the bladder and upper pole of the seminal vesicle. The lumen dilates slightly just posteriorly to the bladder, forming the ampulla. At the base of the prostate, it joins the seminal vesicle to form the ejaculatory duct (Fig. 8-2). Each seminal vesicle is a coiled and sacculated tube that forms much of the protein in the seminal fluid and contracts during ejaculation. The paired seminal vesicles are extraperitoneal and are located between the bladder anteriorly, rectovesical fascia posteriorly, ampulla of the vas deferens medially, and prostatic venous plexus laterally. In men, each seminal vesicle is about 3 cm in length and 1.5 cm in width. The shape of the normal seminal vesicle varies; it can be round, ovoid, or tubular, and in one third of the male population, the seminal vesicles are asymmetric in size or shape. The ejaculatory duct on each side is formed from the union of the seminal vesicle and the vas deferens at the base of the prostate. Each duct is approximately 2 cm in length and ends as a small orifice on the colliculus seminalis, adjacent to the verumontanum and prostatic utricle.

The spermatic cord is composed of the vas deferens and vessels, lymphatics, and nerves. There are three arteries within the spermatic cord; the internal spermatic (testicular) artery, the external spermatic or cremasteric artery (a branch of the inferior epigastric artery), and the artery to the vas deferens (a branch of the vesicular artery). Venous flow from the scrotum is through the pampiniform plexus in the spermatic cord. This plexus drains into the ipsilateral testicular vein. The right testicular vein drains directly into the inferior vena cava just caudal to the renal vein, and the left testicular vein empties into the left renal vein. The cremasteric nerve, genital branch of the genitofemoral nerve, and testicular sympathetic plexus also are constituents of the cord. Four to eight lymphatic vessels ascend in the spermatic cord in the company of the testicular vessels to end in the lateral aortic and preaortic nodes.

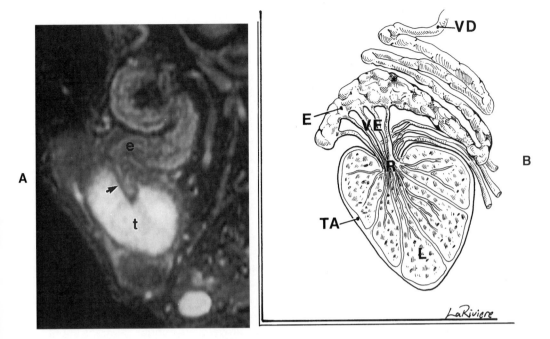

Fig. 8-1   Anatomy of the testis and epididymis. **A,** Oblique sagittal, T₂-weighted MR image of the scrotum in a patient with chronic epididymitis and testicular atrophy. Posterosuperiorly, the spermatic cord enters at the testicle (t) at the mediastinum testis (arrow). The epididymis (e) is tortuous and thickened in this patient; normally, it is 7 to 8 mm in diameter. **B,** The parenchyma of the testis is encased by the tunica albuginea (TA), a thick fibrous capsule. Multiple septa from this capsule divide the parenchyma into several hundred lobules (L). Each lobule contains one or several tortuous seminiferous tubules. At the hilum of the testis (mediastinum testis), these tubules anastomose at the rete testis (R). The tubules of the rete testis empty into 10 or 15 efferent ducts or vasa efferentia (VE), which continue as the upper pole (globus major) of the epididymis (E). This larger, upper pole of the epididymis continues first as the midportion or body and then as the inferior portion or globus minor. The vas deferens (VD) or deferent duct originates at the globus minor of the epididymis.

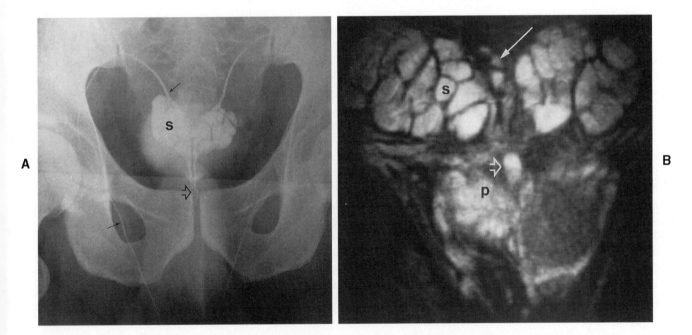

Fig. 8-2   Vasogram **(A)** and coronal T₂-weighted MR image **(B)** demonstrate the normal deferent ducts, seminal vesicles, and ejaculatory ducts. The deferent duct or vas deferens (arrow) is the distal continuation of the epididymis. After crossing the distal ureter, it bends anteromedially to pass between the posterior surface of the bladder and the upper pole of the seminal vesicle (s). It descends to the base of the prostate (p), joining the duct of the seminal vesicle to form the ejaculatory duct (open arrow).

Box 8-1 Prostate Anatomy

Peripheral zone
   Eighty-five percent of prostate cancers
Transitional zone
   Surrounds proximal prostatic urethra
   Benign prostatic hyperplasia
   Ten percent of cancers
Central zone
   Surrounds ejaculatory ducts
Neurovascular bundles
   Posterolateral to prostate (5 o'clock and 7 o'clock
      positions)

The scrotal wall components are derived from the various layers of the abdominal wall. The tunica vaginalis is the lower end of the peritoneal processus vaginalis. Because the tunica vaginalis is reflected on itself, it can be divided into a visceral layer, which is applied directly to the testis, epididymis, and posterior scrotal wall, and a parietal layer, which is in direct contact with the scrotal wall. The visceral layer applies the testis to the posterior scrotal wall by forming an envelope around the testis. A superior and posterior aspect of the testis is the only part that is not in continuity with this covering. The potential space of this serous sac normally is filled with 1 to 2 cc of fluid. Bowel or omentum may herniate into this space, and fluid accumulates in this area to form a hydrocele. The dartos is the highly vascularized outer layer of the scrotum. The appendix testis, or hydatid of Morgagni, is a müllerian duct remnant located on the superior aspect of the testis.

There are 20 to 30 arborizing glands of the prostate (Box 8-1). They drain into the prostatic urethra at and below the verumontanum, the base of which is located midway between the internal and external urethral sphincters. The glandular tissue of the prostate can be subdivided into three discrete zones on the basis of location and patterns of ductular drainage (Fig. 8-3). The peripheral zone is located between the base of the verumontanum and the apex of the gland posteriorly and laterally. It also makes up most of the apex of the prostate. The central zone, which contains more stroma than glandular tissue, is located immediately around the ejaculatory ducts and is indistinguishable from the peripheral zone with most imaging methods. The ducts of the peripheral zone and those of the smaller central zone account for roughly 95% of the glandular tissue of the prostate. The third glandular area is the transitional zone, which surrounds the preprostatic urethra (i.e., that portion of the urethra cephalad to the verumontanum) and accounts for not more than 5% to 10% of the normal glandular prostate in young men. The term *central gland* refers to the central zone, the transitional zone, and the periurethral tissues. The glandular prostate is surrounded by stroma consisting of connective tissue and smooth muscle. The anterior fibromuscular stroma contains smooth muscle, which mixes with periurethral muscle fibers at the bladder neck. Histologically, there is no distinct capsule that surrounds the prostate. Instead, the "capsule" is a blending of the prostatic fibromuscular stroma with endopelvic fascia. There is no prostatic capsule anteriorly or at the prostatic apex.

The prostate gland is surrounded by an exuberant periprostatic venous plexus, which joins the hemorrhoidal and Santorini's plexus to drain into the internal iliac vein. The arterial supply to the prostate derives from the inferior vesical and inferior hemorrhoidal branches of the internal iliac artery. Nerve branches to the seminal vesicles, prostate, urethra, and corpora cavernosa travel together in the neurovascular bundle, which is about 5 to 6 cm in length and is located posteriorly and laterally to the posterior or rectal surface of the prostate (Fig. 8-4). Primary lymphatic drainage of the prostate is provided by the internal iliac lymph node chain.

SELECTED CLINICAL PROBLEMS

Atraumatic Scrotal Pain, Enlargement, or Mass

When confronted with the clinical history of atraumatic scrotal mass, swelling, or pain, it is critical to identify the lesion that involves the testicle primarily (Box 8-2). The major diagnoses to be considered are testicular torsion, epididymitis, orchitis, and testicular neoplasms. Benign disease, frequently inflammatory, is more common in the epididymis and scrotum. Other common nonneoplastic scrotal masses, such as hydrocele or hernia, also involve the extratesticular space. Even the rare extratesticular neoplasm most often is benign. In contrast, a malignant neoplasm must be excluded whenever a focal or diffuse mass of the testicle is detected. Sonography is ideal for the initial examination of the patient with an atraumatic scrotal mass because high-resolution images of the scrotum can be obtained with 7-MHz or 10-MHz transducers. Ultrasonography is accurate for distinguishing a testicular mass from one that originates in the extratesticular space in 95% of patients.

Torsion of the spermatic cord

Torsion refers to an abnormal twist of the spermatic cord that causes testicular ischemia. Although torsion of the cord is possible at any age, it is most common in infants aged less than 1 year and in adolescents. After adolescence, the incidence slowly decreases. In the neonatal period and in infants, the testicle and spermatic

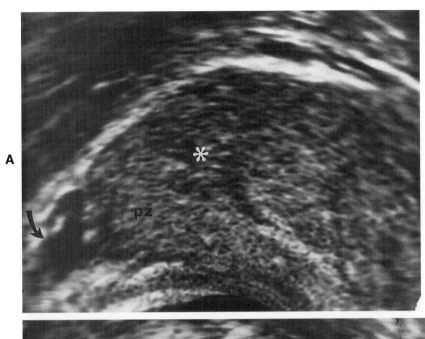

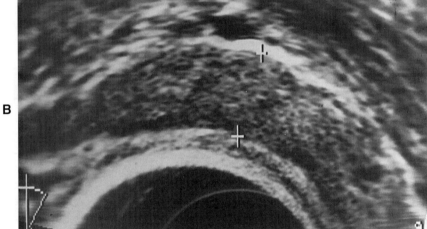

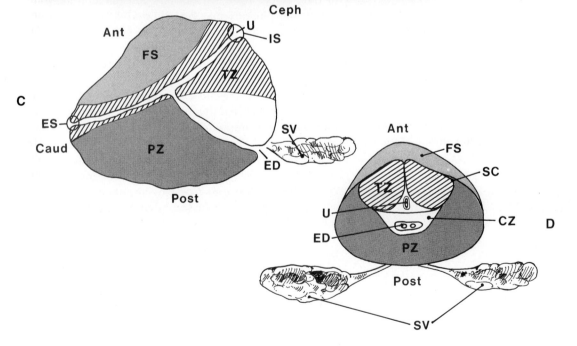

Fig. 8-3 Normal anatomy of the prostate gland. **A,** Peripheral zone tissue (pz) is slightly hyperechoic compared with the central gland (*) of the prostate on an oblique transverse transrectal sonogram (arrow = periprostatic venous plexus). **B,** A transverse sonogram at a more cephalic level shows the normal left seminal vesicle (between electronic markers). **C and D,** Drawings show the glandular anatomy of the prostate in the sagittal and transverse planes. The glandular tissue of the prostate is divided into three zones. The large peripheral zone (PZ) is located posteriorly from the base of the verumontanum to the apex of the prostate gland. The central zone (CZ) is found around the ejaculatory ducts (ED), and the transitional zone (TZ) surrounds the prostatic urethra (U). The surgical capsule (SC) separates the peripheral zone from the central zone, transitional zone, and periurethral tissues, together referred to as the "central gland." The anterior fibromuscular stroma (FS) contains no glandular tissue. IS = internal urethral sphincter; ES = external urethral sphincter; SV = seminal vesicles; Ant = anterior; Post = posterior; Ceph = cephalad; Caud = caudad.

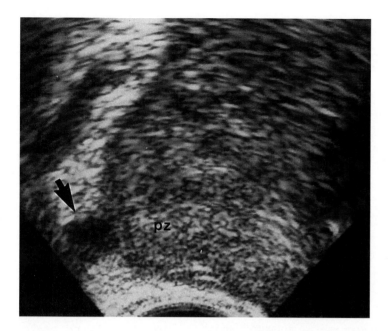

Fig. 8-4 Normal neurovascular bundle. Transverse endorectal sonogram of the prostate demonstrates the normal neurovascular bundle as an extracapsular hypoechoic focus (arrow), posterior and lateral to the peripheral zone (pz) of the prostate.

cord are attached loosely to the scrotum, and the entire cord above the level of the scrotum may undergo torsion (extravaginal torsion). Another anatomic condition that predisposes infants and adolescents to torsion is the anomalous suspension of the testicle within the tunica vaginalis. In this condition, fixation of the testicle to the posterior scrotal wall is incomplete. In addition, the mesenteric attachment of the spermatic cord to the testis is abnormally short, permitting the testis to fall forward and rotate in the tunica vaginalis (intravaginal torsion). This so-called bell-and-clapper deformity involves both testicles in 70% of patients, and simultaneous bilateral torsion occurs in 5% of patients. Therefore, surgical therapy of unilateral testicular torsion calls for contralateral orchiopexy. The undescended testicle also is more likely to torque. Torsion also may occur when the mesorchium, which normally attaches the testis to the epididymis, is abnormally long. This structural anomaly permits the testicle to torque on its own axis, resulting in a less common type of intravaginal torsion. Other structures within the scrotum may undergo torsion and present with a similar clinical picture. The most common of these is the appendix testis, a remnant of the müllerian duct system.

Testicular salvage depends on expeditious diagnosis and prompt surgical detorsion. Torsion may be complete (i.e., a twist of > 360°) but often is incomplete. Spontaneous detorsion and retorsion greatly complicate clinical and radiologic diagnosis. In men with torsion of the spermatic cord of more than 360°, the testicular salvage rate is 80% when detorsion is accomplished within 5 hours, but the rate falls to 20% if torsion is not corrected within 12 hours after the onset of symptoms. Twists of less than 360° may be present for relatively longer periods of time before testicular viability and function are lost irreversibly. Surgery may be indicated if torsion is diagnosed beyond the period of testicular viability ("missed" torsion). Orchiopexy of the opposite testicle may be needed, and several sources suggest that the devitalized testicle should be removed because the liberation of proteins from the necrotic testicle can lead to the formation of autoantibodies that theoretically may compromise the formation or maturation of sperm from the contralateral testicle.

The preferred method of screening for torsion of the spermatic cord is high-resolution ultrasonography with color Doppler (Box 8-3). Comparison studies in children and adults suggest that the sensitivity is comparable with scintigraphy and in the range of 85% to 100%. Sonography may be more sensitive to incomplete torsion and can be repeated when necessary if intermittent torsion is suspected. The acutely torqued testicle may be enlarged and diffusely hypoechoic, or it may contain multifocal areas of decreased echogenicity; however, many patients with acute testicular torsion will have normal testicular

---

Box 8-2 Acute Scrotum

Torsion of the spermatic cord or testicular appendage
Epididymitis
Orchitis
Strangulated hernia
Testicular neoplasm

Box 8-3   Spermatic Cord Torsion—Ultrasound

Torsion may be complete or incomplete
Gray-scale ultrasonography
    Testicle: normal or enlarged, patchy hypoechoic
      areas
    Epididymis: normal or enlarged and hypoechoic
    Scrotal skin: normal or thickened
    Testicle can be small and heterogeneous in chronic
      torsion
Color Doppler ultrasonography
    Establish settings from normal testicle
    No detectable flow, or markedly asymmetric flow
    Incomplete torsion may be falsely normal
    Increased flow in recent detorsion

Box 8-4   Spermatic Cord Torsion—Pertechnetate Scan

Halo sign—round, central photopenic area
Increased dartos flow in mid and late (≥ 24 hours)
    torsion
Nubbin sign—increased activity medial to iliac artery
    at site of twist

Radionuclide imaging with technetium-99m pertechnetate is another radiologic method of imaging testicular torsion (Box 8-4). The radionuclide angiogram may show normal blood flow in the spermatic cord in early, mid, or late torsion. Normal blood flow to the dartos on the radionuclide angiogram may be observed within 5 to 7 hours of torsion, and increased dartos flow with decreased central flow ("halo" sign) is seen in mid and late (> 24 hours) torsion. Static images reveal a round, central photopenic area at the expected site of the testicle in acute, mid, and late torsion. The "halo" sign suggests the diagnosis of testicular torsion but also can be seen in patients with any poorly perfused intratesticular mass, such as an abscess cavity or a hematoma.

Epididymitis and other extratesticular masses

A summary of extratesticular lesions is shown in Table 8-1. In contrast to testicular torsion, the most common acute scrotal process in the postpubertal age group is acute epididymitis. In this age group, acute epididymitis

echogenicity and size. Because the epididymis also is supplied by the testicular artery, it may be enlarged and hypoechoic, and a reactive hydrocele may be seen. Scrotal skin thickening also may be apparent. Torsions that are imaged 12 hours or more after initial torsion may develop a more heterogeneous echogenicity as necrosis occurs. Scrotal skin thickening also may be apparent. On duplex and color Doppler sonography, torsion is suggested when there is no detectable flow to the testis after 1 minute of scanning time or when a single small, intratesticular vessel is seen in the symptomatic testis and readily detectable, diffuse flow is demonstrated in the contralateral testis (Fig. 8-5).

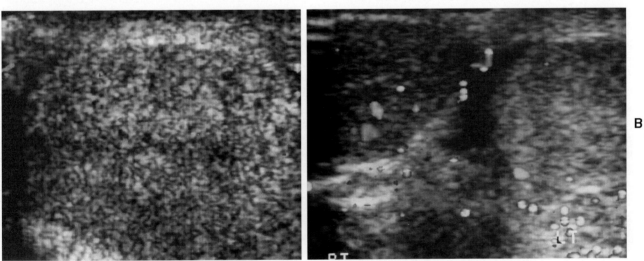

Fig. 8-5   Torsion of the spermatic cord. **A,** Sagittal sonogram shows inhomogeneous echogenicity of the symptomatic testicle. In early stages of torsion, the gray-scale image of the testis often is normal, or there may be only mild enlargement of the testicle. **B,** Transverse color Doppler sonogram demonstrates a normal pattern of flow in the asymptomatic right testicle, confirming adequate Doppler sensitivity. There is no detectable flow in the left testicle. Note also that there is swelling of the left epididymis and a small hydrocele. (Case courtesy of Michael T. Wallach, MD.)

Table 8-1	Extratesticular Lesions	
	Solid	**Cystic**
Epididymis	Epididymis Tumor—rare (adenomatoid tumor)	Epididymal cyst Spermatocele
Tunica vaginalis	Hernia Tumor—rare (mesothelioma)	Hydrocele, simple or complex
Spermatic cord	Tumor—rare (rhabdomyosarcoma)	Varicocele

is nine times as common as torsion. The patient may have acute or subacute pain and fever and may complain of dysuria. On physical examination, there is scrotal erythema, and pyuria is present in more than 90% of patients. Epididymitis is thought to be caused by the retrograde spread of infection from the urethra or prostate.

The cardinal sonographic sign of epididymitis is epididymal enlargement (Box 8-5). In most patients, the epididymis also is of uniformly low echogenicity, but rarely, it can be heterogeneous or of uniformly higher echogenicity (Fig. 8-6). Thickening of the scrotal skin, hydrocele, or both also may be seen. A complex fluid collection around the testicle may indicate complication by pyocele, and an inhomogeneous echogenicity or focal hypoechoic area in the testicle may indicate orchitis, which complicates epididymitis in about 20% of patients, or testicular ischemia. The chronically inflamed epididymis often is enlarged and may be hyperechoic. Color Doppler sonography has been used to diagnose acute epididymitis when the epididymis is not enlarged. The normal epididymis demonstrates no detectable flow, even at the lowest possible flow settings. Hyperemia associated with epididymal inflammation is suggested when there is hypervascularity, i.e., an increase in the absolute number or concentration of vessels (Fig. 8-6D). In as many as 20% of patients, epididymitis may present as hyperemia on color Doppler, and the gray-scale appearance of the epididymis is normal. Hypervascularity can

Box 8-5 Epididymitis—Ultrasonography

Enlarged and hypoechoic epididymis
Hydrocele or pyocele
Scrotal skin thickening
Increased color flow
With or without testicular infarct or orchitis

be focal, sparing the epididymal head or tail, in as many as 25% of patients.

Several rare tumors may present as a solid extratesticular mass. The most common tumor of the epididymis is the adenomatoid tumor, a benign hamartoma often found in the epididymal tail. These tumors can be 5 mm to 5 cm in size and are isoechoic or hyperechoic compared with the testicle. Leiomyoma is the second most common tumor of the epididymis. Benign mesothelioma, which originates from the tunica vaginalis, may present as a small, hyperechoic paratesticular mass associated with a large hydrocele. Primary sarcoma of the spermatic cord may spread into the epididymis or testis (Fig. 8-7). Embryonal rhabdomyosarcoma is the most common malignant spermatic cord sarcoma in boys and young men.

Epididymal cyst, spermatocele, simple and complex hydrocele, and varicocele are among the more common fluid-filled, extratesticular masses. Epididymal cyst and spermatocele are small anechoic cysts that are more common in the head of the epididymis (Fig. 8-8). Unlike an epididymal cyst, a spermatocele contains spermatozoa and may be secondary to previous infection or trauma. A hydrocele is the accumulation of fluid between the visceral and parietal tunica vaginalis. Simple hydrocele may occur in isolation or as a result of epididymitis or orchitis, torsion, trauma, tumor, or a variety of other nonspecific causes. Complex hydroceles may result from pyocele or hematocele. A varicocele is the distended pampiniform venous plexus (Box 8-6). When there are incompetent valves of the internal testicular vein, the varicocele is a compressible, dynamic tangle of vessels measuring more than 2 mm in diameter (Fig. 8-9 on p. 313). Venous distention can be provoked by a standing position or Valsalva maneuver. Rarely, a varicocele may form when the testicular vein is obstructed, for instance, by tumor or thrombus in the left renal vein. These varicoceles may not be compressible or changed by provocative maneuvers. Varicocele occurs in 15% of the population, and more than 95% are on the left side. Some evidence indicates that varicoceles cause a progressive decline in semen quality and may reduce fertility. Because varicoceles are manageable, they should be investigated aggressively in men who are infertile.

Orchitis and testicular abscess

Parenchymal infection of the testicle usually occurs with bacterial epididymitis, but it may occur as a primary infectious process if it results from mumps infection, for example. Orchitis is the most common complication of mumps infection; it occurs in as many as 25% of postpubertal male patients with mumps. In two thirds of patients, it is unilateral, and it usually develops within 7 to 10 days after the onset of parotitis. Although the mumps virus most frequently is responsible, echovirus, group B

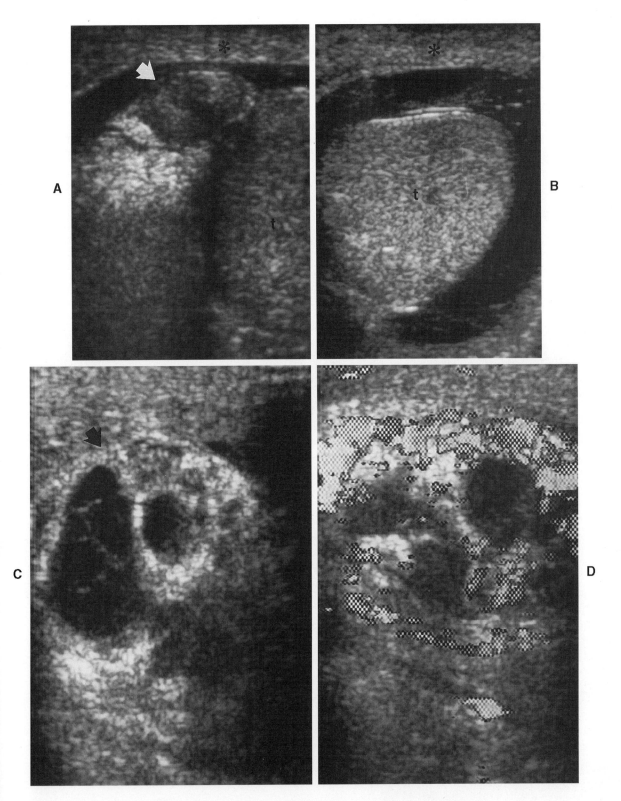

Fig. 8-6   Typical sonographic findings of acute epididymitis and epididymal abscess. **A,** Sagittal sonogram demonstrates marked enlargement of the epididymis (arrow) and thickening of the scrotal skin (*). **B,** There is a complex fluid collection around the testicle, consistent with pyocele (t = testis). **C,** In another patient with an epididymal abscess, a magnified sonogram demonstrates diffuse enlargement of the epididymis (arrow) that contains several hypoechoic areas. **D,** Color Doppler sonogram demonstrates marked hyperemia of the epididymis.

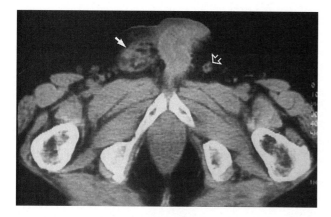

Fig. 8-7   Primary sarcoma of the spermatic cord. CT demonstrates a heterogeneous mass (arrow) containing multiple low attenuation foci that are isodense with fat. Myxoid liposarcoma was removed at surgery (open arrow = normal left spermatic cord).

arboviruses, and lymphocytic choriomeningitis virus also may cause primary infection.

Sonographically, there is diffuse enlargement of the testicle (Box 8-7). The echogenicity of the testicle is homogeneous and usually somewhat decreased, but it can be normal. Color Doppler sonography may demonstrate an increase in the number of visible vessels per unit area of the testicle, especially when compared with the asymptomatic opposite testicle. Coexistent abnormality of the epididymis or scrotal skin may be seen in 40% of patients. When orchitis is a focal process, it can be difficult to distinguish from testicular cancer (Fig. 8-10). Unlike cancer, focal orchitis typically does not distort the otherwise smooth contour of the testicle. Color Doppler ultrasonography may not be helpful in

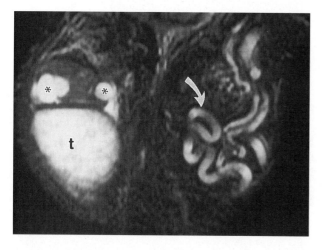

Fig. 8-8   MR imaging of epididymal cysts. Coronal T$_2$-weighted image of the scrotum shows well-defined hyperintense masses (*) in the head of the right epididymis (t = testis; curved arrow = contralateral varicocele). Spermatoceles contain spermatozoa, whereas epididymal cysts do not.

Box 8-6   Varicocele

Dilated pampiniform plexus resulting from spermatic vein valve incompetence
Left side in 95%
Most common manageable cause of male infertility
Compressible, tortuous vessels, > 2 mm in diameter
Distended in standing position or with Valsalva maneuver
Atypical varicocele because of venous obstruction
    Older patient
    Right side
    Unchanged in size with provocative maneuvers

---

distinguishing orchitis from cancer because hypervascularity, compared with normal testicular tissue, can be observed in both diseases, particularly when the focal mass is larger than 1.6 cm. With resolution of the inflammatory process, the testis may return to normal size or may atrophy. Atrophy usually is detectable within 6 months after the orchitis subsides. Unilateral atrophy develops in roughly one third of patients with mumps orchitis, and bilateral atrophy occurs in 10% of patients. A testicular abscess may present as a discrete intratesticular collection of fluid, which typically is complex. In addition, there may be evidence of intrascrotal gas, which appears as a highly reflective interface with "dirty" acoustic shadowing.

Malignant testicular neoplasm

Testicular carcinoma is the most common malignant cancer to afflict the male population in the 15- to 30-year age range. It classically presents as a painless scrotal mass, although about 25% of patients have some discomfort. This diagnosis should be considered in any male patient of appropriate age who presents with a retroperitoneal, mediastinal, or pulmonary parenchymal mass. A well-defined risk factor for testicular carcinoma is cryptorchidism, and there is an increased risk of cancer in the contralateral descended testicle.

Neoplasms of the testicle can be classified as primary

Box 8-7   Orchitis and Testicular Abscess—Ultrasonography

Enlarged and diffusely hypoechoic testicle, or focal hypoechoic area that does not distort the contour
Possible association with scrotal edema or epididymitis
Increased blood flow
Abscess—discrete complex collection with or without gas

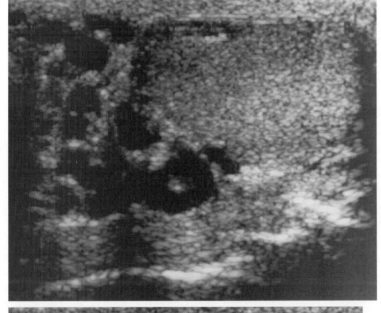

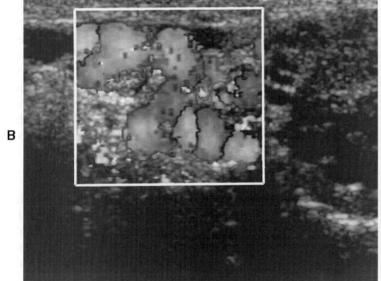

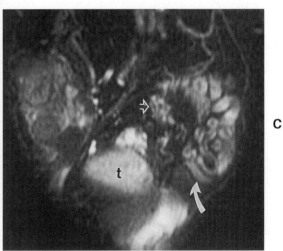

Fig. 8-9   Ultrasound and MR imaging of varicocele. **A,** Superior to the testicle, multiple anechoic spaces of similar size are seen on a scrotal sonogram. **B,** Color Doppler sonogram confirms flow within these spaces and is diagnostic of a varicocele. **C,** Coronal T₂-weighted MR imaging of another patient shows multiple serpentine vessels in the left hemiscrotum (curved arrow), diagnostic of varicocele (t = left testicle; open arrow = normal left epididymis)

germ cell, primary non–germ cell, and secondary or metastatic tumors (Box 8-8). Germ cell tumors are found in about 95% of patients with primary testicular carcinoma. Of these tumors, 40% are seminomas, and an additional 40% have a mixed histologic pattern. The most common of these mixed tumors is teratocarcinoma. Nonseminomatous germ cell tumors (NSGCT) include embryonal cell carcinoma and teratoma and the less common choriocarcinoma and yolk sac carcinoma. Serum alpha fetoprotein concentrations are increased in 60% of patients with testicular cancer, including mixed tumors, embryonal cell carcinoma, and yolk sac carcinoma. Serum β-human chorionic gonadotropin (βHCG) levels are elevated in 50% of patients with testicular carcinoma, including pure seminoma, embryonal carcinoma, and choriocarcinoma. Pure seminomas never cause an increase in alpha fetoprotein, but about 10% have some elevation in the βHCG level. The distinction between seminoma and NSGCT is important because seminomas are exquisitely radiosensitive, unlike their nonseminomatous counterparts. Germ cell tumors may also arise in extragonadal sites; common locations are the retroperitoneum and mediastinum. Non–germ cell tumors account for only about 5% of primary testicular neoplasms. The two most common non–germ cell tumors include the Leydig cell tumor and the Sertoli cell tumor. Some Leydig cell tumors have the capacity to produce testosterone, and 30% are associated with precocious virilization or feminization. One third

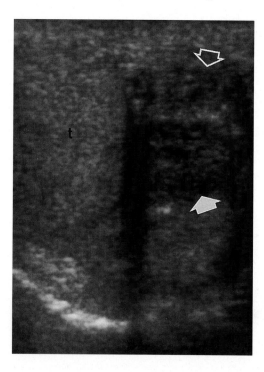

Fig. 8-10 Epididymoorchitis in a 25-year-old man with acute pain and diffuse enlargement of the left hemiscrotum. Transverse sonogram of the scrotum demonstrates a focal hypoechoic mass in the left testicle (solid arrow). In addition, there is diffuse enlargement and decreased echogenicity of the epididymis (open arrow) and thickening of the scrotal skin. In comparison, the right testicle (t) is normal.

of patients with Sertoli cell tumors present with gynecomastia resulting from estrogen or müllerian-inhibiting factor production.

Secondary neoplasms also can occur in the testicle and often are from other genitourinary primaries. Testicular lymphoma is the most common primary and secondary testicular neoplasm in men aged 60 to 80 years. Although the testicle may be the site of disease at presentation, it usually is not the primary site, as clinically occult extratesticular lymphoma usually is found. Because the blood–gonad barrier prevents systemic chemotherapy from reaching it, the testis is a sanctuary for acute leukemia in children and a site for disease relapse. Rarely, lung carcinoma or melanoma may metastasize to the testes.

Although many testicular neoplasms are palpable, sonography may be necessary when clinical suspicion is high, despite a normal physical examination, or if an adequate testicular evaluation is not possible because of tenderness or hydrocele (Box 8-9). Scrotal ultrasonography also is performed in patients who present with extragonadal germ cell tumors. Seminoma presents as an area of uniform decreased echogenicity, which usually is focal but may be diffuse. If focal and peripheral, it may cause the tunica albuginea to bulge. The interface between tumor and normal testicular parenchyma usually is sharp

---

Box 8-8   Testicular Cancer

Risk factors: cryptorchidism, maternal diethylstilbestrol use, testicular atrophy
Germ cell tumors (95%)
  Seminoma—no tumor marker, radiosensitive
  Mixed—teratocarcinoma most common
  Nonseminomatous germ cell tumor—more aggressive than seminoma
    Embryonal carcinoma—positive alpha fetoprotein and human chorionic gonadotropin
    Yolk sac carcinoma—positive alpha fetoprotein
    Choriocarcinoma—positive human chorionic gonadotropin
    Teratoma—positive alpha fetoprotein
Non-germ cell and stromal tumors
  Leydig cell—androgen production
  Sertoli cell—estrogen production
Metastases
  Lymphoma—most common in older men, bilateral
  Leukemia
  Prostate and lung

Box 8-9   Testicular Cancer—Ultrasonography

Predominantly hypoechoic mass is typical of seminoma
  Differential diagnosis—orchitis, abscess, hematoma, contusion, focal infarct
Bulges tunica albuginea
Hyperechoic foci or cysts in mixed histology and nonseminomatous germ cell tumor
Echogenic scar—"burned out" tumor
Diffusely hypoechoic testicle
  Differential diagnosis—ischemia or infarct; orchitis

(Fig. 8-11). Occasionally, diffuse tumor infiltration can lead to a generalized hypoechoic appearance, which may be apparent only by comparison with the contralateral testicle. Lymphoma or metastatic disease usually is seen as a focal hypoechoic mass that is indistinguishable from seminoma (Fig. 8-12). In contrast, mixed histology and NSGCT (particularly embryonal cell carcinoma) can be more heterogeneous in echogenicity because of cystic areas or hyperechoic foci (Figs. 8-13, 8-14). The tumor margin often is less distinct, and the testicular contour can be lobulated. Investigation of testicular neoplasms with color Doppler ultrasonography has shown most lesions larger than 1.6 cm to be hypervascular (i.e., flow is increased to the tumor compared with normal parenchymal flow). In contrast, smaller tumors tend to be

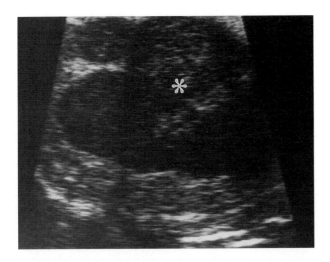

Fig. 8-11 Seminoma. Sagittal sonogram shows a large, lobulated hypoechoic mass (*) in the testicle. The interface between tumor and normal parenchyma of the testis is sharp.

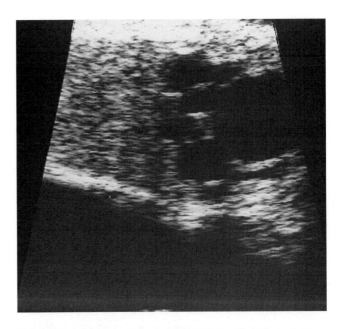

Fig. 8-13 Teratocarcinoma. Sagittal sonogram demonstrates a multiloculated, cystic mass in the left testicle, which is an atypical appearance but may be seen with nonseminomatous germ cell tumors.

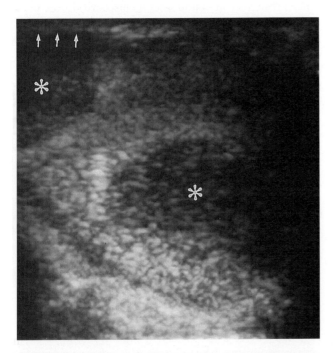

Fig. 8-12 Lymphoma of the testicle in a 57-year-old man presenting with painless enlargement of the scrotum. Sagittal sonogram of the left testicle demonstrates two focal hypoechoic masses (*), one of which bulges the tunica albuginea (arrows).

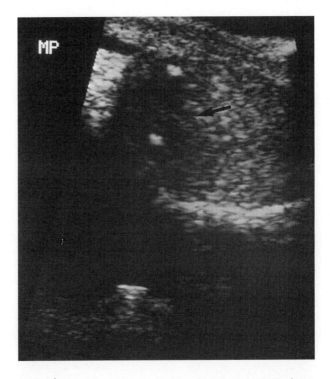

Fig. 8-14 Focal calcifications in a testicular cancer. Sagittal sonogram demonstrates a testicular mass (arrow) containing two echogenic foci, consistent with calcifications. The interface between the tumor and normal parenchyma is poorly defined. At orchiectomy, the echogenic foci were areas of calcification in an embryonal cell carcinoma.

hypovascular. The cell type of the tumor does not correlate with sonographically detectable flow.

The differential diagnosis for a focal intratesticular mass includes orchitis, hematoma, and abscess. A diffuse testicular lesion may be caused by orchitis or infarction and by diffuse neoplasm. Occasionally, distinguishing testicular carcinoma from testicular inflammation may be difficult. Extratesticular findings that may accompany inflammatory processes should be sought; they include enlargement of the epididymis, scrotal skin thickening, and hydrocele. These findings are not associated with testicular neoplasms, although small hydroceles may be present in about 10% of tumors.

Testicular calcifications and microlithiasis

Calcifications in the testes occasionally are identified on scrotal sonograms and have been associated with a variety of diseases. Discrete larger echogenic foci (3 to 9 mm) can be seen with some testicular tumors, including teratocarcinoma, seminoma, embryonal cell carcinoma, and Sertoli cell or Leydig cell tumors (Fig. 8-14). Testicular teratoma often is associated with large, irregular calcifications and mixed cystic and solid areas on sonograms. Treated testicular tumors or "burned out" neoplasms may appear as linear echogenic scars and can contain multiple small (< 3 mm) calcifications. Resolved infection, old hematomas, or small infarcts may result in calcifications, scarring, and contour abnormalities. Multiple, tiny, often diffuse echogenic foci are classified as testicular microlithiasis (Fig. 8-15). These microliths, which are foci of degenerative calcification in seminiferous tubules, measure 1 to 2 mm, and although echogenic, they may not shadow. The condition usually is bilateral but may not be symmetric. Testicular microlithiasis has been seen in cryptorchid or atrophic testes and has been associated with infertility. The clinical significance of this rare disease is its association with testicular cancer; 20% to 45% of occurrences are associated with a focal hypoechoic

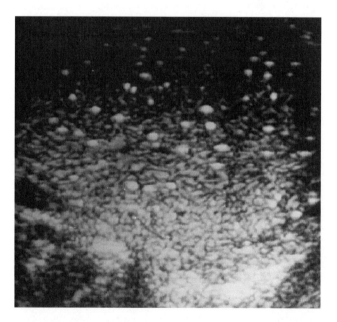

Fig. 8-15 Testicular microlithiasis. Sagittal sonogram demonstrates multiple tiny echogenic foci in the parenchyma of the testis that represent degenerative calcifications in seminiferous tubules. (Case courtesy of Jeffrey M. Brody, MD.)

testicular mass. Although it is not clear whether it is a cause of the associated cancer or the result of another premalignant condition such as intraepithelial germinal cell neoplasm, if testicular microlithiasis is discovered and no intratesticular mass is present, regular clinical follow-up evaluation and surveillance with testicular sonography have been advised.

Staging of Testicular Carcinoma

Primary testicular carcinoma may metastasize by a lymphogenous route, a hematogenous route, or both (Box 8-10). Hematogenous dissemination to the lung, liver, brain, or bones typically does not occur until after there has been lymphatic spread. The lymphatic drainage of the testes follows the course of the testicular or internal spermatic vein. The sentinel lymph node group of a left testicular neoplasm is the left renal perihilar group, located immediately caudal to the left renal vein (Fig. 8-16). A right testicular neoplasm first metastasizes to the paracaval lymph node group at the level of or slightly inferior to the renal vein. Drainage from the right testicle can cross over to the left side of the retroperitoneum, but the opposite is less common. After these initial lymph node stations are involved, the paralumbar nodes inferior to the renal hilum or thoracic sites are affected. Local tumor extension into the epididymis or scrotal skin changes the potential lymphatic drainage of the testicular neoplasm. If the epididymis is involved, drainage to the external iliac node chain may occur, and scrotal involvement may lead to inguinal adenopathy. Abdominal lymphatics drain into the thoracic duct and then into the left brachiocephalic vein. Tumors that spread by this route may involve the lungs, mediastinum, or supraclavicular lymph nodes. A notable exception to the primary lymphatic spread of testicular cancers is choriocarcinoma, which is prone to hematogenous metastases.

Computed tomography (CT) is the conventional method of staging disease in the abdomen and thorax

---

Box 8-10   Staging of Testicular Carcinoma

Three to five percent extragonadal origin (mediastinum, retroperitoneum, sacrococcygeal, pineal)
Metastases at presentation: 15%, seminoma and 33%, nonseminomatous germ cell tumor
"Sentinel nodes": left renal perihilar and right paracaval renal hilar groups
Tumor invading epididymis drains to internal iliac nodes
Tumor invading scrotum drains to inguinal nodes
Hematogenous metastases to lungs and liver

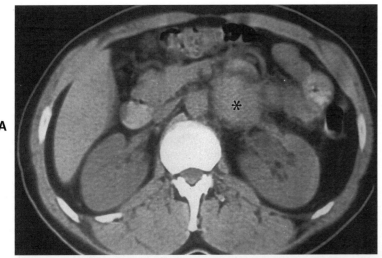

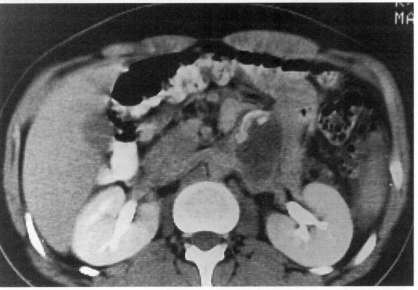

Fig. 8-16 Sentinel lymph node. **A,** In a patient with seminoma of the left testicle, CT demonstrates a paraaortic mass (*) just caudad to the left renal vein. Because the lymphatic drainage of the testicle follows the course of the ipsilateral internal spermatic (testicular) vein, cancer of the left testicle will metastasize to this lymph node group before others. **B,** Infused CT scan in another patient shows a hypodense mass with peripheral calcification at the left renal vein. Low-density nodal metastases can be seen with metastatic testicular neoplasms (particularly teratocarcinoma), lymphoma (usually treated), tuberculosis, squamous cell carcinoma of the genitourinary tract, and rarely, Whipple's disease. This patient had a left testicular mass, surgically proven to be a teratocarcinoma.

(Box 8-11). In patients with Stage I and II disease, abdominal CT is comparable with lymphangiography; its sensitivity is 50% to 60%, and its specificity is approximately 80%. Retroperitoneal lymphadenectomy shows evidence of malignant node involvement in as many as 50% of patients with normal results on abdominal CT scan (lymph node size, 1.5 cm). When compared with CT scanning alone, the addition of lymphangiography to the diagnostic staging work-up improves the sensitivity, but specificity decreases by about 10% to 15%. Lymphangiography may be of value in patients with normal results on CT scans and seminoma because an abnormal result on lymphangiogram may lead to prophylactic mediastinal radiation therapy. Lymphangiography is not used in non-seminomatous tumors because patients who have no evidence of widespread disease on CT scans are candidates for retroperitoneal lymphadenectomy.

Box 8-11	Staging System of Testicular Carcinoma
Stage I	Tumor confined to the testis
Stage IIA	Minimal nodal metastases (usually based on radiologic studies) and limited to the infradiaphragmatic stations
Stage IIB	Bulky retroperitoneal nodal metastases
Stage III	Tumor involving lymphatics above the diaphragm
Stage IV	Extranodal metastases (pulmonary, hepatic, osseous, or central nervous system)

Traumatic Injury to the Scrotum

Violent, blunt scrotal trauma may cause testicular rupture. Pain, nausea, and vomiting may occur, and on physical examination, extreme tenderness, scrotal ecchymosis, and swelling also are frequent symptoms. It is important to remember that an associated neoplasm can be a cause of testicular rupture after rather minor trauma. Early surgical exploration and repair of testicular injuries have reduced morbidity and the need for subsequent orchiectomy. If the tunica albuginea of the testicle has been violated, devitalized seminiferous tubules will be extruded into the potential space between the tunica albuginea and tunica vaginalis, and surgical débridement is indicated. In addition to suspected rupture, the presence of a large scrotal hematoma also is an indication for exploration. The mass effect of a large hematoma can compress the ipsilateral testicle, depriving it of blood. In addition, infection may follow testicular rupture.

Scrotal ultrasonography is the imaging procedure of choice because it helps to determine whether significant parenchymal disruption has occurred, which is essential information when deciding which patients require emergency surgery, and it can assess the size of a scrotal hematoma (Box 8-12). Furthermore, ultrasonography can be used to exclude competing diagnoses, such as epididymoorchitis or torsion, particularly when a history of scrotal trauma is unclear. Ultrasonography correctly predicts the presence of a ruptured testis in 94% of patients with scrotal injury. The most sensitive sign of testicular injury is an irregular or indistinct testicular contour (Fig. 8-17). Focal areas of increased or decreased echogenicity are consistent with contusion. A focal linear or, more often, a complex and multifocal disruption of the normally homogeneous parenchymal echo pattern suggests the diagnosis of testicular fracture (Fig. 8-18). Solid or semisolid collections around the disrupted testicle may represent hematoma and extruded parenchyma; these collections can be mistaken for the ruptured testicle itself. Testicular sonography usually is performed with a high-frequency transducer, which maximizes spatial resolution. If the scrotum is enlarged because of a hematoma, a lower frequency transducer with increased depth of field may be necessary to survey the scrotum for a displaced or compressed testicle.

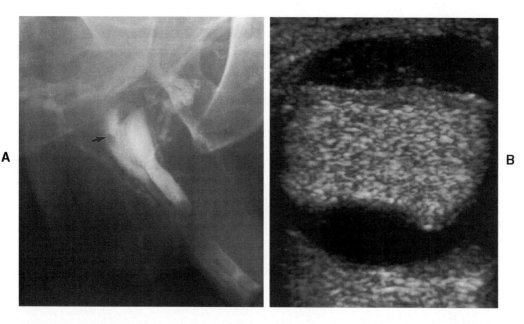

Fig. 8-17   Blunt traumatic injury to the scrotum and urethra. **A,** Retrograde urethrogram demonstrates a complete tear of the bulbar urethra with contrast intravasation into the corpus spongiosum (arrow) and crural veins. **B,** Because of marked swelling of the scrotum, sonography also was performed. A complex hydrocele surrounds a misshapen testicle that has an indistinct contour. At surgery, a large tension hematocele and multiple testicular fractures were found.

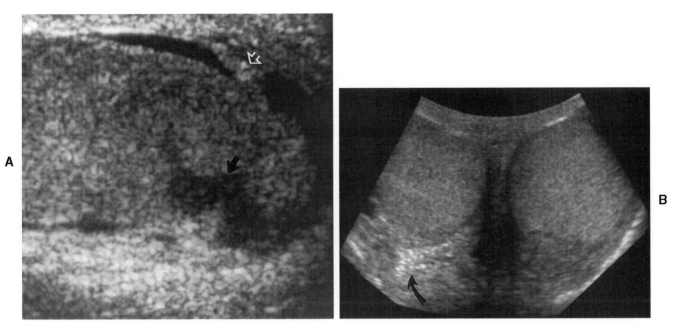

Fig. 8-18   Testicular fracture and scrotal hematoma. **A,** Sagittal sonogram demonstrates a hypoechoic peripheral fracture (arrow) in the lower pole of the testis. At surgery, echogenic debris (open arrow) was extruded seminiferous tubules. **B,** Transverse scrotal sonogram of another patient demonstrates an echogenic, extratesticular mass (curved arrow). Because of marked swelling, surgical exploration was performed, and a hematoma was evacuated.

Undescended Testicle (Cryptorchidism)

Cryptorchidism refers to the condition in which the testicle is not positioned in the base of the scrotum (Box 8-13). Because the testicle originates in the abdominal cavity of the embryo, a cryptorchid testis can be found anywhere along the normal course of testicular descent from the level of the inferior pole of the kidney to the upper scrotum. On the basis of location and in decreasing order of incidence, four types of cryptorchid testis are recognized: (1) retractile, (2) canalicular, (3) abdominal, and (4) ectopic. The retractile testis moves intermittently between the base of the scrotum and the groin and can be observed in up to 80% of patients aged 6 months to 11 years. Retraction, the result of spontaneous or reflexive cremasteric muscle contraction, occurs less commonly after puberty. The canalicular testis is located between the internal and external inguinal rings. The majority of abdominal testes are found immediately proximal to the internal inguinal ring. The rarest type of malpositioned testicle is ectopic cryptorchidism, in which the testicle is found away from the normal pathway of descent. The most common ectopic site is the superficial inguinal pouch, but other described locations include the femoral canal, the suprapubic region, the perineum, and the opposite scrotum (transverse ectopia). Absence, another cause for an impalpable testis, occurs in up to 5% of surgical explorations for cryptorchidism.

Infertility, neoplasia, torsion, and trauma are the major reported complications of cryptorchidism. Irreversible histologic changes occur in the cryptorchid testicle by the age of 2.5 years and are believed to contribute to associated complications of infertility and neoplasia. Testicular maldescent impairs spermatogenesis. Even in unilateral cryptorchidism, a defect in the spermatogenesis of the contralateral scrotal testicle may be present because after surgical correction of cryptorchidism, the mean fertility rate is only 60%. About one-third of undescended testes also have anomalies of wolffian duct-derived structures that may impact on fertility: seminal vesicle cyst, insertion of an ectopic ureter into the vas

---

Box 8-13   Undescended Testicle

Types—canalicular, abdominal, ectopic, retractile
Complications—infertility, neoplasia, torsion, trauma
Higher cancer risk in contralateral testicle
Sonography
   Proximal to inguinal ring
   Testis may be small or diffusely hypoechoic
Computed tomography or MR imaging if ultrasonography results are negative

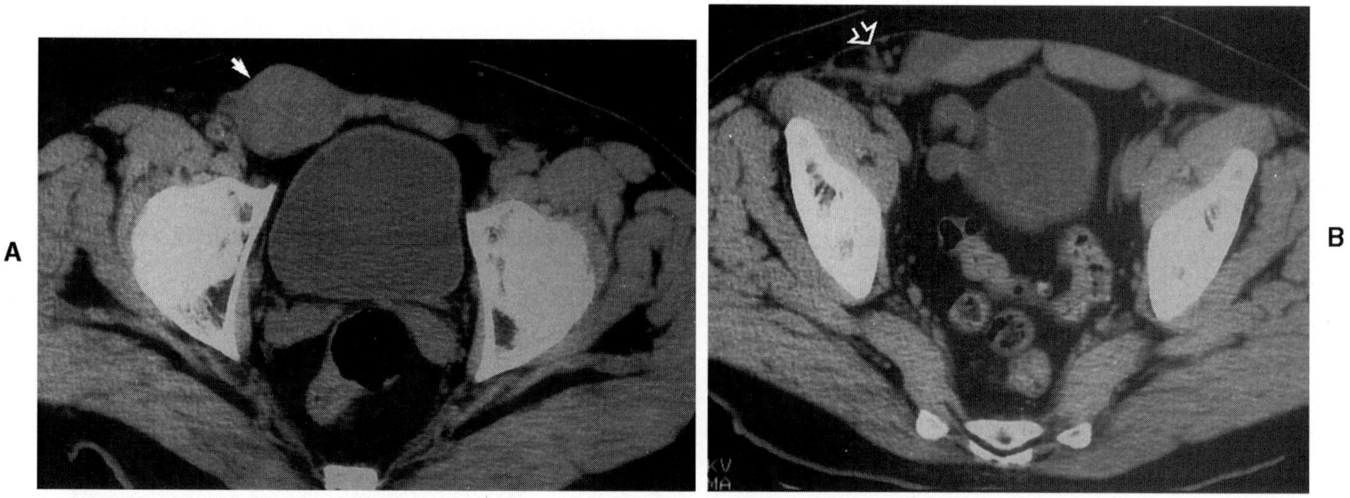

Fig. 8-19 Seminoma originating from a right canalicular testicle. **A,** CT demonstrates a solid mass (arrow) that is medial to the right external iliac vessels and inseparable from the rectus abdominis muscle. **B,** A more cephalic image shows spermatic cord vessels (open arrow) just lateral to the upper margin of the mass.

deferens or seminal vesicle, and agenesis of the epididymis, seminal vesicle, or vas deferens. An estimated 10% of all testicular cancers occur in patients with a history of cryptorchidism, and there is a 40-fold increase in the risk of developing cancer in an undescended testicle. This risk is present only if the undescended testis is unmanaged after the age of 5 years; hence, surgical correction is recommended around the age of 2 years. The most common histologic type of cancer is seminoma, followed by embryonal cell carcinoma (Fig. 8-19). An abdominal testis is four times as likely to undergo malignant degeneration than is an inguinal testis; interestingly, in patients with a unilateral undescended testis, 15% of testicular cancers occur in the contralateral, normally descended testis.

Because about one-fourth of undescended testes are nonpalpable, localization is the main objective of presurgical imaging. The primary imaging methods are ultrasonography and CT. Sonography is the most valuable method for finding the undescended testis when it is located at or caudal to the inguinal ligament. The cryptorchid testicle frequently is small and may be difficult to distinguish from an inguinal node, so it is important to identify the mediastinum of the testicle to identify it as such. CT has been used effectively to establish the location of abdominal testicles, particularly those just proximal to the inguinal canal. A suggested method uses contiguous 5-mm sections beginning at the level of the upper scrotum. Given the characteristic appearance of the normal testicle on T_2-weighted magnetic resonance (MR) images, it is an attractive method for definitively locating the juxtainguinal testis because it does not subject the young patient to ionizing radiation. However, experience

with MR imaging for this purpose is limited. Gonadal phlebography relies on the identification of the pampiniform plexus for localization of the cryptorchid testicle and has fewer associated complications than testicular arteriography. However, it is technically challenging, particularly in the child aged less than 1 year, and should be reserved for the patient whose undescended testicle cannot be located precisely by cross-sectional imaging or surgical exploration.

Prostate Nodule or Enlargement

Carcinoma of the prostate

Cancer of the prostate is the most common malignancy to afflict men and is the second most common cause of cancer-related death in the male population in this country. A paradox exists between the autopsy prevalence and the clinical incidence and mortality of prostate cancer. It is estimated that a 50-year-old man with a 25-year life expectancy has a 42% chance of developing a prostate cancer but only a 9.5% chance of developing the disease clinically, and a 2.5% chance of dying as a direct result of prostate cancer. Therefore, only one of every three to four men with prostate cancer will develop the clinically significant disease.

Pathologists have recognized the importance of tumor differentiation, DNA content, and primary tumor size as important factors for predicting the clinical behavior of prostatic adenocarcinoma. Histopathologic differentiation is graded according to the Gleason system. Pathologists recognize five different malignant glandular patterns of prostatic adenocarcinoma and have designated these patterns as Gleason Grades 1 to 5. Gleason Grade 1 is a malignant glandular pattern that is well differentiated, and Grade 5 is the most poorly differentiated pattern of adenocarcinoma. Prostate cancer of Gleason Grades 1 through 3 rarely involves the regional lymph nodes, whereas Gleason Grades 4 and 5 have the potential for lymphogenous spread. Because it is not uncommon for more than one histopathologic pattern to be present in any single specimen, the grades of the two predominant glandular patterns are summed to yield the Gleason score; tumors are considered to be well differentiated if they have a Gleason score of 2 to 4, moderately differentiated with a score of 5 to 7, and poorly differentiated with a score of 8 to 10. Pathologists also have identified a relationship between tumor size and clinical aggressiveness, which is an observation of potential importance in imaging. Tumors with a volume of 1.5 cc or less (1.3 to 1.4 cm, mean diameter) tend to be associated with local and distant metastases less often than larger primary tumors. Seminal vesicle invasion is more likely to occur after a primary tumor reaches the volume of 2.5 to 3.5 cc (1.7 to 1.9 cm, mean diameter), and lymph node or visceral metastasis usually does not occur until the primary lesion has reached a volume of 4 cc or greater (2.0 cm, mean diameter). It also has been noted that the histologic pattern becomes less differentiated with increasing primary tumor size; hence, as a general rule, the larger the primary cancer, the more aggressive its clinical behavior and, therefore, the more clinically significant it is likely to be.

Historically, the standard method for detecting prostate cancer has been the digital rectal examination (DRE). There is a growing consensus that DRE alone is inadequate because cancers tend to be advanced by the time they are detected with this method. Approximately 30% of cancers detected by DRE have evidence of lymph node or distant metastatic disease, and 35% of the remaining cancers, assumed to be localized, have evidence of extra-

prostatic spread at the time of surgery. At present, two additional tools are available for the early detection of prostate cancer: transrectal ultrasonography and the prostate-specific antigen (PSA) blood test. PSA is a kallikrein-like, serine protease glycoprotein produced exclusively by epithelial cells lining prostatic acini and ducts. In the seminal fluid, PSA is involved directly in the liquefaction of the seminal coagulum. Approximately 85% of men with PSA levels above 10 ng/mL (monoclonal Tandem R and Tandem E [Hybritech, San Diego, CA] or the monoclonal-polyclonal IMX [Abbott Laboratories, Abbott Park, IL]) and 25% with levels between 4 and 9.9 ng/mL have adenocarcinoma of the prostate. Furthermore, some cancers smaller than 1 cm³ or those that are small and poorly differentiated are not associated with elevated PSA levels. PSA levels above normal are not associated exclusively with prostate cancer; they may result from benign prostatic hyperplasia (BPH), acute or chronic prostatitis, prostate intraepithelial neoplasia, or infarcts. Therefore, use of PSA alone as a basis for prostate cancer diagnosis is ill advised. Use of the PSA test result with the DRE, transrectal ultrasound, and biopsy is more valuable. Several groups have attempted to redefine the normal value of PSA relative to the size of the prostate and then to extrapolate abnormal, size-normalized values of PSA that are consistent with prostate cancer. The PSA density is derived by dividing the prostate volume derived from transrectal sonography, in milliliters, into the serum PSA level. Biopsy is recommended when the PSA density exceeds numerical thresholds of 0.1 to 0.14.

The classic appearance of cancer on transrectal ultrasonography of the prostate is a round or oval hypoechoic lesion located in the peripheral zone, where 85% of prostate cancers are found (Fig. 8-20). Approximately 10% of cancers originate in the transitional zone; these are the Stage A cancers that usually are discovered incidentally at the time of transurethral prostatectomy. Transitional

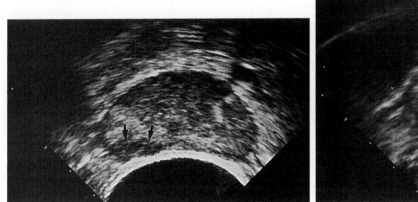 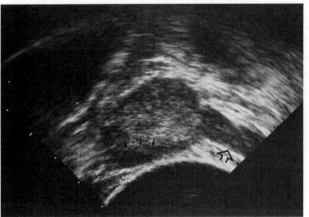

Fig. 8-20 Classic appearance of prostate cancer on transrectal sonography. On transverse (**A**) and sagittal (**B**) sonograms, a focal hypoechoic area (arrows) in the peripheral zone bulges the prostatic capsule (open arrow = left seminal vesicle).

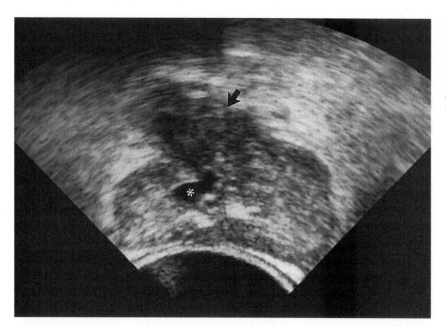

Fig. 8-21 Large prostate cancer originating from the transitional zone. Cancer was found in chips of tissue removed at transurethral prostatectomy. Transverse sonogram demonstrates an exophytic hypoechoic mass (arrow) that grows anteriorly through the fibromuscular stroma and capsule (* = prostatectomy defect).

zone cancers are particularly difficult to detect with sonography because this zone of the prostate often is enlarged and heterogeneous in echogenicity as a result of coexistent BPH (Fig. 8-21). The remaining 5% of prostate cancer originates in the central zone, the parenchymal tissue that surrounds the ejaculatory ducts. Approximately one-third of all prostate cancer is isoechoic with peripheral zone tissue and therefore may be extremely difficult to detect by ultrasonography. Isoechoic cancers may be suspected only when there is an abnormality in the otherwise regular contour of the prostate gland. One percent or less of cancers are hyperechoic, possibly because of the presence of calcifications within the gland, either because the cancer envelops benign calcifications as it grows or because central comedonecrosis is associated with dystrophic calcification.

Transrectal ultrasound is an excellent method for detecting cancers that are 10 mm or larger; however, only about 20% of lesions smaller than 10 mm are detected with this method. About 40% to 50% of prostate cancer is multifocal; that is, two or more foci of cancer are found in the prostate gland during pathologic examination. These accessory foci of cancer frequently are undetectable with ultrasonography when the index cancer is found; the small size or infiltrative growth pattern of these secondary malignant foci may account for this difficulty.

A well-documented problem with cancer characterization by means of transrectal ultrasonography is the nonspecificity of the hypoechoic lesion. In addition to adenocarcinoma, other benign and borderline malignant entities may have a hypoechoic appearance on sonograms (Box 8-14). Several characteristics of the hypo-

echoic lesion can be used to increase the positive predictive value for adenocarcinoma. First, it is important to correlate the findings on transrectal ultrasound with those of DRE. If the hypoechoic lesion corresponds to a palpable abnormality, particularly asymmetric firmness or a discrete nodule, the likelihood of cancer increases. Second, the result of the PSA blood test also is valuable. Lee et al report the positive predictive value of a hypoechoic lesion alone to be only 40%, but the value increases to 50% when the PSA is elevated and increases to 60% when associated with a palpable abnormality. If results of PSA and DRE are abnormal, the positive predictive value of a hypoechoic lesion increases to 70%. The size of the lesion is important: the larger the hypoechoic lesion, the more likely it is to be malignant. Finally, color-coded flow on a Doppler sonogram may represent a secondary finding to initiate biopsy of a lesion. Focal increased flow is associated with a high likelihood of carcinoma or prostatitis at histologic examination; how-

---

Box 8-14 Hypoechoic Lesion in the Peripheral Zone

Adenocarcinoma
Atypical hyperplasia or intraductal dysplasia
Chronic prostatitis
Granulomatous prostatitis
Focal atrophy
Nodules of benign prostatic hyperplasia
Prostatic cyst

ever, this finding has limited sensitivity, and the absence of flow on color Doppler sonography should not preclude biopsy if other signs that suggest malignancy are present.

Body and endorectal surface coil MR imaging also can be used to detect prostate cancer, although MR imaging more commonly is reserved for staging. The presence of a focal hypointense area in the relatively hyperintense peripheral zone on T_2-weighted images is consistent with cancer. Clinically palpable cancers more often are detected by body coil MR imaging (96% sensitivity) than are nonpalpable tumors (58% sensitivity), and nonpalpable posterior cancers are detected more often than anteriorly located tumors. Body coil MR imaging has not been proven to surpass transrectal ultrasound for the diagnosis of prostatic cancer. However, MR imaging performed with an endorectal surface coil increases the accuracy of detection and staging.

MR imaging with an endorectal surface coil enables imaging of the prostate with higher resolution than is achievable with the body coil. Optimal technique includes supine patient position and the use of intramuscular glucagon (1 mg), antialiasing options, and surface coil correction. Through signal filtration, surface coil correction decreases the signal from tissues located near the endorectal coil and is not necessary if endorectal coil imaging is supplemented with anterior phased-array multicoils. In addition, phase and frequency orientation are switched so that phase artifacts are projected left-to-right rather than anteriorly-to-posteriorly on transaxial images. The routine prostate imaging protocol includes T_1-weighted transaxial images of the prostate to assess periprostatic tumor extension and T_2-weighted transaxial and sagittal plane images acquired with a fast spin–echo technique. As with body coil MR imaging, peripheral zone cancers are best detected on T_2-weighted images and most commonly appear as foci of decreased signal intensity in the peripheral zone (Fig. 8-22). However, low-signal foci in the peripheral zone are not always caused by malignancy. Rarely, atypical BPH nodules may appear in the peripheral zone as foci of increased or decreased signal intensity (Fig. 8-23). Microscopically, many of these nodules contain areas of atypical hyperplasia or frank cancer. More commonly, focal hemorrhage from prostate biopsy appears as an amorphous focal area of low or high signal intensity in the peripheral zone on T_2-weighted images. Hemorrhage can persist up to 6 months after biopsy, and if low in signal intensity, it may mimic a peripheral zone cancer. In most patients with intraprostatic hemorrhage, a focal area of high signal intensity is seen in a corresponding area on T_1-weighted images (Fig. 8-24). In some patients, the MR examination is falsely normal in the presence of prostate cancer. Infiltrating cancers, particularly if microscopic, may cause too little signal aberration in the peripheral zone to be detected. Mucinous adenocarcinoma of the prostate, which makes up about 5% of all prostate cancer, also may escape detection because of insufficient signal intensity contrast with the peripheral zone.

Another valuable use of transrectal ultrasound is to direct biopsy of any detected abnormalities. Biopsy of the prostate and seminal vesicles is accomplished readily by this method. Sonographically guided biopsy is performed in the outpatient setting, and routine preparation includes administration of oral antibiotics (ciprofloxacin or norfloxacin) and Fleet's enema; oral antimicrobial therapy usually is continued 24 to 72 hours after the procedure. Routine use of local anesthetic is unnecessary. An automatic-firing spring-loaded biopsy gun facilitates the painless acquisition of core samples with the assistance of a modified transrectal ultrasound transducer and an 18-gauge needle. On average, three to five passes are made through the hypoechoic lesion of interest, and lesions as small as 5 mm are readily sampled. The overall complication rate is acceptably low. Crossover studies have shown that sonographically guided biopsy after negative results of a digitally guided biopsy can increase cancer detection.

Benign prostatic hyperplasia

Because it is relatively unusual in men aged less than 40 years but afflicts approximately 50% to 75% of men aged more than 60 years, BPH primarily is a disease of the senescent prostate. In addition to the major risk factor of age, BPH is more common in blacks and in patients with diabetes or hypertension. Presenting symptoms and signs usually result from prostate-level obstruction of the urethra. Early symptoms can be minimal because hypertrophy of the detrusor compensates for the increase in outflow resistance. With increasing bladder outlet obstruction, the patient may complain of hesitancy, diminution in the force of the urinary stream, postvoid dribbling, and the sensation of incomplete emptying. Irritative symptoms, such as frequency, urgency, and dysuria, are common and may result from uninhibited contractions of the detrusor. With increasing volumes of residual urine, overflow urinary incontinence and nocturia occur, and eventually, the manifestations of chronic urinary retention develop.

Pathologically, BPH is a disease of the glandular tissues that surround the portion of the prostatic urethra that extends from the bladder neck to the verumontanum. The largest and most numerous nodules almost always are situated closer to the proximal end of the verumontanum and originate almost entirely within the transitional zone. These nodules, which are predominantly glandular in type, originate as repeatedly branching ducts that bud off from existing ducts and grow into adjacent stroma; they are responsible for most of the obstructive symptoms attributed to BPH.

A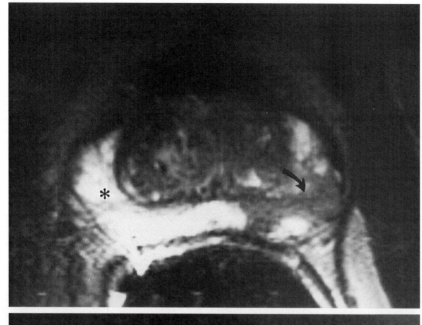

B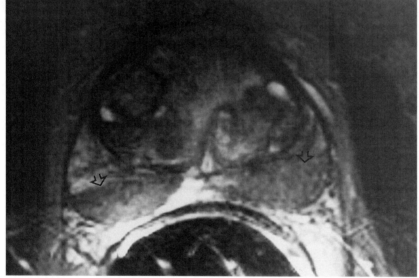

Fig. 8-22 Typical appearance of prostate cancer on MR imaging with an endorectal surface coil. **A,** Fast spin–echo T_2-weighted MR image demonstrates a focal area of decreased signal intensity (curved arrow) in the peripheral zone of the prostate. The capsule of the prostate is intact, and the signal intensity of periprostatic fat is symmetric. The signal intensity of normal peripheral zone tissue (*) is hyperintense on T_2-weighted MR images. **B,** In another patient, fast spin–echo, T_2-weighted MR image shows two separate hypointense foci (open arrows) in the peripheral zone of the prostate. The focus in the left peripheral zone was isoechoic on ultrasonography, but random biopsy results revealed cancer.

Radiologic evaluation of the urinary tract addresses several important clinical issues in the patient with obstructive or irritative symptoms and suspected BPH. The first issue is the status of the upper urinary tract. It is important to ascertain whether elevation of intraurethral resistance has translated into significant ureteral obstruction and obstructive nephropathy. Coexistent disease of the kidneys and ureters, such as congenital anomalies or cancer, also is sought. Bladder compensation is assessed by the radiologic evaluation of bladder size, estimation of postvoiding residual urine volume, bladder wall thickness, the presence of trabeculation, and diverticula formation. Another important objective is to evaluate the prostate for coincidental disease, specifically adenocarci-

noma. Estimation of the absolute size of the prostate is important, particularly if nonsurgical therapy is elected, although there is a poor correlation between absolute prostate size and severity of symptoms related to bladder outlet obstruction.

Intravenous urography (IVU) is performed to evaluate the upper urinary tract and the urinary bladder, but its value in the routine evaluation of prostatism is debated because up to 90% of studies have normal results or clinically insignificant findings. Upper tract malignancy is sought on routine urographic study, but in this population, it is found in only 0.2% of patients. Benign renal cysts, bladder diverticula, some degree of obstruction, and renal stones account for the majority of the abnormal-

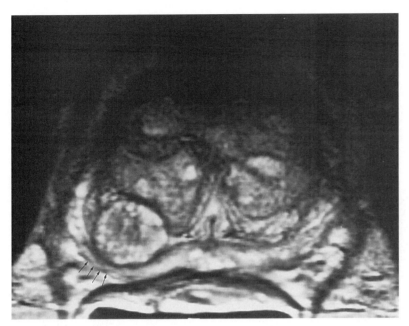

Fig. 8-23 Hyperplastic nodule mimics prostate cancer. The patient was referred for imaging because of a discrete palpable nodule on digital rectal examination. Transverse fast spin–echo T$_2$-weighted image shows a mixed signal intensity nodule in the outer aspect of the transitional zone, which focally thins the adjacent peripheral zone (arrows). The transitional zone of the prostate gland is enlarged and heterogeneous in signal intensity, consistent with glandular benign prostatic hyperplasia.

ities. Enlargement of the prostate elevates the bladder trigone, which results in elevation, straightening, and ultimately a "J-hook" configuration of the distal ureters. With hypoperistalsis of the ureter secondary to mild obstruction of the ureterovesical junction, the entire course of the ureter may be demonstrated on a single film; this is called *ureteral columnation*. Obstruction of the ureterovesical junction of greater severity may result in ureteral dilatation and, if longstanding, ureteral tortuosity (Fig. 8-25). Pelvocalyceal dilation with cortical atrophy can be seen if obstructive nephropathy complicates chronic bladder outlet obstruction caused by BPH.

Bladder size, bladder wall contour, and the prostatic impression are evaluated on the cystographic phase of the IVU. Trabeculation and the presence of bladder wall sacculation or cellule formation correlate with chronic bladder-outlet obstruction and indicate detrusor hypertrophy. Diverticula also can form in this setting, most commonly posterior and superior to the trigone at the ureterovesical junctions, and at the dome. A prominent prostatic impression also is seen on evaluation of the bladder contour. BPH usually results in a smooth, domelike indentation along the floor of the bladder. An irregular or nodular contour can be observed but should raise

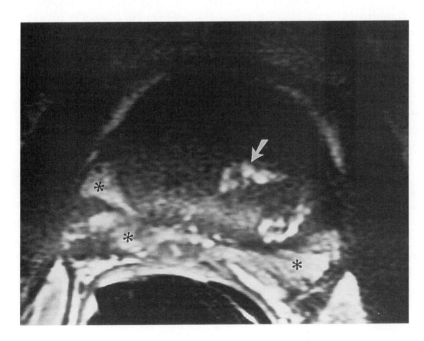

Fig. 8-24 Multifocal hemorrhage related to random prostate biopsy. A T$_1$-weighted image shows multiple foci of increased signal intensity in the peripheral zone (*) and transitional zone (arrow) of the prostate. The normal peripheral zone tissue is isointense compared with muscle on a T$_1$-weighted image. This patient had multiple, random biopsies of the prostate 3 weeks before MR imaging.

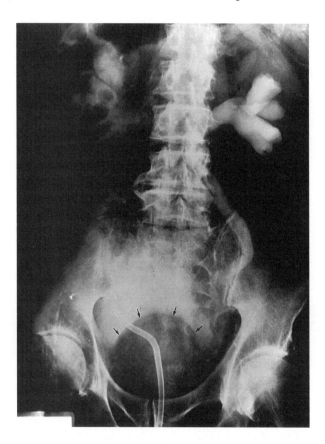

Fig. 8-25   Obstruction of the ureterovesical junction caused by chronic severe benign prostatic hyperplasia. Urogram demonstrates dilatation and tortuosity of the left ureter and minimal opacification of the dilated right intrarenal collecting system. There is a large filling defect at the base of the bladder (arrows) because of marked enlargement of the prostate gland. A catheter drains the obstructed bladder.

the suspicion of prostatic malignancy. A more rounded filling defect that may be seen with so-called median lobe or with Albarran (subcervical) lobe enlargement mimics an intraluminal bladder mass. The absence of a postvoid residual should not be equated with the absence of bladder-outlet obstruction because detrusor hypertrophy may have compensated for increased outlet resistance. Voiding cystourethrography is performed only when vesicoureteral reflux is suspected or when more precise information about the location and size of bladder diverticulation is sought.

Transrectal ultrasonography of the prostate provides information about the size of the prostate, the appearance of the transitional zone, and the presence of coincident prostatic disease. By using the formula for a prolate ellipsoid (the product of $\pi/6$ and the length, width, and height of the prostate), the volume of the prostate gland can be estimated from its orthogonal dimensions on transverse and sagittal images. Because the central gland of

the prostate is distinct sonographically from the peripheral zone in most men aged more than 40 years, the size of the transitional and central zones can be estimated in a similar fashion. An estimate of the weight of the prostate gland can be extrapolated from the prostate volume estimate, assuming the specific gravity of prostate tissue is 1.0 to 1.5 grams per cubic centimeter. Adenomatous nodules may appear as focal hyperechoic or hypoechoic areas in the periurethral prostate, and the distinction from transitional zone cancer is not possible without biopsy. With enlargement of the central gland, the peripheral zone frequently is compressed (Fig. 8-26). In patients with BPH and disproportionate elevations in PSA, transrectal sonography can be used to screen for a synchronous peripheral zone cancer. Regrowth of transitional zone tissue can be demonstrated on transrectal sonography should obstructive symptoms return after transurethral prostatectomy. A precise measurement of the postvoid bladder volume and evaluation of the bladder wall, hydronephrosis, and renal cortical atrophy can be obtained with transabdominal sonography.

MR imaging can be used to demonstrate the changes in the transitional zone that typify BPH, but its value in routine patient imaging is questionable. In patients with BPH, the central gland is enlarged and heterogeneous in signal intensity. Hyperplastic nodules that are predominantly glandular are of increased signal intensity on T_2-weighted images and can be of either low or high intensity on T_1-weighted images (Fig. 8-27). Stromal proliferation tends to produce areas of decreased signal intensity on T_1- and T_2-weighted images (Fig. 8-28). The peripheral zone is thinned and compressed and usually has a higher signal intensity than the enlarged, signal-heterogeneous central gland (Fig. 8-23). Given the distortion of the peripheral zone, it is frequently more difficult to recognize cancer in the peripheral zone on MR images in patients with BPH.

Prostatic and paraprostatic cysts

Focal cystic areas in the prostate most often are found with BPH. Originating from cystic dilatation of transitional zone glands, the proteinaceous cysts are of various sizes and rarely manifest except as an element of BPH itself. Like cystic BPH, acquired prostatic retention cysts originate from dilatation of the glandular acini but are not associated with BPH and can be found in any zone of the prostate. The rare, but potentially serious, prostatic abscess may present as a cystic prostatic mass (see Fig. 8-37A). It occurs as a complication of prostatitis, epididymitis, or surgery. Diabetes is a risk factor.

Other prostatic and paraprostatic cysts are not common but may be important because of associations with infertility or anomalies of the urinary tract. These cysts can be classified by location (Table 8-2). Congenital mid-

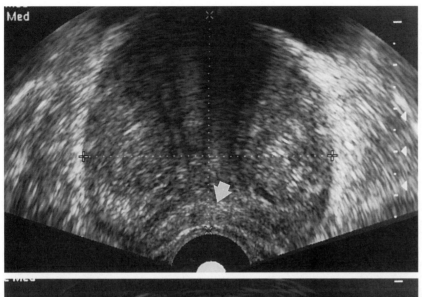

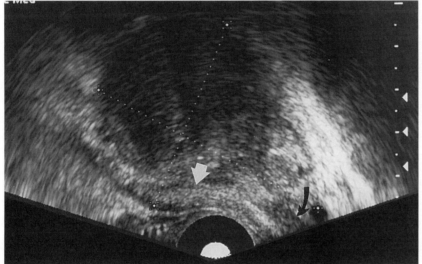

Fig. 8-26 Typical findings of benign prostatic hyperplasia on transrectal sonography. Transverse **(A)** and sagittal sonograms **(B)** show marked enlargement of the central gland. Although compressed, the peripheral zone remains slightly hyperechoic (arrow) compared with the transitional zone and central zone tissues (curved arrow = seminal vesicle).

Table 8-2	Prostatic and Paraprostatic Cysts	
	Intraprostatic	**Extraprostatic**
Midline or paramedian	Utricular cyst Ejaculatory duct cyst	Müllerian duct cyst
Lateral	Congenital prostatic cyst	Seminal vesicle cyst
Any location	Cystic nodule of benign prostatic hyperplasia Acquired retention cyst Abscess	

line or paramedian cysts include the utricular cyst and the müllerian duct cyst. Utricular cysts are intraprostatic, and müllerian duct cysts are located cephalad to the prostate in the retrovesical space. Utricular cysts occur as a result of utricular dilatation and originate from the verumontanum. They can be associated with cryptorchidism and hypospadias. Müllerian duct cysts originate from müllerian duct remnants that do not connect with the prostatic urethra. Müllerian duct cysts may contain stones and can be associated with ipsilateral renal agenesis. If large, these cysts can exert extrinsic mass effect on the bladder outlet or trigone. Ejaculatory cysts can be midline or paramedian in location. Resulting from acquired obstruction of the ejaculatory duct, these cysts may contain calculi or may be associated with ipsilateral seminal vesicle obstruction (Fig. 8-29). Seminal vesicle cysts often occur lateral to the prostate and are secondary to congenital hypoplasia of the ejaculatory duct. Seminal vesicle cysts typically are unilateral and may be associated with ipsilateral renal agenesis (Fig. 8-30 on p. 330). Stones and epididymitis may occur with these cysts.

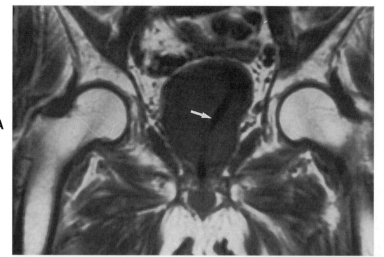

A

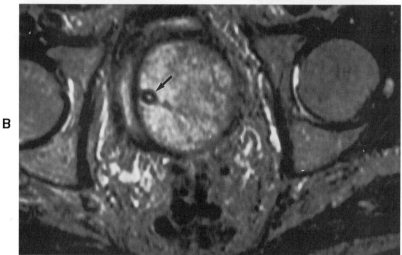

B

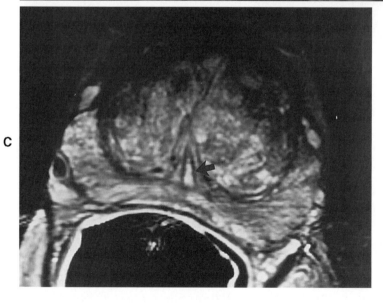

C

Fig. 8-27   MR imaging of benign prostatic hyperplasia (BPH). Coronal T₁-weighted **(A)** and transaxial T₂-weighted **(B)** MR images, obtained with a body coil, demonstrate marked enlargement of the transitional zone in BPH. This case illustrates the eccentric course of the prostatic urethra, denoted by the catheter (arrow), resulting from the hypertrophied glandular tissue of the transitional zone. **C,** In another patient, a transaxial fast spin–echo T₂-weighted image, obtained with an endorectal coil, demonstrates heterogeneous but predominantly hyperintense signal in the central gland. The glandular tissue that hypertrophies is in the transitional zone; there is less involvement of the central zone glands that surround the minimally enlarged left ejaculatory duct (arrow).

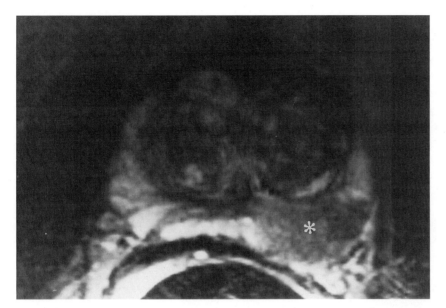

Fig. 8-28 Benign prostatic hyperplasia (BPH) and cancer of the prostate gland. Stromal hyperplasia is diagnosed when there is proliferation of transitional zone tissue that is hypointense on T_1- and T_2-weighted MR images. In addition to stromal BPH, this transaxial fast spin–echo T_2-weighted image demonstrates a typical carcinoma in the left peripheral zone (*).

Staging of Prostatic Carcinoma

The Hopkins modification of the Whitmore-Jewett staging system recognizes four stages of prostate cancer (Box 8-15). In simplified form, Stage A is microscopic prostate cancer, which typically is an incidental discovery in prostate tissue removed during transurethral prostatectomy. Stage B prostate cancer is a macroscopic, palpable tumor that is confined to the prostate gland, whereas Stage C prostate cancer has spread beyond the capsule of the prostate gland but remains clinically localized to the true pelvis. Stage D denotes prostate cancer that is metastatic to either regional lymph nodes, bones, or other distant visceral sites. Accurate staging of prostatic adenocarcinoma is important for two reasons. First, stage at presentation has an important bearing on prognosis. The 5-year disease-free survival rate for patients with Stage B cancer is 80%, but the rate is only 30% for patients with Stage C cancer. Of equal significance is that clinical staging determines available treatment options for the patient. Stage A1 prostate cancer usually is managed by watchful waiting. Patients with Stage A2 or Stage B cancer

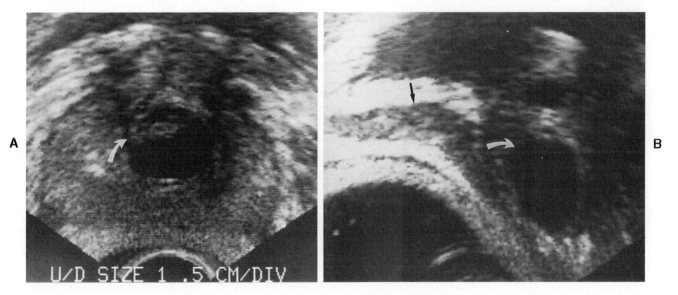

Fig. 8-29 Midline prostatic cyst in a 42-year-old man with hematospermia. Transverse (**A**) and sagittal transrectal (**B**) sonograms show a 2.5-cm prostatic cyst (curved arrow) containing debris. It does not extend above the base of the prostate gland. Normal spermatozoa were recovered from an aspirate of this large ejaculatory cyst (black arrow = normal seminal vesicle).

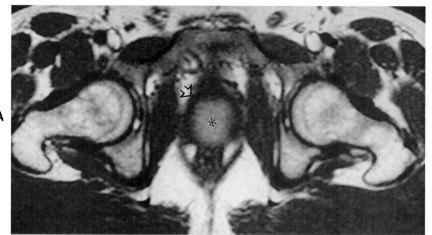

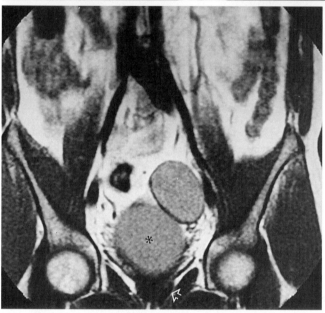

Fig. 8-30   Large pelvic cyst in a patient with dysuria, hematospermia, and congenital absence of the left kidney. Transaxial **(A)** and coronal **(B)** T₁-weighted images demonstrate a large bilobed cystic mass (*) that originates from the base of the prostate gland (open arrows). At surgery, proteinaceous and hemorrhagic fluid was aspirated from this seminal vesicle cyst.

Box 8-15   Prostate Cancer Staging System (Hopkins Modification of the Whitmore-Jewett Staging System)

Stage A—Microscopic, not palpable
  A1—Cancer in < 5% of tissue, low grade
  A2—Cancer in multiple areas, or Gleason Grade higher than 4
Stage B—Macroscopic, palpable
  B1—≤ 1.5 cm in diameter, only in one lobe
  B2—> 1.5 cm or in several lobes
Stage C—Extracapsular extension
  C1—Seminal vesicles but not pelvic sidewall
  C2—Fixed to pelvic wall
Stage D—Metastatic disease
  D1—Three or fewer nodes, confined to pelvis
  D2—More extensive nodal or extrapelvic disease

---

are candidates for radical prostatectomy or definitive radiation therapy. Stage C cancer patients generally are offered radiotherapy, although radical prostatectomy is considered when extracapsular extension is focal, the tumor is of low grade, and negative surgical margins are achievable. Patients with metastatic prostate cancer are treated with palliative therapy, which includes various forms of hormonal therapy, such as orchiectomy or total androgen blockade.

The conventional staging practice in the patient with newly diagnosed prostate cancer begins with measurement of the blood PSA and radionuclide bone scanning (Box 8-16). Osseous metastases from prostate adenocarcinoma involve, in descending order of frequency, the pelvic bones, lumbar spine, femur, thoracic spine, and ribs. Five percent of bone metastases are purely lytic, and about 10% are mixed osteolytic and osteoblastic; the overwhelming majority of bony lesions are predominantly osteoblastic. Bone scan results that are consistent

Box 8-16 Evaluating Stage C and D Prostate Cancer

Extracapsular spread
   Transrectal prostate ultrasonography with biopsy
   Endorectal coil MR imaging
Nodal metastases
   Computed tomography (or MR imaging)
   Percutaneous needle biopsy if nodes are larger than
      10 mm
   Laparoscopic or surgical dissection
Bone metastases
   Prostate-specific antigen blood test first, then bone
      scan

patients with prostatic carcinoma have intrathoracic metastases when first examined. As many as 25% of patients with Stage D cancer have lung or pleural involvement, and lymphangiitis carcinomatosa is a more common pattern of metastatic prostate adenocarcinoma than multiple pulmonary nodules.

The prognostic significance of tumor spread to the lymph nodes is clear; more than 80% of patients with lymphogenous spread of prostate cancer develop metastases to bone within 5 years. In contrast, the chance is less than 20% that patients with negative lymph node results will develop metastases to bone. The most frequent pelvic sites of lymphatic spread are the surgical obturator, internal iliac, and external iliac nodal groups (Fig. 8-31). Prostate cancer also can extend directly into the seminal vesicles, bladder base, and perivesical fat (Fig. 8-32); however, it infrequently spreads posteriorly to the rectum through Denonvilliers' rectovesical fascia. CT and body coil MR imaging demonstrate lymph node involvement on the basis of nodal enlargement. The sensitivity and specificity of CT and MR imaging for evaluating lymphadenopathy, defined as nodes larger than 1.5 cm in diameter, range from 25% to 90% and from 85% to 95%, respectively. Hence, CT is deficient in the diagnosis of lymph node metastasis because of a high percentage of false-negative results. Furthermore, the transverse axial plane is particularly inaccurate for detecting direct extension of prostatic carcinoma into the seminal vesicle and bladder base. Lymphangiography is one method for identifying metastatic foci in lymph nodes of normal size, but this technique has fallen into disfavor because of its variable accuracy of 50% to 80% and because it does not opacify the internal iliac or presacral lymph nodes,

with metastatic disease, together with a corroborative PSA level, identify the prostate cancer as Stage D2. False-negative bone scan results are unusual but have been reported in as many as 8% of patients. Results of bone scans almost always are negative for metastatic disease when the PSA level is 10 ng/mL or less, and no more than 4% of scans have abnormal results with PSA levels between 10 ng/mL and 20 ng/mL. Conversely, PSA levels in excess of 58 ng/mL frequently are indicative of bone metastases, irrespective of plain film or bone scan findings. If the bone scan is inconsistent with metastatic disease, the status of the pelvic and retroperitoneal lymph nodes is evaluated, typically with abdominal and pelvic CT or at surgery before prostatectomy. A chest radiograph also is recommended, although only about 6% of

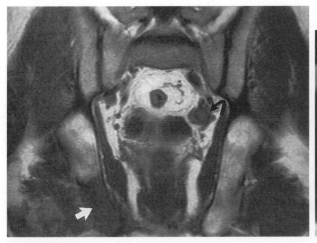 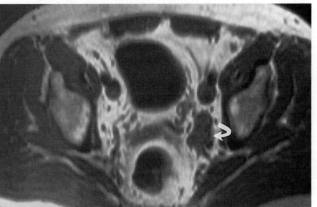

Fig. 8-31 Lymph node metastases from prostate cancer. Coronal (**A**) and transaxial (**B**) T_1-weighted MR images were performed as part of a staging evaluation. The lymph nodes of the internal iliac group (curved arrows) are enlarged; these nodes sometimes are called the *surgical obturator nodes*. In addition, abnormal signal in the marrow of the right ischium (arrow) is consistent with bone metastasis.

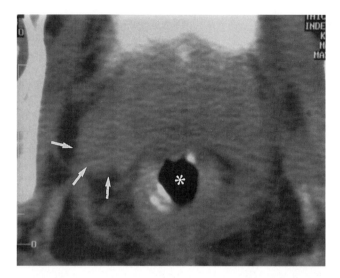

Fig. 8-32 CT findings of extraprostatic spread of cancer. A large tongue of tissue (arrows) extends superolaterally from the base of the prostate and obliterates the normal plane of fat between the prostate and the seminal vesicle. It is unusual for prostate cancer to grow posteriorly into the rectum (* = air within the rectum).

relatively common sites of prostatic cancer spread. As a result, laparoscopic or surgical pelvic lymphadenectomy plays an important role in staging. Transperitoneal laparoscopic dissection of pelvic lymph nodes has gained popularity for staging prostatic cancer and cancers of the bladder, cervix, and penis. The boundaries of the laparoscopic node dissection are identical to those of a limited open lymphadenectomy and include the lymph node groups encompassed by the common iliac vessels superiorly, the internal iliac vessels posteriorly, the external iliac vessels anteriorly, and the prostate medially. Laparoscopic and open lymphadenectomy remove about 12 lymph nodes, and either procedure is undertaken at the same time a radical prostatectomy is planned. If the frozen section sample of any lymph nodes is positive for tumor, curative radical prostatectomy should not be attempted, because recurrence is common, even with minimal lymph node involvement. Between 10% and 25% of patients with clinical Stage A2 or B1 prostatic cancer and 30% of those with stage B2 prostate cancer have positive lymph nodes at staging lymphadenectomy. Metastases to the liver and adrenal glands also occur, but usually occur late in the course of prostate cancer. These sites are evaluated routinely and adequately with abdominal CT.

Recent interest has focused on the use of transrectal ultrasonography and MR imaging to improve the accuracy of staging of prostate cancer. Specifically, it was hoped that either or both of these imaging modalities would improve the detection of extraprostatic spread of cancer into the periprostatic fat and seminal vesicles. Several observations about the extraprostatic spread of prostate cancer, which were discovered from rigorous

evaluation of anatomic specimens removed at radical prostatectomy, are worthy of review. There is no true capsule enclosing the prostate. The prostate capsule is simply a loose blending of prostatic fibromuscular stroma with the endopelvic fascia. There is no capsule covering the anterior or apical parts of the prostate. Prostate cancers that originate in the transitional zone (Stage A) spread beyond the capsule less frequently than those that originate in the peripheral zone, and when they do, the anterior or anterolateral margin of the gland is the site of transgression (Fig. 8-21). In contrast, peripheral zone cancers (Stage B) have a greater tendency to spread beyond the prostate along the posterior or posterolateral surface. The likelihood that a cancer will transgress the prostatic capsule is correlated with the size of the primary tumor and tumor grade. The neurovascular bundles are important structures because preservation of one of these structures is necessary for potency-sparing prostatectomy. In addition, it has been shown that the majority of advanced peripheral zone cancers spread beyond the prostate along these perineural pathways or contiguous with their site of origin. Each neurovascular bundle is approximately 5 to 6 cm in length and is located posteriorly and laterally to the rectal surface of the prostate gland. Both neurovascular bundles can be seen on transrectal ultrasound in about 50% of patients, and in another 30% to 35% of patients, one of the neurovascular bundles can be seen as a distinct round or oval hypoechoic structure (Fig. 8-4). The hypoechoic appearance results from the vascular component of the bundle.

Criteria for the extraprostatic spread of prostate cancer have been established for transrectal ultrasonography and for MR imaging (Box 8-17). The accuracy of the sonographic detection of extraprostatic spread depends on the location of the primary cancer and its size. Ultrasonographic signs of tumor spread include irregularity or interruption of the periprostatic fat line or a local bulge or distortion of the prostatic contour (Fig. 8-33). Body coil MR imaging criteria for tumor transgression of the prostatic capsule include interruption of the low-signal intensity prostatic margin, irregular gland contour, and abnormal low-signal intensity areas in the periprostatic veins or fat contiguous to a hypointense peripheral zone lesion. Signs that suggest capsular transgression also have been described for MR imaging of the prostate with an endorectal coil. In addition to gross capsular transgres-

---

Box 8-17 Extraprostatic Spread of Prostate Cancer

Interruption or irregularity of the prostatic contour
Focal bulge or distortion
Abnormal signal in periprostatic fat

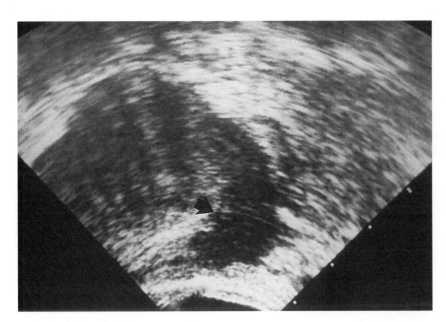

Fig. 8-33 Extraprostatic spread of cancer on transrectal sonography. Transverse image demonstrates a hypoechoic area in the peripheral zone (arrow) with an irregular, serrated capsular margin.

sion, transcapsular spread is suggested when there is a focal distortion of the capsular margin adjacent to the neurovascular bundle or when there is bulge and deformity of the capsular contour contiguous with a focal, asymmetric area of low-signal intensity in the peripheral zone (Fig. 8-34).

There are three pathoanatomic routes by which prostate cancer secondarily spreads to the seminal vesicles. In the majority of patients, cancer spreads around or through ejaculatory ducts to the seminal vesicles. Direct spread into the seminal vesicles from a cancer in the peripheral zone also can occur, and, least commonly, de novo noncontiguous involvement of the seminal vesicles is observed. With respect to seminal vesicle invasion on transrectal sonography, several signs are valuable for making this diagnosis. These signs include diffuse or patchy hyperechogenicity of the seminal vesicle relative to the echopattern of the bladder wall, enlargement of the anteroposterior dimension of the seminal vesicle more than 1 cm, anterior displacement of the seminal vesicles of more than 1 cm from the rectal wall, cystic dilatation of the seminal vesicles of more than 1 cm in the anteroposterior dimension, and marked asymmetry in size or configuration (Fig. 8-35). Hyperechogenicity combined with any two other signs has a reported sensitivity of 71% and specificity of 94%. MR imaging with the body coil and the endorectal coil also has been used to stage prostate cancer with respect to seminal vesicle invasion. Decrease in the signal intensity of the seminal vesicles on T_2-weighted images, asymmetric enlargement resulting from obstruction, and the presence of high signal caused by hemorrhage within the seminal vesicles on T_1-weighted images have been described as useful signs (Fig. 8-36 on p. 336). Foci of low-signal intensity

in the seminal vesicles on T_2-weighted images are nonspecific; occasionally, these signal-intensity changes result from biopsy-related hemorrhage, senile amyloidosis, or compression of the seminal vesicles by a hyperplastic prostate gland.

Initial enthusiasm for MR imaging in staging the local spread of cancer has been tempered by the findings of a multiinstitutional collaborative trial reported by Tempany et al in 1994 that found low accuracy for body coil and endorectal coil MR imaging. In that study, no statistically significant difference was determined in the staging accuracy of these modalities; overall accuracy with conventional body coil, fat-suppressed body coil, and endorectal coil MR imaging was 61%, 64%, and 54%, respectively. In addition to the overall inaccuracy of these techniques, considerable interreader variability was reported.

Fever and Prostatodynia

Prostatitis

Prostatitis is a clinical syndrome in which inflammation of the prostate gland manifests as pelvic or perineal pain or as irritative symptoms referable to micturition or ejaculation. Prostatitis is classified conventionally as acute prostatitis, chronic prostatitis, and prostatodynia. Supportive evidence for the diagnosis derives from clinical evaluation and Gram's stain of expressed prostatic secretions and from culture of the urine, prostatic secretions, or semen. Acute prostatitis frequently causes fever, chills, dysuria, frequency, and pain in the rectal area or perineum. DRE reveals a swollen ("boggy") gland, which is firm, warm, and tender. *Escherichia coli*, *Pseudomonas* species, and enterococci can be recovered from the

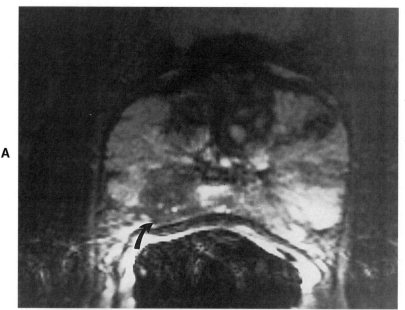

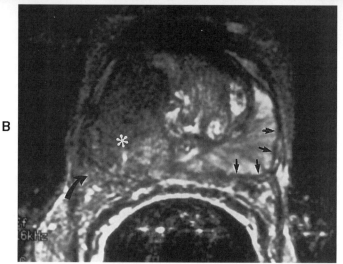

Fig. 8-34   Extraprostatic spread of cancer on MR imaging with an endorectal surface coil. **A,** Transaxial fast spin–echo T$_2$-weighted image shows a focal bulge of the capsule (curved arrow) adjacent to a hypointense lesion in the peripheral zone. **B,** In another patient, there is gross transcapsular spread of prostate cancer. There is abnormal signal in the periprostatic fat (curved arrow) and distortion of the capsular margin adjacent to a large prostate cancer (*). The tumor also has spread anteriorly into the transitional zone of the prostate. Note the normal capsule (small arrows) around the contralateral peripheral zone.

urine or expressed prostatic secretions. Acute bacterial prostatitis typically responds to antibiotic therapy. The development of a prostatic abscess is an infrequent complication of acute prostatitis in the era of antibiotics, but immunosuppressed patients and patients with diabetes continue to be susceptible. In contrast, chronic prostatitis is an indolent disease marked by relapses of dysuria, urgency, and pain. Often, results of DRE are normal, and the diagnosis rests on the finding of leukocytes (> 10 per high-power field) in expressed prostatic secretions. It is postulated that *Chlamydia, Ureaplasma, Mycoplasma,* or *Trichomonas* may be important causative agents in chronic nonbacterial prostatitis. Nonspecific granulomatous prostatitis is a form of focal prostatitis that can mimic carcinoma clinically and on transrectal sonograms. Results of biopsy reveal either caseating or noncaseating granulomas. The most common form of specific granulomatous prostatitis is caused by Calmette-Guérin bacillus, which is used for immunotherapy of superficial bladder cancer. Chronic prostatitis is a cause of recurrent urinary tract infection and epididymitis. Recurrent prostatitis also may be the consequence of infected prostatic calculi. Prostatodynia is a diagnosis reserved for the patient with clinical symptoms referable to the prostate but with no microscopic or microbiologic evidence of prostatic inflammation. The complaints of these patients should not be minimized because symptoms may be caused by cystitis or carcinoma of the bladder.

Transrectal sonography is a valuable adjunct to the clinical examination of the patient with prostatodynia and suspected prostatitis. In the patient with acute pros-

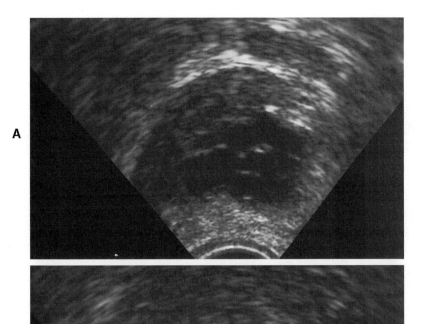

Fig. 8-35   Seminal vesicle invasion on transrectal sonography. A hypoechoic mass was seen in the peripheral zone of the base of the prostate gland. **A,** Oblique transverse image demonstrates marked enlargement (anteroposterior dimension more than 1 cm) and cystic dilatation of the right seminal vesicle. **B,** In comparison, the left seminal vesicle (arrow) is normal in size and echogenicity. Results of needle biopsy of the right seminal vesicle revealed prostate cancer.

tatitis, the gland is enlarged and may be diffusely hypoechoic. Increased through transmission of sound may be observed because of interstitial edema. Heterogeneous echo patterns can be found in many patients with acute prostatitis, and a hypoechoic halo in the periurethral region has been reported. The capsule may be irregular or thickened. Solitary or diffuse prostatic calculi also are more common in this disease. A more discrete hypoechoic mass containing midrange echoes should raise the possibility of abscess (Fig. 8-37A). As a general rule, normal results of sonographic evaluation are valuable in excluding the diagnosis of acute prostatitis. Occasionally, CT or MR imaging is used to demonstrate the enlarged, inflamed prostate, epididymitis, or an obstructed, dilated, thin-walled bladder (Fig. 8-37B). Chronic prostatitis cannot be diagnosed specifically with ultrasonography, and its diagnosis relies primarily on clinical parameters.

Erectile Dysfunction

Erectile dysfunction is defined as ''the inability to either obtain or maintain a penile erection that is sufficient for vaginal penetration in 50% or more attempts during intercourse.'' At a consensus conference of the National Institutes of Health, it was agreed that ''erectile dysfunction'' should replace the term ''impotence.'' In certain groups of patients, such as those with longstanding diabetes, the incidence of erectile dysfunction has been estimated to be as high as 40% to 50%. Early reports suggested that psychogenic causes accounted for an overwhelming majority of cases and that organic factors contributed to only about 5% of all causes of erectile dysfunction. As the physiology of erection was delineated and more intricate tests of penile tumescence were implemented, various series have reported that 50% to 80% of cases can be attributed to organic causes (Box 8-18). Of the organic etiologies, vasculogenic erectile dysfunction is the most common. Specifically, the most frequent organic abnormalities that are associated with erectile dysfunction are lack of adequate venous occlusion, hypogastric cavernosal arterial atherosclerosis and other vasculopathies, diabetes, peripheral neuropathy, endocrinopathy, and major pelvic trauma.

Selection of the appropriate management of erectile

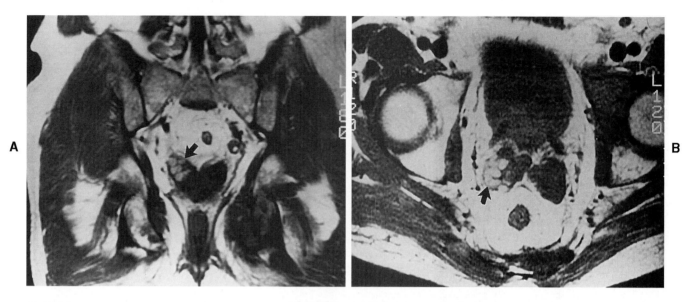

Fig. 8-36 MR imaging of the seminal vesicle hemorrhage resulting from invasive prostate cancer. Coronal **(A)** and transverse axial **(B)** T₁-weighted images of the pelvis (repetition time = 600 msec; echo time = 20 msec) demonstrate abnormal increased signal intensity in the right seminal vesicle (arrow). Hemorrhage related to recent biopsy is the most common explanation for this abnormality. Note that there is a metastasis to the left ischium.

dysfunction begins with the delineation of its causes. For instance, if erectile dysfunction is multifactorial but potentially drug-related, a trial of pharmacologic substitution is indicated before more invasive alternatives are tried. The interventional radiologist may be called on to perform angioplasty, which is more successful when occlusive atherosclerotic disease is focal. In patients with venous leakage, successful occlusion of the dorsal vein of the penis and crural veins has been reported using sclerosing agents, coils, and detachable balloons. In patients with diffuse atherosclerotic disease, arterial reconstruction, bypass, or penile prosthesis may be necessary.

Anatomy of the penis

The erectile components of the penis consist of the paired corpora cavernosa and the corpus spongiosum. The corpus spongiosum surrounds the anterior urethra and forms the glans penis distally. The corpora cavernosa, which are the main structures for penile erection, consist of multiple interconnecting lacunar spaces or sinusoids that are lined by vascular endothelium. In the flaccid penis, the lacunae are collapsed, whereas in the erect penis, the lacunae are engorged with blood. In the perineum, the corpora cavernosa diverge to form the crura, which attach to the inferior aspect of the ischiopubic rami. The corpora cavernosa are enclosed by a rigid, fibrous covering, the tunica albuginea.

Vascular anatomy

The arterial supply of the penis is routed through the right and left internal pudendal artery and branches of the internal iliac arteries. Each internal pudendal artery gives off a perineal branch, a bulbar artery, and a small urethral artery before continuing as the artery of the penis. The artery of the penis enters the base of the penis and branches into the deep penile or cavernosal artery and the dorsal artery of the penis. The cavernosal artery lies near the center of each corporal body and is the primary source of blood flow to erectile tissue. Numerous corkscrew-shaped helicine arteries originate from each cavernosal artery and communicate with the sinusoidal spaces. The lacunar spaces are drained by small venules, which coalesce to form larger emissary veins. These emissary veins pierce the tunica albuginea at oblique angles and anastomose to form the circumflex veins, which eventually drain into the deep dorsal vein of the penis. The venous drainage from the proximal crura is distinct from that of the rest of the penis; its course is primarily through the cavernosal and crural veins. Sinusoidal distention in the erect penis is maintained by a venoocclusive mechanism, which consists of the mechanical compression of emissary veins against the unyielding tunica albuginea and can occur only when the sinusoids are expanded completely.

Innervation

Peripheral innervation of the penis consists of sympathetic nerves originating from T11 to L2 and parasympathetic and somatic nerves originating from S2 to S4. Cholinergic autonomic nerves and nonadrenergic or noncholinergic autonomic nerves cause smooth-muscle relaxation. In contrast, adrenergic neural activity causes smooth-muscle contraction.

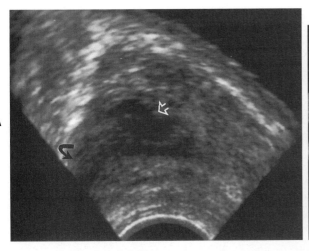
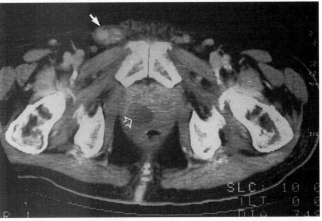

Fig. 8-37   Prostatic abscess. **A,** Sagittal transrectal sonogram demonstrates an ill-defined, hypoechoic mass (open arrow) in the prostate. The capsule of the prostate gland is indistinct, and the distance between the rectum and the prostate is increased because of periprostatic inflammation (curved arrow = seminal vesicle). **B,** CT confirms a hypodense mass (open arrow), consistent with an abscess, in a swollen prostate gland. The periprostatic fat planes are obliterated because of inflammation around the prostate. Note the enlarged and edematous right spermatic cord (arrow); this prostatic infection was secondary to epididymoorchitis.

Box 8-18   Causes of Erectile Dysfunction

Endocrinologic
    Diabetes mellitus, hyperprolactinemia, hypogonadism
Neurogenic
    Spinal cord injury, multiple sclerosis, peripheral neuropathy, cerebrovascular accident, idiopathic or temporal lobe epilepsy, Alzheimer's disease, cervical spondylosis, primary autonomic insufficiency
Pharmacologic
    Alcohol, anticonvulsants, antihypertensives, narcotics, psychotropic agents
Postsurgical
    Radical prostatectomy, cystectomy, or proctocolectomy
Psychogenic
Vasculogenic
    Venous incompetence, atherosclerotic disease, diabetes, trauma, structural alterations of the corporal body sinusoids (cavernosal fibrosis or cavernous muscle myopathy)

Mechanism of erection and detumescence

Erection begins with the relaxation of lacunar and arterial smooth muscle. Relaxation of cavernosal and helicine smooth muscle effects an increase in arterial diameter and blood flow to the lacunae. Relaxation of the smooth muscle that surrounds the lacunar spaces of the corpora cavernosa facilitates arterial inflow through a decrease in peripheral vascular resistance. In addition, dilatation of the lacunae causes passive compression of the emissary veins against the relatively noncompliant tunica albuginea, facilitating engorgement of the penis with blood (i.e., the venoocclusive mechanism).

Detumescence follows penile smooth-muscle contraction. Sympathetic neural activity causes an increase in smooth-muscle tone of the helicine arteries and the lacunae. As a result, arterial inflow decreases, and the lacunae collapse.

Evaluation of erectile dysfunction

There is no universally accepted algorithm for the work-up of the patient with erectile dysfunction. However, the first important objective is to determine if there could be a vasculogenic cause. The most common examinations available to the radiologist for the evaluation of vasculogenic erectile dysfunction include duplex and color Doppler sonography, dynamic infusion cavernosometry and cavernosography, nuclear blood flow and wash-out studies, and selective pudendal pharmacoangiography.

Gray-scale real-time sonography with a 7.5- to 10-MHz linear-array transducer has been used to assess the architecture of the corporal bodies. In addition, duplex and color Doppler sonography are used to assess the patency of the cavernosal arteries and the competency of the penile veins. On transverse gray-scale images, the corpora cavernosa are paired, round, or oval structures encom-

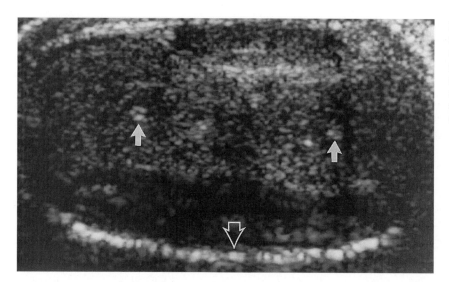

Fig. 8-38 Normal transverse sonogram of the flaccid penis. The tunica albuginea (open arrow) encircles the corporal bodies. The corpora cavernosa and spongiosa are homogeneous and hypoechoic. The corpora cavernosal arteries are hyperechoic interfaces (solid arrows) in the middle of each corpus cavernosum.

passed by the tunica albuginea, which is highly echogenic. The septum of the penis is an extension of the tunica albuginea and appears as an echogenic line between the corpora cavernosa. Each cavernosal artery is located centrally or eccentrically toward the septum within the corpora cavernosa and usually can be identified by echogenic walls and visible pulsations (Fig. 8-38). Fibrotic areas adjacent to or within the tunica albuginea

may cause pain during erection (Peyronie's disease). Focal areas of scarring or fibrosis in the corpora cavernosa prevent lacunar dilatation and filling. Sonographically, these fibrotic plaques are seen as focal areas of increased echogenicity, which may be associated with posterior acoustic shadowing when calcified (Fig. 8-39).

Several measurable parameters have been used to quantify penile blood flow by means of duplex Doppler

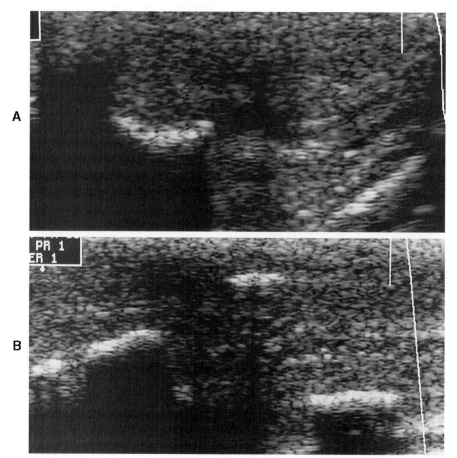

Fig. 8-39 Peyronie's disease. Transverse **(A)** and sagittal **(B)** sonograms of the penis demonstrate multiple linear echogenicities that cast an acoustic shadow. These thick plaques are related to abnormal collagen deposition in the tunica albuginea.

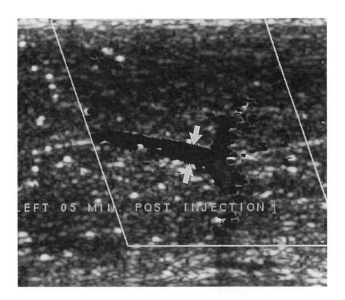

Fig. 8-40 Normal response after intracavernosal injection of papaverine. The diameter of the cavernosal artery measures 1.3 mm (arrows); it should increase by approximately 75% from the baseline measurement.

sonography; these parameters include peak flow velocity, resistive index, arterial dilatation, pulsatility of the cavernosal artery, and increase in penile volume. The first stage of the Doppler sonographic examination evaluates the flaccid penis. Color Doppler imaging can be used to identify the cavernosal artery and to determine its location and flow direction. The transverse internal diameter of each cavernosal artery is measured. The Doppler sample gate then is placed on the cavernosal artery at the base of the penis, and an angle-corrected spectral waveform is recorded for analysis.

The second stage of the evaluation involves measur-

Box 8-19	**Spectral Analysis of the Cavernosal Artery in Vasculogenic Erectile Dysfunction**

Arteriogenic cause: peak systolic velocity < 25 cm/sec
Arteriogenic cause: asymmetric peak systolic velocity of >10 cm/sec
Venous incompetence: end diastolic velocity ≥ 3 cm/sec

ing Doppler signals from the cavernosal artery before and after the intracorporal injection of vasodilating medications. Pharmacologic enhancement of erection is achieved by the intracavernosal injection of papaverine, a nonspecific smooth-muscle relaxant. Several minutes after the cavernosal injection of 30 mg of papaverine, the diameter of the cavernosal arteries is measured again. Systolic and diastolic velocity measurements are recorded 5, 10, 15, and 20 minutes after this pharmacologic intervention (Box 8-19). Flow velocity within the superficial and dorsal penile veins also can be measured.

The normal cavernosal artery before pharmacologic erection may range from immeasurably small to 0.6 mm in diameter; the average diameter is about 0.4 mm. The diameter of the cavernosal artery in the erect penis increases more than 75% or in average size to a diameter of about 1 mm (Fig. 8-40); however, because of the small size of the cavernosal arteries, the potential error in measurement of size is substantial. The normal peak systolic velocity in the erect penis ranges from 35 to 60 cm/sec (Fig. 8-41). A mean peak velocity of 25 cm/sec or less is

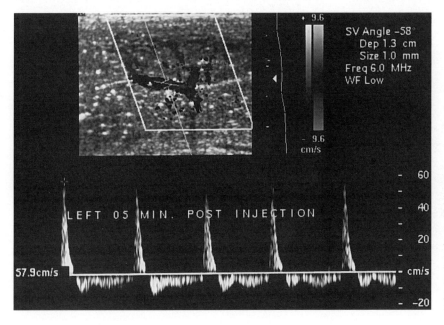

Fig. 8-41 Normal spectral pattern after intracavernosal injection of papaverine. Sagittal sonogram of the erect penis shows the Doppler gate positioned in the cavernosal artery. The normal spectral pattern consists of a peak systolic velocity that is more than 35 cm/sec; there is no end diastolic flow. In this patient, the peak systolic velocity is 58 cm/sec, and there is reversed flow at end diastole.

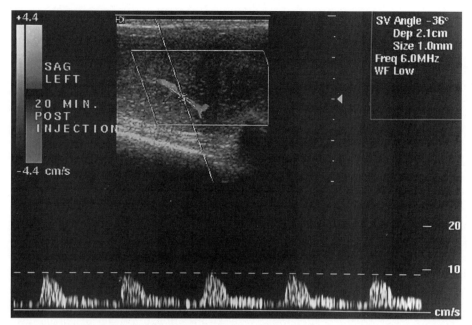

Fig. 8-42   Arteriogenic cause of erectile dysfunction. Sagittal sonogram of the cavernosal artery obtained 20 minutes after the intracavernosal injection of papaverine demonstrates a peak systolic velocity of only 9 cm/sec and an end diastolic velocity of 4 cm/sec.

seen in patients with significant arterial disease (Fig. 8-42). Asymmetric peak systolic velocity between the two cavernosal arteries of 10 cm/sec suggests the presence of unilateral arterial disease of the penis. Patients with arterial inflow disease should be referred for definitive examination with selective internal pudendal arteriography.

Doppler sonography also can be used to evaluate the competence of the venoocclusive mechanism. At full rigidity and with adequate arterial inflow, the venoocclusive mechanism is most functional, and the cavernosal artery spectral pattern should display a high resistance pattern (i.e., no or little end diastolic flow). A persistent high diastolic flow suggests inadequacy of the venoocclusive mechanism. When measured 15 to 20 minutes after intracavernosal injection of papaverine, an end diastolic

flow of 3 cm/sec or more suggests abnormal venous leakage despite normal arterial inflow (Fig. 8-43).

If dysfunction of the venoocclusive mechanism is suggested by duplex Doppler studies, cavernosometry and cavernosography are performed to confirm and further delineate suspected abnormalities. The details of this evaluation have been summarized by Rosen et al, and only the fundamental components of the test are presented here. Small butterfly needles (25-gauge) are placed in both of the corpora cavernosa. One needle is used for pressure measurements, and the other needle is used for infusion of warm saline and low osmolar contrast material. Baseline intracorporal pressure and penile circumference are recorded first. Vasoactive medication is injected into the corpora cavernosa, and the rise in pres-

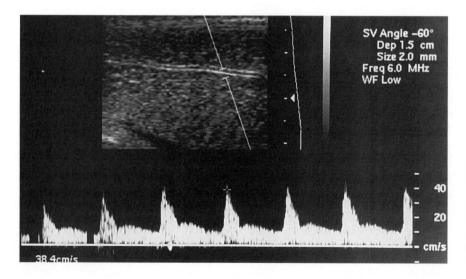

Fig. 8-43   Venous incompetence. Sagittal sonogram of the cavernosal artery obtained 15 minutes after the intracavernosal injection of papaverine shows an abnormally elevated end diastolic velocity of 10 cm/sec (normal, < 3 cm/sec). The peak systolic velocity is 38 cm/sec (normal, > 35 cm/sec).

sure in the corpora cavernosa and the change in penile circumference are monitored for at least 10 minutes or until an equilibrium is reached. If no erection is produced or maintained after pharmacologic intervention, heparinized saline is infused to produce and maintain an erection. The infusion rate required to maintain the erect penis up to an intracavernosal pressure of 150 mm Hg is recorded; this finding is related directly to venoocclusive function. An infusion rate of less than 30 mL is considered normal. Venous outflow resistance also can be assessed by infusing saline to a suprasystolic intracavernosal pressure and determining the rate of the fall in pressure after the infusion is discontinued. If corporal venoocclusive dysfunction is present, intracavernosal pressure falls rapidly. Cavernosography entails infusing approximately 100 to 150 mL of contrast material while the intracavernosal pressure is maintained at 90 mm Hg. Fluoroscopy and spot films of this portion of the evaluation may reveal the site of venous leakage and may provide anatomic information useful for surgical or interventional radiologic management.

Selective internal pudendal pharmacoarteriography usually is reserved for the patient who is being considered for arterial reconstructive surgery or angioplasty and whose sonographic examination suggests the presence of significant arterial disease. The arteriographic evaluation of the penile vascular supply begins with standard aortoiliac arteriography to evaluate for a proximal atherosclerotic lesion and to evaluate the patency of the inferior epigastric arteries, which commonly are used in surgical revascularization. Selective internal pudendal arteriography then is performed to evaluate fully the branches of the artery. The intracavernosal injection of pharmacologic agents, such as nitroglycerine, papaverine, or prostaglandin E1, is required to dilate the cavernosal artery to allow better assessment of this vessel.

Atherosclerosis, which usually is a diffuse process, can affect any part of the relevant arterial vascular anatomy from the aorta to the cavernosal artery. In patients aged more than 50 years, vasculogenic erectile dysfunction usually is diagnosed on the basis of atherosclerosis affecting the iliac or internal pudendal arteries. In contradistinction, traumatic focal stenosis or occlusion of the common penile artery occurs because this artery follows a course directly over the ischiopubic rami, which more likely is the site of an arterial lesion that causes erectile dysfunction in younger patients. Vascular changes associated with perineal radiation therapy also can affect the common penile artery, which lies close to the prostate gland.

SUGGESTED READINGS

Benson C, Doubilet P, Richie J: Sonography of the male genital tract, *AJR Am J Roentgenol* 153:705-713, 1989.

Bretton P, Evans N, Borden J, et al: The use of PSA density to improve the sensitivity of PSA in detecting prostate carcinoma, *Cancer* 74:2991-2995, 1994.

Catalona W, Smith D, Ratliff T, et al: Measurement of prostate-specific antigen in serum as a screening test for prostate cancer, *N Engl J Med* 324:1156-1161, 1991.

Doble A, Carter S: Ultrasonographic findings in prostatitis, *Urol Clin North Am* 16(4):763-772, 1989.

Fournier G, Laing F, McAninch J: Scrotal ultrasonography and the management of testicular trauma, *Urol Clin North Am* 16(2):377-385, 1989.

Gittes R: Carcinoma of the prostate, *N Engl J Med* 324(4):236-245, 1991.

Hamper U, Sheth S, Walsh P, et al: Stage B adenocarcinoma of the prostate: transrectal US and pathologic correlation of nonmalignant hypoechoic peripheral zone lesions, *Radiology* 180:101-104, 1991.

Hodge K, McNeal J, Stamey T: Ultrasound guided transrectal core biopsies of the palpably abnormal prostate, *J Urol* 142:66-70, 1989.

Horstman W, Middleton W, Melson G: Scrotal inflammatory disease: color Doppler ultrasound findings, *Radiology* 179:55-59, 1991.

Horstman W, Middleton W, Melson G, et al: Color Doppler ultrasound of the scrotum, *RadioGraphics* 11:941-957, 1991.

Jeffrey RB, Laing F, Hricak H: Sonography of testicular trauma, *AJR Am J Roentgenol* 141:993-995, 1983.

Krane R, Goldstein I, deTejada I: Impotence, *N Engl J Med* 321:1648-1659, 1989.

Lee F, Torp-Pederson S, Littrup P, et al: Hypoechoic lesions of the prostate: clinical relevance of tumor size, digital rectal examination, and prostate-specific antigen, *Radiology* 170:29-32, 1989.

McClennan B: Diagnostic imaging evaluation of benign prostatic hyperplasia, *Urol Clin North Am* 17(3):517-536, 1990.

McNeal J: Normal anatomy of the prostate and changes in benign prostatic hypertrophy and carcinoma, *Semin Ultrasound CT MRI* 9(5):329-334, 1988.

Middleton W, Siegel B, Melson G, et al: Acute scrotal disorders: prospective comparison of color Doppler ultrasound and testicular scintigraphy, *Radiology* 177:177-181, 1990.

Mueller S, Lue T: Evaluation of vasculogenic impotence, *Urol Clin North Am* 15(1):65-76, 1988.

Pantelides, M, Bowman S, George N: Levels of PSA that predict skeletal spread in prostate cancer, *Br J Urol* 70:299-303, 1992.

Patriquin H, Yazbeck S, Trunh B, et al: Testicular torsion in infants and children: diagnosis with Doppler sonography, *Radiology* 188:781-785, 1993.

Quam J, King B, James E, et al: Duplex and color Doppler sonographic evaluation of vasculogenic impotence, *AJR Am J Roentgenol* 153:1141-1147, 1989.

Rifkin M, Zerhouni E, Gatsonis C, et al: Comparison of magnetic resonance imaging and ultrasonography in staging early prostate cancer, *N Engl J Med* 323:621–626, 1990.

Rosen M, Schwartz A, Levine F, et al: Radiologic assessment of impotence: angiography, sonography, cavernosography, and scintigraphy, *AJR Am J Roentgenol* 157:923–931, 1991.

Tempany C, Zhou X, Zerhouni E, et al: Staging of prostate cancer: results of RDOG project comparing three MR imaging techniques, *Radiology* 192:47–54, 1994.

Terris M, McNeal J, Stamey T: Invasion of the seminal vesicles by prostatic cancer: detection with transrectal sonography, *AJR Am J Roentgenol* 155:811–815, 1990.

Villers A, McNeal J, Redwine E, et al: The role of perineural space invasion in the local spread of prostatic adenocarcinoma, *J Urol* 142:763–768, 1989.

Wasserman, N, Lapointe S, Eckmann D, et al: Assessment of prostatism: role of intravenous urography, *Radiology* 165:831–835, 1987.

Cross-sectional imaging plays a major role in the evaluation of adrenal gland disease. In many patients, not only can adrenal gland pathology be identified, but a specific diagnosis can be offered. However, despite the impressive advances in imaging technology, there are numerous instances in which imaging suffers from poor specificity, and invasive procedures must be performed. The appropriate selection and accurate interpretation of adrenal imaging and interventional studies are the subject of this chapter, which is divided into three sections. In the first section, the embryology, physiology, anatomy, and imaging of the adrenal gland are reviewed. Mass lesions of the adrenal gland are discussed in the second section. The third section reviews the approach to several common clinical problems in which adrenal imaging plays an integral role.

EMBRYOLOGY, PHYSIOLOGY, ANATOMY, AND IMAGING

Embryology

The embryology of the adrenal gland reflects its physiologic and anatomic separation into the cortex and medulla. The adrenal cortex develops from the coelomic mesoderm in the fourth to sixth weeks of life as a cluster of cells between the root of the mesentery and the genital ridge. The adrenal medulla is of neural crest origin and therefore is derived from neuroectoderm. The development of the adrenal gland is independent from that of the kidney, and the ipsilateral adrenal gland is positioned normally in more than 90% of patients with agenesis or malposition of the kidney.

Physiology

Adrenal cortical tissue, which makes up approximately 90% of the adrenal gland by weight, synthesizes cholesterol-derived steroid hormones. Adrenal steroids contain either 19 or 21 carbon atoms. Steroids with 21 carbon atoms, or C21 steroids, have either glucocorticoid or mineralocorticoid activity, and the C19 steroids have androgenic activity predominantly.

The major glucocorticoid produced by the adrenal gland is cortisol, which plays an important role in the regulation of protein, carbohydrate, lipid, and nucleic acid metabolism. In addition, cortisol has potent anti-inflammatory properties. Adrenal synthesis and secretion of cortisol are stimulated by corticotropin (ACTH), a peptide produced in basophilic cells of the anterior pituitary gland. The important factors that influence release of corticotropin include the sleep–wake cycle, stress, plasma cortisol concentration, and corticotropin-releasing hormone (CRH), which is produced in the hypothalamus. Thus, a negative feedback servomechanism involving cortisol, corticotropin, and CRH regulates adrenal secretion of glucocorticoids.

The renin system has a pivotal role in the regulation of extracellular fluid, largely through its action on the adrenal mineralocorticoid, aldosterone. Renin is an enzyme produced and stored in the granules of the juxtaglomerular cells, which surround the afferent arterioles of the renal glomerulus. Renin is released in response to reduced renal perfusion as signaled by reduced afferent arteriole perfusion pressure, increased delivery of filtered sodium to the distal tubule, and increased sympathetic nerve stimulus. Renin acts on angiotensinogen to form angiotensin I, and the converting enzyme forms angiotensin II from angiotensin I. Angiotensin II is a potent stimulator of aldosterone production by the adrenal cortex. Increasing blood levels of aldosterone lead to sodium retention and an expansion of the extracellular fluid volume. In addition, aldosterone is an important regulator of potassium metabolism.

The major androgen secreted by the adrenal cortex is dehydroepiandrosterone (DHEA), which is the main precursor of the urinary 17-ketosteroids. The relatively weak adrenal androgens exert a greater effect after conversion in extraadrenal tissues to the more potent androgen, testosterone. Corticotropin regulates the production of DHEA and other weak androgens by the adrenal cortex.

Physiologically, the adrenal medulla is best thought of as an endocrinologic homologue with the postganglionic sympathetic neuron. The medulla maintains high concentrations of catecholamines, of which 85% is epinephrine. In contrast to the regulation of adrenal cortical steroid secretion by hormones or enzymes, release of catecholamines into the blood stream in response to systemic stress follows from stimulation by the preganglionic sympathetic nerves. The medulla is composed of chromaffin cells, so named because these cells stain brown with chromic acid salts, which oxidize intracellular catecholamines.

Anatomy

The right adrenal gland is suprarenal in location and is first imaged 1 to 2 cm cephalad to the upper pole of the right kidney. Its inferior extent can be seen anterior and medial to the upper pole. The right adrenal gland is posterior to the inferior vena cava, lateral to the right crus, and medial to the right lobe of the liver. The left adrenal gland is located at or caudal to the level of the right adrenal gland. It more often is imaged anteromedially to the upper pole of the left kidney and frequently

extends to the level of the left renal hilum. The left adrenal gland is lateral to the aorta and left crus and posterior to the pancreas and splenic vessels. The anatomic relationship of the right and left adrenal glands to the inferior vena cava and the splenic vein, respectively, is important because it may suggest an adrenal origin for a large upper quadrant mass.

At birth, the adrenal glands are almost one third the size of the kidneys, whereas in adults, they are about one thirtieth the size of the kidneys. The cephalocaudal length of the adrenal gland varies from 4 to 6 cm and the width varies from 2 to 3 cm. Because of this variation, these dimensions infrequently are used as criteria for the assessment of adrenal gland size. This variation also explains why endocrinologically hyperfunctioning and pathologically hyperplastic adrenal glands may appear normal in size at imaging and surgery (Fig. 9-1). Depending on the transverse level, the adrenal gland may have a variety of configurations, varying from oblique linear to an inverted-Y, -V, or -T shape. The constituents of the inverted-Y shape may be referred to as the single anteromedial ridge and two posterior or posterolateral limbs. The width of a normal adrenal limb, when measured perpendicularly to the long axis in the transverse axial plane, has a range of 4 to 9 mm.

Each adrenal gland typically is supplied by three arteries: the inferior, middle, and superior adrenal arteries. The inferior adrenal artery most often is a branch of the proximal, ipsilateral renal artery and usually is the major artery to the adrenal gland. Each adrenal gland is drained by a single central adrenal vein. From the right adrenal gland, three segmental veins join to form a short central vein that enters the posterior inferior vena cava. From the left adrenal gland, a long, single adrenal vein enters the superior aspect of the left renal vein opposite the gonadal vein.

Imaging

Imaging of the enlarged adrenal gland or adrenal mass can be accomplished with a variety of modalities, including plain film tomography, ultrasonography, computed tomography (CT), magnetic resonance (MR) imaging, nuclear scintigraphy, and angiography. CT probably is the most readily available and consistently effective means of imaging the healthy and the abnormal adrenal gland. However, in the investigation of a large upper-quadrant mass, the multiplanar imaging capabilities of MR imaging and ultrasonography particularly are valuable when the relationship of a mass to the kidney or to other retroperitoneal organs or vessels needs to be determined. Angiography and nuclear scintigraphy have limited and specific roles in the evaluation of adrenal gland abnormalities.

The normal adrenal gland can be imaged in nearly all but the leanest patients by CT. Most adrenal masses are

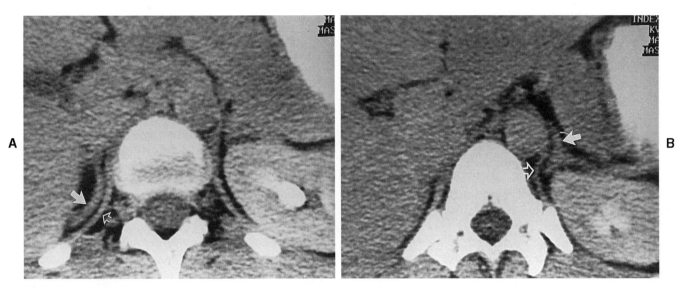

Fig. 9-1   CT of adrenal hyperplasia in a hirsute female with elevated concentration of dehydroepi-androsterone in the urine. CT scans demonstrate normal shape and size of the right (solid arrow in **A**) and left adrenal glands (solid arrow in **B**). The ipsilateral diaphragmatic crus (open arrows) commonly is used as an internal standard for normal adrenal size. The measured width of the normal adrenal limb ranges from 4 to 9 mm, and because of this variation, adrenal hyperplasia may not be distinguished from a normal adrenal gland at imaging or at surgery.

identified adequately with 10-mm collimated, contiguous sections. However, small masses may be difficult to detect unless 5-mm or thinner sections are used. Dilute oral contrast medium is administered routinely. Intravenous contrast enhancement of the kidney, liver, or pancreas may be helpful to distinguish an adrenal mass from these organs. In addition, intravenous contrast enhancement may be a valuable adjunct for characterizing an adrenal mass. CT guidance also is commonly used for percutaneous needle biopsy of an adrenal mass. Biopsy of an adrenal mass can be accomplished with the patient in a prone position, but often this necessitates steep needle angulation to avoid transgressing the pleural space in the posterior sulcus. The transhepatic approach, which avoids the pleural space and the need for cephalocaudal needle angulation, is an effective method for biopsy of a right adrenal mass. A useful alternative to the prone position is the ipsilateral decubitus position, particularly when a left adrenal mass is to be sampled. This position elevates the dependent diaphragm and reduces respiratory excursion of the ipsilateral thorax and upper abdomen, thereby reducing the risk of pleural entry by the biopsy needle.

Routine MR imaging of the adrenal gland should include T_1- and T_2-weighted images. A multiple slice, spin-echo sequence with 192 or 256 y-lines and a slice thickness of 5 to 7 mm demonstrates both adrenal glands in more than 90% of patients. Chemical-shift imaging can be performed with T_1-weighted, gradient–echo pulse sequences (spoiled gradient–echo or fast low-angle shot; repetition time [TR] = 70 to 160 msec; echo time [TE]

for in-phase image of 4.2 to 4.9 msec and for opposed-phase images of 2.1 to 2.9 or 6.3 msec; flip angle 90°). Although surface coils have been used, the body coil provides a larger field of view and makes the evaluation less cumbersome. The transverse imaging plane is the one used principally to evaluate the healthy or abnormal adrenal gland. With respect to demonstrating the healthy adrenal gland and masses exceeding 1 to 2 cm in diameter, MR imaging is comparable with CT. A practical advantage of MR imaging is that images in the coronal and the sagittal plane can be obtained without the need for image reformatting and are useful in the evaluation of the origin and extension of a large upper-quadrant mass. Normal adrenal tissue has a uniform, intermediate signal intensity on T_1-weighted images that is slightly less intense than that of normal liver and renal cortex. On T_2-weighted images, the healthy adrenal gland may be difficult to distinguish from adjacent retroperitoneal fat.

Ultrasonography can be used to evaluate the normal adrenal gland, but it is variably successful because of the small size of the adrenal gland and its frequent obscuration by retroperitoneal fat. One method to image the right adrenal gland uses a lateral or anterior approach with the patient in a supine or left lateral decubitus position. Scanning through the ninth to tenth intercostal spaces is performed. An imaginary line connecting the center of the right kidney and the inferior vena cava should pass through the right adrenal gland in either the sagittal or transverse plane. The left adrenal gland is imaged in a coronal plane by scanning in the posterior axillary line with the patient in the right lateral decubitus position. An imaginary line drawn through the spleen or the left kidney to the aorta should intersect the left adrenal gland. Normally, the adrenal gland appears as a hypoechoic triangular or semilunar structure, but often only echogenic retroperitoneal fat is seen. Ultrasonography plays a greater role in the examination of the patient with a known or suspected adrenal mass lesion. It is particularly valuable when there is a need to distinguish an adrenal mass from one originating from the upper pole of the kidney, the liver, or the pancreas. In some patients, an adrenal mass can be characterized accurately sonographically, e.g., when the fat content of an adrenal myelolipoma is recognized.

Imaging of the adrenal glands with radiopharmaceuticals provides functional information that is unavailable from other imaging modalities. I^{131} 6 beta-iodomethyl-19-norcholesterol (NP-59) is a cholesterol analogue that accumulates in adrenocortical tissues. Adrenal uptake of NP-59 is affected by circulating levels of corticotropin and inversely is related to the size of the body cholesterol pool. Exogenous corticosteroid administration suppresses pituitary secretion of ACTH, decreasing baseline adrenal uptake of this radiotracer. In the presence of a known hyperfunctioning adrenal lesion, administration of a potent corticosteroid, such as dexamethasone, before an NP-59 scan permits assessment of the autonomy of the adrenal lesion. Furthermore, the distribution of adrenal radioactivity after dexamethasone suppression distinguishes between abnormal lesions that are unilateral (i.e., neoplasm) from those that are bilateral (i.e., hyperplasia). Despite its continued investigational status, this radiopharmaceutical has been shown to be useful in the examination of patients with biochemical evidence of adrenal hyperfunction. Functional lesions of the adrenal medulla can be imaged using I^{131} meta-iodobenzylguanidine (I^{131}-mIBG), a radiopharmaceutical that bears a structural similarity to norepinephrine. I^{131}-mIBG scanning has been used effectively in the assessment of patients with suspected extraadrenal or recurrent pheochromocytomas. It also may be used to evaluate sites of metastases in patients with malignant pheochromocytoma and to follow patients with multiple endocrine neoplasia syndrome.

There are several specific indications for angiography in the evaluation of the adrenal gland. Patients may undergo adrenal arteriography as part of a comprehensive arteriographic examination to determine the organ of origin of a large abdominal mass if this remains unclear despite adequate evaluation by cross-sectional imaging. Adrenal venography and venous sampling are reserved for patients with primary aldosteronism or, more rarely, Cushing's syndrome; in these patients, adenoma must be distinguished from adrenal hyperplasia. Total body venous sampling also can be used effectively when the

site of recurrent or persistent pheochromocytoma is sought. Complications of adrenal venography include extravasation, venous thrombosis, adrenal infarction, and minor retroperitoneal hemorrhage.

MASSES OF THE ADRENAL GLAND

Adenoma

Adenomas are common, benign tumors of the adrenal cortex. Adenomas larger than 0.5 cm in diameter are found in 1.5% of autopsy cases and in 1% of patients who undergo abdominal CT examinations. The majority of these tumors are nonfunctional and are discovered as an incidental finding. Most nonhyperfunctioning adenomas consist of large cells containing abundant cytoplasmic lipid. Functional adrenal adenomas may be the cause of Cushing's syndrome, primary hyperaldosteronism, virilization, or feminization.

Size, contour, consistency, and growth are features that frequently are used to characterize adrenal masses by cross-sectional imaging (Table 9-1). Most adrenal adenomas are 3 cm or smaller in diameter at the time they are discovered, and it is rare for these tumors to measure 6 cm or larger when initially detected. The contour of these tumors usually is well defined and smooth. The typical appearance is a solid and homogeneous mass with an attenuation that is lower than that of adjacent muscle. Attenuation coefficients of less than 0 Hounsfield units (HU) are specific for adrenal adenoma, and the majority of masses with measured attenuation less than 15 HU are adenomas (Fig. 9-2). Calcification and central necrosis are decidedly unusual (Fig. 9-3). These tumors may enhance to some degree (i.e., less than a 20 HU increase in attenuation is measured when compared with the noncontrast CT density). An important feature of an adrenal

Table 9-1   Differentiation of Adenoma and Metastasis

	Adenoma	Metastasis
Size at presentation	Often < 3 cm	Variable
Change in size over time	No	Yes
Measured CT attenuation	≤ 15 HU	> 15 HU
Signal intensity*	Iso- to hypointense to liver	Hyperintense to liver
Calculated T_2 time	< 60 msec	≥ 60 msec
Out-of-phase image†	Decreased	Same or increased

*On a conventional T_2-weighted image.
†Out-of-phase image refers to the signal intensity of the mass on a T_1-weighted gradient–echo out-of-phase image compared with an in-phase image.

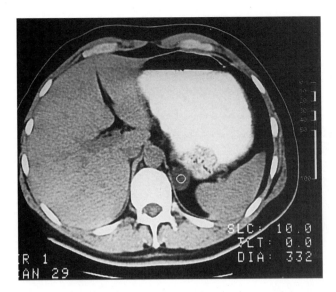

Fig. 9-2 Attenuation coefficient measurement to characterize adrenal adenoma. The typical adrenal adenoma is a well-circumscribed, solid mass with homogeneous low attenuation; most are smaller than 3 cm in diameter. Three attenuation measurements of this mass were −3.1 HU, 0.2 HU, and −0.2 HU.

adenoma is that this tumor is stable in size at serial imaging for intervals of up to 2 years.

Adenomas larger than 1 to 1.5 cm in diameter can be evaluated with MR imaging. Although the signal intensity of this tumor on T_1- and T_2-weighted images may be useful in characterization, unfortunately it is not always specific. Nonfunctional adenomas usually are isointense with normal adrenal tissue on T_1- and T_2-weighted images. These tumors are isointense to liver on T_1-weighted images and

isointense-to-slightly hyperintense to liver on T_2-weighted images (Fig. 9-4A). A number of techniques have been investigated to distinguish adenomas from other adrenal masses on high-field MR imaging, including calculated T_2 relaxation time, dynamic contrast-enhanced imaging, and chemical-shift gradient–echo imaging.

Chemical-shift imaging has become the standard MR imaging method of characterizing adrenal adenomas. The chemical-shift family of pulse sequences is based on the difference in resonance frequency between the two major constituents of the hydrogen resonance spectrum: water and triglyceride protons. This difference translates to a frequency shift of 224 Hz on a 1.5-T system, and at this field strength, fat and water cycle in and out of phase approximately every 2.1 to 2.3 msec. If the echo is sampled when water and fat are in phase, the fat and water combine to generate a larger signal than an echo collected when they are out of phase. With gradient–echo sequences and short echo times, the signal intensity of an adrenal mass can be evaluated by using in-phase and out-of-phase pulse sequences. Adrenocortical adenomas consist of large, lipid-laden cells similar to those of the zona fasciculata, and they are unlike most adrenal metastases and pheochromocytomas, although some malignant tumors may contain cytoplasmic lipid (e.g., hepatocellular carcinoma, renal cell carcinoma, liposarcoma, and well-differentiated adrenocortical carcinoma). Postulating that the cancellation of signal in masses containing water and fat (i.e., adenomas) would result in a relative decrease in signal intensity on opposed-phase images, chemical-shift imaging can characterize adrenal masses with a sensitivity of 80% to 90% and a specificity of 95% to 100% (Fig. 9-4B, Fig. 9-4C, and Fig. 9-5). In contrast,

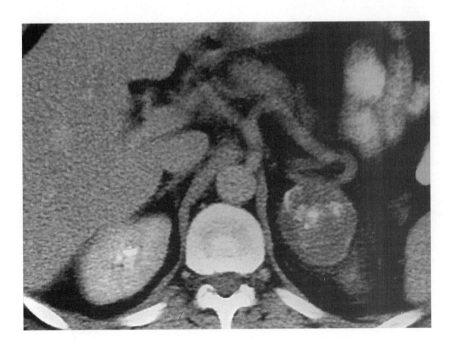

Fig. 9-3 Nodular and linear calcification in a left adrenal adenoma.

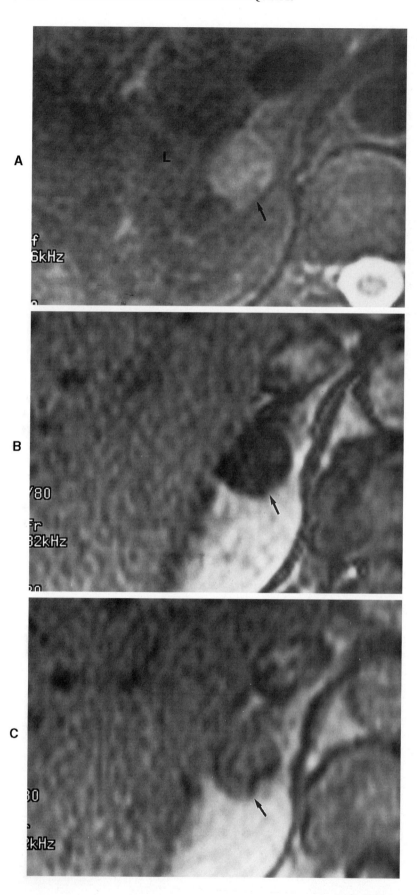

Fig. 9-4   MR imaging of an adrenal adenoma. **A,** A right adrenal mass (arrow) is hyperintense compared with liver (L) on a magnified fast spin-echo, T$_2$-weighted image (repetition time [TR] = 3600 msec; effective echo time [TE] = 102 msec). **B and C,** On the opposed-phase, T$_1$-weighted gradient-echo image (flip angle = 80°; TR = 91 msec; TE = 2.7 msec) of the mass, there is marked loss of signal intensity when compared with the in-phase gradient-echo image (flip angle = 80°; TR = 108 msec; TE = 4.2 msec).

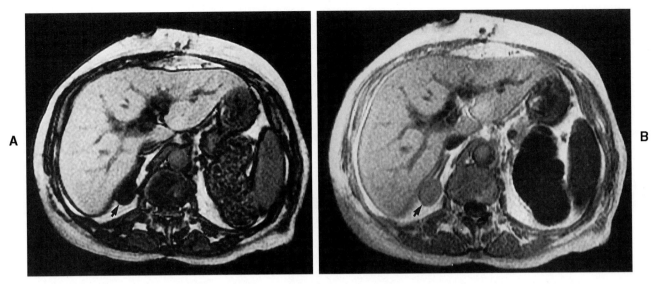

Fig. 9-5   Typical appearance of adrenal adenoma on chemical-shift MR imaging. Opposed-phase, T_1-weighted gradient–echo MR image (**A**) demonstrates marked loss of signal intensity in a right adrenal mass (arrow) compared with its appearance on an in-phase image (**B**). Notice that there is no significant change in signal intensity of the liver, spleen, or muscle. (From Mayo-Smith WW, Lee MJ, McNicholas MMJ, et al: Characterization of adrenal masses by use of chemical shift MR imaging: observer performance versus quantitative measures, *AJR Am J Roentgenol* 165:91–95, 1995.)

other adrenal masses (most metastases and pheochromocytomas) and reference tissues, such as muscle and spleen, do not contain fat and should not demonstrate significant change in signal intensity between in-phase and opposed-phase sequences. False-negative results may be caused by unusually small amounts of fat in adenomas; false-positive results could be explained by the presence of small amounts of fat reported rarely in masses other than adenomas.

Adrenal Metastases

If surgery is contemplated in the patient with a history of a primary malignancy, particularly lung, breast, kidney, or melanoma, metastasis must be excluded when an adrenal mass is discovered. Adrenal metastasis occurs in 10% to as many as 30% of patients early in the course of non–small cell lung cancer, and the autopsy incidence is as high as 40%. Similarly, as many as 30% of patients with breast cancer may have adrenal metastasis at the time of radiologic staging. Despite these statistics, the prevalence of adrenal metastasis in a patient with an adrenal mass and history of cancer ranges from 33% to 75%. Therefore, even when bilateral adrenal masses are discovered, one cannot assume they are metastatic in origin (Box 9-1; Fig. 9-6).

Although no specific radiologic signs of adrenal metastasis have been identified, the suspicion of malignancy should be raised when several observations are made. Change in size on serial imaging studies may be a more valuable parameter than absolute size on any given study. Although malignant adrenal tumors grow more rapidly and therefore generally are larger at detection, metastases to the adrenal gland can be as small as 1 cm or as large as 10 cm when discovered. If an adrenal mass grows during a 4- to 6-month period of observation or if it clearly decreases in size during systemic treatment of the primary malignancy, it is reasonable to assume that it is a metastatic lesion (Fig. 9-7). When small, metastasis can have a radiologic appearance similar to that of adrenal adenomas (i.e., a well-circumscribed mass with homogeneous attenuation). However, several features of small tumors (i.e., < 5 cm) suggest malignancy, including an irregular or poorly defined margin, moderately-to-markedly inhomogeneous attenuation, and an enhancing thick rim or nodular margin. Invasion of local viscera or bone suggests malignancy. Finally, metastasis to the adrenal

---

Box 9-1   Bilateral Adrenal Masses

Common
    Adenoma
    Metastases
Uncommon
    Hemorrhage—10% neonates, 20% adults
    Lymphoma—up to 50%
    Granulomatous infection, subacute stage
    Pheochromocytoma—10%

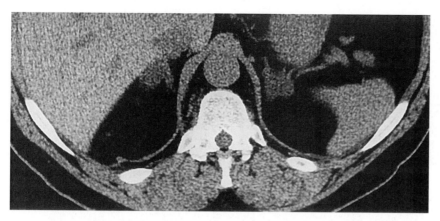

Fig. 9-6   Bilateral adrenal masses in a patient with carcinoma of the lung. Although these masses have a lobulated contour, each had a measured CT attenuation of less than 0 HU. A biopsy of the left adrenal mass was taken and was proven to be an adenoma. At 2 years of follow-up evaluation with serial CT scans, there has been no change in size.

glands often is accompanied by evidence of widespread metastases to other organs, particularly liver, retroperitoneal nodes, or lung.

When the cause of an adrenal mass must be determined in a patient with a known primary malignancy, percutaneous needle biopsy is a safe and accurate alternative to additional or follow-up imaging. Because this invasive procedure is not without risk, it is important to establish before biopsy is taken that determining the nature of the adrenal mass will have a significant impact on therapy or prognosis. The positive and negative predictive value of image-guided needle biopsy in patients with a history of lung cancer is 100% and 90%, respectively. However, the negative predictive value is only

approximately 80% when the adrenal biopsy specimen is nondiagnostic; false-negative adrenal biopsy results have been reported. Therefore, in patients with a history of cancer in whom the a priori probability of adrenal metastasis is high, repeated aspiration or biopsy of an adrenal mass should be considered when the pathology report is nondiagnostic.

In the patient with no known history of malignancy, it is unusual for an incidentally discovered adrenal mass to be the initial presentation of a distant primary. In these patients, a role may exist for MR imaging or serial imaging studies to assess for change in size. When imaged on midfield-strength magnets, adrenal metastases tend to be of higher signal intensity than liver parenchyma on T$_2$-

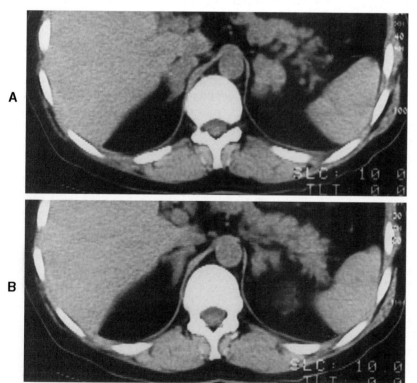

Fig. 9-7   Adrenal metastases. **A,** Uninfused CT demonstrates bilateral nodular adrenal masses. Percutaneous needle biopsy of the left adrenal gland showed metastatic lung cancer. **B,** After chemotherapy, the adrenal masses are smaller.

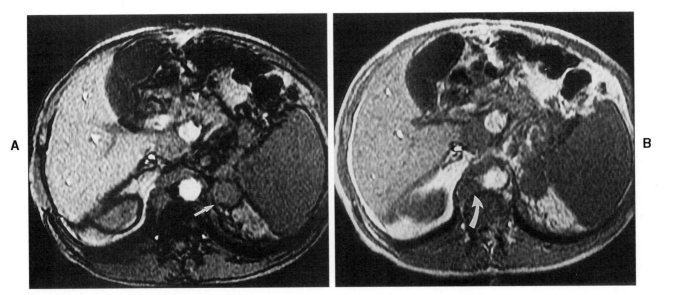

Fig. 9-8   Chemical-shift MR imaging of adrenal metastasis. **A,** Opposed-phase, T_1-weighted gradi-ent–echo MR image shows a left adrenal mass (arrow) that is isointense relative to spleen. When compared with the in-phase gradient–echo MR image **B,** the signal intensity of the adrenal mass is unchanged. Note that retrocrural lymphadenopathy (curved arrow) also is unchanged in signal intensity. (From Mayo-Smith WW, Lee MJ, McNicholas MMJ, et al: Characterization of adrenal masses by use of chemical shift MR imaging: observer performance versus quantitative measures, *AJR Am J Roentgenol* 165:91–95, 1995.)

weighted images. On T_1-weighted images, the signal in-tensity of adrenal metastases typically is lower than that of liver and retroperitoneal fat. Metastases also tend to have a longer calculated T_2-relaxation time (> 60 msec when measured on a 1.5-T magnet), a different dynamic enhancement pattern than that of adrenal adenomas, and the same signal intensity on opposed-phase compared with in-phase gradient–echo T_1-weighted images (Fig. 9-8).

Pheochromocytoma

Pheochromocytoma, a neoplasm of chromaffin cells, has the capacity to store and release catecholamines (Box 9-2). Although these tumors account for only 0.1% of causes of hypertension, pheochromocytomas are im-portant as a cause of reversible hypertension and may cause sudden death resulting from hypertensive crisis, shock, or both. Despite their importance, as many as 60% of tumors identified during autopsy were unsuspected during the patient's life.

The majority of pheochromocytomas occur sporadi-cally, but in approximately 5% of patients, pheochromo-cytoma is inherited as an autosomal dominant trait, either alone or combined with other abnormalities. Pheochro-mocytoma may occur as a part of the multiple endocrine neoplasia (MEN) syndromes. Sipple's syndrome, or MEN

IIA, consists of pheochromocytoma, medullary carci-noma of the thyroid, and hyperparathyroidism; pheo-chromocytoma occurs in about 50% of affected kindred. The MEN IIB syndrome consists of medullary carcinoma of the thyroid, pheochromocytoma, and multiple muco-sal neuromas. Pheochromocytomas associated with the MEN syndromes often are multicentric and frequently bilateral (Fig. 9-9). Approximately 10% of patients with retinal cerebellar hemangioblastomatosis (von Hippel-Lindau syndrome) and fewer than 1% of patients with Type I neurofibromatosis also have a pheochromocy-toma. There is also an increased prevalence of pheochro-

---

Box 9-2   Pheochromocytoma

Five percent inherited: multiple endocrine neoplasia IIA and IIB, von Hippel-Lindau, Type I neurofibro-matosis
Ten percent: bilateral, extraadrenal, malignant
''Ps'': high blood pressure (90%), palpitations, perspiration, pain (headache)
Computed tomography: 2 cm or more in diameter, homogeneous attenuation, rarely cystic
Magnetic resonance imaging: hyperintense on conventional T_2-weighted image

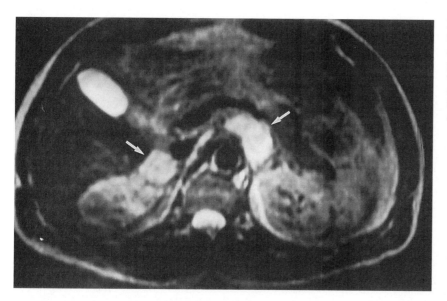

Fig. 9-9 Bilateral pheochromocytomas. On CT, bilateral noncystic adrenal masses were seen in a patient with multiple endocrine neoplasia syndrome. A conventional spin–echo, T_2-weighted image (repetition time = 2500 msec; echo time = 80 msec) demonstrates hyperintense adrenal masses consistent with pheochromocytomas.

mocytoma in patients with Carney's syndrome (triad of pheochromocytoma, pulmonary chondroma, and gastric leiomyoma), Sturge-Weber syndrome, or tuberous sclerosis.

In adults, 90% of sporadic pheochromocytomas originate in the adrenal medulla, and 10% are extraadrenal in origin (paraganglioma). Bilateral adrenal pheochromocytoma occurs in 7% of adults with a pheochromocytoma. In children, 30% of pheochromocytomas are extraadrenal, and bilateral adrenal pheochromocytoma occurs in 25% of patients. The majority of extraadrenal pheochromocytomas are located within the abdomen and originate in chromaffin cells of paravertebral sympathetic nerves or nerve plexi. The most common single location of an extraadrenal retroperitoneal paraganglioma is the organ of Zuckerkandl, which encompasses all chromaffin cell-bearing tissue along the lower abdominal aorta from the origin of the inferior mesenteric artery to the aortic bifurcation and into the iliac vessels.

The majority of pheochromocytoma tumors are benign. Although nuclear atypia, pleomorphism, and multinucleation are suggestive, malignancy often is difficult to determine based on histopathologic criteria alone. The diagnosis of malignant pheochromocytoma depends heavily on documenting local invasion or distant metastases. Malignant tumors tend to be slow-growing and to metastasize to liver, bone, regional lymph nodes, and lung. Between 6% and 10% of adrenal pheochromocytomas and approximately 15% of extraadrenal pheochromocytomas are malignant.

The majority of the clinical manifestations of pheochromocytoma result from the known physiologic effects of catecholamine release. The classic clinical feature ascribed to pheochromocytoma is the paroxysm or crisis consisting of headache, palpitations, and diaphoresis;

about 60% of patients experience one or more of these symptoms weekly, and the remainder usually have one or more daily. Although these paroxysms are distinctive, hypertension is the most common feature; it occurs in more than 90% of patients. The biochemical diagnosis of pheochromocytoma can be made based on a 24-hour collection of urine, provided the patient is symptomatic or hypertensive during the collection period. Collected urine is analyzed for levels of free catecholamines and catecholamine metabolites.

Computed tomography is the preferred initial imaging choice because the majority of adrenal pheochromocytomas are 2 cm or larger in diameter at diagnosis. When smaller than 3 to 4 cm, these tumors typically are well defined and of homogeneous soft-tissue attenuation (Fig. 9-10). Larger tumors are more likely to contain areas of central necrosis and can simulate a cystic adrenal mass (Fig. 9-11). Calcification, which may be conglomerate or curvilinear, has been reported, but it is unusual. Extraadrenal pheochromocytomas or paragangliomas usually are larger than adrenal pheochromocytomas; the average diameter in one series was 8.6 cm. The location of abdominal paragangliomas is related closely to the distribution of the aorticosympathetic chain; 60% are at or above the kidneys, and 40% are below the kidneys.

Some advocate the routine use of MR imaging in the search for a pheochromocytoma or paraganglioma, but as a general rule, CT is equally accurate, readily available, and less expensive. The classic description of benign adrenal pheochromocytoma on T_2-weighted MR images is a well-defined, hyperintense adrenal mass, with signal intensity greater than that of liver and muscle and greater than that of fat. The signal intensity on long TR sequences is higher consistently than the signal intensity of adenomas, regardless of the size of the pheochromocytoma;

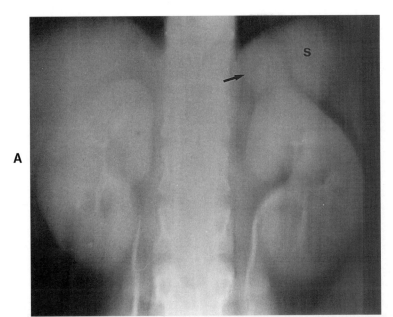

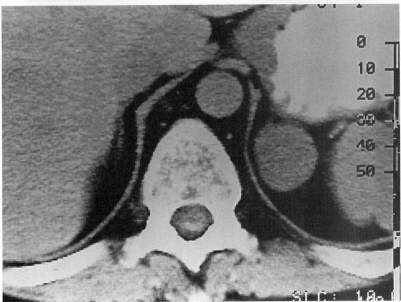

Fig. 9-10 Pheochromocytoma in a 34-year-old patient with sustained hypertension. **A,** Nephrotomogram demonstrates a 3-cm mass (arrow) cephalad to the upper pole of the left kidney (s = fundus of the stomach). **B,** On uninfused CT, a well-defined left adrenal mass with homogeneous soft-tissue attenuation is seen.

however, on fast or turbo spin-echo imaging, these tumors may not be as hyperintense as on a conventional spin-echo sequence. The presence of blood products also may reduce the signal intensity of a pheochromocytoma on T_2-weighted images. Other tumors that are predominantly cystic or primary adrenal cysts may have a similar appearance. MR imaging may have an advantage over CT in the postoperative patient with suspected recurrence of pheochromocytoma when metallic clips and anatomic distortion complicate imaging of the surgical bed.

Angiography and adrenal medullary scintigraphy also can be used to localize pheochromocytomas and paragangliomas, although their role is subordinate to that of CT

and MR imaging. Pheochromocytomas are hypervascular masses on arteriograms in 80% of patients, but avascular regions can be seen in 20% of tumors because of central necrosis. Adrenergic blockade is indicated before adrenal arteriography because of the risk of precipitating a fatal hypertensive crisis. Total body venous sampling can be an effective, albeit tedious, way to search for a recurrent pheochromocytoma that is occult on CT scans. In this procedure, venous blood samples are collected at multiple sites in the chest, abdomen, and pelvis and are analyzed for catecholamine concentration. A site with a markedly elevated level of catecholamines in the venous effluent harbors the tumor. The search for an occult, recurrent, or extraadrenal pheochromocytoma also can

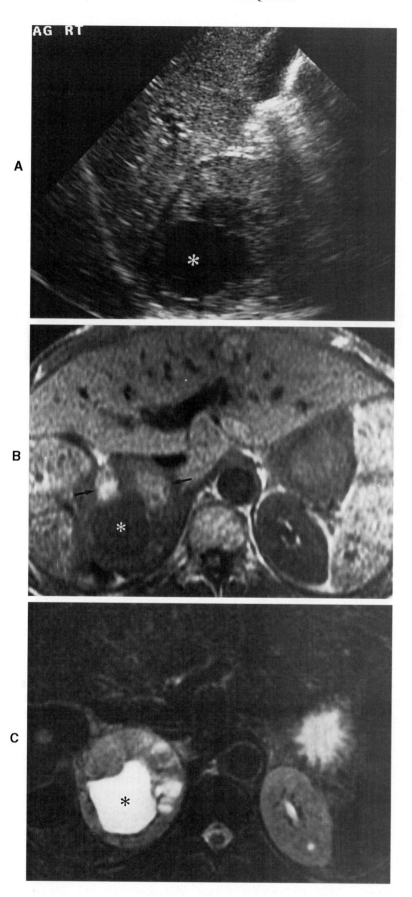

Fig. 9-11 Pheochromocytoma with areas of hemorrhage and cystic necrosis. **A,** A right suprarenal mass with a central cystic area (*) was seen on a sagittal sonogram. **B and C,** Spin-echo T_1-weighted and fast spin-echo T_2-weighted images demonstrate a large central cystic area (*) in the adrenal mass. Foci of increased signal intensity on the T_1-weighted image (arrows) were attributable to hemorrhage.

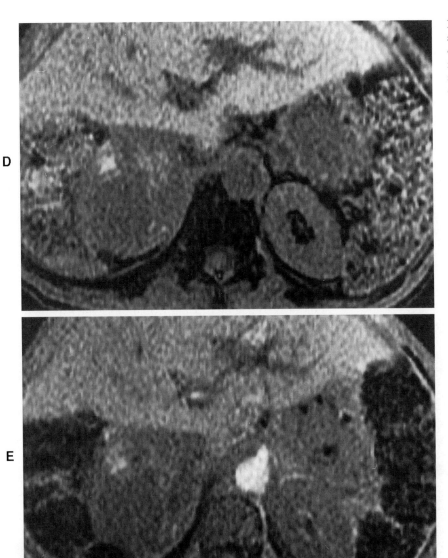

Fig. 9-11   D and E, Chemical-shift MR images demonstrate no change in signal intensity of the mass between opposed-phase **(D)** and in-phase **(E)** T_1-weighted gradient–echo images. At surgery, a large, necrotic pheochromocytoma was removed.

be accomplished by adrenal scintigraphy with the radiopharmaceutical I^{131} mIBG. This evaluation is a more practical way of examining the entire body than venous sampling and is of value in the localization of extraadrenal pheochromocytomas. Preliminary investigations suggest that a somatostatin analogue, indium-111 pentetreotide, shows promise as a scintigraphic method for localizing pheochromocytoma and paraganglioma.

Adrenal Cortical Carcinoma

Adrenal carcinoma is a tumor of adrenal cortical tissue with a cancer registry incidence of 0.0006% (Box 9-3). With aggressive searching, as many as 40% of these tumors are found to be functional; an elevated concentration of 17-ketosteroids measured in a 24-hour urine col-

lection is the most sensitive endocrinologic test for adrenal hyperfunction. Cushing's syndrome, with or without prominent virilizing effects, is the most common clinical manifestation of adrenal function associated with these tumors. Adrenal cortical carcinoma may metasta-

---

Box 9-3   Adrenal Cortical Carcinoma

Very rare primary adrenal malignancy
Forty percent hyperfunctional: elevated urine 17-ketosteroid
Often 6 cm or larger, heterogeneous attenuation, foci of calcification in 30%
Locally invasive, metastases to liver, lung, and bone

size to lung, liver, peritoneum, regional lymph nodes, and bone. Histopathologic evidence of frank malignancy often is lacking, and therefore pathologists frequently rely on radiologic or surgical descriptions of size and invasiveness to make the diagnosis.

Several distinguishing features of adrenal cortical carcinoma can be observed on IVU, ultrasonography, or CT. These tumors usually are large when discovered. The majority of adrenal carcinomas are 6 cm or larger at presentation, although smaller tumors have been reported. It is important to remember that the radiologic appearance of these smaller tumors may be indistinguishable from other tumors, especially metastasis to the adrenal gland. However, adrenal cortical carcinomas smaller than 5 cm almost always are functional, a fact that underscores the need for a thorough endocrinologic evaluation. Tumor margins often are irregular, ill defined, or nodular. Large tumors are more likely to be inhomogeneous in attenuation or to contain central areas of low density caused by necrosis. Foci of calcification are found

in as many as 30% of adrenal carcinomas. After administration of contrast material, the tumor typically enhances inhomogeneously, or a thick, nodular enhancing rim may be seen. These radiologic signs suggest the diagnosis of carcinoma, but they are not specific for malignancy; pheochromocytoma may have an identical appearance.

Local invasion of adjacent organs or bone, one of the radiographic signs of malignancy, should be carefully sought. It also is important to seek evidence of metastatic spread to regional lymph nodes, liver, or venous tributaries (i.e., left renal vein or inferior vena cava). Evidence of metastatic disease can be found at presentation in up to 50% of patients with adrenal carcinomas and is the other clue to the diagnosis of a malignant tumor.

On T_1-weighted MR imaging, adrenal carcinomas usually are isointense to liver. These tumors are hyperintense to liver on T_2-weighted images, and central areas of necrosis appear isointense to other body fluids (Fig. 9-12). The multiplanar imaging capability of MR imaging may be of value in demonstrating the adrenal origin of these large

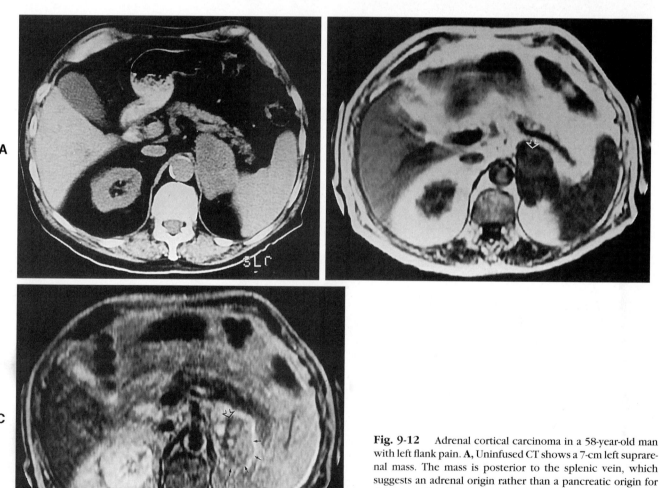

Fig. 9-12 Adrenal cortical carcinoma in a 58-year-old man with left flank pain. **A,** Uninfused CT shows a 7-cm left suprarenal mass. The mass is posterior to the splenic vein, which suggests an adrenal origin rather than a pancreatic origin for the tumor. **B and C,** Conventional spin–echo T_1-weighted and T_2-weighted images demonstrate areas of hemorrhage (open arrow) and microcyst formation in parts of the mass. On the T_2-weighted image, the solid part of the mass (small arrows) is hyperintense compared to liver.

tumors and direct invasion of tumor into liver or kidney. In addition, flow-sensitive sequences may be used to supplement routine spin–echo sequences to demonstrate inferior vena cava or renal vein invasion by tumor thrombus.

Adrenal Hemorrhage

Acute adrenal hemorrhage in adults can be spontaneous or can be associated with blunt trauma, anticoagulant use, or adrenal venography. Spontaneous adrenal hemorrhage may occur in the setting of septicemia (Waterhouse-Friedrichsen syndrome), recent surgery, severe burn injury, or an adrenal neoplasm. Metastatic melanoma particularly is prone to spontaneous adrenal hemorrhage. In adults, adrenal hemorrhage is bilateral in up to 20% of patients and may result in acute adrenal insufficiency (adrenal apoplexy), which frequently evades clinical recognition.

Adrenal hemorrhage most often appears as a well-defined round or oval mass lesion, ranging in size from 1 to 5 cm. Although focal or diffuse areas of increased attenuation (50 to 90 HU) are most consistent with acute hemorrhage on CT scans, it is more common for hemorrhage to be isodense to liver, nonenhanced renal cortex, or muscle (Fig. 9-13). On sonograms, acute hemorrhage

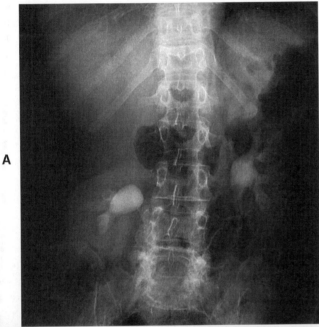

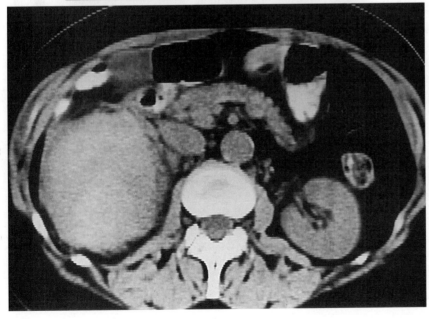

Fig. 9-13 Acute adrenal hemorrhage in a 67-year-old man with severe flank pain. **A,** 15-minute film from an intravenous urogram shows marked inferior displacement of the right kidney. The cortical margin of the right kidney appears normal. **B,** Uninfused CT demonstrates a large, hyperdense suprarenal mass. At surgery, there was hemorrhage into an adrenal metastasis.

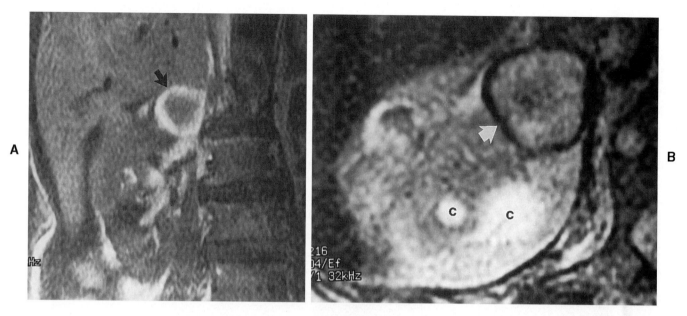

Fig. 9-14   Ring pattern of idiopathic subacute adrenal hemorrhage on MR imaging. **A,** Coronal spin–echo T₁-weighted image (repetition time [TR] = 650 msec; echo time [TE] = 11 msec) demonstrates hyperintense signal along the periphery of a right suprarenal mass. **B,** The transaxial fast spin–echo T₂-weighted image (TR = 4216 msec; effective TE = 104 msec) shows marked hypointensity along the peripheral margin of the mass (arrow) and relatively decreased signal in the center of the mass. The signal intensity pattern of the periphery of this mass is consistent with methemoglobin (c = renal cortical cysts).

appears as a mildly hyperechoic mass with a brightly echogenic center. Subacute hemorrhage (i.e., 1 to 2 months or older) is less echogenic and may appear more cyst-like (adrenal pseudocyst). One characteristic of adrenal hemorrhage is that it will decrease progressively in size during a 6-month period of observation, when the inciting cause of hemorrhage is removed.

Evolving hemorrhage in the adrenal gland may be diagnosed on MR images. Focal areas or a "ring pattern" of high-signal intensity on T₁-weighted images are attributed to the presence of methemoglobin in subacute hemorrhage. Low-signal intensity areas, typically seen in a ring pattern around the periphery of subacute and chronic hemorrhage on T₂-weighted images, result from the magnetic susceptibility effect of methemoglobin or hemosiderin (Fig. 9-14). Although it may be easier to perform ultrasonography or CT on the clinically ill patient, the potential for making a specific diagnosis makes MR imaging the preferred method for imaging suspected adrenal hemorrhage.

brous tissue-lined cysts). Pseudocysts most often are the sequelae of chronic adrenal hemorrhage.

When compared with renal cysts, adrenal cysts have more variability in their appearance. Consistent with endocrinologic nonfunction, adrenal cysts tend to be large (6 cm or larger) at clinical presentation. Mass effect on adjacent organs may be prominent. Large adrenal cysts can be difficult to distinguish from exophytic upper pole renal cysts, and in these patients, multiplanar imaging methods like ultrasonography or MR imaging are most valuable (Fig. 9-15). Although an imperceptible or thin (6 mm or less) wall commonly is observed, pseudocysts may have a thick or lobulated wall and internal septations. Occasionally, it may be difficult to distinguish an adrenal cyst from a tumor that has undergone extensive necrosis. Peripheral or curvilinear calcification is seen in as many as 15% of patients (Fig. 9-16). Percutaneous needle aspiration can be used effectively to confirm the adrenal origin of these cysts and to exclude the presence of malignant

Adrenal Cyst

Primary cyst of the adrenal gland is a rare, benign, and usually nonfunctional lesion (Box 9-4). Sixty percent of adrenal cysts are subclassified pathologically as either lymphangiomatous, epithelial, or infectious types. The remaining 40% of adrenal cysts are pseudocysts (i.e., fi-

Box 9-4   Cystic Adrenal Mass
Primary adrenal cyst Pheochromocytoma Melanoma metastases

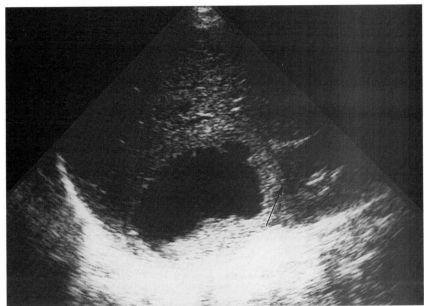

A

Fig. 9-15 Imaging of a large adrenal cyst in the sagittal plane. On a urogram (not shown), it was not certain whether a large mass originated from the right kidney or adrenal gland. **A,** A sagittal sonogram demonstrates a thick-walled cystic mass, and the upper pole of the right kidney (arrow) appeared normal. **B,** Sagittal proton density-weighted image (repetition time = 2000 msec; echo time = 20 msec) confirms the suprarenal location of the mass. Fine-needle aspiration revealed cholesterol crystals consistent with an adrenal cyst.

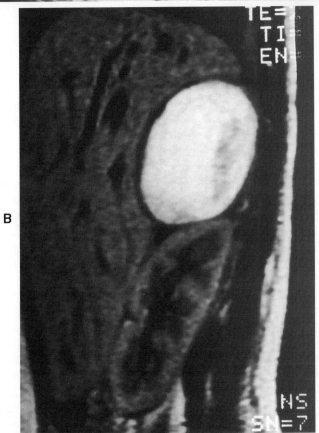

B

cells. Adrenal cyst fluid, unlike the renal cyst aspirate, contains higher concentrations of adrenal steroid hormone precursors, such as DHEA or 11-deoxycortisol. In addition, this fluid may appear turbid as a result of the presence of cholesterol crystals. The fluid generally is acellular, although occasional benign lymphocytes or macrophages may be identified. Complete evacuation of cyst fluid may eliminate symptoms, making surgery unnecessary for management.

Lymphoma

Adrenal gland infiltration by lymphoma most often occurs with retroperitoneal or ipsilateral renal lym-

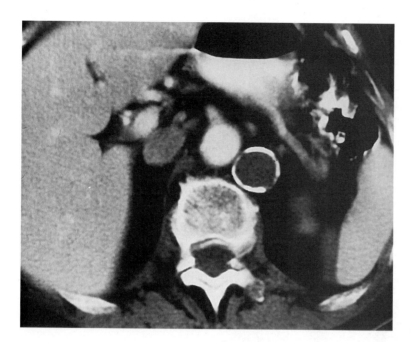

Fig. 9-16 Infused CT demonstrates rim calcification of a left adrenal cyst.

phoma. Adrenal involvement occurs more frequently with non-Hodgkin's lymphoma than with Hodgkin's disease and is bilateral in as many as 50% of patients.

Lymphoma of the adrenal glands may be imaged as a mass lesion or as diffuse enlargement of the gland. Like lymphoma in other locations, adrenal lymphoma may appear on sonograms as a somewhat hypoechoic mass compared with the hepatic parenchyma. Small tumors may be round or oval and homogeneous in attenuation on CT scans, typically between 40 and 60 HU. Lymphoma usually enhances less intensely than adjacent renal cortical tissue. Necrotic adrenal lymphoma may appear like a complex cystic mass with a thick and irregular wall, but necrosis is not common unless the patient has been treated or the tumor is growing rapidly. Other clues to the diagnosis of adrenal lymphoma are the presence of concurrent retroperitoneal lymphadenopathy or a change in size with management in accordance with other sites of lymphoma (Fig. 9-17). The few reported cases of adrenal lymphoma imaged with MR imaging have been of higher signal intensity than liver parenchyma on T_2-weighted images like other malignant adrenal masses.

Myelolipoma

Myelolipoma is a benign, nonfunctioning tumor of the adrenal cortex (Box 9-5). Such tumors are not common; the autopsy incidence of myelolipoma is 0.08% to 0.20%. Pathologically, mature adipose and hematopoietic tissues are found in addition to variable foci of hemorrhage. Myelolipomas usually are silent clinically, and most often they present as incidental adrenal masses. Symptoms may

occur with large tumors because of mass effect or with intratumoral hemorrhage.

The presence of mature adipose tissue gives this tumor a characteristic appearance on plain films, sonograms, CT scans, and MR images. On a plain film or nephrotomogram, a radiolucent suprarenal mass that displaces the renal axis may be seen, especially when a myelolipoma is large. Ultrasound images show a suprarenal mass of increased echogenicity, commensurate with the fat content of these tumors. On CT scans, myelolipomas are well defined but are heterogeneous in attenuation because of the mixed adipose and myeloid constituents (Fig. 9-18). Although adenomas also may be of lower attenuation than soft tissue, myelolipomas usually are more heterogeneous than adrenal adenomas (Fig. 9-19). Most myelolipomas are smaller than 5 cm at presentation, but tumors larger than 20 cm have been reported. Foci of calcification also may be seen, particularly when hemorrhage has occurred. The adipose tissue or methemoglobin within

---

Box 9-5 Adrenal Mass Lesions That Contain Fat

Common
  Adenoma (measured attenuation < 10 HU)
  Myelolipoma
Uncommon
  Renal cell carcinoma
  Adrenal cortical carcinoma (well differentiated)
  Pheochromocytoma

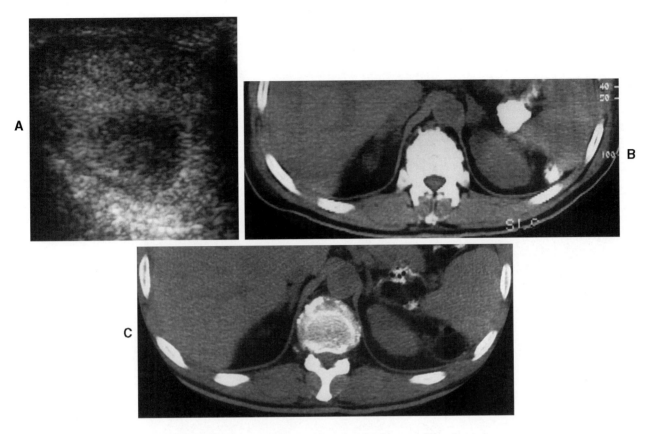

Fig. 9-17   Adrenal and testicular lymphoma in a 57-year-old man with a history of lymphoma in remission. **A,** Three hypoechoic masses were seen on a sagittal sonogram of the right testicle. **B,** CT scan demonstrates nodular enlargement of both adrenal glands. **C,** After chemotherapy for lymphoma, the masses decreased in size, but the adrenal glands still are slightly enlarged.

a myelolipoma appears as a focus of high-signal intensity on T_1-weighted MR images. Angiography of these tumors may show compressed normal adrenal tissue as a vascular rim around hypovascular or avascular areas corresponding to foci of fat. Percutaneous needle biopsy occasionally may be needed to make a definite diagnosis of myelolipoma. If biopsy is performed, it is important that fat and myeloid elements be represented in the tissue specimen because the finding of adipose tissue alone may result from the sampling of retroperitoneal fat rather than tumor.

SELECTED CLINICAL PROBLEMS IN ADRENAL IMAGING

Incidental Adrenal Mass

An adrenal mass often is discovered incidentally during the examination of a patient for an unrelated medical problem. Unsuspected adrenal masses have been detected on up to 1% of upper abdominal CT studies. Another common setting in which an adrenal mass is first detected is in the staging process in patients with a known malignancy. A rational approach to the evaluation of this common problem is essential and can be used to guide consultation with the referring physician and additional work-up, if necessary (Box 9-6 on p. 364).

In addition to the systematic selection and analysis of radiologic studies, it is important to ascertain several pieces of clinical information. Knowledge of a primary extraadrenal malignancy that can metastasize to the adrenal gland is critical. Primary malignancies of the lung, breast, and kidney as well as melanoma and lymphoma most frequently are associated with adrenal metastases; however, it also is important to note that between one third and two thirds of adrenal masses are benign, nonfunctioning adenomas in patients with a known history of cancer. In the patient with no known history of cancer, the most common cause of an adrenal mass lesion is an adenoma. Although an incidentally discovered adrenal mass may be the initial presentation of a distant primary malignancy, this situation is distinctly unusual. It also is important to determine if there are signs, symptoms, or biochemical evidence of the overproduction of adrenal hormones. Therefore, patients with incidentally discovered adrenal masses should have a complete endocrino-

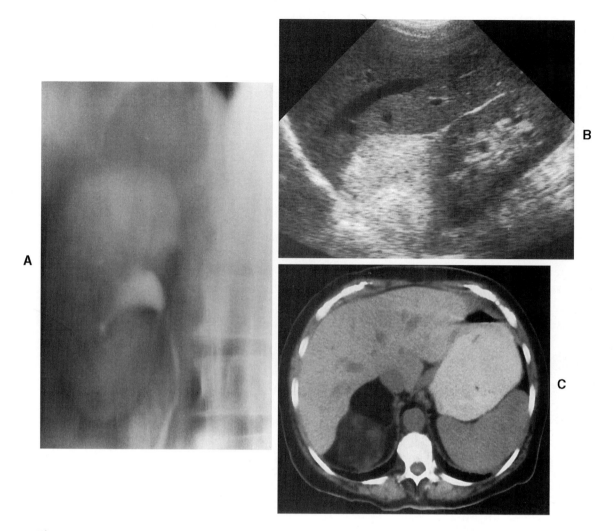

Fig. 9-18   Typical appearance of adrenal myelolipoma. **A,** Coned-down view from a nephrotomo-gram demonstrates a large radiolucent mass, which indents the upper pole of the right kidney. **B,** Sagittal sonogram shows a suprarenal mass of markedly increased echogenicity. **C,** The heterogeneous adrenal mass is dumbbell-shaped on uninfused CT. The mixed attenuation pattern reflects a pure fatty component anteriorly and a mixed adipose–myeloid component posteriorly.

logic work-up that should include, but should not be limited to, a 24-hour urine collection for 17-hydroxycorti-costeroids and 17-ketosteroids. If hyperfunction is documented, the adrenal mass should be removed surgically, regardless of its appearance on cross-sectional imaging.

The radiologic features of an adrenal mass that are useful in separating benign from malignant lesions include size at presentation, change in size, absolute value and homogeneity of attenuation, margin, and enhancement pattern. In addition, the presence of local tissue or venous invasion by an adrenal mass or metastases to the lungs, liver, or regional lymph nodes has been equated with malignancy.

Size of the adrenal mass most often is cited as the critical discriminating factor for distinguishing adrenal adenoma from carcinoma. Although adenomas as large as 10.5 cm have been reported, adenomas 6 cm or larger are rare. The majority of adenomas measure 3 cm or smaller when discovered incidentally. Metastases to the adrenal gland vary in size; one study reported a range of 1 to 10 cm. The majority of adrenal cortical carcinomas are 6 cm or larger at presentation; combining the data from six series, 73% of 144 adrenal cortical carcinomas were larger than 6 cm at presentation. Carcinomas occasionally are discovered when they are smaller than 6 cm, but they tend to be associated with adrenal hyperfunction, and, therefore, surgical removal would be indicated on that basis. Other radiologic features, such as attenuation, contour, and enhancement, also should be considered when analyzing an adrenal mass; these features were discussed in the section on individual adrenal lesions.

Chemical-shift MR imaging currently is the most accurate imaging method for characterizing adrenal adenomas; Mitchell et al have characterized adrenal adenomas accurately in 95% to 100% of patients. In contrast, analyses of relative signal intensity suggest that there is a 20% to 30% overlap between benign and malignant adrenal lesions on conventional T_1- and T_2-weighted spin–echo images without fat suppression.

Percutaneous needle biopsy is a safe and effective means of distinguishing metastases to the adrenal gland from primary adrenal tumor; however, pathologists frequently are unable to distinguish adenoma from carcinoma based on cytology or biopsy alone. The decision to perform needle biopsy should be discussed with the full knowledge of its potential benefits and risks to the patient. In the cancer patient with widespread metastatic disease, it is relatively unimportant to determine the nature of the adrenal mass by biopsy. In addition to the risk of pneumothorax and hemorrhage, needle biopsy also carries the small, but potentially fatal, risk of precipitating hypertensive crisis in a patient with an occult pheochromocytoma. Finally, given the possibility, although small, of false-negative results, repeat needle biopsy should be considered if the a priori likelihood of adrenal metastasis is high.

Recommendations are summarized as follows:

(1) From an endocrinologic standpoint, if the mass is associated with evidence of adrenal hyperfunction, it should be removed.
(2) Size, measured attenuation on CT, and appearance on chemical-shift MR imaging also should influence management decisions. Disagreement persists as to the size of an adrenal mass that mandates surgical removal. Size thresholds above which surgery is recommended vary from 3.5 cm to 6 cm. A measured attenuation of the mass of 15 HU or

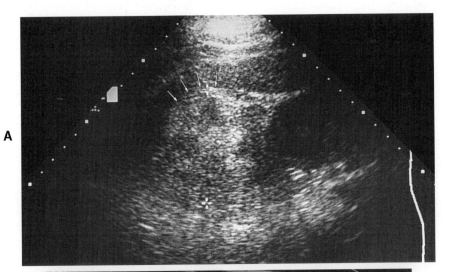

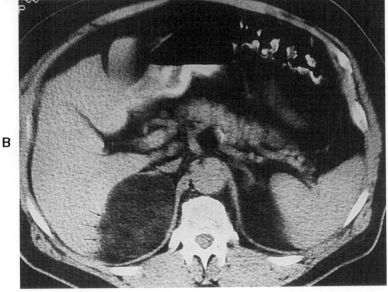

Fig. 9-19 Adrenal myelolipoma. **A,** Sagittal sonogram shows a suprarenal mass (electronic markers) with hyperechoic and isoechoic components. There is mass effect on the liver capsule (white arrows). **B,** Uninfused CT demonstrates the typical mottled appearance of a myelolipoma; this appearance would be atypical for an adenoma (arrows = mass effect on liver capsule).

Box 9-6 Evaluation of an Incidental Adrenal Mass

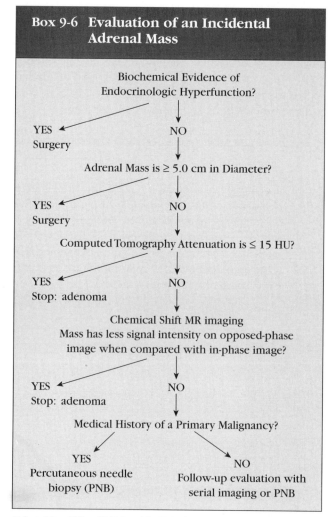

Biochemical Evidence of
Endocrinologic Hyperfunction?

YES → Surgery   NO

Adrenal Mass is ≥ 5.0 cm in Diameter?

YES → Surgery   NO

Computed Tomography Attenuation is ≤ 15 HU?

YES → Stop: adenoma   NO

Chemical Shift MR imaging
Mass has less signal intensity on opposed-phase
image when compared with in-phase image?

YES → Stop: adenoma   NO

Medical History of a Primary Malignancy?

YES   NO
Percutaneous needle   Follow-up evaluation with
biopsy (PNB)   serial imaging or PNB

(Adapted from Bilbey JH, McLoughlin RF, Kurkjian PS, et al: MR imaging of adrenal masses: value of chemical shift imaging for distinguishing adenomas from other tumors, *AJR Am J Roentgenol* 164:637–642, 1995.)

less is predictive of an adenoma; the obverse is not true. Another specific sign of adenoma is loss of signal intensity on opposed-phase gradient–echo T_1-weighted imaging. Masses that are interpreted as being consistent with a benign tumor based on imaging, or those found to be "benign" after biopsy, should be followed closely with serial imaging for interval growth at 2, 6, and 18 months. Well-documented growth mandates surgical removal. If a mass is stable in size at 18-month follow-up evaluation, it may be left in place.

(3) If there is a medical history of cancer, particularly lung, breast, renal cell, or melanoma, and provided the tissue diagnosis of metastases to the adrenal gland would influence management, a percutaneous biopsy of the adrenal mass should be undertaken if it has features on CT or chemical-shift MR imaging that are not typical for adenoma. Biopsy should be repeated if the initial pathology report is nondiagnostic.

Localization of Pheochromocytoma

Given biochemical evidence for a catecholamine-secreting tumor, the next objectives in the work-up of the suspected pheochromocytoma are to localize and characterize the tumor. Not only is establishing its adrenal or extraadrenal location important, but the tumor also must be characterized with respect to multiplicity, tissue invasion, and presence of metastases.

Computed tomography of the abdomen and pelvis is the imaging procedure of choice. Because pheochromocytomas usually are 2 cm or larger at presentation, unenhanced CT is an effective imaging method; its detection rate equals or exceeds 90%. The administration of intravenous contrast material to improve characterization usually is not necessary, particularly when there is biochemical evidence for a catecholamine-producing tumor, and the small risk of hypertensive crisis associated with intravenous contrast material administration can be avoided. If the adrenal glands and upper abdomen are normal, the remainder of the abdomen and pelvis should be imaged to search for a retroperitoneal paraganglioma.

Evaluation of Cushing's Syndrome

In 1932, Harvey Cushing described a clinical syndrome characterized by truncal obesity, fatigue, weakness, abdominal striae, amenorrhea, hirsutism, hypertension, glycosuria, and osteoporosis. Cushing's syndrome is a result of increased production of cortisol by the adrenal gland (Box 9-7). Eighty percent of cases are caused by bilateral adrenal hyperplasia, the result of adrenocortical stimulation by hypersecretion of corticotropin (corticotropin-dependent Cushing's syndrome). The remaining 20% of cases result from the overproduction of cortisol by an adrenal neoplasm or, more rarely, from nodular adrenal hyperplasia (Fig. 9-20), which results in the suppression of corticotropin production by the pituitary gland (corticotropin-independent Cushing's syndrome).

Appropriate management requires the accurate distinction between corticotropin-dependent and corticotropin-independent causes of Cushing's syndrome. In-

Box 9-7 Cushing's Syndrome

Corticotropin-dependent in 80%
  Pituitary adenoma (Cushing's disease)—70%
  Corticotropin-producing tumor (ectopic
    corticotropin syndrome)—10%
Corticotropin-independent in 20%
  Adrenal adenoma—10%
  Adrenal cortical carcinoma—8%
  Bilateral micro- or macronodular hyperplasia—2%

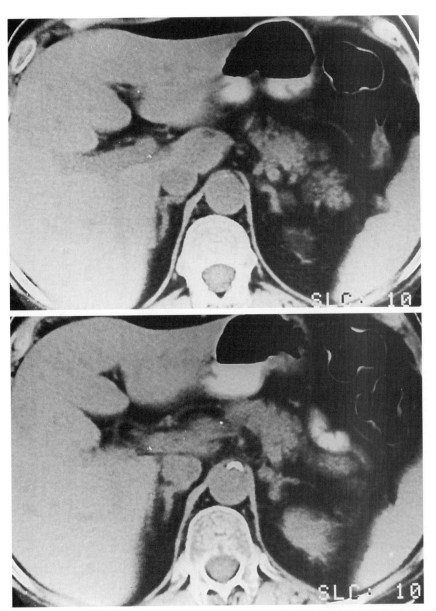

Fig. 9-20   Corticotropin-independent Cushing's syndrome caused by macronodular adrenal hyperplasia. Uninfused CT shows enlargement of both adrenal glands, and in particular, there is nodular enlargement of the left adrenal gland.

creased production of corticotropin by a pituitary adenoma, also known as Cushing's disease, accounts for 85% of patients with corticotropin-dependent Cushing's syndrome. Cushing's disease can be evaluated with contrast-enhanced MR imaging of the pituitary and petrosal venous sampling. A minority of cases of corticotropin-dependent Cushing's syndrome are caused by the autonomous production by nonendocrine tumors of polypeptides that are biochemically and immunologically indistinguishable from corticotropin. Most of these cases of ectopic corticotropin syndrome have been associated with small cell carcinoma of the lung, but carcinoid tumors of the bronchus, pancreas, and thymus, medullary carcinoma of the thyroid, pheochromocytoma, and other neuroendocrine tumors have been reported to cause Cushing's syndrome by this mechanism. Adrenal tumors

that are associated with overproduction of cortisol invariably are unilateral. Adrenal adenomas account for two-thirds of the cases of ACTH-independent Cushing's syndrome. Adrenocortical carcinoma, which accounts for the remainder of cases, commonly produces excessive amounts of more than one adrenal steroid hormone; therefore, overlapping clinical features, such as Cushing's syndrome with virilization syndrome in the female patient, are not uncommon.

The radiologist should be aware of several nonradiologic tests to distinguish corticotropin-dependent and corticotropin-independent Cushing's syndrome, and to distinguish pituitary from ectopic causes of excess corticotropin production. These tests include (1) plasma concentration of corticotropin as measured by radioimmune assay, (2) high-dose dexamethasone suppression test, and

(3) corticotropin-releasing hormone stimulation test. In particular, low or undetectable plasma corticotropin levels provide strong evidence of a primary adrenal neoplasm. These tests may be valuable particularly when imaging results are equivocal or inconsistent with clinical impressions.

Imaging of the adrenal glands is indicated when there is a need to confirm primary adrenal cause for Cushing's syndrome. Because of its availability and accuracy, thin-section CT is the method of choice for imaging the adrenal glands in the patient with corticotropin-independent Cushing's syndrome. Adrenal adenomas that cause Cushing's syndrome usually are 2 cm or larger and should be identifiable on thin-section CT images. An incidental, nonfunctional adrenal adenoma or cortical nodular hyperplasia in an otherwise normal or hyperplastic adrenal gland may mimic a primary adrenal cause for Cushing's syndrome. Although an autonomous adrenal tumor should be associated with atrophy of nonneoplastic adrenal cortical tissue because corticotropin levels are suppressed, this finding may not always be evident with CT.

If the clinical suspicion of an adrenal neoplasm remains after a normal, thin-section CT evaluation, adrenal vein sampling or functional imaging with adrenal cortical scintigraphy should be performed. Adrenal vein sampling is done to localize the site of a small adrenal neoplasm by measuring the concentration of cortisol from each adrenal vein. If a functional adrenal tumor is present, cortisol levels from the ipsilateral adrenal vein will be at least twice that in the contralateral vein or peripheral blood. NP-59 scintigraphy also can be useful if an adequate CT evaluation cannot be performed or if false-negative CT results are suspected. This adrenal cortical radiotracer will localize to one adrenal gland in the case of an autonomous adrenal tumor, but it will be symmetri-

cally distributed in both glands if adrenal hyperplasia is the cause of Cushing's syndrome.

Evaluation of Hyperaldosteronism

Aldosteronism is a syndrome associated with hypersecretion of the major adrenal mineralocorticoid, aldosterone. Clinically, patients present with polyuria, diastolic hypertension, hyponatremia, and signs of total-body potassium depletion. Primary aldosteronism suggests that the stimulus for aldosterone overproduction occurs within the adrenal gland and is independent of the renin–angiotensin system, whereas in secondary aldosteronism, the stimulus originates from an extraadrenal source. Primary aldosteronism is distinguished from secondary aldosteronism by the lack of suppression of aldosterone secretion during blood volume expansion. Once primary aldosteronism is established, the aldosterone-producing stimulus must be identified radiologically (Box 9-8).

Approximately 70% of primary hyperaldosteronism is caused by a solitary adrenal adenoma (Conn's syndrome). Bilateral adrenal glomerular hyperplasia (idiopathic hyperaldosteronism) accounts for about 30% of cases. Aldosterone-producing adenomas frequently are smaller than 2 cm at presentation (Fig. 9-21). Adrenocortical carci-

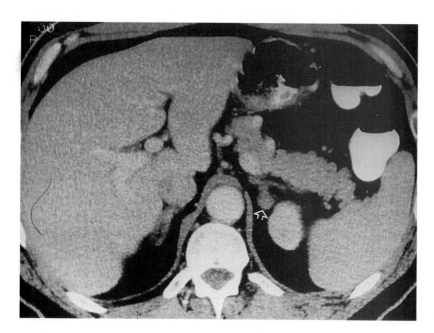

Fig. 9-21 Aldosterone-producing adenoma. Infused CT demonstrates a 1-cm enhancing nodule (open arrow) in the posteromedial limb of the left adrenal gland. In contrast with nonfunctional adenomas, aldosteronomas almost always are less than 2 cm at clinical presentation.

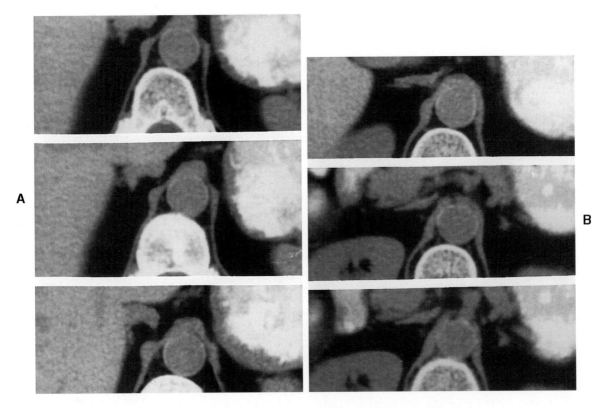

Fig. 9-22   Idiopathic atrophy of the adrenal glands in a patient with adrenocortical insufficiency and lymphocytic thyroiditis. **A and B,** Serial noninfused CT scans demonstrate marked atrophy of both adrenal glands. This appearance also might indicate chronic tuberculous infection.

noma causes aldosteronism in less than 1% of patients, and when it does, there usually is evidence for hypercortisolism. As a general rule, the biochemical abnormalities observed in patients with primary aldosteronism caused by adrenal hyperplasia are less pronounced than in those with aldosteronism caused by adenoma, but the overlap is too great to be of diagnostic value. Primary aldosteronism associated with adenoma is managed with surgery, whereas that associated with hyperplasia is managed medically with the aldosterone antagonist spironolactone.

The importance of the radiologic evaluation is clear because appropriate management critically depends on an accurate determination of the cause of primary aldosteronism. Thin-section CT, in search of an adrenal adenoma, is the preferred method of testing. However, because adrenal adenomas that cause hyperaldosteronism may be as small as 0.8 cm, adrenal hyperplasia cannot be assumed to be the cause of hyperaldosteronism when the adrenal glands appear normal on CT scans. Therefore, the patient should undergo adrenal venography with venous sampling when the adrenal glands are normal on CT. The rationale for venous sampling is that venous blood from the adrenal gland harboring an adenoma has a relative concentration of aldosterone 20 times greater than the unaffected adrenal gland. In adrenal hyperplasia,

the concentration of aldosterone should be the same in blood samples obtained from both adrenal veins. In general, CT accurately localizes an adenoma in about two-thirds of patients with primary hyperaldosteronism, but venography with venous sampling localizes a unilateral cause for hyperaldosteronism in close to 90% of patients.

Evaluation of Adrenocortical Insufficiency

The diagnosis of adrenocortical insufficiency is made when characteristic clinical signs and symptoms are presented, and when corticotropin stimulation test results are abnormal (Table 9-2). Primary adrenocortical insufficiency, or Addison's disease, occurs when 90% or more of the adrenal cortex is destroyed. Secondary adrenal insufficiency most commonly results from the suppression of the hypothalamic–pituitary axis by exogenously administered steroids, but it also may result from panhypopituitarism.

Idiopathic atrophy is the most common cause of subacute and chronic adrenal insufficiency in developed countries. Adrenal atrophy likely is the result of an autoimmune process because circulating autoantibodies to adrenal cortical tissue are found in nearly 50% of patients. In addition, many of these patients have other diseases

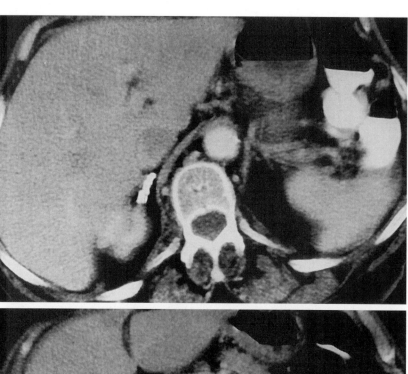

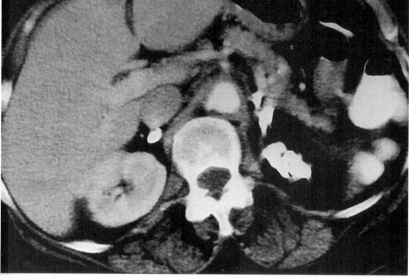

Fig. 9-23 Chronic tuberculous infection of the adrenal glands. Infused CT demonstrates linear and nodular calcifications of both adrenal glands.

Table 9-2 Causes of Adrenocortical Insufficiency

	Acute onset	Subacute–chronic
Common	Withdrawal of exogenous steroids	Idiopathic (autoimmune) atrophy
	Bilateral adrenal hemorrhage	Granulomatous adrenal infection (tuberculosis, histoplasmosis)
Uncommon		Metastases or lymphoma

thought to be autoimmune in pathophysiology. Adrenocortical destruction also may occur after chronic granulomatous infections, particularly tuberculosis. Disseminated histoplasmosis, North American and South American blastomycosis, and coccidioidomycosis infections also may result in adrenocortical insufficiency. Despite the prevalence of metastatic disease to the adrenal glands, it is a relatively uncommon cause of adrenal insufficiency. In contrast to subacute and chronic insufficiency, acute adrenal insufficiency most often results from the rapid withdrawal of steroids from patients with adrenal atrophy caused by chronic steroid use. Fulminant hemorrhagic destruction of both adrenal glands, usually associated with overwhelming septicemia, is another cause of acute adrenocortical insufficiency. It is not uncommon for signs and symptoms of adrenal insufficiency

Box 9-9 Focal or Diffuse Calcification in an Adrenal Mass

Common
  Chronic hemorrhage
  Tuberculous infection
  Adrenal cyst (15%)
Uncommon
  Adrenal cortical carcinoma (30%)
  Pheochromocytoma
  Neuroblastoma

to become apparent days to weeks after the actual episode of adrenal hemorrhage.

Insight into the cause of adrenocortical insufficiency can be gained by cross-sectional imaging. Thin-section CT of the adrenal glands is the test of choice, and scans should be scrutinized for adrenal size, shape, and the presence of calcifications. The finding of adrenal glands that clearly are decreased in size is consistent with either idiopathic atrophy or chronic tuberculous infection (Fig. 9-22 on p. 367). Calcification of small adrenal glands, if present, is more in keeping with tuberculous infection than with idiopathic atrophy (Fig 9-23; Box 9-9). However, the absence of calcifications does not exclude a diagnosis of tuberculosis. Adrenal glands that are clearly enlarged are consistent with tuberculosis or, more rarely, histoplasmosis or metastatic disease. Most patients with adrenal tuberculosis and enlarged adrenal glands have a history of adrenocortical insufficiency of less than 2 years' duration. Patients with metastatic disease of the adrenal glands that results in adrenal insufficiency typically have evidence of generalized metastatic disease.

Evaluation of Virilization or Feminization

Female virilization may be a manifestation of an androgen-secreting adrenal tumor or a congenital enzymatic defect of steroid hormone synthesis that results in adrenal hyperplasia (Fig. 9-24). In patients with adrenal neoplasm, many tumors are malignant, and the majority have reached sufficient size at presentation that detection with CT is likely. Virilization also may be caused by an ovarian tumor, and therefore evaluation of the pelvis is indicated when results of CT scan of the adrenal glands are normal.

Feminizing effects in male patients almost always sug-

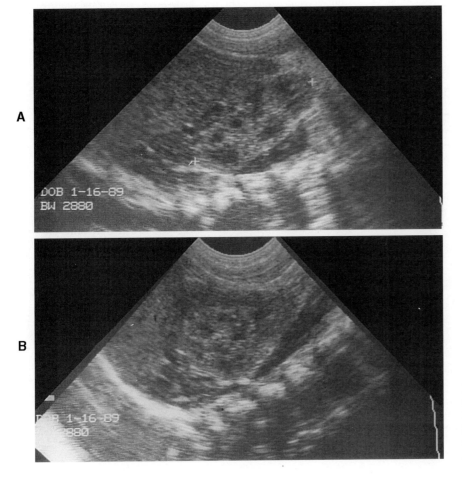

Fig. 9-24 Congenital adrenal hyperplasia in a patient with male pseudohermaphroditism. Sagittal sonograms demonstrate mass-like enlargement of the right (**A**) and left (**B**) adrenal glands in a newborn with ambiguous external genitalia.

gest the diagnosis of adrenal cortical carcinoma, although adenomas also have been reported to cause feminization. As in the virilized female patient, thin-section CT and MR imaging of the adrenal glands are the imaging modalities of choice.

SUGGESTED READINGS

Baker ME, Blinder R, Spritzer C, et al: MR evaluation of adrenal masses at 1.5 T, *AJR Am J Roentgenol* 153:307–312, 1989.

Belldegrun A, Hussain S, Seltzer SE, et al: Incidentally discovered mass of the adrenal gland, *Surg Gynecol Obstet* 163(3):203–207, 1986.

Berland LL, Koslin DB, Kenney PJ, et al: Differentiation between small benign and malignant adrenal masses with dynamic incremented CT, *AJR Am J Roentgenol* 151:95–101, 1988.

Bilbey JH, McLoughlin RF, Kurkjian PS, et al: MR imaging of adrenal masses: value of chemical shift imaging for distinguishing adenomas from other tumors, *AJR Am J Roentgenol* 164:637–642, 1995.

Chezmar JL, Robbins SM, Nelson RC, et al: Adrenal masses: characterization with T_1-weighted MR imaging, *Radiology* 166:357–359, 1988.

Copeland PM: The incidentally discovered adrenal mass, *Ann Intern Med* 98:940–945, 1983.

Doppman J, Gill JR Jr., Nienhuis AW, et al: CT findings in Addison's disease, *JCAT* 6(4):757–761, 1982.

Fishman EK, Deutch BM, Hartman DS, et al: Primary adrenocortical carcinoma: CT evaluation with clinical correlation, *AJR Am J Roentgenol* 148:531–535, 1987.

Hayes WS, Davidson AJ, Grimley PM, et al: Extraadrenal retroperitoneal paraganglioma: clinical, pathologic, and CT findings, *AJR Am J Roentgenol* 155:1247–1250, 1990.

Kier R, McCarthy S: MR characterization of adrenal masses: field strength and pulse sequence considerations, *Radiology* 171:671–674, 1989.

Korobkin M, Lombardi TJ, Aisen AM, et al: Characterization of adrenal masses with chemical shift and gadolinium-enhanced MR imaging, *Radiology* 197:411–418, 1995.

Krestin GP, Steinbrich W, Friedmann G: Adrenal masses: evaluation with fast gradient-echo MR imaging and Gd-DTPA-enhanced dynamic studies, *Radiology* 171:675–680, 1989.

Lee MJ, Hahn PF, Papanicolaou N, et al: Benign and malignant adrenal masses: CT distinction with attenuation coefficients, size, and observer analysis, *Radiology* 184:38–43, 1991.

Ling D, Korobkin M, Silverman PM, et al: CT demonstration of bilateral adrenal hemorrhage, *AJR Am J Roentgenol* 141:307–308, 1988.

Mitchell DG, Crovello M, Matteucci T, et al: Benign adrenocortical masses: diagnosis with chemical shift MR imaging, *Radiology* 185:345–351, 1992.

Miyake H, Maeda H, Tashiro M, et al: CT of adrenal tumors: frequency and clinical significance of low-attenuation lesions, *AJR Am J Radiol* 152:1005–1007, 1989.

Oliver TW Jr, Bernardino ME, Miller JI, et al: Isolated adrenal masses in nonsmall-cell bronchogenic carcinoma, *Radiology* 153:217–218, 1984.

Reinig JW, Stutley JE, Leonhardt CM, et al: Differentiation of adrenal masses with MR imaging: comparison of techniques, *Radiology* 192:41–46, 1994.

Silverman SG, Mueller PM, Pinkney LP, et al: Predictive value of image-guided adrenal biopsy: analysis of results in 101 biopsies, *Radiology* 187:715–718, 1993.

Tsushima Y, Ishizaka H, Matsumoto M: Adrenal masses: differentiation with chemical shift, fast low-angle shot MR imaging, *Radiology* 186:705–709, 1993.

Vita JA, Silverberg SJ, Goland RS, et al: Clinical clues to the cause of Addison's disease, *Am J Med* 78:461–466, 1985.

Welch TJ, Sheedy PF III, van Heerden JA, et al: Pheochromocytoma: value of computed tomography, *Radiology* 148:501–503, 1983.

CHAPTER 10

Interventional Genitourinary Radiology

In the genitourinary system, as in other organ systems, radiologically guided interventional procedures have grown in popularity and usage over the past two decades. Interventional genitourinary radiology procedures are widely used, and familiarity and experience with these procedures are necessary in most clinical settings. Growth in the use of these procedures results from the minimally invasive nature of percutaneous procedures. Advantages include shortened hospital stay, diminished need for anesthesia, lower costs, and rapid recuperation after the procedures. Also driving the increase in popularity for interventional procedures have been improvements in equipment, including imaging equipment improvements and catheter and guidewire technology advances. Along with the advancing technology and increasing experience with minimally invasive procedures, the applications of interventional genitourinary procedures also have grown.

PERCUTANEOUS INTERVENTIONAL URINARY TRACT PROCEDURES

Patient Selection and Preparation

Before percutaneous puncture of the urinary system is undertaken, basic coagulation profile (prothrombin time [PT], partial thromboplastin time [PTT], and platelet count) should be obtained (Box 10-1). Abnormalities should be reversed whenever possible. In patients with thrombocytopenia, platelet transfusion can be performed before and during percutaneous urinary tract procedures. A platelet count more than 50,000 is desirable before percutaneous renal puncture, although lower platelet counts may be acceptable if the procedure is considered extremely urgent.

Antibiotics should be administered before urinary tract puncture (Box 10-2). If no urinary infection is suspected, a broad-spectrum antibiotic (usually a cephalosporin) can be administered immediately before the procedure and every 8 hours while the patient is hospitalized, for as long as 24 hours. Antibiotic administration can be discontinued after the procedure if the patient has no evidence of infection when discharged. If urinary tract infection is suspected but no specific organism has been cultured, the combination of an aminoglycoside and ampicillin or a similar penicillin derivative should be administered immediately before the procedure. Patients in this category include those with evidence of ongoing urinary tract infection and those with a high risk of asymptomatic urinary tract infection, e.g., patients with urinary conduit diversions or with infection-based stones. Ideally, culture-specific antibiotics should be given before percutaneous urinary intervention in patients with known urinary tract infection. In addition, a bladder catheter should be placed in most patients, because procedures may be protracted and urination with the patient in the prone position will be difficult. Finally, signed informed consent should be obtained before the procedure, with its indications and risks explained to the patient.

Imaging Guidance

Most percutaneous urinary tract procedures involve transrenal puncture, which usually is performed with fluoroscopic guidance. However, initial localization of the kidney can be performed with the guidance of ultrasonography. In rare cases, computed tomography (CT) guidance can be used for transrenal urinary tract procedures. CT is especially useful to ensure a safe transrenal puncture in patients whose congenital urinary tract anomalies or abnormalities of surrounding organs can be visualized only with CT guidance. Almost all procedures can be performed with standard fluoroscopic guidance. Although a fluoroscopic system that allows angulation of the image intensifier is ideal for percutaneous transrenal procedures, these procedures can be performed readily with most fluoroscopic equipment.

Antegrade Pyelography and the Whitaker Test

Antegrade pyelography, which entails simple percutaneous puncture and opacification of the collecting system and ureter, is performed for radiographic evaluation of the ureter and collecting system. Antegrade pyelography may be useful for patients with suspected urinary tract abnormalities who have contraindications to intravascular administration of contrast material or for those who have poorly functioning or obstructed kidneys. This

procedure also may be performed as a prelude to percutaneous nephrostomy drainage or Whitaker testing. The Whitaker test is used to evaluate and quantify suspected ureteral obstruction (Box 10-3). The Whitaker test is an extension of antegrade pyelography. Both require fine-needle puncture and opacification of the intrarenal collecting system. With Whitaker testing, active infusion of dilute contrast material is used to evaluate the capacitance of the urinary system to transmit varying fluid volumes. After or during dynamic infusion, pressure gradients are measured between the renal pelvis and the bladder, and obstructions, when present, can be quantified. The Whitaker test is the most objective measure of the urodynamic significance of areas of ureteral narrowing or of collecting system dilatation. The Whitaker test yields objective, reproducible data that can be essential for management planning. Specifically, Whitaker testing commonly is used to evaluate ureteropelvic junction (UPJ) strictures or other ureteral strictures to determine the need for percutaneous or open surgical repair. In addition, percutaneous pyelography and Whitaker testing often are useful in the evaluation of a hydronephrotic transplant kidney. Because of the potential nephrotoxicity of intravascular contrast material and the minimal risk associated with antegrade pyelography, this procedure often is selected to evaluate transplanted kidneys in patients with suspected obstructive uropathy.

Antegrade pyelography and the Whitaker test are performed after fine-needle puncture of the intrarenal collecting system. A 21- or 22-gauge thin-wall needle is adequate for these procedures. Fine-needle puncture of the kidney is associated with low risk of vascular injury and sepsis. Numerous transrenal punctures with a 21- or 22-gauge needle may be performed with relative impunity because of the low risk of significant complications.

When the bladder has been catheterized and the patient is in prone position on the fluoroscopy table, the flank is cleansed and draped according to standard sterile techniques. The kidney is localized with either fluoroscopy or ultrasonography. Sometimes a previously obtained abdominal radiograph can be used as a reference for identifying renal position. If the kidney is not readily visible, a puncture site can be selected empirically 2 to 3 cm lateral to the top of the L2 vertebral body. Before puncture, local anesthetic should be administered. For

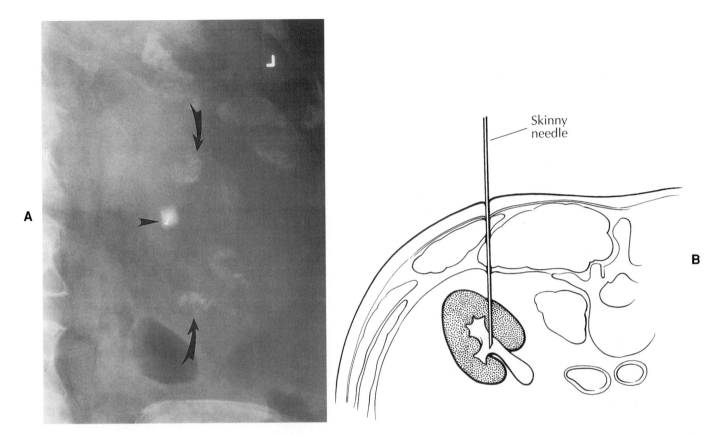

Fig. 10-1 Percutaneous needle puncture of the kidney for antegrade pyelography. **A,** A prone radiograph of the left kidney in a patient with numerous stone fragments (curved arrows) in calyces after extracorporeal lithotripsy. Antegrade pyelography is being performed before percutaneous nephrostomy drainage. A skinny needle has been passed (arrowhead) in a vertical direction in the region of the renal pelvis with the patient in a prone position. **B,** Diagram of skinny needle puncture of the right kidney in a patient in the prone position. The needle is passed in a vertical direction into the region of the renal pelvis.

transrenal puncture, the skinny needle is passed in a vertical direction (Fig. 10-1) while the patient suspends respiration. In patients with normal body habitus, the needle should be advanced 10 to 12 cm with a single pass. The needle stylet then should be removed, and a syringe is attached to the needle. The needle then can be withdrawn while continuous aspiration is applied. When aspiration returns urine, withdrawal is halted. The urine aspirate should be saved for culturing. Iodinated contrast material then can be injected into the urinary system via the skinny needle. Once satisfactory needle position has been confirmed fluoroscopically with opacification of the intrarenal collecting system, more contrast material may be injected under intermittent fluoroscopic monitoring. Overdistension of the collecting system should be avoided to minimize the risk of sepsis. Overdistension can lead to pyelovenous backflow of urine, carrying along any pathogens contained in the urine. To avoid overdistension, a "transfusion" technique should be used. With this technique, an equal volume of pure

contrast material is injected after the withdrawal of a volume of urine and dilute contrast material via the needle. With this procedure, opacification of the urinary system is slower, but overdistension is avoided because the volume of contrast material injected matches the volume of urine withdrawn.

For antegrade pyelography, spot films are obtained as needed to demonstrate the entire pelvocalyceal system and ureter, with particular attention to the sites of suspected abnormality. If significant obstruction is identified, a percutaneous nephrostomy drain can be placed. Alternatively, if no significant obstruction is seen or if a drain is not required, antegrade pyelography can be terminated, and the needle withdrawn. If no obstruction is encountered and if a drain is not placed during this procedure, antibiotics should be continued for at least 24 hours after the procedure is terminated.

The Whitaker test is performed after opacification of the collecting system for antegrade pyelography. Opacification is performed to ensure that the needle is in the

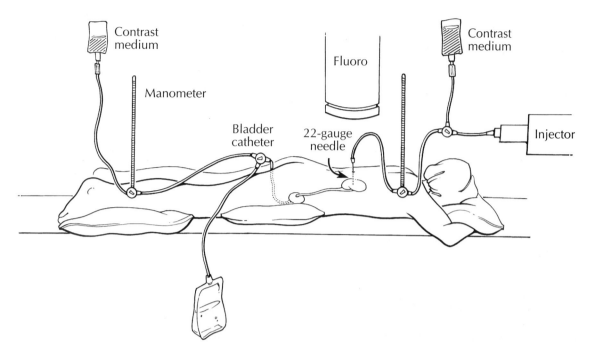

Fig. 10-2 Equipment set-up for urodynamic (Whitaker) test of ureteral capacitance.

correct position without extravasation outside the urinary tract. The equipment needed for the Whitaker test is somewhat complex (Fig. 10-2). With the needle in place, the bladder is emptied, and manometers, infusion lines, a power infusion pump, and a bladder drainage conduit are connected. The two manometers should be placed at an equal height above the floor. Bladder and renal pelvic pressures are measured before and immediately after each timed infusion. For the Whitaker test, dilute contrast material is infused into the renal pelvis at a rate of 5 mL per minute for 10 minutes. Pressures are measured and recorded. The second infusion is performed at a rate of 10 mL per minute for 10 minutes, and, finally, a third infusion is performed at a rate of 15 mL per minute for 10 minutes. Infusions should be discontinued immediately if adjusted renal pelvis pressure exceeds 40 cm of water, if severe flank pain develops, or if significant contrast material extravasation occurs. If results are equivocal from this initial series of infusions, the test is repeated with the bladder filled. On occasion, mild obstruction may become evident with increased pressure only with a full bladder. The patient should be instructed to notify personnel during the procedure if symptoms are reproduced during infusion of contrast material. The reproduction of symptoms, such as flank pain, supports the presence of urodynamically significant obstruction.

Adjusted renal pelvic pressures are calculated by subtracting the bladder pressure from the renal pelvic pressure, thereby removing the component of general intraabdominal pressure from the measurements. Table 10-1 outlines a system for classifying the numeric results of the Whitaker test and converting them to degree of ureteral obstruction.

Percutaneous Nephrostomy Drainage

Indications for percutaneous nephrostomy (PN) drainage are numerous. The most common indications are decompression of an obstructed kidney, urinary diversion for management of urinary tract fistula or perforation, decompression of an infected urinary tract, or as a prelude to additional urinary tract interventions, such as stent placement or endoscopy. The risks of PN (Table 10-2) include septicemia (2%), life-threatening hemorrhage (1% to 2%), and adjacent organ injury (1%). The only absolute contraindication is the presence of an uncorrected bleeding disorder.

With this procedure as with other percutaneous

Table 10-1 Interpretation of Whitaker Test Results	
Differential pressure (cm H$_2$O)	Degree of obstruction
0–12	None
13–20	Mild
21–34	Moderate
More than 34	Severe

Table 10-2   Major Complications of Percutaneous Nephrostomy Drainage

Complication	Rate (%)
Sepsis	2
Hemorrhage requiring transfusion	2
Adjacent organ injury	1

transrenal procedures, antibiotics should be preadministered. The choice of antibiotics has been outlined previously in this section (Box 10-2). Selection of the transrenal puncture site is important to avoid unnecessary vascular injury. Ideally, the nephrostomy tract should traverse the kidney near the junction of the ventral two thirds and the dorsal one third of the kidney. This area is known as Brodel's line or the avascular plane (Fig. 10-3) of the kidney. It represents a watershed zone that is supplied by only small vessel ramifications from the anterior and posterior renal artery branches (Fig. 10-4). This plane has been used for renal surgical procedures to minimize renal atrophy after surgery. The location of

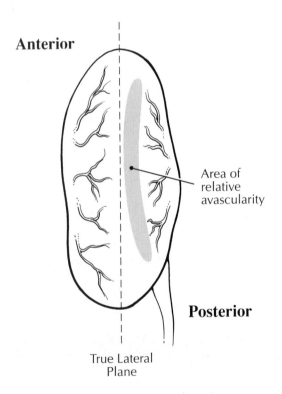

Anterior

Area of relative avascularity

Posterior

True Lateral Plane

Fig. 10-3   Diagram demonstrating the area of relative avascularity in the kidney. It is most desirable to perform transrenal puncture of the kidney through this region of the renal parenchyma. This area represents a watershed zone between the distributions of the anterior and posterior divisions of the renal artery. There are no large blood vessels in the renal parenchyma in this plane.

the avascular plane can be estimated by using real time sonography, CT, or fluoroscopy. In most cases, the simplest technique for guiding transrenal puncture is fluoroscopy with opacification of the collecting system, which can be performed via antegrade pyelography through a skinny needle, with intravenous urography (IVU), or with retrograde injection of contrast material via a stent or through a urinary conduit diversion. Posterior calyces should be identifiable with opacification. These calyces usually are positioned more medially than anterior calyces. In addition, they generally are seen en face when imaged in the anteroposterior plane (Fig. 10-5). Identification of posterior calyces can be enhanced in patients in the prone position by injecting small volumes (5 to 10 mL) of room air into the calyces; the air will flow to fill these dorsally oriented structures. Once the posterior calyces have been identified, selection of the exact calyx to be punctured will depend on position of the calyx and intention of the procedure. If the procedure is being performed to divert urine or decompress an obstructed system, a posterior calyx located below the twelfth rib should be selected for transrenal puncture. If additional interventions, such as stent placement, are likely, puncture of a calyx in the upper pole will make access to the ureter or to specific areas of the kidney more easily achieved. The selected posterior calyx should be punctured from a posterior obliquity of 25° to 30° from the vertical position (Figs. 10-6, 10-7), which can be achieved by leaving the patient in the prone position and angling the fluoroscopy tube 25° to 30°. The kidney then can be punctured along the axis of the fluoroscopic beam, assuring an appropriate approach. Alternatively, the patient's ipsilateral flank can be elevated 25° to 30° when vertical fluoroscopy is used. After the puncture site is identified with fluoroscopic localization, the area of skin in line with the planned site of calyceal entry should be anesthetized with lidocaine, 1%, without epinephrine. Superficial and deep skin anesthetization should be performed along the anticipated puncture tract before transrenal puncture. A small skin incision is made with a scalpel at the site of intended puncture. The calyx then is punctured with an 18- to 22-gauge needle under continuous fluoroscopic monitoring while the patient suspends respiration (Fig. 10-8 on p. 378). Use of a radiolucent needle holder (Fig. 10-9 on p. 378) allows fluoroscopic needle guidance while avoiding radiation exposure to and obscuration by the operator's hand. Actual puncture of the calyx can be seen fluoroscopically (Fig. 10-10 on p. 379). Urine can be aspirated to confirm needle position. An angiographic guidewire (0.035 to 0.038 inch) then should be advanced into the collecting system. Once an adequate length of guidewire has been placed within the intrarenal collecting system, the needle is removed, and an angiographic catheter can be advanced along the guidewire (Fig. 10-11 on p. 379). The catheter

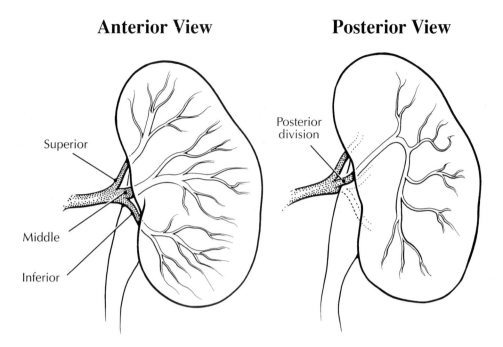

Anterior View   **Posterior View**

Superior

Middle

Inferior

Posterior
division

Fig. 10-4   Normal renal artery anatomy. This diagram shows standard renal artery anatomy. There is a single posterior renal artery branch supplying the dorsal one-third of the renal parenchyma. The anterior renal artery branch trifurcates into three major divisions. The distribution of this artery supplies the ventral two-thirds of the kidney.

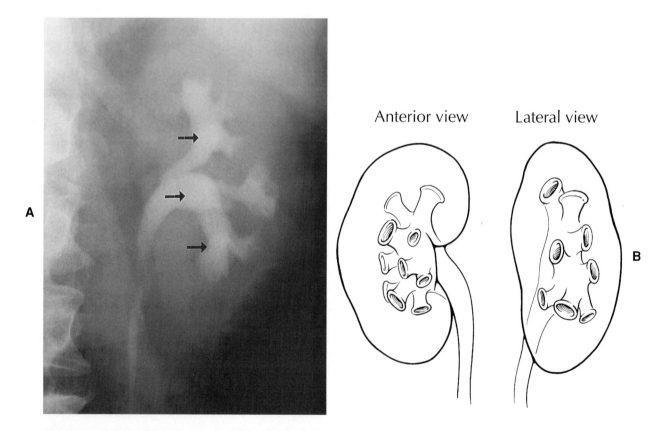

A

B

Anterior view   Lateral view

Fig. 10-5   Normal calyceal anatomy. **A,** This radiograph from a urogram and the accompanying diagram, **B,** demonstrate normal calyceal anatomy. Calyces that are seen in profile on an anterior view usually are anterior calyces. The calyces seen en face as circles (arrows) are posteriorly oriented calyces. Posterior calyces are preferred for puncture for percutaneous drainage procedures.

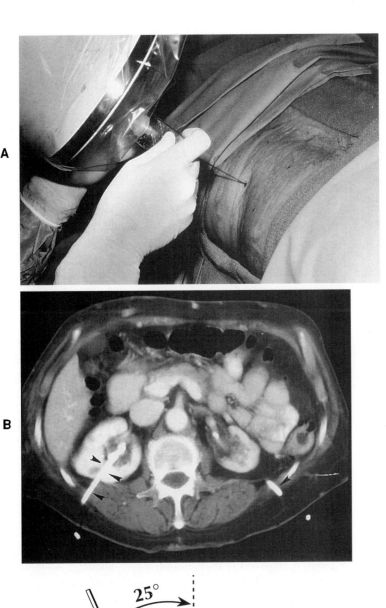

Fig. 10-6 Posterior oblique percutaneous transrenal puncture. **A,** With the patient in a prone position, the fluoroscopic image intensifier can be rotated 25° from vertical. The percutaneous needle then is passed into the kidney along the axis of the image intensifier to ensure proper angulation of the entry tract. **B,** CT of a different patient with bilateral nephrostomy tubes. The oblique transrenal tract (arrowheads) goes through the relatively avascular region of the kidneys.

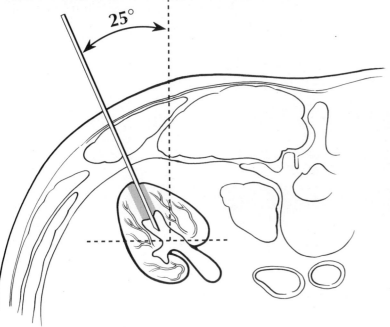

Fig. 10-7 Transrenal puncture technique. Diagram depicting ideal transrenal puncture location. Puncture of a posterior calyx from a 25° angle should traverse the zone of relative avascularity and avoid large renal artery branches.

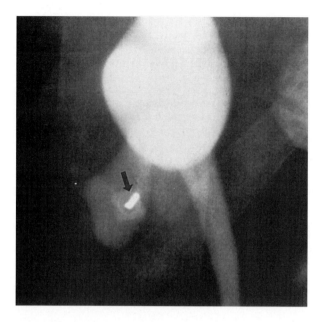

Fig. 10-8 Fluoroscopic image of the posterior oblique puncture technique of a calyx. This fluoroscopic image taken from a 25° posterior oblique angle demonstrates the needle (arrow) in line with the axis of the image intensifier and the calyx to be punctured.

selected will depend on the operator's preference, but a standard catheter shaped like a hockey stick works well with most patients. The catheter steers the guidewire into a stable position for additional tract dilatation. Ideally, the guidewire can be advanced well into the ureter to decrease the risk of dislodging the guidewire during additional manipulations. Once the guidewire is positioned, the catheter is removed, and the tract is dilated over the guidewire to an appropriate size for nephrostomy tube placement (Fig. 10-12). For simple urine drainage, an 8-

to 10-F tube is adequate. For a solitary kidney or for drainage of viscous urine, i.e., infected or hemorrhagic urine, tubes 12 to 14 F in diameter are recommended. To avoid unnecessary accidental dislodgment of the PN tubes, only self-retaining nephrostomy tubes should be used (Fig. 10-13). Before terminating the procedure, contrast material should be injected through the PN tube to confirm satisfactory position and function of the drainage catheter.

A patient who remains in the hospital should be visited daily for approximately 3 days to ensure adequate PN tube function. Urine output should be monitored carefully while the patient is hospitalized. Some hematuria is expected for up to 72 hours after PN tube placement. In addition, bacteriuria occurs in nearly all patients with prolonged PN drainage. This bacteriuria is of no clinical significance if urinary drainage is adequate; i.e., the nephrostomy tube is patent. Nephrostomy tubes should be changed prophylactically every 4 to 8 weeks to avoid tube obstruction. Shorter tube-change intervals may be required in some patients, but intervals more than 8 weeks should be avoided because tube occlusion can lead to dramatic and rapid onset of significant clinical problems. Obstructed urinary outflow coupled with bacteriuria can lead to rapid development of pyonephrosis and septicemia, and exchange of an obstructed PN tube is technically more demanding than exchanging a patent PN tube.

Ureteral Stenting

Ureteral stents can be placed for the maintenance of ureteral patency in patients with urolithiasis and in those with benign or malignant strictures. In addition, ureteral stents can enhance ureteral healing while minimizing risk

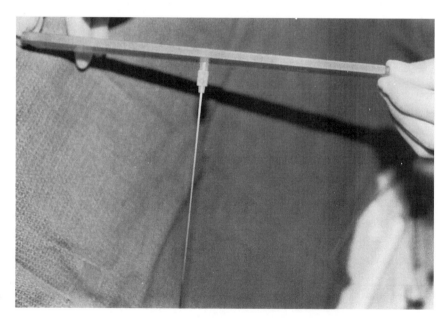

Fig. 10-9 Radiolucent needle holder for percutaneous transrenal puncture. A lucite needle holder can be used so that the needle can be passed under continuous fluoroscopic monitoring and avoid exposure to the operator's hands.

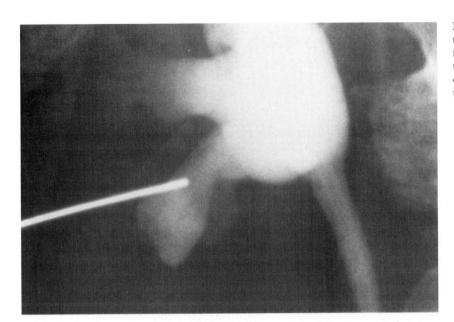

Fig. 10-10   Calyceal puncture. Following transrenal advancement of the needle, the fluoroscopic tube is replaced to a vertical position. Calyceal puncture can be seen easily fluoroscopically with the image intensifier in this position.

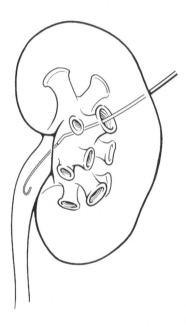

Fig. 10-11   Using a steerable catheter to advance the guidewire into a stable position. This diagram demonstrates standard catheter and guidewire technique to steer the guidewire into a stable position for additional manipulation before placing a percutaneous nephrostomy drain. Ideally, the guidewire should be advanced down the ureter.

of stricturing in patients with ureteral fistulas or in those who have undergone endoluminal ureteral manipulations, including endopyelotomy, which entails transmural incision of the ureteral wall, and ureteral balloon dilatation.

The risks associated with placement of percutaneous antegrade ureteral stents are similar to those associated with placement of PN tubes. Ureteral perforation occa-

sionally occurs during attempts at ureteral stent placement. Although ureteral perforation may interfere with completion of stent placement, the perforations are self-limited and of little clinical significance if adequate renal drainage is maintained after the procedure.

Usually, percutaneous ureteral stent placement is requested after PN drainage. Transrenal percutaneous puncture and tract dilatation should be performed as outlined previously for PN drainage procedures. For stent placement, transrenal access via a mid or upper calyx is preferred to provide the most favorable approach down the ureter. Before additional manipulation, two guidewires should be placed. This task can be accomplished by using a sheathed dilator (Fig. 10-14). One of these wires will be used as a working wire, and the other should remain in place as a safety guidewire for use if the working wire becomes dislodged or kinked. With standard angiographic techniques, the working wire then can be steered through the UPJ. Often, use of a hydrophilic guidewire facilitates these manipulations. The angiographic guidewire should be advanced down the length of the ureter and into the bladder. An angiographic catheter could be advanced over the guidewire so that its tip reaches the bladder lumen. The next step, determining the correct stent length, can be achieved with various methods, but the most direct uses the bent-guidewire technique (Fig. 10-15 on p. 382). With the catheter tip within the bladder, a guidewire is advanced so that its tip is within the catheter just below the ureterovesical junction. This guidewire then is kinked at its exit from the catheter hub outside the patient's flank. The guidewire then is retracted further until the tip, which is within the angiographic catheter, is in the renal pelvis. Its location is visible readily with fluoroscopy. A second kink is made where the guidewire exits the catheter hub outside

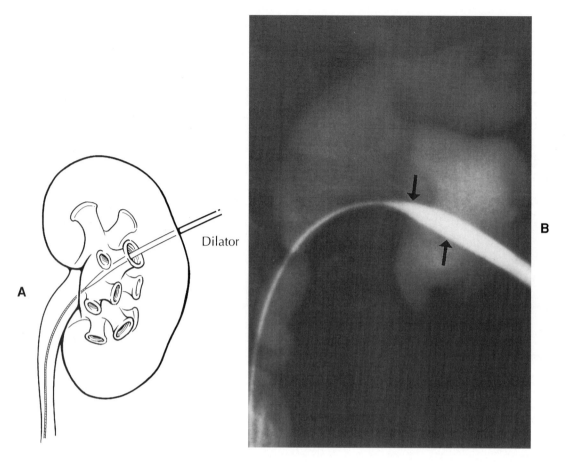

Fig. 10-12 Nephrostomy tract dilatation. **A,** Diagram of a fascial dilatator being advanced over the guidewire to dilate the transrenal nephrostomy tract. **B,** Radiograph demonstrating a dilator (arrows) being advanced transrenally over the working guidewire.

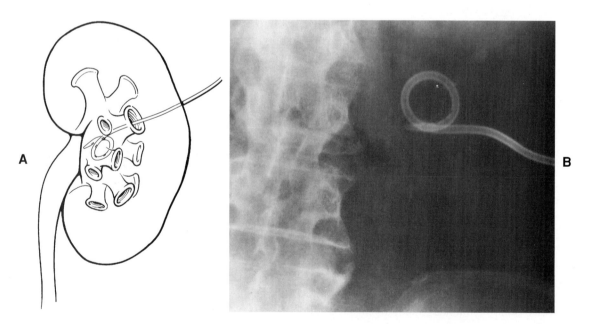

Fig. 10-13 Self-retaining nephrostomy tube in place. **A,** Diagram of a standard self-retaining nephrostomy tube in place with the tip coiled in the renal pelvis. This catheter has a string that forces it to maintain its pigtail configuration. **B,** Radiograph demonstrating the typical radiographic appearance of a standard self-retaining percutaneous nephrostomy catheter.

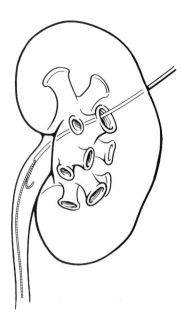

Fig. 10-14   Placement of a safety guidewire for complex transrenal manipulations. This diagram demonstrates the technique for placing a second guidewire through the existing nephrostomy tract. A sheathed dilator is advanced over the working guidewire. The dilator segment is removed, leaving the sheath in place through which additional guidewires can be advanced.

the patient's flank. The guidewire then is removed completely, and the catheter is left in place. The distance between the two guidewire kinks provides an exact measurement between the ureterovesical junction and the renal pelvis and therefore determines the length of the straight segment of the ureteral stent to be placed. A new working guidewire then should be advanced into the catheter. A stiff angiographic guidewire is preferred for stent placement. The catheter then is removed, and the stiff working guidewire is left in place. A tapered 8-F angiographic catheter then is advanced over the guidewire into the bladder. This catheter is used to test for stenotic areas that might impede placement of the ureteral stent. If no resistance is encountered, a stent, 8 F or smaller, can be placed without additional manipulation. If resistance is encountered, the 8-F catheter is removed and replaced over the guidewire with a 9-F sheathed dilator. This sheath should be advanced as close to the bladder as possible to facilitate stent placement. The dilator segment then is removed, and the ureteral sheath is left in place over the working guidewire. With or without the sheath, the stent then is advanced over the guidewire until the tip of the stent is well within the bladder. If an adequate length of stent has been advanced into the bladder, then on retracting the working guidewire, the lower loop of the ureteral stent will form within the bladder lumen. If the length is inadequate, the guidewire should be readvanced through the stent, followed

by additional advancement of the stent itself. If ureteral stenosis prevents adequate advancement of the stent, balloon dilatation of the stenotic ureter should be performed. Balloons 6 to 10 mm in diameter routinely are used for ureteroplasty. The entire stenotic segment should be dilated with a balloon before an attempt is made to replace the ureteral stent. High-pressure balloons often are required to dilate malignant or chronic benign ureteral strictures.

After advancing an adequate length of the stent into the bladder, the guidewire is retracted, and the lower coil of the stent is reconstituted within the bladder. Fluoroscopy of the renal end of the stent then is performed to estimate whether an adequate length of stent remains to allow reconstitution of the upper loop within the renal pelvis. If the stent has been advanced too far distally, it can be retracted by applying traction to the suture threaded through its proximal end. Once positioned for final stent placement, the introducer sheath, if used, is removed. The retracting suture then is removed while the stent is maintained in a stable position with gentle pressure on the pusher catheter. After removal of the suture, the guidewire is retracted further so only the flexible portion of the guidewire remains within the proximal end of the ureteral stent, which allows the upper loop to begin to reconstitute and avoids inadvertent advancement of the stent into an unsatisfactorily low position. With only the floppy portion of the guidewire in the stent, the pusher is used to advance the stent through the remaining segment of the nephrostomy tract and into the renal pelvis while the guidewire is withdrawn simultaneously. This technique causes the upper loop of the stent to form within the renal pelvis.

Once the stent has been placed, the safety guidewire can be used to position a small-bore nephrostomy catheter for temporary maintenance of the nephrostomy tract. The nephrostomy catheter should be left in place for 12 to 24 hours to confirm that the ureteral stent is functional. If no symptoms of ureteral occlusion develop, the nephrostomy tube can be removed after a nephrostogram demonstrates satisfactory position and function of the ureteral stent. The nephrostomy tube should be removed under fluoroscopic guidance to ensure that the ureteral stent is not dislodged inadvertently during tube removal. The nephrostomy tract will close spontaneously during the next 4 days.

In some patients, a ureteral stent may be desirable, but the nephrostomy tract should be maintained for future percutaneous procedures or stent changes. In these patients, an alternative method of stenting is placement of an internal and external ureteral stent. This technique uses a single catheter that extends from the patient's flank through the kidney, down the ureter, and into the bladder (Fig. 10-16). These catheters are available commercially, or they may be tailored from an extra-length

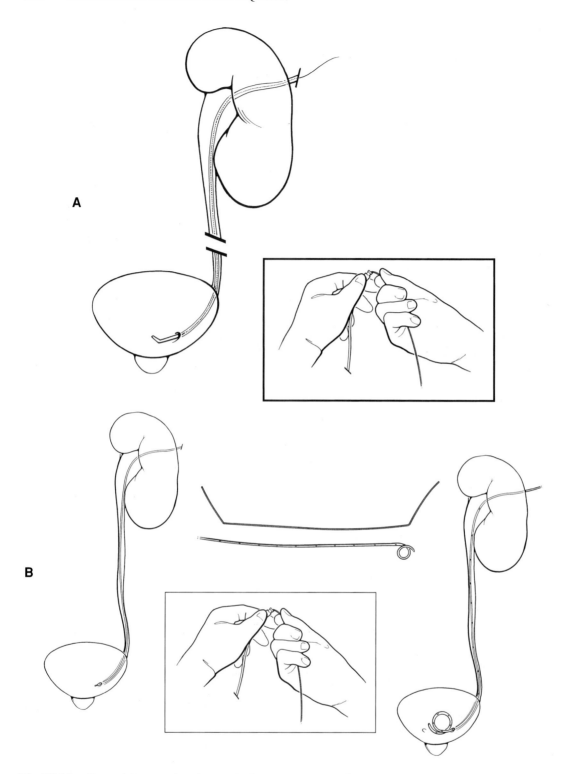

Fig. 10-15   Determining stent length using the bent-guidewire technique. **A,** This diagram demonstrates the bent-guidewire technique used to determine stent length. Through a catheter advanced beyond the ureterovesical junction (UVJ), a guidewire is advanced so that its tip is at the UVJ. The guidewire is kinked externally at the hub of the catheter. **B,** The guidewire then is retracted until its tip is in the renal pelvis as seen fluoroscopically. The external portion of the guidewire again is kinked at the hub of the catheter. The guidewire then is removed, and stent length is determined by the distance between the two kinks. That length is exactly the length from the UVJ to the renal pelvis.

Internal/external

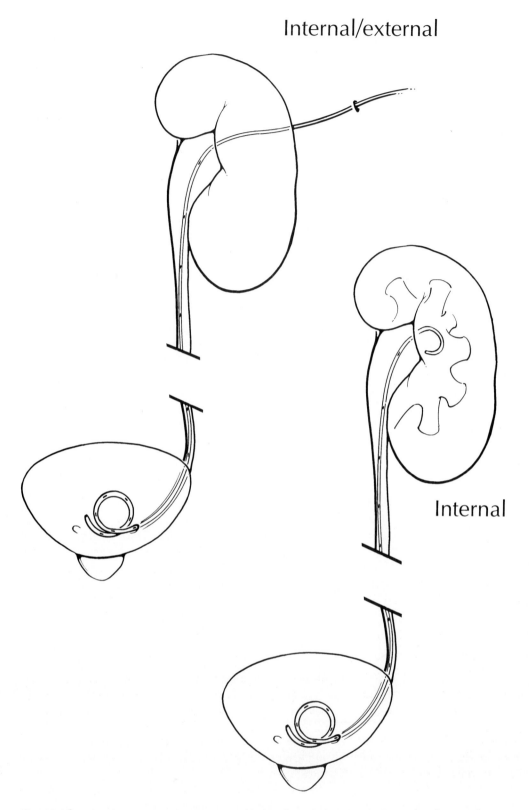

Internal

Fig. 10-16 Two basic types of percutaneously placed ureteral stents. An internal and external ureteral stent can be used to stent the ureter and maintain percutaneous access via the transrenal tract. Alternatively, an internal ureteral stent can be placed via the percutaneous tract.

nephrostomy tube. Varying numbers of side holes may be placed along the length of this catheter, extending from the renal pelvis to the bladder. For management of ureteral fistulas or perforations, side holes should be placed above and below the site of ureteral injury, and placement of side holes in the area of ureteral leakage should be avoided. This facilitates healing of the ureteral wall and supplies adequate urinary drainage. These internal and external ureteral stents should be used when ureteral stenting is indicated but prolonged percutaneous renal access is desired. Once placed, the external limb of these catheters may be capped, and the catheter functions as an internal ureteral stent but with preservation of the transrenal tract. This type of catheter routinely is used for management of ureteral fistulas and perforations and following ureteral dilatation because follow-up imaging studies, such as pyelography, and repeated dilatation procedures usually are required.

The procedure for placement of these stents closely parallels placement of internal ureteral stents. The bent-wire technique is used to determine the location of the side holes to be placed in the catheter for drainage. Modification of these standard nephrostomy catheters entails fashioning side holes along the desired length of the catheter shaft.

Long-term management of internal ureteral stents is assumed by urologists. Once these stents are placed, they can be removed or replaced in a retrograde fashion by means of a cystoscope. Internal and external ureteral stents should be changed prophylactically every 4 to 6 weeks to avoid stent occlusion. Pyelography should be performed whenever a stent is replaced to assess the status of the ureter and to confirm that the new ureteral stent is positioned appropriately. A new internal and external ureteral stent must be placed so that side holes in the catheter are advanced beyond the renal parenchyma. If not, parenchymal bleeding will persist and lead to premature tube occlusion.

Percutaneous Nephrolithotomy and Other Transrenal Endoscopic Procedures

Transrenal endoscopy is used for fragmentation and removal of urinary tract calculi, for endoscopic surgical procedures such as endopyelotomy, and for inspection and possible biopsy of the urothelium. Transrenal urinary tract endoscopy requires larger transrenal tracts; for rigid endoscopes, a percutaneous transrenal tract 10 mm in diameter is created.

Approximately 80% to 90% of kidney stones can be managed nonsurgically with extracorporeal shock wave lithotripsy (ESWL), although some renal calculi and ureteral stones are refractory to ESWL management and require percutaneous fragmentation and removal. Percutaneous stone removal procedures are preferred to other

---

Box 10-4 Indications for Percutaneous Nephrolithotomy

Large stone volume
   Single stone >2 to 2.5 cm in diameter
   Multiples stones with >2.5 to 3 cm in aggregate
    diameter
   Staghorn calculus
Stones refractory to extracorporeal lithotripsy
Partial or complete ureteral obstruction
Patient unsuitable for extracorporeal lithotripsy

---

techniques when renal stones are larger than 25 mm in diameter, are branched in configuration, are composed of cystine, or are associated with ureteral obstruction (Box 10-4). In addition, some patients may exceed the weight limitations of a lithotripsy device, eliminating ESWL as an option for stone management. Finally, in some patients, complete and unequivocal stone removal absolutely is essential; in these settings, percutaneous stone removal is preferred.

Large-bore tracts may be created for other endoscopic procedures. Most common in this group are the endoscopic surgical procedures, such as endopyelotomy. Endopyelotomy is used to manage benign strictures of the ureter, most of which are located at the UPJ and are thought to be congenital in origin. Endopyelotomy is an alternative to open surgical pyeloplasty for management of primary ureteral strictures or strictures that recur after initial surgical repair. Under endoscopic visualization, the stenotic segment of ureter is incised longitudinally. The incision is transmural and is considered adequate when periureteral fat is visualized endoscopically. After incision, the stenotic segment is balloon-dilated and stented. The advantages of endopyelotomy are those inherent in minimally invasive surgical procedures, including decreased cost, shortened hospitalization, and shortened recuperative period. Also, the effectiveness of endopyelotomy as management for primary ureteral strictures is comparable with that of open surgical procedures. Finally, endopyelotomy has an advantage over open surgery in the management of secondary strictures, for which follow-up open surgical procedures are complex and less commonly result in adequate resolution of strictures.

Other endoscopic procedures that are less commonly performed include transrenal inspection and biopsy of the renal collecting system and the ureter, which are performed generally on patients with filling defects or strictures when the underlying tissue diagnosis is unknown. Endoscopic procedures can be performed as an alternative to open surgical inspection or surgical procedures for biopsy access. A transrenal approach seldom is used for this application because most ureteral and pyelocalyceal lesions can be reached in a retrograde fashion with a flexible ureteroscope, avoiding the need to create a transrenal tract.

The risks associated with large-bore nephrostomy tract creation are similar to those for standard PN tube placement, including renal hemorrhage necessitating blood transfusion (up to 10% of patients), sepsis (2%), and adjacent organ injury (1%). The only absolute contraindication for this procedure is an uncorrected coagulopathy. In addition, if rigid nephroscopy is planned, large-bore tract creation is subject to length limitations. Most standard rigid endoscopes have a working length of 20 cm or less, which is slightly longer than the standard nephrostomy sheaths supplied by manufacturers. In large patients, the skin-to-calyx distance may exceed 20 cm. In these patients, flexible endoscopy can be performed through a nephrostomy tract that has been allowed to mature by keeping a large-bore PN drainage tube after initial tract creation. This tube should be left in place at least 7 days before attempting transrenal endoscopy without a nephroscopic sheath. If excessive skin-to-calyx length is anticipated, a limited CT scan at the level of the kidney should be performed with the patient in a prone position to estimate tract length before initiating the nephrostomy procedure.

Before the procedure, antibiotics should be administered as outlined in the section concerning placement of the PN tube (Box 10-2). Because many patients with a large stone burden will harbor infection-based stones, antibiotic prophylaxis is crucial. A posterior calyx should be selected for transrenal puncture and tract creation. Because access to a certain area within the pyelocalyceal system or the ureter is desired, site selection for puncture is crucial. For nephrostolithotomy, an upper pole calyx generally allows endoscopic access to the largest segment of the intrarenal collecting system. To minimize complications, transrenal puncture should be performed below the twelfth rib. For the upper pole, puncturing between the eleventh and twelfth ribs often is required and should be considered safe. Because the pleural reflection commonly extends to the eleventh rib or lower, puncturing above the eleventh rib should be avoided because of the high risk of transpleural tract passage and resulting pneumothorax, hemothorax, and empyema. Calyceal puncture technique is outlined previously in this chapter, and the initial steps for large-bore nephrostomy tract creation are the same (Fig. 10-17). However, after placement of a heavy-duty guidewire and a safety guidewire, the tract is dilated to 9 F with a fascial dilator. The next dilatation can be performed with a high-pressure balloon dilatation catheter (Fig. 10-17). The inflated diameter should be 10 mm, and the balloon length should be 10 to 12 cm. This length will allow dilatation of the entire tract with one or two balloon inflations. After dilatation of the tract, the balloon catheter is removed, and placement of a 10-mm sheathed dilator is attempted (Fig. 10-17). If balloon dilatation incompletely dilates the entire tract, smaller semirigid fascial dilators may be used to dilate the tract gradually to the maximum diameter of 10 mm. The sheathed dilator then can be placed over the guidewire, the dilator removed, and the guidewires and nephroscopy sheath left in place (Fig. 10-17). Endoscopy can be performed through this sheath immediately, or a drainage catheter can be passed through the sheath if endoscopy is deferred. Placing a safety catheter over the safety guidewire is advisable after placement of a large-bore drainage catheter. A standard 5-F angiographic catheter can serve as a "safety" catheter; it should be advanced over the safety wire so that its tip is in a stable position, preferably within the bladder. At the end of the procedure, both nephrostomy catheters should be sutured to the skin, and the large-bore tube should be left to external drainage to allow outflow of urine and residual blood clot. The patient should be visited daily for at least 3 days, if hospitalized, to assure tube function and to identify possible nephrostomy complications early. Possible tube-related complications include kinking, retraction, and occlusion. Urine output should be monitored carefully. Hematuria routinely lasts as long as 72 hours, but hematocrit levels should be monitored if hematuria is excessive. If large-bore PN drainage catheters are left in place, they should be changed prophylactically every 6 to 8 weeks.

With meticulous and thorough endoscopic techniques, stone-free rates of 85% or higher can be achieved with percutaneous nephrolithotomy. In patients with complex-shaped stones, multiple transrenal nephrostomy tracts may be required to reach fragments clustered in isolated segments of the kidney. In addition, adjunctive procedures, such as ESWL or chemolysis, may be required to complete stone removal after percutaneous debulking when stones with very complex shapes are present. Chemolysis infusion systems easily are placed via the percutaneous nephrostomy tracts, which initially were used for stone removal. These infusion systems use an inflow and outflow catheter for the infusion of agents that bathe and slowly dissolve the residual stone fragments. Large-bore PN drainage catheters also are useful after adjunctive ESWL because they serve as a low-resistance outflow pathway for stone fragments.

In performing endopyelotomy, care must be taken because UPJ strictures sometimes form as a result of chronic ureteral compression by aberrant renal arteries or veins. Because these accessory vessels nearly always cross anteriorly to the ureter, the transmural incision should be performed posterolaterally through the wall of the ureter (Fig. 10-18) to avoid vascular injury. In addition, preoperative identification of anomalous vessels

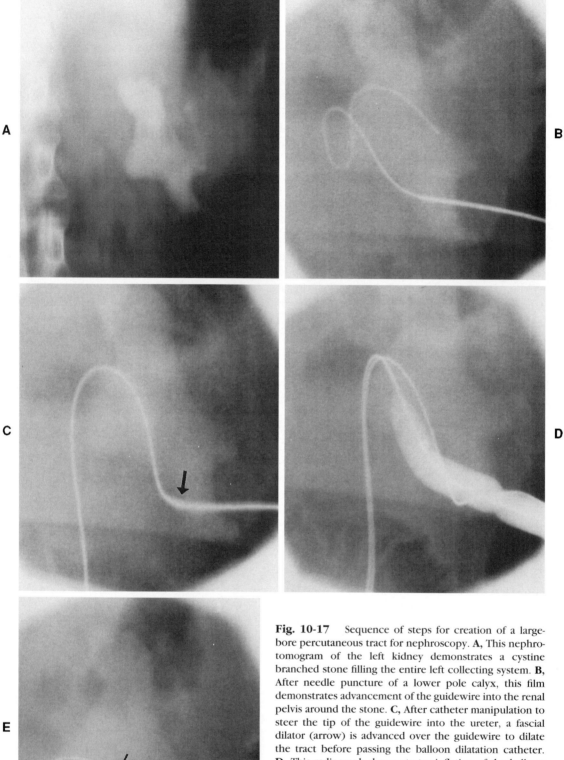

Fig. 10-17 Sequence of steps for creation of a large-bore percutaneous tract for nephroscopy. **A,** This nephrotomogram of the left kidney demonstrates a cystine branched stone filling the entire left collecting system. **B,** After needle puncture of a lower pole calyx, this film demonstrates advancement of the guidewire into the renal pelvis around the stone. **C,** After catheter manipulation to steer the tip of the guidewire into the ureter, a fascial dilator (arrow) is advanced over the guidewire to dilate the tract before passing the balloon dilatation catheter. **D,** This radiograph demonstrates inflation of the balloon dilator. With the balloon dilator, the tract can be dilated rapidly from 8 F to 30 F with a single inflation. This radiograph also demonstrates a second safety guidewire through the nephrostomy tract, which was placed as a precaution. **E,** After balloon dilatation, the working sheath is advanced into the kidney. The sheath (arrows) has been advanced into the renal pelvis. The sheath can be used for endoscopy, stone fragmentation, and removal.

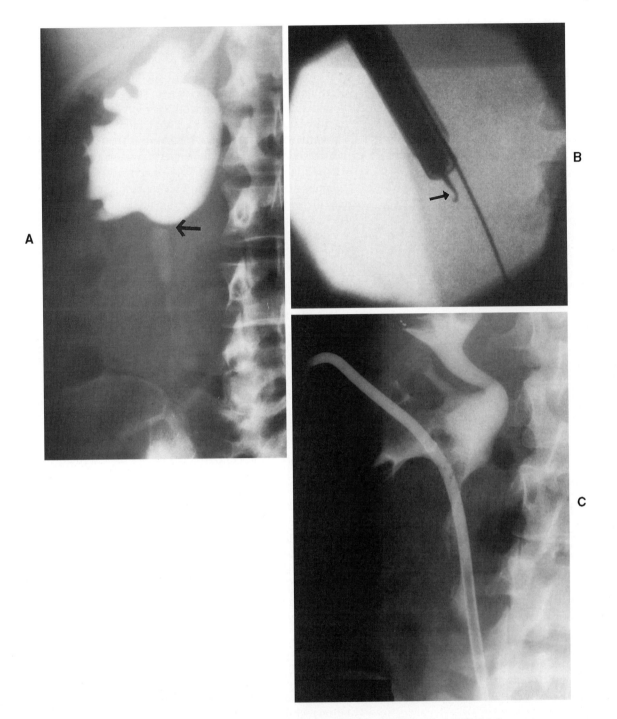

Fig. 10-18   Sequence of radiographs demonstrating endopyelotomy technique. **A,** A radiograph from an intravenous urogram of the right kidney demonstrates an appearance typical for ureteropelvic junction (UPJ) stricture. The renal pelvis is hugely dilated with narrowing at the UPJ (arrow) and a normal caliber ureter. **B,** Intraoperative radiograph after creation of a large-bore percutaneous tract with a sheath in place. A cold knife (arrow) is used to make a longitudinal transmural incision of the UPJ. **C,** A nephrostogram performed 6 weeks after endopyelotomy demonstrates marked decrease in the renal pelvic dilatation compared with the preoperative appearance.

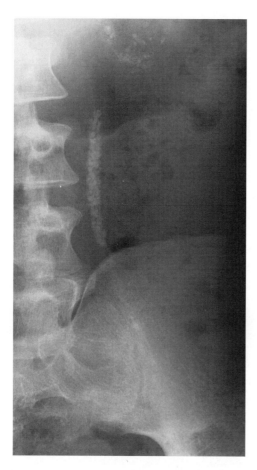

Fig. 10-19 Steinstrasse. This abdominal radiograph taken after extracorporeal shockwave lithotripsy of a large renal stone demonstrates the typical appearance of a steinstrasse, which is a collection of stone fragments lodged in the ureter. The formation of steinstrasse often heralds the development of ureteral obstruction.

may influence a surgeon to choose open surgical stricture repair rather than endopyelotomy. Aberrant vessels can be identified before surgery with helical CT scanning and CT angiography procedures. The identification of aberrant vessels of significant size (at least 4 mm in diameter) implies a substantial risk of massive bleeding if the vessel is incised inadvertently during endopyelotomy.

Extracorporeal Shock Wave Lithotripsy

During the 1980s, ESWL became widely available in the United States for management of urinary tract stones. As many as 85% of patients with urolithiasis can be treated successfully with ESWL alone. Although standard ESWL does not require percutaneous interventional uroradiology procedures, complications that necessitate intervention occur in up to 10% of patients treated with ESWL. Examination of patients before ESWL does require medical imaging and should include identification of stones, estimation of overall stone burden, and evaluation of the

urinary system with a contrast study. This last technique is used to ensure the absence of ureteral obstruction, which could impede passage of stone fragments after ESWL. Guidance for ESWL is provided by either fluoroscopy units or ultrasound systems. The patient is positioned so that the imaged stone lies in close proximity to the focus of the shock wave generated by the ESWL equipment. Once targeted, the stone is treated with repeated shockwave bursts generated extracorporeally, but focused internally, on the stone. Successful ESWL management results in complete fragmentation of the stone into pieces no larger than 2 to 3 mm in diameter. Abdominal radiographs taken after ESWL are useful to assess success of stone fragmentation and passage. The stone fragments generally pass spontaneously in an antegrade fashion with voided urine. Some stones, such as cystine stones, are refractory to ESWL management; these are best removed percutaneously. In addition, larger stones, when fragmented with ESWL, commonly cause complications such as ureteral obstruction, or they may fail to pass completely and lead to fragment reaggregation and stone reformation. Most centers use percutaneous nephrostolithotomy rather than ESWL as the primary tool for managing these larger stones. In 5% to 10% of patients with uncomplicated stones, ureteral obstruction develops after ESWL. This obstruction usually results from a number of stone fragments coalescing in the ureter (Fig. 10-19). This coalescence of fragments is described as a "steinstrasse," translated as *stone street*. These stone collections usually pass spontaneously, but in approximately 25% of patients with steinstrasse, retrograde stenting or PN drainage catheters may be required to manage the ureteral obstruction until the fragments become dislodged and pass. Rarely, more complex interventions are required to manage these obstructing stone casts. These interventions include ureteral dilatation, stone flushing, or long-term ureteral stenting.

Transluminal Ureteral Dilatation

Although UPJ strictures usually are managed endoscopically with endopyelotomy, other benign ureteral strictures can be managed successfully with balloon dilatation techniques that are analogous to angioplasty procedures used in the vascular system. Complete discussion of these techniques is beyond the scope of this chapter, but the essential components will be described.

Access to the ureteral stricture can be obtained via percutaneous transrenal tracts or in a retrograde fashion via retrograde cannulation of the ureter. A guidewire should be advanced through the stricture and into a stable position. Angiographic catheters are useful in steering guidewires through tortuous or severely narrowed strictures. In addition, hydrophilic guidewires are extremely useful in traversing difficult ureteral strictures. Before balloon dilatation, a heavy-duty stiff guidewire should be advanced through the stricture. For tight strictures, before balloon dilatation, an 8-F tapered angiographic catheter should be advanced through the stricture to predilate the stricture and allow for easy passage of the uninflated balloon catheter. This catheter then is removed, and the balloon dilatation catheter positioned across the stricture. High-pressure balloons often are needed to dilate ureteral strictures successfully. For standard ureteroplasty procedures, 8- to 10-mm balloon dilatation catheters should be used. After successful balloon dilatation, as demonstrated by absence of residual narrowing with the balloon inflated, the ureter should be stented for 4 to 8 weeks while the dilated segment heals. For antegrade balloon dilatation, an internal and external ureteral stent is advisable because repeated dilatations often are required for satisfactory long-term ureteral patency rates.

Success rates for balloon ureteroplasty depend on the cause, the extent, and the chronicity of the stricture. In the ideal setting, which consists of a focal, acute stricture without associated ureteral devascularization, success rates are 90% or more. This type of stricture commonly is seen in association with inadvertent ureteral ligation, which most often occurs during vaginal hysterectomy. On the opposite end of the spectrum of prognoses are strictures that occur at the junction of the ureter and a urinary bowel conduit. Some ureteral devascularization commonly occurs during the creation of urinary conduit diversions. Balloon ureteroplasty of strictures at the anastomotic sites usually has poor long-term patency rates. Long-term patency is achieved in only approximately 20% of patients after balloon dilatation of these strictures, even with multiple dilatations. Other strictures associated with poor ureteroplasty success rates include those caused by radiation therapy or neoplasms; however, because postoperative and postirradiation patients also are difficult surgical cases, percutaneous ureteroplasty may be attempted to preclude the need for complex open surgical procedures.

Renal Cyst Aspiration and Sclerosis

Renal cyst aspiration, once commonly used to distinguish benign cysts from renal neoplasms, rarely is indicated today because ultrasound, CT, and MR imaging are extremely accurate in diagnosing simple cysts. Cystic lesions that do not meet the imaging criteria of simple cysts are considered indeterminate. Cyst aspiration may be used in additional evaluation of these lesions; however, imaging follow-up or surgical excision often are the procedures of choice. However, a cystic renal mass that when aspirated yields clear fluid with negative cytology and normal lactate dehydrogenase should be diagnosed as a benign simple cyst. More complex aspirated fluid, including hemorrhagic fluid, suggests the possibility of an underlying malignancy. Many cyst aspirations are indeterminate because of the presence of hemorrhage and the absence of malignant cells. These aspirates suggest an entity other than a benign simple cyst, and surgery often will ensue. Therefore, cyst aspiration rarely is used, and thorough cross-sectional imaging should be performed before cyst aspiration is considered for diagnosis.

Cyst aspiration can be performed with standard fine-needle (21- or 22-gauge) techniques. Ideally, aspirations should be performed in a fluoroscopic room under ultrasonographic guidance. After cleansing of the skin and injection of local anesthetic at the site of puncture, the needle is advanced into the cyst under continuous sonographic monitoring or intermittent ultrasound guidance. Once the cyst is punctured, the cyst fluid should be evacuated, and its volume should be recorded. Specimens of fluid should be sent for culture, cytology, and chemical analysis.

A minority of simple renal cysts cause symptoms. Larger simple cysts may cause flank pain from compression of renal parenchyma, stretching of the renal capsule, or obstruction to urine outflow caused by mass effect. In these patients, cyst ablation can be used therapeutically. Cyst ablation is a simple technique that can be performed on an outpatient basis. As with other transrenal procedures, routine coagulation factors should be analyzed, and an appropriate antibiotic given before the procedure. Using standard sterile technique, the cyst is punctured with a fine (21- or 22-gauge) needle. As with cyst aspiration, the cyst should be evacuated, and the fluid sent for analysis after its volume has been measured. Before ablation, a 4-F or 5-F catheter should be placed within the cyst over a guidewire that can be inserted through the skinny needle. Before ablation can be undertaken, water-soluble contrast material should be injected into the cyst, and fluoroscopic evaluation should be performed. Ablation should not be undertaken if there is extravasation outside the cyst or communication between the cyst and the intrarenal collecting system or blood vessels.

Numerous agents have been advocated for ablation of renal cysts. Absolute alcohol is effective, readily available, and easy to use. For cyst ablation, a volume of absolute alcohol equal to 25% to 50% of the volume aspirated from the simple cyst is injected back into the cyst via the catheter. The sclerosant should be left within the cyst for approximately 10 minutes, during which time the patient should change position every 2 minutes to better distribute the alcohol around the entire lining of the cyst. After the 10-minute interval, the alcohol should be aspirated, and the catheter removed. Cyst ablation usually causes minimal discomfort to the patient and can be performed safely as an outpatient procedure. More than 50% of cysts can be ablated sucessfully with a single treatment. Larger cysts may require repeated ablation to induce complete cyst involution.

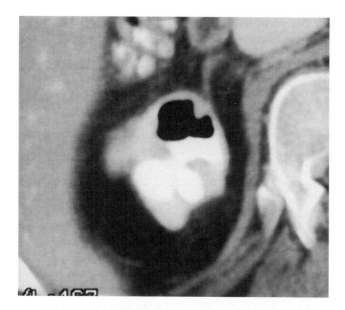

Fig. 10-20   Localized emphysematous pyelonephritis. This contrast-infused CT scan demonstrates a focal gas and fluid collection in the upper pole of the right kidney, typical of emphysematous pyelonephritis. This type of emphysematous pyelonephritis may be managed with percutaneous drainage and systemic antibiotic administration.

Perinephric and Renal Abscess Drainage

Management of retroperitoneal abscesses with percutaneous drainage has become routine in most radiology departments. Similarly, renal and perinephric abscesses are managed readily with a combination of percutaneous drainage and systemic administration of antibiotics. This combination usually obviates the need for open surgical decompression. Renal and perirenal abscesses usually are identified with CT or ultrasound. These usually have the appearance of complex fluid collections with surrounding enhancement on CT and internal echoes with ultrasound. Extensive perinephric stranding often is co-existent because of surrounding inflammation and congestion. On some occasions, gas may be seen within the fluid collection (Fig. 10-20); if so, it is indicative of ongoing infection. These abscesses are best drained under ultrasound or CT guidance. Initially, a 21- or 22-gauge needle is used to puncture the collection, aspirate a sample of material, and provide access for catheter placement. In equivocal cases, puncture and fluid aspiration can be performed for diagnosis and as a prelude to drain placement, if necessary. If the initial aspirate is not clear fluid, a drain should be placed definitely. Additionally, the aspirate should be saved for culture and analysis. Drainage catheters are placed in a routine fashion. An 0.018-inch guidewire is inserted through the skinny needle and advanced into the abscess cavity. The tract is dilated initially with a small dilator, and an 0.035- to

0.038-inch guidewire is advanced into the abscess cavity. The tract then is dilated further. A drainage catheter, 8 F or larger, should be placed within the cavity for adequate drainage of the often viscous abscess contents. Once the catheter is placed, the abscess cavity should be evacuated by manually applying aspiration to the drainage catheter with a syringe. The catheter then should be connected to passive external drainage and sutured in place. The drainage catheter should be left in place until there is no output from the drainage catheter for at least 12 hours and until the patient has recuperated without evidence of continued infection. In some patients, multiple drains and transcatheter irrigation may be required to evacuate these abscesses completely.

Focal emphysematous pyelonephritis is a special situation that can be managed with percutaneous drainage. Traditionally, all patients with emphysematous pyelonephritis were thought to require surgical nephrectomy; however, recent studies have suggested that a subgroup of these patients may be treated nonsurgically. If gas is detected within the kidney in a patient with sepsis, CT scanning of the kidney should be performed. Based on the CT scan, emphysematous pyelonephritis can be classified as either diffuse or localized, and appropriate management can be planned. The localized form of emphysematous pyelonephritis represents a focal parenchymal abscess attributable to a gas-producing organism. This condition can be managed successfully with percutaneous drainage combined with systemic antibiotic administration. With percutaneous management of localized emphysematous pyelonephritis, it is essential that coexisting ureteral obstruction, if present, also be remedied to ensure infection resolution. If ureteral obstruction is present, a PN drainage catheter or ureteral stent should be placed in addition to the abscess drainage catheter. Early management of localized emphysematous pyelonephritis can lead to complete resolution of the infection and normalization of function of the involved kidney. Alternatively, diffuse emphysematous pyelonephritis indicates irreversible damage to the majority of the kidney and is best managed with nephrectomy when the patient's condition allows.

Percutaneous Renal Biopsy

Percutaneous renal biopsy usually is performed for one of two reasons. First, biopsies are performed to obtain a tissue sample of a renal mass. Because most renal masses can be accurately diagnosed with modern cross-sectional imaging techniques, biopsy rarely is necessary before treatment. Simple renal cyst, the most common renal mass, can be diagnosed readily with CT or ultrasound evaluation. Biopsies of these cysts should not be taken. Alternatively, renal cell carcinomas, the most common primary malignancy of the kidney, usually are diagnosed easily with cross-sectional imaging. In addition, angiomyolipomas, the most common solid benign tumor of the kidney, can be diagnosed in approximately 90% of patients with CT imaging as fat is visible within the tumor. In any of these settings, percutaneous biopsy should not be performed. Biopsy of a solid renal mass should be avoided when possible because biopsy poses a risk of confounding other diagnostic information and carries some risks itself. For instance, renal cell carcinomas can contain oncocytic cells. Thus, when percutaneous biopsy of a renal mass yields histologic evidence of an oncocytoma, a benign renal adenoma, malignancy still is a possibility. For this reason, surgical excision is required, regardless of the results of the biopsy, and the biopsy therefore is pointless. Also, renal cell carcinomas, oncocytomas, and angiomyolipomas may be vascular lesions, and the risk of significant hemorrhage resulting from percutaneous biopsy must be considered. Biopsy of geographic infiltrating renal masses, which often are transitional cell carcinomas, also poses a risk of seeding the biopsy tract with metastatic deposits.

When should percutaneous biopsy be used in the diagnosis of renal masses? If a patient has a known extrarenal malignancy and a solitary renal mass and if surgical nephrectomy would be considered a treatment option if this were a renal cell carcinoma, biopsy should be performed. Typically, this scenario relates to patients with lymphoma because renal lymphoma is not rare. Solitary metastasis may occur with renal lymphoma. Also, renal lymphoma responds to chemotherapy and is not considered a surgical lesion. For these reasons, biopsy of a solitary renal mass in a patient with renal lymphoma is performed to distinguish a renal metastasis from a primary renal malignancy. In one other unusual situation, renal mass biopsy may be somewhat helpful. A small number of patients have a propensity to develop multiple oncocytomas of the kidney. If a patient has had a renal oncocytoma surgically removed and if he or she develops other solid renal lesions, the excision of which would endanger the patient's renal functional status, then biopsy may provide evidence to support a nonsurgical approach. Although a biopsy of these new masses that yield benign oncocytes does not exclude malignancy definitively, it does support strongly the diagnosis of benign lesions. These patients should be followed closely with cross-sectional imaging at intervals no longer than 6 months. Any rapidly progressing lesions or lesions that develop imaging features atypical of oncocytomas should be considered highly suspicious for malignant tumors.

The second group of patients who commonly undergo percutaneous biopsy are those with medical renal disease that requires tissue diagnosis. These biopsies usually are performed without imaging guidance or with only ultrasound guidance. CT guidance can be used in especially difficult cases. Typically, the renal biopsy should be obtained from the posterolateral aspect of the lower pole of either kidney. Core biopsies should be obtained, and the core should include some of the cortex of the kidney so numerous glomeruli will be present in the sample. Automated biopsy guns or manually operating cutting needles can be used to obtain adequate samples. Routinely, 14-gauge needles are used to obtain these core samples for classification of the underlying type of medical renal disease.

Percutaneous Cystostomy

To expand on other percutaneous drainage techniques, radiologists also may perform percutaneous cystostomy with standard radiologic techniques learned from other interventional radiology applications. Either a small-bore or a large-bore catheter may be used for cystostomy drainage. For short-term drainage, a small-bore (8 to 14 F), self-retaining drainage catheter can be used. Standard nephrostomy catheters with the tip coiled within the bladder lumen are used. For long-term drainage, 24- to 30-F catheters should be used.

Percutaneous cystostomy catheters are placed in patients with intractable incontinence, severe bladder outlet obstruction, or urethral laceration. In most of these patients, percutaneous cystostomy catheters are used as a temporizing means before definitive surgical repair.

The risks of percutaneous cystostomy placement are similar to those of other percutaneous drainage procedures and include a small risk of hemorrhage or infection. Percutaneous cystostomy is performed via a suprapubic needle puncture of the bladder, which is performed near the midline. The puncture site is several centimeters above the pubic symphysis. Ideally, the bladder should be distended before puncture. The bladder can be localized with fluoroscopy or ultrasound. Once the puncture is performed, a small aliquot of urine should be aspirated to confirm transvesical puncture. A guidewire then is advanced into the bladder lumen, and the tract is dilated to an appropriate size for placement of the drainage catheter. For large-bore drain placement, a balloon dilatation catheter should be used to dilate the tract rapidly from 10 F to 24 F with one balloon dilatation. This technique also minimizes the risk of dislodging the guidewire during repeated fascial dilatations. Once the tract is dilated, a sheath is placed through the tract over the guidewire, and a large-bore drainage catheter can be advanced into the bladder lumen. A Malecot, or standard bladder catheter with balloon retention device, can be used for drainage. The catheter should be sutured in place at the skin and left to external drainage. Follow-up cystography or voiding cystourethrography can be performed in an antegrade fashion via the percutaneous cystostomy catheter.

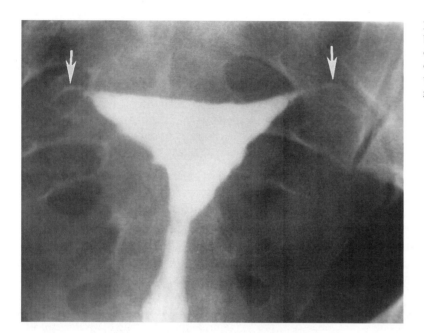

Fig. 10-21   Occlusion of the interstitial segment of both fallopian tubes. This hysterosalpingogram demonstrates bilateral occlusion of the interstitial segment of the fallopian tube (arrows). This type of fallopian tube occlusion often is amenable to radiologically guided recanalization.

INTERVENTION IN FEMALE INFERTILITY

Radiology plays a small but important role in the management of female infertility. Radiologists can be helpful in identifying female factors responsible for infertility, including uterine anomalies such as septate uterus, other uterine abnormalities including synechiae, and tubal factors including hydrosalpinx, salpingitis, isthmica nodosa, or tubal occlusion. These diseases are discussed in more detail in Chapter 7.

Interventional radiology techniques can be used to treat some women with obstructed fallopian tubes. Radiologically guided transvaginal fallopian tube recanalization is a safe and effective technique for restoring patency to fallopian tubes that are blocked near their junction with the uterus. Proximal tubal occlusion presents a unique opportunity for radiologists to assist in the management of female infertility. Blockages of the fallopian tubes that occur within the first 1 to 2 cm of the fallopian tube os (Fig. 10-21) are problematic for gynecologists. Because this interstitial segment of the fallopian tube is surrounded by myometrium, it is inaccessible to laparoscopic visualization. In addition, surgical studies of resected fallopian tubes have demonstrated that the most common cause of interstitial fallopian tube obstruction is debris blocking an otherwise normal segment of tube. This fact has led radiologists to perform recanalization procedures in which catheters and guidewires are used to dislodge these blocking debris plugs. This technique, a modification of standard guidewire and catheter technique, can be performed as an outpatient procedure with minimal risks. Recanalization of an interstitial tubal blockage is successful in nearly 90% of patients, and up to 50% of patients can achieve conception after fallopian tube recanalization.

Detailed description of fallopian tube recanalization techniques is beyond the scope of this chapter; however, in brief, fallopian tube recanalization usually is guided fluoroscopically after contrast material hysterosalpingography. After confirmation of proximal fallopian tube occlusion with the contrast study (Fig. 10-22), a 6-F angiographic catheter is advanced through the cervical canal and maneuvered until it engages the fallopian tube os (Fig. 10-22). The fallopian tube actually is recanalized by using a coaxial system comprising a 3-F catheter and an 0.018-inch guidewire. This catheter and wire system is advanced through the lumen of the 6-F catheter and into the lumen of the fallopian tube (Fig. 10-22). Gentle guidewire probing usually leads to successful fallopian tube recanalization. A selective salpingogram then is performed to confirm successful recanalization and to assess the status of the entire fallopian tube (Fig. 10-22). If necessary, the procedure then can be repeated to recanalize the contralateral tube.

Potential complications of fallopian tube recanalization include tubal perforation. Although perforation occurs in approximately 15% of patients, it is self-limited and rarely leads to morbidity or sequelae. Clinically significant infection or bleeding also is rarely caused by fallopian tube recanalization. As with other interventional procedures, intraprocedural vasovagal reactions occur occasionally. The cause appears to be psychological stress, and these reactions are reversed readily with infusion of intravascular fluid and atropine, when necessary.

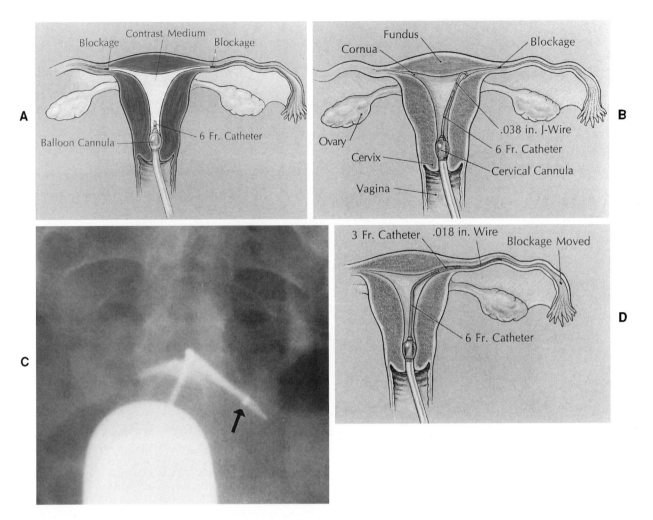

Fig. 10-22   Sequence of steps used for fallopian tube recanalization. **A,** Diagram of bilateral interstitial fallopian tube occlusion confirmed with hysterosalpingography as the first step in the recanalization procedure. **B,** Diagram demonstrating advancement of a curved catheter to the left fallopian tube os. **C,** Radiograph demonstrating selective catheterization of the left fallopian tube os. A radiopaque line (arrow) marks the end of the angiographic catheter at the origin of the fallopian tube. **D,** Diagram demonstrating the process of recanalizing the occluded fallopian tube. The recanalization is performed using coaxial technique to dislodge the blockage.   *Continued*

INTERVENTION IN MALE INFERTILITY

Radiologists also have a role in the treatment of male infertility patients. The major role of the interventional radiologist is in the diagnosis and treatment of some patients with erectile dysfunction and for occlusion of varicoceles. The majority of men with nonpsychogenic impotence have vascular disorders of the arteries or the veins of the penis. Normally, there must be minimal venous outflow from the penis to maintain an erection (Fig. 10-23). Excessive venous outflow, also known as venous leak, is the most common vascular abnormality causing erectile dysfunction. Once diagnosed, venous leak can be managed surgically with venous ligation or arterial-venous bypass grafting. As an alternative to surgery, veins draining the penis can be occluded percutaneously after catheterization of the dorsal vein of the penis. Draining veins then are catheterized selectively, followed by ablation of these veins with intravascular sclerosants.

A minority of patients with vascular-based erectile dysfunction suffer from arterial insufficiency. In most of these patients, atherosclerotic disease is the underlying cause. In a small percentage of patients, arterial occlusions develop after focal trauma to the pelvis and perineum. Results of angioplasty of stenoses or occlusion of the pudendal artery or its branches, including the penile artery and the cavernosal branches, have been disappointing. Long-term patency of these vessels has not been achieved in most patients treated with transluminal an-

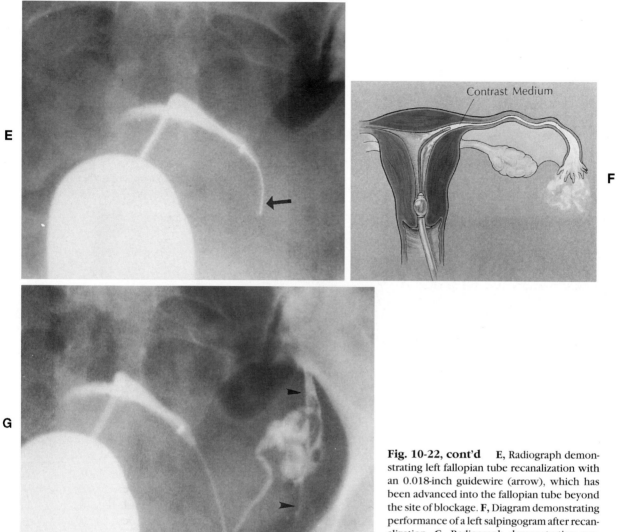

Fig. 10-22, cont'd **E,** Radiograph demonstrating left fallopian tube recanalization with an 0.018-inch guidewire (arrow), which has been advanced into the fallopian tube beyond the site of blockage. **F,** Diagram demonstrating performance of a left salpingogram after recanalization. **G,** Radiograph demonstrating successful recanalization of the left fallopian tube. The fallopian tube is patent with free spillage (arrowheads) into the peritoneal cavity.

gioplasty. Alternatively, focal stenosis of one or both hypogastric arteries can be managed successfully with angioplasty. Compared with the smaller arteries supplying the penis, the hypogastric artery has a larger caliber and higher flow rates; these factors likely account for high patency rates with angioplasty management.

Angioplasty of the hypogastric artery can be performed after diagnostic angiography. Typically, the artery to be treated is approached via puncture of the contralateral femoral artery. Standard angiographic guidewires and angioplasty balloon catheters are used for management. The size of the angioplasty balloon depends on the diameter of the blood vessel as measured during the diagnostic studies.

In addition, management of other causes of male infertility is being explored at some institutions. Techniques used for fallopian tube recanalization have been extended to treat men with ejaculatory duct occlusion. Bilateral ejaculatory duct occlusion or stenosis is a cause of azoospermia. In some instances, this condition can be managed with radiologic recanalization techniques. Transrectal seminal vesicle puncture can be achieved under ultrasonic guidance. A catheter and guidewire can be steered through the seminal vesicle and into the ejaculatory duct. Once the guidewire has traversed the ejaculatory duct orifice, it can be advanced into the urethra. This guidewire can be retrieved and used for retrograde balloon dilatation or incision of the ejaculatory duct orifice. This minimally invasive technique confirms that no orifice in the body is safe from the radiologist's probing.

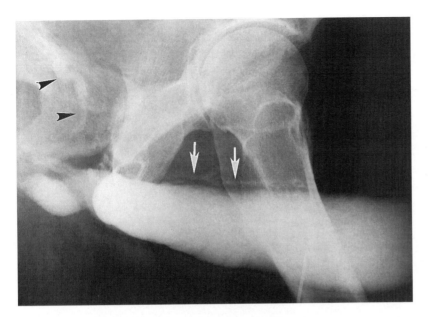

Fig. 10-23 Cavernosogram. This left posterior oblique radiograph demonstrates contrast opacification of the corpora cavernosa of the penis during chemically induced erection. Normal cavernosography demonstrates opacification of the entire corpora cavernosa bilaterally with minimal, if any, venous filling. There is filling of the dorsal vein of the penis (arrows) and minimal venous filling of periprostatic veins (arrowheads) on the right. This periprostatic vein opacification indicates a minimal venous leak in this patient.

PERCUTANEOUS TRANSLUMINAL ANGIOPLASTY

Percutaneous transluminal angioplasty in the urinary tract is limited to management of renal artery stenoses and hypogastric artery stenoses as described previously. Percutaneous transluminal angioplasty is an accepted technique for the management of focal stenoses of the renal arteries. Angioplasty is used to improve perfusion to the kidney and to manage renovascular hypertension and renal insufficiency resulting from renal underperfusion. Renal artery angioplasty is performed after demonstration by diagnostic arteriography of lesions amenable to percutaneous management with standard angiographic and angioplasty techniques. The best results with

transluminal angioplasty have been achieved in managing focal areas of fibromuscular dysplasia (Fig. 10-24). Atherosclerotic lesions away from the origin of the renal artery also respond well to angioplasty. Ostial atherosclerotic lesions, however, respond poorly to primary angioplasty techniques. Currently, there is evidence that angioplasty augmented with endovascular stenting improves patency rates with management of ostial renal artery stenoses.

Renal artery angioplasty requires careful and meticulous techniques. Particular care must be taken when crossing a stenotic lesion with a guidewire. Plaques are undermined easily, and the result can lead to dissection, distal embolization, and renal artery occlusion. Vasodilators should be administered concurrently with renal angioplasty procedures to avoid excessive arterial spasm and resulting thrombosis.

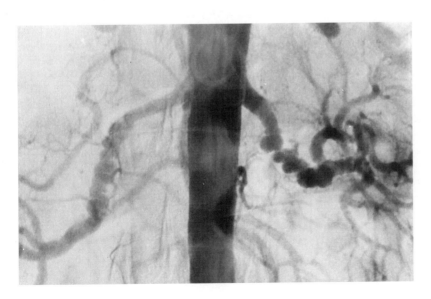

Fig. 10-24 Renal artery fibromuscular dysplasia. This digital subtraction arteriogram demonstrates the typical appearance of renal artery fibromuscular dysplasia bilaterally. This type of renal artery stenosis usually is amenable to percutaneous transluminal angioplasty.

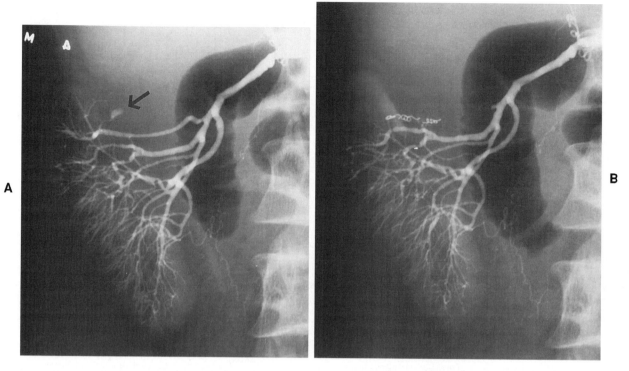

Fig. 10-25   Percutaneous transcatheter embolization of active renal hemorrhage. **A,** This trauma patient was hemodynamically unstable and extensive perinephric hemorrhage was diagnosed with CT. This selective right renal arteriogram demonstrates active bleeding (arrow) from an upper pole renal artery branch. **B,** After selective catheterization of this branch, metal coils were used to occlude the bleeding artery, leading to rapid stabilization of this patient's condition.

PERCUTANEOUS VASCULAR OCCLUSION

Complete discussion of this topic is beyond the scope of this chapter; however, the radiologist should be aware of some applications in which percutaneous arterial occlusion techniques are useful in genitourinary radiology. Arterial occlusion is useful in genitourinary radiology to manage active arterial bleeding and arterial venous malformations, to devascularize hypervascular tumors for nonsurgical renal ablation, and to manage intractable uterine bleeding.

Active renal hemorrhage usually occurs after renal trauma, including iatrogenic trauma. With the increased use of percutaneous renal biopsy and transrenal procedures, iatrogenically induced artery injury is not rare. Regardless of the cause, active bleeding from branches of the renal artery may be managed with percutaneous transcatheter embolization (Fig. 10-25) in many patients. Ideally, superselective catheterization of the bleeding artery should be performed, followed by transcatheter delivery of embolic materials (Table 10-3), such as Gelfoam particles and metal coils to occlude the bleeding end-artery branches. Superselective catheterization and embolization minimize damage to normal renal parenchyma

and prevent additional bleeding and avoid the risk of collateral arteries supplying the bleeding focus. Superselective catheterization usually can be achieved with coaxial systems that are available commercially. Arteriovenous malformations are managed similarly (Fig. 10-26). In these patients, careful selection of the size of embolic materials is important because arterial–venous shunting will be prominent, and systemic embolization can occur as a complication. Gelfoam pledgets can be used initially to devascularize the majority of these arteriovenous malformations. Devascularization should be followed with a permanent occlusive agent, such as polyvinyl alcohol.

Table 10-3 Suggested Materials for Renal Embolization	
Lesion	**Embolic material**
Arterial bleeding	Gelfoam and coils
Vascular malformation	Polyvinyl alcohol and coils
Renal ablation	Ethanol
Renal neoplasm	Polyvinyl alcohol, Gelfoam, and ethanol

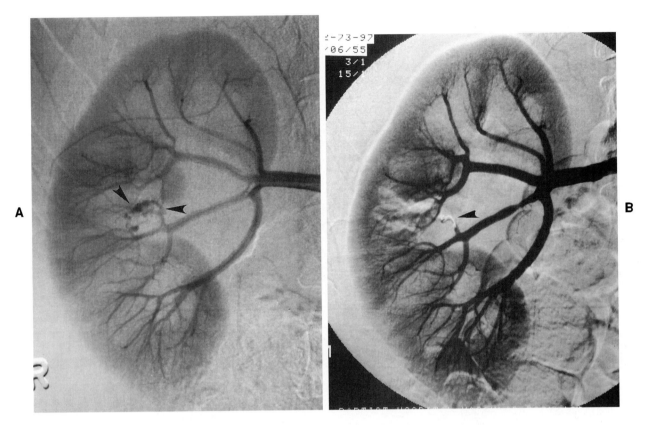

Fig. 10-26   Percutaneous embolization of a renal arteriovenous malformation. **A,** This young man suffered from intermittent episodes of severe gross hematuria. This selective right renal arteriogram demonstrates a focal, vascular malformation (arrowheads). **B,** After superselective catheterization with a coaxial catheter system, a metal coil (arrowhead) was used to occlude the feeding artery and obliterate the vascular malformation.

Embolization techniques for renal ablation or devascularization of renal malignancy require slightly different techniques. Therapeutic renal ablation usually is performed in patients with chronic renal failure who develop symptoms secondary to problems related to their native kidneys. These problems can include intractable hematuria, hypertension, or proteinuria. In these patients, devascularization requires widespread, permanent occlusion of all renal artery branches (Fig. 10-27), including tiny cortical branches. Devascularization of renal malignancies is performed as a palliative measure or to lessen intraoperative bleeding in surgical candidates. In patients with advanced-stage renal cell carcinomas, palliative treatment is used for symptoms such as intractable hematuria or pain related to the primary or metastatic tumor. For renal ablation, a liquid sclerosant, such as absolute alcohol, should be used so that renal ablation is complete and irreversible, leaving no functioning renal parenchyma. To ensure that injected alcohol is limited to the kidney, precautions must be taken during ablation. After catheterization of the renal artery, a latex balloon occlusion catheter is placed selectively in the renal artery. With the balloon inflated to occlude blood flow in the

renal artery, contrast material is injected through the lumen of the catheter and into the renal artery branches. With fluoroscopy, the volume of sclerosant needed to ablate the kidney can be estimated. Usually, 2 to 5 mL of alcohol are adequate to ablate a single kidney completely. Once the needed volume has been estimated, the balloon is deflated for several minutes to allow the kidney to reperfuse. The balloon then is reinflated, and the alcohol or other sclerosant is injected gradually into the renal artery. Balloon inflation is maintained for 10 additional minutes. After the balloon is deflated, a follow-up renal arteriogram is obtained (Fig. 10-27). If ablation is incomplete, the procedure can be repeated. For renal tumor ablation, particulate sclerosants, such as polyvinyl alcohol, are ideal. After feeding vessels are catheterized, a slurry of polyvinyl alcohol is injected slowly through the catheter to occlude vessels supplying the renal tumor. Follow-up arteriography is used to gauge adequacy of tumor devascularization. Absolute alcohol and Gelfoam can be used as secondary agents for kidney tumor ablation. After significant devascularization and absence of significant arterial–venous shunting have been achieved with the particulate sclerosing agents, alcohol may be

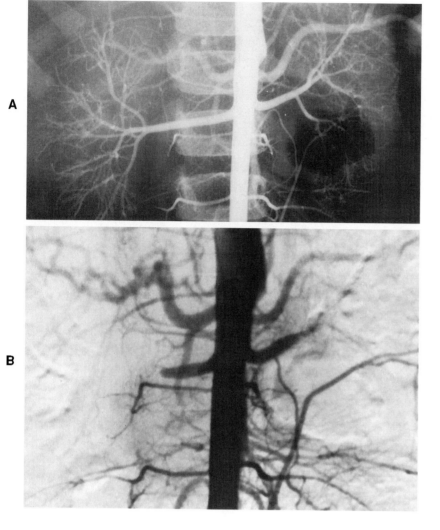

Fig. 10-27   Renal artery ablation. **A,** This midstream aortogram demonstrates normal renal arteries bilaterally. This dialysis-dependent child with chronic renal failure had intractable hypertension. This arteriogram was done as a prelude to renal ablation therapy. **B,** Arteriogram taken after ablation of the renal artery and its branches with injection of alcohol. There is complete occlusion of the main renal arteries and no flow to the renal parenchyma, indicating successful renal ablation.

injected sparingly for additional devascularization. Occluding devices, such as metallic coils or occlusion balloons, should be avoided when attempting to ablate renal tumors or native kidneys. These agents are excellent for large-vessel occlusion or to occlude terminal branch vessels; however, numerous collateral networks can potentially supply the kidney, and these may enlarge if the major renal arteries are occluded therapeutically. The result is not only inadequate devascularization, but also possible compounding of the problem because repeated catheterization and embolization are extremely difficult, or even impossible, when only collateral pathways provide the major perfusion to the kidney.

SUGGESTED READINGS

Banner MP: Extracorporeal shock wave lithotripsy: selection of patients and long-term complications, *Radiol Clin North Am* 29:543–556, 1991.

Beckmann CF, Roth RA, Bihrle W III: Dilation of benign ureteral strictures, *Radiology* 172:437–441, 1989.

Bennett LN, Voegeli DR, Crummy AB, et al: Urologic complications following renal transplantation: role of interventional radiologic procedures, *Radiology* 160:531–536, 1986.

Carson CC III, Danneberger JE, Weinerth JL: Percutaneous lithotripsy in morbid obesity, *J Urol* 139:243–245, 1988.

Cassis AN, Brannen GE, Bush WH, et al: Endopyelotomy: review of results and complications, *J Urol* 146:1492–1495, 1991.

Chaussy C, Schmiedt E: Shock wave treatment for stones in the upper urinary tract, *Urol Clin North Am* 10:743–750, 1983.

Coptcoat MJ, Webb DR, Kellett MJ, et al: The complications of extracorporeal shockwave lithotripsy: management and prevention, *Br J Urol* 58:578–580, 1986.

Cussenot O, Desgrandchamps F, Ollier P, et al: Anatomical bases of percutaneous surgery for calculi in horseshoe kidney, *Surg Radiol Anat* 14:209–213, 1992.

Dickinson IK, Fletcher MS, Bailey MJ, et al: Combination of percutaneous surgery and extracorporeal shockwave lithotripsy for the treatment of large renal calculi, *Br J Urol* 58:581–584, 1986.

Dunnick NR, Carson CC, Braun SD, et al: Complications of percutaneous nephrostolithotomy, *Radiology* 157:51-55, 1985.

Dyer RB: Percutaneous nephrostomy. In Harrison LH, Kandel LB, editors: *Techniques in urologic stone surgery*, Mount Kisco, NY, 1986, Futura.

Dyer RB, Zagoria RJ, Auringer ST, et al: Radiologic contribution to the management of patients undergoing extracorporeal shock wave lithotripsy, *Crit Rev Diagn Imaging* 28:295-330, 1988.

Earthman WJ, Mazer JM, Winfield AC: Angiomyolipomas in tuberous sclerosis: subselective embolotherapy with alcohol, with long-term follow-up study, *Radiology* 160:437-441, 1986.

Evanoff GV, Thompson CS, Foley R, et al: Spectrum of gas within the kidney: emphysematous pyelonephritis and emphysematous pyelitis, *Am J Med* 83:149-154, 1987.

Ferral H, Stackhouse DJ, Bjarnason H, et al: Complications of percutaneous nephrostomy tube placement, *Sem Intervent Radiol* 11:198-206, 1994.

Fritzsche P: Antegrade pyelography: therapeutic applications, *Radiol Clin North Am* 24:573-586, 1986.

Gerber GS, Lyon ES: Endopyelotomy: patient selection, results, and complications, *Urology* 43:2-10, 1994.

Grossman HB, Schwartz SL, Konnak JW: Ureteroscopic treatment of urothelial carcinoma of the ureter and renal pelvis, *J Urol* 148:275-277, 1992.

Hollowell JG, Roth RA, Beckmann CF: Radiologic technique to mark ureteral calculi for extracorporeal shock-wave lithotripsy, *Urology* 30:127-129, 1987.

Hopper KD, Yakes WF: The posterior intercostal approach for percutaneous renal procedures: risk of puncturing the lung, spleen, and liver as determined by CT, *AJR Am J Roentgenol* 154:115-117, 1990.

Kletscher BA, Segura JW, LeRoy AJ, et al: Percutaneous antegrade endoscopic pyelotomy: review of 50 consecutive cases, *J Urol* 153:701-703, 1995.

Lang EK: Percutaneous nephrostolithotomy and lithotripsy: a multi-institutional survey of complications, *Radiology* 162:25-30, 1987.

Lang EK, Glorioso LW III: Antegrade transluminal dilatation of benign ureteral strictures: long-term results, *AJR Am J Roentgenol* 150:131-134, 1988.

Lee WJ, Badlani GH, Karlin GS, et al: Treatment of ureteropelvic strictures with percutaneous pyelotomy: experience in 62 patients, *AJR Am J Roentgenol* 151:515-518, 1988.

LeRoy AJ, Segura JW: Extracorporeal shock-wave lithotripsy, *Radiol Clin North Am* 24:623-631, 1986.

Lingeman JE, Coury TA, Newman DM, et al: Comparison of results and morbidity of percutaneous nephrostolithotomy and extracorporeal shock wave lithotripsy, *J Urol* 138:485-490, 1987.

Lowe LH, Zagoria RJ, Baumgartner BR, et al: Role of imaging and intervention in complex infections of the urinary tract, *AJR Am J Roentgenol* 163:363-367, 1994.

Michaels EK, Fowler JE Jr: Extracorporeal shock wave lithotripsy for struvite renal calculi: prospective study with extended followup, *J Urol* 146:728-732, 1991.

Papanicolaou N: Renal anatomy relevant to percutaneous interventions, *Sem Intervent Radiol* 12:163-172, 1995.

Pfister RC, Newhouse JH: Interventional percutaneous pyeloureteral techniques. I. Antegrade pyelography and ureteral perfusion, *Radiol Clin North Am* 17:341-350, 1979.

Platts AD, Dick R: Negative contrast pyelography prior to nephrostomy insertion, *J Intervent Radiol* 4:36-38, 1989.

Rickards D, Jones SN: Percutaneous interventional uroradiology, *Br J Radiol* 62:573-581, 1989.

Riedy MJ, Lebowitz RL: Percutaneous studies of the upper urinary tract in children, with special emphasis on infants, *Radiology* 160:231-235, 1986.

Sacks D, Banner MP, Meranze SG, et al: Renal and related retroperitoneal abscesses: percutaneous drainage, *Radiology* 167:447-451, 1988.

Schmeller NT, Kersting H, Schüller J, et al: Combination of chemolysis and shock wave lithotripsy in the treatment of cystine renal calculi, *J Urol* 131:434-438, 1984.

Segura JW: Role of percutaneous procedures in the management of renal calculi, *Urol Clin North Am* 17:207-216, 1990.

Segura JW, Patterson DE, LeRoy AJ: Combined percutaneous ultrasonic lithotripsy and extracorporeal shock wave lithotripsy for struvite staghorn calculi, *World J Urol* 5:245-247, 1987.

Spies JB, Rosen RJ, Lebowitz AS: Antibiotic prophylaxis in vascular and interventional radiology: a rational approach, *Radiology* 166:381-387, 1988.

Taha SA, Al-Mohaya S, Abdulkader A, et al: Prognosis of radiologically non-functioning obstructed kidneys, *Br J Urol* 62:209-213, 1988.

Tegtmeyer CJ, Kellum CD, Jenkins A, et al: Extracorporeal shock wave lithotripsy: interventional radiologic solutions to associated problems, *Radiology* 161:587-592, 1986.

Thurmond AS: Selective salpingography and fallopian tube recanalization, *AJR Am J Roentgenol* 156:33-38, 1991.

Thurmond AS, Rösch J, Patton PE, et al: Fluoroscopic transcervical fallopian tube catheterization for diagnosis and treatment of female infertility caused by tubal obstruction, *Radiographics* 8:621-640, 1988.

Voegeli DR, Crummy AB, McDermott JC, et al: Percutaneous management of the urological complications of renal transplantation, *Radiographics* 6:1007-1022, 1986.

Zagoria RJ, Dyer RB, Harrison LH, et al: Percutaneous management of localized emphysematous pyelonephritis, *J Vasc Interv Radiol* 2:156-158, 1991.

Index